A NEW FIELD IN MIND

MCGILL-QUEEN'S/ASSOCIATED MEDICAL SERVICES STUDIES
IN THE HISTORY OF MEDICINE, HEALTH, AND SOCIETY

SERIES EDITORS: J.T.H. CONNOR AND ERIKA DYCK

This series presents books in the history of medicine, health studies, and social
policy, exploring interactions between the institutions, ideas, and practices of
medicine and those of society as a whole. To begin to understand these complex
relationships and their history is a vital step to ensuring the protection of a fundamental human right: the right to health. Volumes in this series have received
financial support to assist publication from Associated Medical Services, Inc.
(AMS), a Canadian charitable organization with an impressive history as a catalyst
for change in Canadian healthcare. For eighty years, AMS has had a profound
impact through its support of the history of medicine and the education of
healthcare professionals, and by making strategic investments to address critical
issues in our healthcare system. AMS has funded eight chairs in the history of
medicine across Canada, is a primary sponsor of many of the country's history
of medicine and nursing organizations, and offers fellowships and grants through
the AMS History of Medicine and Healthcare Program (www.amshealthcare.ca).

A New Field in Mind

*A History of Interdisciplinarity
in the Early Brain Sciences*

FRANK W. STAHNISCH

McGill-Queen's University Press
Montreal & Kingston • London • Chicago

ISBN 978-0-7735-5932-5 (cloth)
ISBN 978-0-2280-0050-1 (ePDF)
ISBN 978-0-2280-0051-8 (ePUB)

Legal deposit second quarter 2020
Bibliothèque nationale du Québec

Printed in Canada on acid-free paper that is 100% ancient forest free
(100% post-consumer recycled), processed chlorine free

This book has been published with the help of a grant from the Canadian
Federation for the Humanities and Social Sciences, through the Awards to
Scholarly Publications Program, using funds provided by the Social Sciences
and Humanities Research Council of Canada.

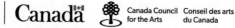

Funded by the   Financé par le
Government   gouvernement   Canada   Canada Council Conseil des arts
of Canada   du Canada   for the Arts   du Canada

We acknowledge the support of the Canada Council for the Arts.

Nous remercions le Conseil des arts du Canada de son soutien.

Library and Archives Canada Cataloguing in Publication

Title: A new field in mind: a history of interdisciplinarity in the early
    brain sciences/Frank W. Stahnisch.

Names: Stahnisch, Frank, author.

Series: McGill-Queen's/Associated Medical Services studies in the history
    of medicine, health, and society; 52.

Description: Series statement: McGill-Queen's/Associated Medical Services studies
    in the history of medicine, health, and society; 52 | Includes bibliographical
    references and index.

Identifiers: Canadiana (print) 20190197366 | Canadiana (ebook) 20190197420 |
    ISBN 9780773559325 (cloth) | ISBN 9780228000501 (ePDF) |
    ISBN 9780228000518 (ePUB)

Subjects: LCSH: Neurosciences—History.

Classification: LCC RC338.S73 2019 | DDC 612.809—dc23

This book was typeset by Marquis Interscript in 10.5/13 Sabon.

This book is dedicated to my wife, Katharina, for all the love, continued support, and endless understanding that accompanied the extensive period in which the manuscript was conceived and written, as well as for keeping up her spirit and smile during the many transitions we had to go through, now as a family and in the period that led to the appearance of this monograph.

Contents

Illustrations

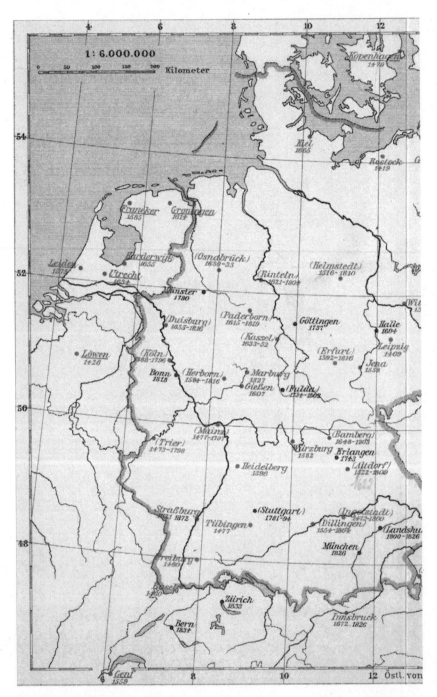

Map of the German universities in 1906 (on a scale of 1: 6,000,000). The years refer to opening or closing years, while universities, which are given in curved brackets, had been closed, from Franz Eulenburg: "Die Frequenz der deutschen Universitaeten von ihrer Gruendung bis zur Gegenwart." *Abhandlungen der Koeniglich-Saechsischen*

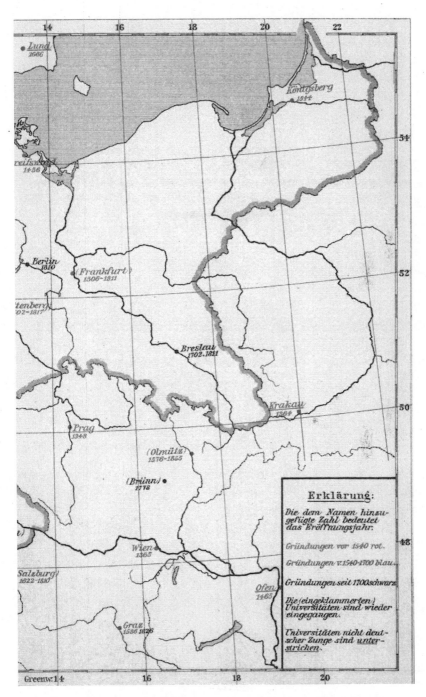

Gesellschaft der Wissenschaften 53, no. 2 (1906): 1–16, and esp. 325. / Map courtesy of the Saechsische Landesbibliothek – State and University Library, Dresden, Saxony, Germany (SLUB; http://digital.slub-dresden.de/id301424497/344)

Preface

Over recent decades, "neuroscience" as a research field has been broadly discussed in academia and in the public media, and even introduced into seemingly unrelated areas of social discourse in the domains of politics, law, and economics.[1] Within these discourses, the very existence of the "neurosciences" is now largely taken for granted and rarely linked back to the explicit social, cultural, and historical contexts from which they originated. This book looks at the making of this expanding field, particularly in the early interdisciplinary research centres in German-speaking countries, while unearthing and presenting the cultural and scientific dimensions that led to the emergence of "neuroscience" in its modern meaning.[2]

A New Field in Mind: A History of Interdisciplinarity in the Early Brain Sciences has been conceived and written somewhat as an archaeological exploration of one of the most important interdisciplinary areas of medicine and biology: the modern neurosciences – their epistemic and institutional precursor developments, as well as their multiple international contexts.[3] The topic and scope of this book will be particularly useful beyond the genuine interest of professional historians of science and medicine, to the extended neuroscience and psychiatry communities, especially in North America. It transcends many well-entrenched traditional views that scientific research was primarily associated with specialized and thus "disciplined" institutes, organized in pyramidal hierarchical fashion and circumscribed as specific knowledge communities for each academic discipline (such as anatomy, pathology, clinical neurology, and so forth). While putting the above-mentioned theoretical considerations to work within the historiographical framing of the book, I explore both the role and the scope of interdisciplinary projects within the German-speaking tradition of neuromorphology, from the creation of the

"Neurological Institute" in Vienna in 1882 to the eventual foundation in 1962 of the "Neuroscience Research Program" in the United States as a new core for the international, modern neuroscience community.

This book can further be seen as a historiographical attempt to examine the theoretical as well as cultural developments that led to the expansion of the distinct new research field of the neurosciences as we know it today. My focus particularly on interdisciplinarity in the relations among neuroanatomy, neuropathology, laboratory histology, and morphological applications in the academic medical and psychiatric clinics reveals much about the historical impact of three different political and cultural systems – German Imperialism, the social experiment of the Weimar Democracy, and later the horrific developments of National Socialism – on the emergence of the brain sciences. This broad historiographical perspective on the development of interdisciplinary working contexts in early twentieth-century neuromorphology allows us to map transformations in vastly divergent political, social, and cultural arenas and makes possible a culturally rich and thoroughly comparative analysis of developments in the area of brain sciences during times of political and social unrest between the 1880s and the 1960s. With these goals in mind, I trace these perspectives in the early evolution of modern neuroscience *avant la lettre*, as it were; that is, before "neuroscience" had even been coined as a distinct technical term for this new field.[4]

The research presented here is based on extensive archival work in numerous historical collections and libraries in Germany, Austria, Switzerland, France, Poland, Canada, and the United States. My monograph thus fills a lacuna in historiographical knowledge about the modern life sciences, while also marking out the distinctly complex historical development of "interdisciplinarity"[5] in the German-speaking neurosciences themselves. Likewise, I offer a complementary perspective, so as to view the significant impact of this tradition on subsequent research developments as they emerged on both sides of the Atlantic during the postwar period.

Certain chapters of the book are based on material from earlier articles and chapters that I have published in journals and edited collections in recent years. These are here respectively acknowledged: "Die Neurowissenschaften in Strassburg zwischen 1872 und 1945. Forschungstaetigkeiten zwischen politischen und kulturellen Zaesuren" (*Sudhoffs Archiv. Zeitschrift fuer Wissenschaftsgeschichte* 100, no. 2, 2016, 227–62); "Transforming the Lab: Technological and Societal Concerns in the Pursuit of De- and Regeneration in the German Morphological Neurosciences, 1910–1930" (*Medicine Studies. An International Journal for History, Philosophy, and Ethics of Medicine & Allied Sciences* 1, no. 1,

2009, 41–54); (with Thomas Hoffmann), "Kurt Goldstein and the Neurology of Movement during the Interwar Years: Physiological Experimentation, Clinical Psychology and Early Rehabilitation" (*Was bewegt uns? Menschen im Spannungsfeld zwischen Mobilitaet und Beschleunigung.* Bochum, Germany: Projektverlag, 2010, 283–311); "Psychiatrie und Hirnforschung. Zu den interstitiellen Uebergaengen des staedtischen Wissenschaftsraums im Labor der Berliner Metropole – Oskar und Cécile Vogt, Korbinian Brodmann, Kurt Goldstein" (*Psychiater und Zeitgeist. Zur Geschichte der Psychiatrie in Berlin.* Berlin, Germany: Pabst Science Publisher, 2008, 76–93); "Ludwig Edinger (1855–1918): Pioneer in Neurology" (*Journal of Neurology* 255, no. 1, 2008, 147–8); "The Early Eugenics Movement and Emerging Professional Psychiatry: Conceptual Transfers and Personal Relationships between Germany and North America, 1880s to 1930s" (*Canadian Bulletin of Medical History* 31, no. 1, 2014, 17–40); "'Abwehr,' 'Widerstand' und 'kulturelle Neuorientierung': Zu Re-Konfigurationen der Traumaforschung bei zwangsemigrierten deutschsprachigen Neurologen und Psychiatern" (*Trauma und Wissenschaft.* Goettingen, Germany: Vandenhoeck & Ruprecht, 2009, 29–60); "German-Speaking Émigré-Neuroscientists in North America after 1933: Critical Reflections on Emigration-Induced Scientific Change" (*Oesterreichische Zeitschrift fuer Geschichtswissenschaften* 21, no. 3, 2010, 36–68); as well as "Des gens comme moi étaient désignés comme des 'psychiatres vétérinaires': Les relations germano-américaines en recherches biomédicales dans la période de l'immédiat après-guerre, 1948-1973" (*Neuroscience et Psychiatrie.* Paris, France: Éditions Hermann 2019, 81–117). I very gratefully acknowledge the permission and generosity of all my publishers: Franz Steiner Verlag, Springer Europe, Projektverlag Bochum, Pabst Science in Switzerland and Germany; the University of Toronto Press in Canada; Vandenhoeck & Ruprecht in Germany; Studienverlag Innsbruck in Austria; as well as Éditions Hermann in France.

Furthermore, I have benefited immensely from numerous invitations to make presentations at research universities and independent centres for the neurosciences and humanities in Europe, North America, and Australia, along with papers delivered at national and international conferences. By way of these activities I have been able to share my analyses with many colleagues and students in the field, leading to continuous and enriching intellectual exchanges. These experiences are here also gratefully acknowledged, as they were of tremendous help in shaping the thought processes toward this monograph on the early brain sciences in German-speaking countries and their respective cultural influences on research styles, academic norms, and community behaviours.

Acknowledgments

Throughout the research period for this book, I was inspired, construc-
tively provoked, and supported by various mentors, colleagues, family
members, and friends, and to a significant extent by the graduate and
undergraduate students in my classes. I am extremely pleased to have the
opportunity here to express my gratitude to all of them, even if many will
no longer recollect our meetings, my earlier visits, and the exciting conversations that we shared. Some of these took place at academic conferences, in classes, and in workshops during the day, but many were held
in institute offices, departmental libraries, and cafés late into the night. I
mention most of them here by name, as an expression of my sincere
gratitude: Fred Andermann (†), Heijko Bauer, Ingo Bechmann, Antonio
Bergua, Christian Bonah, Cornelius Borck, Daniel Boyer, Bob Brain, Andy
Bulloch, Alison Bumstead, Alberto Cambrosio, Steven T. Casper, Tricia
Close-Koenig, Brianne Collins, David R. Colman (†), Michael Cowan,
Claude Debru, Chris Degeling, Rolando Del Maestro, Glenn Dolphin,
Wolfgang U. Eckart, Karl Max Einhaeupl, Paul Eling, Eric Engstrom, Tom
Feasby, Bill Feindel (†), Patrick Feng, Stan Finger, Paul Foley, Aravind
Ganesh, Delia Gavrus, Bill Ghali, Bob Gordon, Helmut Groeger, Anne
Harrington, Anke Hemmerling, Peter C.W. Hoffmann, Thomas Hoffmann,
Bernd Holdorff, Russell Johnson, Ingrid Kaestner, Axel Karenberg,
Christopher G. Kemp, Peter J. Koehler, Rudolf Koetter, Hendrik Kraay,
Alan M. Kraut, Georg W. Kreutzberg (†), Werner F. Kuemmel, Erna
Kurbegović, Paula Larsson, Aleksandra Loewenau, Marjorie Lorch, Kelsey
Lucyk, Chris Lyons, Massimo Mazzotti, Laurence H. McFalls, Pamela
Miller, Winfried Neuhuber, Granville H. Nickerson, Robert Nitsch, Anzo
Nguyen, Tom Noseworthy, Jesse Olszynko-Gryn, Matt Oram, Maggie
Osler (†), Philipp Osten, Buhm Soon Park, Scott Patten, Juergen Peiffer (†),

Stephen Pow, Will Pratt, Hans-Joerg Rheinberger, Iris Ritzmann, Volker Roelcke, Guel A. Russell, Milagros Salas-Prato, David Satin, Helga Satzinger, Alan N. Schechter, Steffen Schlee, Thomas Schlich, Martina Schluender, Florian Schmaltz, Bill Seidelman, Michel C.F. Shamy, Keith Sharkey, Allan L. Sherwin (†), Michael I. Shevell, Ned Shorter, Bill Shragge (†), Helmut Siefert (†), Barbara Simmel, Ted Sourkes (†), Hank Stam, Darwin Stapleton, Ian Steele-Russell (†), Holger Steinberg, Steve Sturdy, Jason Szabo, Jessica Tannenbaum, Peter Toohey, Sascha Topp, Rogelio Velez-Mendoza, Fernando Vidal, Diana Wear, Matthias M. Weber, Paul J. Weindling, George Weisz, Renate Wittern, Gregor Wolbring, Eberhard Wolff, Megan Wolff, Stephen Yearley, Allan Young, Karl Zilles, and Stephan Zuechner.

A substantial part of the book was written while I was the recipient of a Feodor Lynen Award of the Alexander von Humboldt Foundation and held tenure as a visiting assistant professor at McGill University. There, my colleagues read earlier drafts and graciously supported my research. The Department of Social Studies of Medicine provided a stimulating working milieu that has been unparalleled thus far. In Calgary, my new colleagues – especially in the Hotchkiss Brain Institute, the O'Brien Institute for Public Health, the History and Philosophy of Science Program, and the Science, Technology, Environment and Medicine Studies Laboratory – have provided a fertile environment for me to complete this project. It has been my pleasure to work with Beth Cusitar, Mikkel Dack, Keith Hann, Erna Kurbegović, Brenan Smith, and Donna Weich, all of whose research assistance, editorial advice, and meticulous correction of the English language have fostered the writing process.

A number of academic institutions and foundations have supported my extensive research process over the past decade. At the Charité Medical School's Institute of Anatomy in Berlin, its previous director, Robert Nitsch, nurtured my early interests in the subject, while Renate Wittern, the director-emeritus of the University of Erlangen-Nuernberg's Institute of the History of Medicine and Medical Ethics, gave me the pleasure of my first position in the history of medicine. I was fortunate to have been affiliated with Associated Medical Services (formerly known as the Hannah Foundation) in Toronto; the Cumming School of Medicine at the University of Calgary; the Office for History of Science and Technology at the University of California, Berkeley; the Montreal Neurological Institute and the Osler Library for the History of Medicine; Departments I and III of the Max Planck Institute for the History of Science; the Archives of the Max Planck Society; the Department for History and Ethics of

Medicine at Ruprecht Karls University in Heidelberg; the Department for History, Philosophy, and Ethics of Medicine at Gutenberg University in Mainz; the Laboratoire d'épistémologie des sciences de la vie et de la santé, Université de Strasbourg; the Driburger Kreis of the German Society for the History of Medicine, Science, and Technology; the Deutsche Gesellschaft fuer Geschichte der Nervenheilkunde; the International Society for the History of the Neurosciences; the Canadian Society for the History of Medicine; the American Academy of Neurology; the Office of History of the National Institutes of Health; the Becker Medical Library at Washington University in St Louis; the Neuroscience History Archives of the University of California's Louise M. Darling Biomedical Library; the Calgary History of Medicine Society; and the Mackie Family Collection in the History of Neuroscience.

The archivists, librarians, and assistants of so many libraries and archives provided crucial support for collecting the historical material. I am grateful for their professionalism and have benefited from their knowledge in finding sources, archival holdings, people, and contextual information. As they are so many, I cannot mention them here by name; yet I would like to acknowledge the institutions to which I owe so much. I am extremely grateful for the help that I received in Europe from: the Zweigbibliothek fuer Wissenschaftsgeschichte and Institutsbibliotheken fuer Anatomie, Neurologie, and Medizingeschichte of the Humboldt University of Berlin; the Medizinische Zentralbibliothek and the Library of the Humboldt University; the Library of the Max Planck Institute for the History of Science; the Staatsbibliothek Preussischer Kulturbesitz; the Bundesarchiv; the Bayerische Staatsbibliothek and Hauptstaatsarchiv; the Library and Archives of the Ludwig-Maximilians-University; the Aussenarchiv of the Max Planck Institute for Psychiatry; the Library of the Max Planck Institute for Neurobiology; the Leipziger Archiv zur Psychiatriegeschichte; the University Archives of the University of Cologne; the Institute for the History and Ethics of Medicine in Frankfurt am Main; the Edinger Institute; the Library of the Max Planck Institute for Brain Research; the Archives and the Senckenbergische Bibliothek of the Johann Wolfgang Goethe University as well as the German National Library in Frankfurt am Main; the C. and O. Vogt Institute for Brain Research at Heinrich Heine University; the Libraries of the Institute for Anatomy and the Psychiatric Clinic of the Friedrich Alexander University in Erlangen; the private collection of Juergen Peiffer (†); the Archives Bas-Rhin and Services des Archives of the Université Pasteur de Strasbourg; the University Library and Archives, the Psychiatriearchiv and the

Handschriftenabteilung as well as the Karl Sudhoff Institute at Leipzig University; the Archives of the University of Wrocław and the State Archives of Wrocław; the Bodleian Libraries at the University of Oxford, the National Library of Scotland/Leabharlann Nàiseanta na h-Alba, along with the Archives of the Institute for the History of Medicine and Medical Museum at the University of Zurich.

In North America, I worked in the following institutional libraries and archives: the Wilder Penfield Archives of the Osler Library; the Redpath University Library, the University Archives, and the Library of the Montreal Neurological Institute at McGill; Le centre canadien des études allemandes et européennes at the Université de Montréal and the Hans Selye Archives; the Archives of Nova Scotia; the University Library and the Special Collection of Medical History, Dalhousie University; the Canadian Museum of Immigration at Pier 21 in Halifax; Library and Archives Canada; the Smithsonian Institution and Archives of the Library of Congress in Washington, D C; the National Library of Medicine and the History Office of the National Institutes of Health; the Becker Medical Library and Rare Books Division; the University Library and Archives and the Viktor Hamburger Collection of Washington University in St. Louis; the University Library and Archives of the University of Calgary; the Archives of the University of California, Berkeley; San Francisco's Holocaust Memorial Institute; the University Library and the Neuroscience History Rare Books Collection of the University of California; Texas A&M University's Melbern G. Glasscock Center for Humanities Research; the Department of Psychiatry of Weill Medical College of Cornell University in New York; the University Archives of Drexel University and the Muetter Museum of the College of Physicians of Philadelphia; the Countway Library at Harvard University; the Leo-Baeck Institute, Columbia University Library, and the Rockefeller Archive Center in New York; the Library of Congress, the National Archives, and the United States Holocaust Memorial Museum in Washington, D C.

I am further indebted to the following bodies that supported my research during particular phases: the Deutsche Forschungsgemeinschaft; the Alexander von Humboldt-Foundation, Gerda Henkel Foundation; Deutscher Akademischer Austauschdienst; the Social Sciences and Humanities Research Council of Canada; the Canadian Institutes of Health Research; the Alberta Medical Foundation; Associated Medical Services; a John J. Pisano Award of the National Institutes of Health; an H. Richard Tyler Award of the American Academy of Neurology; the Dean of the Medical Faculty and Department of History at McGill; the

Montreal Neurological Institute; a Mary Louise Nickerson Fellowship in Neuro-History of the Osler Library; the Dean of the Cumming School of Medicine; enhancement grants through the University of Calgary; and the Awards to Scholarly Publications Program of the Canadian Federation for the Humanities and Social Sciences. I also thank McGill-Queen's University Press for the encouragement and invitation to submit this manuscript to them and wish to particularly include Kyla Madden, Casey Gazzelone, Finn Purcell, Kathleen Fraser, and my fabulous Toronto-based copy-editor Jane McWhinney, as well as the three anonymous reviewers who commented painstakingly on my earlier manuscript. My gratitude goes further to Jim Connor and Erika Dyck, for having included my book as series editors with the McGill-Queen's/Associated Medical Services Studies in the History of Medicine, Health, and Society. Finally, I extend my special gratitude to my colleagues in the University of Calgary's History of Neuroscience Interest Group, who gave me the comforting feeling of an intellectual home, even if I was sometimes away for longer stretches of time to pursue my research and writing.

FRANK W. STAHNISCH
University of Calgary &
University of California, Berkeley

Abbreviations

ADAS	Archives départementales [du Bas-Rhin] à Strasbourg
AMUW	Archiv der Medizinischen Universitaet Wien
BA KO	Bundesarchiv Koblenz
Bay HSta	Bavarian Main State Archive
CIOS	Combined Intelligence Operative Sub-Committee Reports [of the United States VII Army]
CNS	Central Nervous System
DFA	Deutsche Forschungsanstalt [later: Kaiser Wilhelm Institut] for Psychiatry
DGN	Deutsche Gesellschaft fuer Neurologie
DGR	Deutsche Gesellschaft fuer Rassenhygiene [German Society for Racial Hygiene]
DZfNhlk	*Deutsche Zeitschrift fuer Nervenheilkunde*
GDR	German Democratic Republic
GeStapo	Geheime Staatspolizei
HAMPG	Historisches Archiv der Max-Planck-Gesellschaft
HAMPIP	Historisches Archiv des Max-Planck-Instituts fuer Psychiatrie
K & K	(*"Kaiserliche und Koenigliche"*) Official institutions and communications within the Austro-Hungarian double monarchy
KWI	Kaiser Wilhelm Institute
KWIBR	Kaiser Wilhelm Institute for Brain Research [in Berlin-Buch]
KWG	Kaiser Wilhelm Society (Kaiser Wilhelm Gesellschaft)
MIT	Massachusetts Institute of Technology
MPI	Max Planck Institute

NIH	National Institutes of Health
NS	National Socialism
NSDAeB	Nationalsozialistischer deutscher Aerztebund
NSDAP	Nationalsozialistische deutsche Arbeiterpartei
NSLB	Nationalsozialistischer deutscher Lehrerbund
PNS	Peripheral Nervous System
RAC	Rockefeller Archive Center [Sleepy Hollow, New York State]
RF	Rockefeller Foundation
SA	Sturmabteilung [Storm Troopers]
SDGGN	*Schriftenreihe der Deutschen Gesellschaft fuer Geschichte der Nervenheilkunde*
SS	Schutzstaffel [Defence Corps]
T4	Tiergartenstrasse 4 [Berlin headquarters of the Nazi euthanasia program]
UAF	Universitaetsarchiv Frankfurt am Main
UAHUB	Universitaetsarchiv der Humboldt Universitaet Berlin
UAL	Universitaetsarchiv Leipzig
UK	United Kingdom
US	United States [of America]
WUSM	Washington University School of Medicine, St Louis
WWI	World War I
WWII	World War II
ZBfNP	*Zentralblatt fuer Nervenheilkunde, Psychiatrie und gerichtliche Psychopathologie* [after 1890: *Zentralblatt fuer Nervenheilkunde und Psychiatrie*]
ZfN	*Zeitschrift fuer Neurologie*

A NEW FIELD IN MIND

I

Introduction

Neuropathology was a basic science for neurosurgeons, as well as for neurologists and psychiatrists. It would always have to be a subject of further investigation and for teaching in any neurological institute, generation after generation.

Wilder Penfield[1]

The new research field of "the neurosciences" has attracted immense recognition and concern in the wider public over the past two decades largely thanks to its enormous developments in research technologies and breathtaking methodologies. In parallel, there have been great medical and social hopes that the underlying research progress would soon translate into new treatment options for neurological and mental diseases as well as into forms of advanced knowledge in biomedicine. At the same time, scholars and the public alike have continuously emphasized that this translation was unlikely – because of the complexity of the research topics themselves and the difficulty of integrating new findings into adequate health and social uses. Better causal models and neurological and psychiatric treatment options are also needed.[2] In the nearer future, both the advances and the impasses of modern clinical and basic neuroscience will prospectively affect our ways of thinking about new diagnostic classifications, refined clinical nosologies, and the pathological aetiologies related to the brain and the spinal cord in unanticipated dimensions. This includes our understanding of, and treatment options toward, mental health and mental disorders for the individuals concerned.[3] It is striking to see that among such debates about the progress and reach of this research field, the very notion of the term "neurosciences" goes uncontested and is hardly examined in its intricate historical, social, and organizational origins. In this book I look at the motivations and the making of this burgeoning field in the early interdisciplinary research centres in Germany,

Austria, and Switzerland, particularly between 1882 and 1962, while laying bare the groundbreaking cultural and scientific dimensions that led to the emergence of "neuroscience" in its very modern meaning. The book thus presents an instructive example that will, I hope, help deepen our understanding of the scientific necessities in brain research. At the same time, it calls for leaving the ivory towers of the universities in order to review and examine the effects of "pure knowledge" in its connection with the applied approaches and economic interests of the social and *public sphere* at large.[4] Furthermore, the field of neuromorphology around the turn of the twentieth century also experienced a number of new challenges from within the scientific community itself – the technologies used, for example, the experimental questions asked, and the new diagnostic potentials revealed through its research results.[5] As such, the book is of multiple importance to the historiographical, epistemological, philosophical, and methodological aspects of the science studies.

I also present a specific analysis of an important yet hitherto neglected field in the historiography of biomedical science. In the latter sections I compare the fate of émigré neuroscientists in Canada and the United States as political developments in Nazi Germany led to the expulsion of almost a third of all neurologists and psychiatrists from Central Europe, most of whom were received into North American research and teaching institutions. One of the many consequences of the reintegration of differing communities of neuromorphologists into the pre-existing scientific culture on the other side of the Atlantic was the gradual though effective transformation of this field into one of most prolific areas of knowledge production in the post–World War II period,[6] a process that I compare with the earlier advances and developments in the German-speaking research community.

The narrative account of this monographic book therefore offers an almost archaeological account of some of the foundations and multiple paths that led to development of one of the most powerful interdisciplinary areas of the life sciences. In this attempt at historiography, I explore and analyze the theoretical as well as the cultural developments that fostered the growth of the neurosciences as we know it today. A close focus on the problem of interdisciplinarity in the neuromorphological sciences in German-speaking countries from the 1880s to the early 1960s, especially the impact of three different historical political and cultural systems (German Imperialism, the social experiment of the Weimar Democracy, and the devastating influences of National Socialism) allows us to scrutinize the emergence and growth of the modern neurosciences and connect them to the respective chronologies and effects of the three contextual political systems.[7] The narrative of my book will give further hints as to how this important interdisciplinary work has been perceived in the neurosciences along with the very organization of its research institutions, programs, and locales.

Having had the opportunity of exchanging impressions and experiences with North American neuroscientists over the past decade – although many reluctantly asked what a historian of medicine actually does – I learned that it is a commonly held belief (by neuroscientists as well as historians of science and medicine, both in Central Europe and in North America) that there had not been a unified landscape of the neurosciences in the first decades of the last century. This belief completely contradicted my earlier research observations, which had evoked rather strong and systemic relationships between technical developments, contemporary institutions, and the people such as researchers, assistants, contractors, and administrators who worked in those institutions and thus influenced and shaped their institutional cultures. The first personal reaction among my North American colleagues was often one of complete astonishment: Why would it be of interest to know how the neuroscientific pursuit was historically determined in the first place? Are the questions and hypotheses that a neuroscientist raises not found in neuroscientific research problems themselves? Yet when I presented them with historical instances, spanning more than a hundred years, in which philosophers, psychologists, internists, surgeons, serologists, pathologists, and many others had worked together on neuroscientific problems, my accounts were often met by surprise, increasingly giving way to genuine curiosity about the rather unknown early history of modern neuroscience: Why did contemporary philosophers attend the lectures of influential neuroanatomists on the locus of consciousness? Why did neurologists approach *Gestalt* psychologists for diagnoses and therapies of war-wounded soldiers? Why would pathologists in the 1940s still act as diagnostic "guiding lights" for neurosurgeons, converting their knowledge into useful clinical tools for the topological planning processes of surgical interventions in their operation theatres?

These and other related historical questions became interesting for me to explore. In 1882 – 137 years ago – the first institute dedicated completely to brain research was created in Vienna.[8] Today, American neuroscientists often ask: How is it that we don't know about these origins of neuroscience? Why did we think that such centres were invented on US soil? The Central European echo is much the same: How can it be that a scientific tradition that had its origins and heyday in Vienna and the other German-speaking metropolises of Berlin, Munich, and Zurich disappeared and was reimported from the United States only recently?

It is important to appreciate that what appears to have been a revolutionary development in twentieth-century biomedical science was not "a purely American affair."[9] The interplay between such discipline-based knowledge centres and differing local practices in early brain research has yet to be explored explicitly from a science and technology studies perspective. Also, the historical question of "interdisciplinary research approaches" remains to be investigated with regard to modern biomedical science in general and neuroscience in particular. However, to this day we have not had an encompassing historical account of what caused the emergence of interdisciplinary research programs such as MIT professor Francis O. ("Frank") Schmitt's (1903–1995) Neuroscience Research Program to begin with (see also figure 8.1).[10]

I want to start by addressing some of the hallmark characteristics that current scholarship has brought out since it has been dealing with the question of interdisciplinarity in the biomedical sciences from an in-depth theoretical perspective.[11] Current interest in the morphological research sphere of the German neurosciences between the 1880s and the early 1960s has revealed that historical concepts, practices, and organizational patterns were widely used in early brain research centres. This context legitimizes the use of the term of "neuroscience" as a descriptor to identify contemporary research traditions that manifested as a largely interdisciplinary *problem field*.[12] While scholars have only recently begun to investigate the development of interdisciplinary research projects in the biomedical sciences, studies into similar developments in the physical and chemical sciences have already been in process for a longer while.[13] The development of the German-speaking neuroscience field thus marks an important research desideratum that will enable readers to appreciate and value the scientific, organizational, and also cultural innovations that influenced the course of biomedical research so profoundly from the beginning of the century to after World War II.[14]

I will here emphasize particularly the relationship of interdisciplinary work with different *national research styles* in the time period under study.[15] "National styles" are commonly understood as differences in medical practices that can be attributed to differing cultural and intellectual traditions and are shaped by corresponding norms, perceptions, and actions.[16] I am particularly interested in the influences of neighbouring fields and disciplines on German-speaking neuromorphologists and in how such contextual developments altered pre-existing experimental and clinical traditions:[17] What were the factors that triggered changes in the views of neuromorphologists on the rigidity of the brain's structure? How did they accommodate for plastic phenomena as these forms of biological regeneration became criticized within the clinical arena? And in what ways did neuromorphologists try to bypass "electrophysiological threats,"[18] which indicated that somatic localizationism could not be sufficiently aligned with interpretations of disease dynamics? As applied and theoretical knowledge became further integrated into political spheres, social and psychological considerations within neuromorphology also appeared increasingly relevant. Neurological and psychiatric sciences were becoming involved in *biopolitical discourses* especially between the 1910s and the late 1940s, most notably in discussions on eugenics in the Weimar period and the euthanasia program in Nazi Germany.[19] What has until now still been lacking, however, is a detailed analysis of how particular research assumptions of the nineteenth century influenced the biopolitical discourses of the first half of the twentieth.[20]

The area delineated by the term "neuromorphology" is conceived here as the study of the structure of the brain as it was practised during the period from the 1880s to the early 1960s, when that study became the focus of many research programs in the contemporary neurosciences. The neuromorphological tradition marked an important segment of what was considered at the time as "brain research" (or *Hirnforschung* – in German parlance). It was a central research subject in the combined field of clinical and research neurology and psychiatry (*Nervenheilkunde*).[21] My decision to focus particularly on the structural aspects of the brain and the central nervous system is a necessary downsizing strategy that is not intended to exclude the physiological areas of the field.[22] Despite these methodological limitations, there still remains ample material for an analysis of the contemporary neuromorphological sciences, making this a promising endeavour in exploring the important intersections among neuroanatomy, neuropathology, brain psychiatry, aspects from clinical neurosurgery, and neurology, neuroradiology, and neuroserology.[23] (The latter constituted a research subfield that studied the properties of serum and other body fluids in their connection with infections and diseases of the brain and spinal cord.[24]) These "disciplines" can be perceived as constitutive elements in the making of the interdisciplinary research field in twentieth-century German-speaking neuroscience.

The timeframe from the 1880s to the early 1960s expediently allows us to address the political and cultural contexts of three major articulations of German cultural and political history while exploring the geographical area of the German-speaking countries as being crucial to the emergence of this new research field. What I mean in this regard is that the changes in the organization and pursuit of the neurosciences from the Wilhelminian period (perceived here as the *status quo ante* deriving from the nineteenth-century, discipline-centred, and full-professor-oriented *Ordinarienuniversitaet*) throughout the Weimar Republic and the National Socialist period.[25] The Weimar period represented a nearly fifteen-year interim of protracted experiments both in the scientific and social domains of institutional reform and later in the subsuming of much of the interdisciplinary endeavours into the politically dominated scientific and educational frameworks of the National Socialist regime.[26] These period histories will be interpreted with an analytic focus on process-oriented, social-contextual, and comparative evidence. The resulting narrative gives us answers and insights as to why neuroscientific research emerged at the beginning of the twentieth century, and why the German-speaking context was such an important social environment and cultural catalyst for these processes to occur.[27] Historians of science have made tentative conjectures for ways of tying this picture to the later differentiation of the field; one thinks, for example, of Michael Hagner's publication *Homo cerebralis*,[28] which features the earlier psychiatric tradition introduced by Wilhelm Griesinger (1817–1868) based on the use of neuroanatomical brain models for enhancing the understanding of mental functions and diseases, or Max Stadler's work *Assembling Life*, which is concerned with the intricate relationship between biophysics and the neurosciences in the postwar period.[29]

From a historiographical perspective, I will discuss important guiding principles, background philosophies, and substantive research programs that oriented, altered, and shaped the outlook on the sciences of the brain and nerves – neuroscience even before the term was actually introduced in early 1962.[30] As for theoretical question about the organization of "neuroscientific theories" from a philosophy of science perspective,[31] I need to add some caveats here. As a medical historian, I do not intend to present an explicit logic of the neurosciences; nor will I address the structure of neuroscientific theories in a way in which an early Thomas Nagel (b. 1937) might philosophically have thought about the structure of the natural sciences.[32] Nor is it my intention to provide an exclusive history of the ideas of early twentieth-century neuroscience reminiscent of the way Arthur Oncken Lovejoy (1873–1962) and others understood the history of science to be guided by group-thought, individual reasoning, and preconceived research ideas.[33]

I have a more practical and socializational interest that stemmed from personal exchanges with contemporary neuroscientists through my work in clinical neuroscience for three years in my early professional career. When I spoke to modern German neurologists, for instance, mentioning my historical interest in the early development of interdisciplinary centres in the neurosciences, the use of this organizational concept often became associated with the recent foundation of neuroscience research institutes and centres in the 1990s, such as those at the Georg August University of Goettingen, the Charité Medical School in Berlin, and at the Friedrich Wilhelms University of Bonn. Many of the neuroscientists I met believed that the creation of such centres was a direct import to Germany of an organizational model that had developed in twentieth-century American neuroscience, only gradually trickling into German academia since the 1980s.[34] Mention was often made, in particular, of such research centres as the Washington University in St Louis Program in Neuroscience, Missouri; the previous Salk Institute in LaJolla, California; the Kavli Institute for Neuroscience at Yale, New Haven in Connecticut; the National Institute of Mental Health in Bethesda, Maryland; or the Montreal Neurological Institute in Quebec.[35]

When I found myself asking senior neuroscientists in Germany directly what they perceived as the substantial differences between modern American institutions and their former German counterparts such as the Edinger Institute in Frankfurt am Main, the Deutsche Forschungsanstalt for Psychiatry in Munich, or the Brain Research Institute of the Kaiser Wilhelm Gesellschaft, most of them shrugged their shoulders.[36] Conversely, historians of medicine have often related the developments of interdisciplinary research centres to the local contexts of their respective universities and cities (the universities of Frankfurt, Berlin, or Leipzig, for instance),[37] or have looked at non-university research institutions such as the former Kaiser Wilhelm Institutes, as separate and independent creations.[38] My narrative thus somewhat parallels that of the French historian of medicine Jean Paul Gaudiellière and his work on biomedical cancer research in France and the United States:[39]

> [The] post-war period saw the growth of biomedical complexes characterized by the intensification of research in the life sciences, the hunt for novel molecules, and a new alliance between biologists and the state ... Although biomedicine has, above all, been dominated by experimental medicine, other sets of practices have persisted alongside those employed by the experimenter, including molecular

modelling ... and biomedical scientists have developed complex relationships with hospital clinicians and public health officials, which
have varied *from arm's-length distance, to mutual interdependence,
and – more rarely – to outright collaboration.*[40]

The historiographical problem has now become more circumscribed:
as is often the case, new theories and practices arise from a changing
disciplinary makeup in the organization of scientific institutions and
research pursuits. This has, for example, previously been shown by the
American historian of science Derek DaSolla Price (1922–1983) and
British historian of medicine Jonathan Harwood (b. 1942) for the field
of biophysics and experimental biology.[41] Breaking out from the disciplinary composition of anatomy, physiology, pathology, neurology, and psychiatry in the nineteenth century also fostered new trends toward
group-oriented neuroscientific activities more frequently seen since the
1910s and 1920s. This trend is exhibited by prominent medical scientists
such as the Vienna neuroanatomist Heinrich Obersteiner (1847–1922)
(see figure 1.1), the Breslau clinical neurologist Otfrid Foerster (1873–
1941), the neuropathologist Ludwig Edinger (1855–1918) in Frankfurt
am Main, the Munich brain psychiatrist Emil Kraepelin (1856–1926),
and the neuroanatomist Oskar Vogt (1870–1959) in Berlin.[42]

These approaches antedated many later interdisciplinary research centres in Central Europe in several ways and also served as important
templates for a number of influential brain researchers on the western
side of the Atlantic; one thinks of such scholars as Canadian neurologist
Wilder Penfield (1891–1976) in Montreal, neurosurgeon Harvey Cushing
(1869–1939) at Yale, and St Louis–trained neurophysiologist Frank
Schmitt, who subsequently transformed biomedical research in the later
twentieth century.[43]

Yet so far, we lack an appropriate historical explanation as to what
initially triggered these developments and how the research field of neuroscience became envisaged and crafted with particular *leitmotifs* in mind.
I hope that a narrative approach to the contemporary research on the
structure of the brain and spinal cord will help us to scrutinize the conceptual determinants, laboratory practices, and interchanges between tacit
knowledge and organizational patterns in neuromorphological research.[44]
I shall also explore the social experiences and the individual background
knowledge of contemporary neuromorphologists regarding the "cultural
embeddedness" of their programs, while putting German-American soci-
ologist Karin Knorr-Cetina's notion of an "intensification of society in

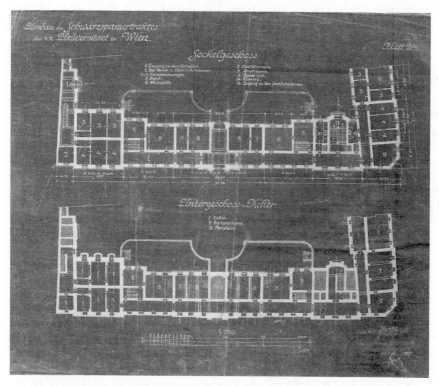

1.1 Reconstruction of the *Schwarzpaniertrakt* of the University of Vienna: Architectural plan of the raised ground floor of the Neurological Institute of Dr H. Obersteiner (upper and lower floors) before its remodelling, in 1905 (Bildersammlung Josephinum; MUW-AS-002461-0022+0023 Neurological Institute). © Courtesy of Josephinum, Ethics, Collections and History of Medicine of the Medical University of Vienna, Austria.

the laboratory" (*Verdichtung von Gesellschaft im Labor*) to work.[45] Knorr-Cetina sees the development of modern biomedical science as influenced, if not driven, by sociocultural changes, which are often woven into patterns of research organization.[46] In this survey of the historiography of the neuromorphological sciences between the 1880s and the early 1960s, I also tackle larger interdisciplinarity narratives. I visited several archives at major German-speaking sites of neuroscientific research, archives investigated regionally by other scholars as well.[47] Further examination of North American sources has enabled me to investigate how particular scientific networks and internationally oriented institutions acted as cultural hosts for many of the émigré neuroscientists arriving in the United States and Canada in the 1930s and 1940s.[48] Our attention here is thus focused on the organizational arrangements out of which

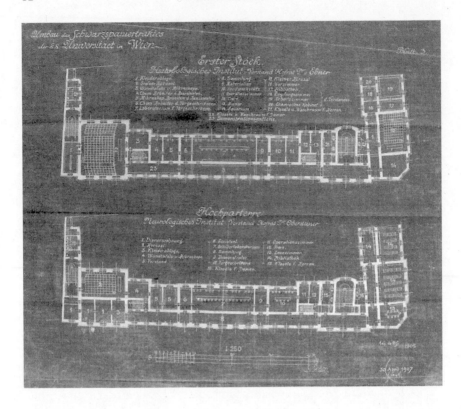

these new *epistemic cultures* emerged in early twentieth-century German-speaking neuroscience.[49]

VIENNA – THE LANDMARK!

As the "institutional birthday" of modern brain research efforts around the *fin de siècle*, we could highlight 14 December 1882. It marks the date when Vienna neuroanatomist Heinrich Obersteiner received full approval for the creation of the Institute for the Anatomical and Physiological Study of the Central Nervous System (Institut zur Anatomischen und Physiologischen Erforschung des Nervensystems) (see figure 1.1). This moment in time set the stage for the formation of a research department that became devoted exclusively to the study of the brain and nerves from both clinical and basic research perspectives.[50] Before Obersteiner assumed the professorship of physiology and pathology of the nervous system at the University of Vienna in 1900, he had practised as a consultant in the Doeblinger Mental Asylum on the outskirts of the

Austro-Hungarian capital, where he had already promoted research in the field of Theoretical Neurology. In a letter to the Austro-Hungarian minister of education and cultural affairs, Graf Leo von Thurn und Hohenstein (1811–1888), dated 27 March 1883, Obersteiner described the productivity of his new institute:

> Although probably not accounting for a fully comprehensive compilation, nearly 98 publications have come out of my institute, which are distributed as follows to the contributing disciplines:
>
> | | |
> |---|---|
> | Normal Anatomy | 16 |
> | Comparative Anatomy | 7 |
> | Pathological Anatomy | 66 |
> | Physiology | 7 |
> | Microscopic Technology | 2 |
>
> Currently, all branches of theoretical neurology are represented, including pathological anatomy.[51]

Obersteiner was educated in the conventional "disciplinary" tradition of neurology, yet had frequently changed his assistant positions in neurophysiology, neuroanatomy, and clinical neurology. He was the grandson in a family dynasty of Viennese physicians and, like his father and grandfather before him, had studied at the university of his native city.[52] Among his teachers were the anatomical educator and textbook author Joseph Hyrtl (1811–1894), and one of the most important founders of anatomical pathology, Carl von Rokitansky (1804–1878). While still in his early student years, Obersteiner had been invited to work with Austria's foremost experimental physiologist, Ernst Wilhelm von Bruecke (1819–1892), joining the latter's laboratory as a research assistant. Before he even received his doctorate, Obersteiner in 1869 published his first neurological work on the structure of the cerebellar cortex.[53] His clinical interests were fostered in addition through the influence of his father-in-law, the notable psychiatrist and neurologist Theodor Meynert (1833–1892) from the University of Vienna, who had also supervised Sigmund Freud's (1856–1939) doctoral thesis.[54] Obersteiner then received his *Habilitation* (licence in postsecondary teaching) for anatomy and pathology of the nervous system in 1873 and was appointed associate professor to the Vienna Medical Faculty in 1880. This process involved a great deal of personal networking, influential dynastical relationships, and nepotistic weight-pulling, all of which spoke to the particular local Vienna milieu and its research community.

Although the family resources on which Obersteiner could draw were considerable, the beginnings of his institute were rather humble. When he applied to the medical faculty to create a small workshop-style laboratory in November 1882, the dean, Richard Heschl (1824–1881), responded by stating that his proposal was "unnecessary," since the relevant activities were already being undertaken in the pre-existing departments. Obersteiner was told that if he wished to store a few instruments for his investigations, he could put them in a wooden box under the pathologists' dissection tables.[55] Despite this personal embarrassment and the evident resentment of his plans on the part of the established *Ordinarien* professors and department heads, Obersteiner did not give up on the idea of creating a specialized institute for brain research. With the help of some of his influential teachers in the basic research community and his *Nervenaerzte* colleagues from the clinical field of neurology and psychiatry, he prepared the ground for the eventual acceptance of his plans. The cornerstone of this history was, however, a matter of chance: on 14 December 1882 a munitions factory that had just been abandoned by the Austro-Hungarian Army was made available to him.[56] Advantageously positioned near the Vienna General Hospital and the Josephinum College for Military Surgeons, the building was larger than many of the existing university institutes. Obersteiner had now received an ideal venue for his specialized institute, which he was to differentiate further into several brain research divisions: normal anatomy, comparative anatomy, pathological anatomy, physiology, and microscopic technology.

Obersteiner's institute in Vienna was still very much a local foundation, driven by a prominent entrepreneurial individual and largely dependent on private financial contributions. However, the creation of the Emergency Council for German Science in 1920 (the Notgemeinschaft Deutsche Wissenschaft – since 1929 known as the Deutsche Forschungsgemeinschaft) marked a decisive moment for early research in the neurosciences. This was a turning point in the sociopolitical funding structure of science – and, of course, medicine – which greatly influenced future investigations of the brain and nervous system in German-speaking countries.[57] Additional research grants from abroad through organizations such as the American Rockefeller Foundation helped stabilize early neuroscientific research programs after World War I and its disastrous effects on German science at large.[58]

When asking which notions of the benefit, necessity, and epistemic value of interdisciplinarity prevailed historically in *avant-garde* neuroscientists, it is crucial that we also take a close look at contemporary experimental efforts. These efforts were particularly associated with public health and community service projects (*Gemeinschaftsaufgaben*), crucial research demands (*Forschungsanstrengungen*), and collaborative work endeavours (*Zusammenarbeiten*), which figured strongly in the informal letters and official research proposals of the time.[59] An additional aspect of this question, as American historian of science Timothy Lenoir emphasizes in his seminal book *Instituting Science: The Cultural Production of Scientific Disciplines* (1997), is that historiographical work on the formation of scientific disciplines in the nineteenth century has led to a historiographical preoccupation with and bias toward university institutes and medical research clinics. In fact, earlier scholarship blended cross-institutional and extra-university forms of research organization and scientific programs, and these forms became typical for many areas in later technology-driven research fields. Nevertheless, Lenoir called attention to the need to "depict universities as participants in a situated knowledge community, and in effect, to treat the disciplinary structure of the university as part of a regional knowledge economy."[60] The concept of such *regional knowledge economies* will be particularly useful for my historiographical perspective, since it transcends the traditional view that research is associated with specialized and thus "disciplined" institutes,[61] organized in pyramidal hierarchical structures, and circumscribed as distinct knowledge communities for each scientific discipline.

While putting some of these theoretical considerations to work, I further explore in this book the role and the scope of interdisciplinary projects within the German tradition of neuromorphology between 1882 and 1962. This book can therefore be viewed a prototypical case for the new and emerging neuroscientific field to open up from the pursuit of "pure knowledge" (in the contemporary German meaning of *reine Wissenschaft*) and connect with broader "applied ideas," social practices and financial interests in the wider economic and public spheres (*anwendungsbezogene Wissenschaft*). Furthermore, neuromorphology at this time experienced a number of challenges from within the scientific field itself, stemming from the technologies used, the experimental questions stimulated, and the new diagnostic potentials of its research results.[62]

Accordingly, I hope to scrutinize the experiences and work profiles of some of the key players involved in shaping and transforming the emerging field of German-speaking neuromorphology at the beginning of the twentieth century and provide a group biographical and institutional framework for further in-depth analyses of the formation and design of the essential *topoi* in contemporary neuromorphological research. I approach these biographical profiles from a perspective of historical epistemology, considering the interrelation of practice and theory, the organization of mutual research trends, and cultural differences in the identification of research priorities. I have therefore relied on materials from various archives *on* and *of* the neurosciences at universities and other research centres within the borders of the German Empire after 1871 – including, for example, Strasburg and Breslau – thereafter expanding my analysis to the interwar period, the "Third Reich," and the postwar period after 1945.

"GROUP RESEARCH ACTIVITIES": IN AND BEYOND THE KAISER WILHELM SOCIETY

When the Deutsche Forschungsgemeinschaft was inaugurated on 30 October 1920 in Berlin right after the end of World War I as an emergency council to support German scholarship and science, a remarkable personal, philanthropic, and political interest in the institution's activities was immediately stimulated. This rise in public awareness resulted notably in a flow of money *in* and *for* international research exchanges, successfully orchestrated by the organization's first president, Friedrich Schmidt-Ott (1860–1956), a former minister of the Prussian Ministry of Science, Arts, and Culture and assistant to the notorious architect of leading nineteenth-century Prussian research facilities Friedrich Althoff (1839–1908).[63] A similar influence of public attention was also seen in the engagement of the American Rockefeller Foundation in German neuroscience from the 1920s to the 1940s. In fact, big science endeavours (*Grossforschungsanstrengungen*) in Weimar Germany can hardly be understood without taking the foundation's major financial contributions into account. The Rockefeller Foundation thereby sought to "help Germany out of its continued scientific isolation," as the foundation's Europe officer Edwin R. Embrée (1883–1950) stated in a November 1922 letter responding to John V. Van Sickle (1862–1939), when "war and inflation had destroyed a large part of local endowments and the public authorities had to step in." Embrée's assessment was later echoed by his officer colleague during the latter's own visit to Frankfurt am Main on 15 May 1931.[64]

The Rockefeller Foundation's engagement was manifold and complex, since this international funding body supported noteworthy university departments and research units alike. Soon afterward it became a primary stakeholder in the reshaping of the German Kaiser Wilhelm Society and many of its research institutes. Through the mediation of its Paris office and the strategic planning of Alan Gregg (1890–1957), section chair of the Rockefeller Foundation's funding program for psychiatry, psychosomatics, and brain research (see also figure 5.3), it became highly influential in the initiation and growth of German-speaking neuroscience at large.[65] North American money became a substantial funding source that deeply invigorated research ties among the institutes, which formed Germany's "Brain Triangle," as I like to describe it. This structure was constituted primarily by the Deutsche Forschungsanstalt for Psychiatry in Munich, Bavaria, headed by Emil Kraepelin; the Kaiser Wilhelm Institute (KWI) for Brain Research in Berlin, which Oskar and Cécile Vogt (1875–1962) had inaugurated; and Otfrid Foerster's Neurological Institute at the University of Breslau, in Lower Silesia (see figure 1.3).

Yet, rather than offering an altruistic engagement in the German-speaking medical sciences, the large sums of foreign money supplied through the American Rockefeller Foundation particularly were intended to rebuild the transatlantic exchange relationships between researchers in all stages of their education. (I expand further on the details of the administrative mechanics and the specific local and networking effects of the Rockefeller Foundation's role in funding German neuroscience between 1921 and 1942 below, in chapter 4.) North American science administrators, research trainees, and visiting professors arrived, for example, to work in the KWI for Brain Research in Berlin with Oskar Vogt, Cécile Vogt, Maximilian Rose (1883–1937), and Max Bielschowsky (1869–1940), where they set out to study the "psychology of the 'Neurosen' [neuropathies], and ... the peculiar *characteristics connected with the problem of heredity*" of the brain.[66] The forms of collaborative work in extended groups which subsequently became necessary initiated a complete move away from the autonomous research disciplines with their nineteenth-century origins.[67]

Even though the "neurosciences" could not have been singled out among the respective community research projects themselves, a number of working groups were nevertheless supported by the Deutsche Forschungsgemeinschaft in related areas such as cancer research, which bordered strongly on current investigations in neuropathology, neuroanatomy, clinical neurology, and brain psychiatry.[68] Through this process, step by step, the corresponding disciplines gradually drifted into quite a primary nexus of political and public attention.[69] The longevity of such innovative science policies, which the Deutsche Forschungsgemeinschaft had adopted since the middle of the 1920s, also needs to be highlighted. The general process itself can be understood as *a highly political form of funding concentration*. It was carried out in order to establish politically oriented and mandated research institutions involving highly acclaimed researchers and preselected sites in the vicinity of major research universities. The funding process to support such politicized community research projects was realized mainly through the close interrelation of leadership personnel both in the Deutsche Forschungsgemeinschaft and in pre-war extra-university institutes. The most prominent institution was certainly the Kaiser Wilhelm Society with its fifteen Nobel laureates, which had been founded in Berlin on 11 January 1911 under the chairmanship of the Prussian minister of education and cultural affairs, August von Trott zu Solz (1855–1938), with the declared political intent of forming a "German Oxford" in the sciences – notably in the southwest quadrant of the capital, Berlin.[70]

An instance of the rising politicization of the process of reorganizing science and technology after the late 1910s can be found in the continuing creation throughout the 1930s of Deutsche Forschungsgemeinschaft working groups (*Arbeitsgemeinschaften*), which formed important networks and collaborative relationships among researchers and clinicians from all over Germany. One such group was the Working Group II for Racial Hygiene and Racial Politics. Representatives from all major neuroscience and biological psychiatric institutions took part in the proceedings of this specific working group. Its tasks were meticulously laid out in the founding policy paper; they included programs for public education, basic brain research, clinical psychiatric investigations, postgraduate training, research into practices of sterilizing individuals with inherited neurological and psychiatric disorders, demographic disease statistics, and patient and family counselling activities.[71] Members of the Advisory Committee of the Working Group II met on 22 February 1930. Among them were, for example, the infamous Berlin racial anthropologist Eugen Fischer (1874–1967); the director of the KWI for Brain Research, Oskar Vogt; the surgeon and Prussian privy councillor August Bier (1861–1949); Munich psychiatrist and ardent eugenicist Ernst Ruedin (1874–1952); the Freiburg military pathologist Ludwig Aschoff (1866–1942); the Munich public hygienist Friedrich von Mueller (1858–1941); the racial hygienist Ludwig Schmidt-Kehl (1891–1941) from Wuerzburg; venereal hygienist Ernst von Duering (1858–1944); and the president of the Kaiser Wilhelm Society, Friedrich Glum (1891–1974).[72]

The organizational network and manifold funding activities were not limited to the self-declared racial anthropologists who made use of the enormous funding opportunities offered through the Working Group II, as Volker Roelcke and Matthias M. Weber have shown in their publications.[73] Conversely, Ruedin, director of the demographic division at the

Deutsche Forschungsanstalt for Psychiatry, wrote to the minister of state, Friedrich Schmidt-Ott, on 16 January 1930, detailing the future impact of his new community research projects "of counting and *identifying the mentally ill and handicapped* as well as the respective disease prevalence in the individual regions of Germany."[74] Other credulous brain researchers shared the values and promoted the ideals of the new Deutsche Forschungsgemeinschaft, as did the highly renowned Oskar Vogt, himself a human cortex researcher and likewise the director of the KWI for Brain Research in Berlin-Buch (see also figure 4.3). In a letter to the president of the Deutsche Forschungsgemeinschaft, Friedrich Schmidt-Ott, on 2 December 1930, Vogt tried to position the emerging brain research activities as a valuable contribution to the large-scale science programs in public health and racial hygiene, while helping to move them into the Deutsche Forschungsgemeinschaft's institutional awareness and funding portfolio:

Your Excellency has shown in his invitation from 3 Nov[ember 1930] that the anthropological research endeavours in the German "population" [*Bevoelkerung*] will take place on a much broader basis ... [However,] when regular and constant hereditary factors were studied in the past, it was found that not all hereditary modes applied to human reproduction, making it necessary to conduct new animal experiments. My collaborator N[icolai]. Timofeeff-Ressovsky [1900–1981] in particular has developed this important field of study and begun to elucidate the inconstantly manifested hereditary factors in (neurological) disease.[75]

As with many other negotiations with major funding agencies, Vogt promoted his collaborators and offered research aid through associates in his department at the KWI for Brain Research – as it emerges from the above excerpt from his letter to the Deutsche Forschungsgemeinschaft related to neurogenetics activities. In order to support the community service projects that the Deutsche Forschungsgemeinschaft had singled out as primary areas for its research support, Vogt also advocated for the scientific promises of the new interdisciplinary makeup of his own institute and made a point of emphasizing the great progress that had been made in the institute since its inception as the small Neurobiological Laboratory in the private apartment of Vogt and his wife, Cécile, at 12, Magdeburger Strasse in Berlin (see figure 3.3).[76]

The new KWI for Brain Research was built as a close analog to Obersteiner's institute in Vienna and was supported by funding from the influential Krupp family of steel industrialists, which became available after Friedrich Alfred Krupp's (1849–1902) wife had been a neurological hypnosis patient of Vogt, who had apparently treated her ailment with relatively good success. With the continued engagement of the Rockefeller Foundation in German brain science, and the additional provision of a free building lot offered by the city of Berlin, it became possible to secure the foundation of a new cutting-edge KWI for Brain Research in Berlin-Buch. Altogether, the institute cost 1.5 million Reichsmark, 200,000 of which was provided by the German Reich and 300,000 by the Krupp family, the State of Prussia having originally proposed adding another 205,000 Reichsmark.[77] Yet this seeming beneficence was by no means represented in the way the development originally unfolded, as officer Alan Gregg wrote back to the New York head office on 6 November 1928. He called the Vogts' private apartment laboratory "a surprising show," in which they had admirably managed to study the central nervous system from comprehensive anatomical, physiological, and embryological perspectives over three decades "with poor equipment and inadequate space." And Gregg saw fit to mention that Oskar Vogt was "still under 60."[78]

It was not astonishing, however, that the government of the State of Prussia eventually ceased its support of the project, since the Ministry of Education and Cultural Affairs had realized that its engagement in the university sector had already been too extensive. This happened exactly at the critical point in time when the Vogts' "apartment laboratory," as it was often called, had become so cramped that it had "metastasized" into adjacent buildings on Magdeburger Strasse, creating much trouble with the neighbours and the police.[79] Nevertheless, when Vogt personally threatened to cancel the whole endeavour of creating the KWI for Brain Research in Berlin – by publicly announcing that he would accept an offer as the new director of the Deutsche Forschungsanstalt for Psychiatry in Munich – the academic, political, and economic stakeholders immediately rejoined forces and, in combination with renewed financial support of the Rockefeller Foundation, rescued the institute. The KWI for Brain Research was soon built in the northeast of Berlin according to the advice of the city physician and hygienist Wilhelm von Drigalski (1871–1950). Drigalski drew attention to the fact that the Berlin community of Buch already had several larger mental asylums and rehabilitation sanatoria in place.[80] The new location thus promised "enough patient material" (in the language of the time) for the purposes of extensive brain research for the institute to be built. In addition to the eight research divisions, which had been anticipated in the original plan for the institute's organization – divisions for neuropathology, neuroanatomy, neurophysiology, neurogenetics, microscopy, radiology, demographics, and psychopathology – Vogt also applied for the creation of a smaller division and research ward for clinical psychiatry. It would contain forty beds, which he eventually received, to fulfill the institute's clinical mandate within the municipal masterplan.[81]

Vogt now could announce publicly that the new Berlin brain research institute of the Kaiser Wilhelm Society, was "the first European" institute of its kind.[82] In this new institute, the Vogts and their collaborators, such as the highly innovative neurophysiologist Korbinian Brodmann (1868–1918)[83] – who provided a still much-used map of the cerebral cortex in primates (see the cover image of this book), which was based on neurophysiological experiments and clinical observations in human patients – began to investigate the histological basis of neuropsychiatric diseases (*Pathoklisenarchitektur*). This program relied on the investigation of serial microscopic slices through whole brains, in conjunction with evidence from pathological, physiological, and genetic studies of brain development, which were published in the institute's own journal as well as in separate textbooks such as their publication *Experiences Regarding the Pathological Changes in the Striatum and the Pallidum as well as the Pathophysiology of the Related Disease Phenomena* in 1919 (*Zur Kenntnis der pathologischen Veraenderungen des Striatum und des Pallidum und zur Pathophysiologie der dabei auftretenden Krankheitserscheinungen*) (see also figure 3.4).[84]

Vogt hastened to promote the contributions of his KWI for Brain Research to a variety of large-scale research-funding programs in the German state of Prussia. His proposal eventually ended up in the Working Group II (supported by the national Deutsche Forschungsgemeinschaft), offering to add to the new science of racial anthropology in which the "KWI for Brain Research should receive widest possible credit and funding for its contributions."[85] Vogt only later changed his mind after frictions occurred with Nazi officials, who wanted to force him into retirement because of what was perceived as a "Jewish" and "Bolshevik" stronghold in German leading-edge biomedicine – alluding to the high number of Jewish physicians and Russian researchers, and to the Vogts' own contribution to the study of the brain of the leader of the Russian revolution, Vladimir Ilyich Uljanov Lenin (1870–1924).[86] Regarding the external social perceptions of contemporary neuroscience, it is also interesting to note that the very large and functionally suited modern concrete building of the KWI – as it had been designed by the internationally acclaimed Polish architect Jakub Lewicki (1886–1953) – was itself rejected by the

Nazis, as they believed that it displayed "Bolshevist architecture," while conversely, at the end of World War II in 1945, the advancing Russian troops saw it as displaying a purely bourgeois "American Style"[87] (see figure 4.3).

"BRAIN RESEARCH DIVISIONS":
IN THE AFTERMATH OF THE OBERSTEINER MODEL

I want to expand here a bit more on the specific organization of the research groups, the scientific institutions, and their interchanges in German-speaking neuromorphology during the decades of the 1920s and 1930s. This will prepare us to better address the historical problem field regarding new forms of interdisciplinary research organization. The early decades of the twentieth century, in general, mark a period of increased preoccupation with the subject of de- and regenerative processes in various areas of the neurosciences, psychiatry, and society at large.[88] Initial approaches – such as the Frankfurt neurophysiologist Albrecht Bethe's (1872–1954) *New Experiments on the Regeneration of the Nerve Fibers* of 1907 (*Neue Versuche ueber die Regeneration der Nervenfasern*), Ludwig Edinger's *Investigations Regarding New Formations in Dislocated Nerves* (1908b) (*Untersuchungen ueber die Neubildung des durchtrennten Nerven*), or Max Bielschowsky's work *On the Traumatic Regeneration Processes in the Central Nerve Fibers* published in 1909 (*Ueber Regenerationserscheinungen an Zentralen Nervenfasern*) – emerged from the many experiments in the intimate privacy of laboratories and encapsulated in the departments of anatomy, biology, and pathology of the traditional German research university style.[89] With the visible exception of Obersteiner's institute in Vienna, the research organization of the foregoing units and laboratories was primarily hierarchical. The institutes were led predominantly by a single director, who often controlled the research approaches and venues in all the subordinate divisions.[90]

What is most important for my narrative, however, is that the scientific methods that were used often remained "pure" in the sense that related technologies, machines, and even experimental practices were kept strictly within the confines of specialized departments. These departments would then emerge as the central "go-to place" at each university for other departments needing some research steps to be carried out for them, which would then be incorporated into the research processes and products of those "other" departments. It must be noted, though, that individual departments ran naturally at their own speed, setting their own directions and implementing their own policies – microtomes, for instance, were found only in anatomy departments and galvanizing electro-machines only in physiology ones. Research activities were predominantly organized in advance from the student research assistant level upward to the collaborating *Privatdozenten* (as adjunct faculty and rather cheap research labourers).[91] However, the scientific output that was published from each of these institutes was, in most cases, (co-)authored together with the directing *Professor ordinarius* (full professor and chair). This practice often symbolized the subordinate assistants' sheer gratitude to the eminent chief of the institution for precious laboratory and seminar room space, as well as for the academic positions themselves, which provided the necessary basis for contemporary researchers to produce their scientific work.[92]

For clinical psychiatrists and neurologists, in comparison to those of basic research institutes within the German-speaking university system, existing methodological boundaries did not appear to be clear-cut. If we take the significant clinical departments of psychiatry and neurology of Leipzig and Strasburg as examples (see further in chapter 2), it must be conceded that they were equipped with their own pathomorphological laboratories at the beginning of the first decade of the twentieth century; the department at the University of Leipzig opened its laboratory for brain research in 1906, while the Strasburg laboratory came into existence in 1910.[93] While on the one hand, this emphasis on the clinical department's possession of its "own" laboratory might be seen as an inclusion strategy to guarantee disciplinary diversification, on the other, it was often just a primitive reflex to circumvent problematic exchanges between the clinical departments and research institutes with all their administrative quarrels. For a brief period during the first two decades of the twentieth century, neurological clinics even found themselves losing out against their competitors from the basic sciences. At that point, they simply did not want to be "the only institutions ... without a scientific laboratory," as the director of the Strasburg Clinic, Friedrich Jolly (1844–1904) frankly remarked in 1895 in an insightful letter to the brain psychiatrist Carl Fuerstner (1848–1906) at the same university.[94]

Yet such far-reaching demands often did not compare well with the actual reality of scientific and medical research: in contrast to the institutional organization of neurological and psychiatric clinics, the general course of career development in neuromorphology was not specifically "lined up." To a certain extent, the future scientific elite remained severely exposed to job restrictions and many sought to leave the institutional hierarchy at their earliest opportunity. This critical situation resulted in a rather precarious social and political organization of the brain research community in the German-speaking countries, which in this respect differed little from the situation that Harwood has singled out for the emerging field of experimental genetics at the same time:[95]

> One consequence of this policy [the exclusive funding of pre-existing university institutes] was that although the number of professors grew by only about 40 percent between 1870 and 1914, the number of junior posts (*Privatdozenten* and *Extraordinarien*) increased by threefold to fourfold, thus keeping pace with the growth of the student body. For young biologists, however, the situation was much worse, since there was no net increase in the number of tenured posts between 1900 and 1910 [and] most of these posts were untenured and many were unsalaried.[96]

A close look into the institutional files of prominent research universities further reveals that intellectual migration rates were high during this period. About 60 percent of the novices and young researchers (*Hilfsassistenten* and *Unterassistenten*) studied at a minimum of three different universities, and about 50 percent of the middle-rank assistants had held two earlier positions before entering other services in psychiatry, anatomy, or pathology. This overview serves to illustrate a *free-floating culture of ideas*, practical experiences, and organizational skills which strikingly prevailed as the organizational context of the early neuromorphological field.[97] As noted at the beginning of this introduction, the ensuing research approaches in neuronal regeneration paired well with innovative advances, such as the demonstration of fibre outgrowth (the notion of "nerve fibres" has become obsolete today, while the modern term of nerve axons was used very rarely at the end of the nineteenth and beginning of the twentieth century), the depiction of the growth cone, and the temporary cultivation of *in vitro* nerves, at the very fringes of the experimental field.

This situation likewise represented new types of institutional conditions that instigated numerous methodological advances regarding leading-edge research on the attracting and repelling factors of nerve growth, for instance, or the relationship between physical training effects and neuroplastic phenomena. In research presentations, in publications, and in academic lectures, the views of neurologists and brain psychiatrists – such as those by psychiatrist Carl Wernicke (1848–1905) at the University of Breslau, Emil Kraepelin as the director of the newly formed Deutsche

Forschungsanstalt for Psychiatry, and Oswald Bumke (1871–1950), chief of the Department of Psychiatry at the University of Munich – reflected recent developments in the sociocultural context. Public discourse at the time, in fact, witnessed passionate debate on such topics as the health consequences of urbanization, industrialization, and the medical implications of the labour question. Particularly, "degenerative" views in psychiatric and neurological theory underpinned widespread cultural beliefs about what German historian Joachim Radkau has called *The Age of Nervousness* in German history, extending from the dominance of Reich chancellor Otto von Bismarck (1815–1898) to the period of National Socialism.[98] These beliefs closely echoed social and clinical assumptions associated with the quest for hereditary "neuropathic dispositions":[99]

On the whole, the researcher gets the impression that neurasthenia stems much more from the medical consultation room than from neurological theory. Experience much more than science is at the roots of neurasthenia, though science is not without importance. But the endeavors to localize neurasthenia according to the question of the famous [Rudolph] Virchow [1821–1902] Ubi est morbus? were thwarted by the plethora of patients' experiences.[100]

With the advent of World War I and subsequently during the Weimar Republic, neuroanatomical and histopathological methods began to rise to acceptance as standard methodologies in programs on nervous de- and regeneration. These programs were aimed particularly at analyzing the growth forms of nervous tissue, discerning the structural origins of axonal outgrowth, and investigating the relation of the nerves within singular architectures of the brain and spinal cord.[101]

As with any other biomedical research field, these innovative laboratory-based technologies played a decisive role in enabling further understanding, in this case of hereditary and traumatic neurodegenerative diseases.[102] Psychiatrists, neurologists, and clinical pathologists all used the new staining methods, even though they were working in quite different experimental settings. Yet the common denominator of all these endeavours was researchers' mutual interest in investigating observable clinical phenomena in human patients in what they considered adequate laboratory models. In return, clinical symptoms were related back to the pathological findings in *post-mortem* analyses and general morphological diseases – as seen in the works of Oswald Bumke, Walther Spielmeyer (1879–1935), and Otto Binswanger (1852–1929). Scientific discourse on what were defined as de- and regeneration phenomena now essentially became deferred to a privileged place of medical knowledge production: the neuromorphological laboratory. At the same time, discourse further diversified in what became new *regional knowledge economies*, such as the integrated laboratories of the psychiatric and neurological clinics of the time. As eminent Spanish experimentalist Santiago Ramón y Cajal (1852–1934) observed, "no histologist has been able to demonstrate with absolute certainty the reality of regenerative phenomena in the white matter" of the motor cortex.[103] Similar statements, directed at colleagues in the neuromorphological field, resonated well with many contemporary working groups in brain research.[104] And this epistemic indeterminacy also gave rise to the practice of interdisciplinary bridge-building or epistemic *incorporations*, as in the assimilation of knowledge derived from nutrition physiology and social assumptions about neurodegenerative diseases and brain injuries, for instance.[105] From here, a major theoretical perspective crystallized in the prominent views of the Frankfurt neurologist Ludwig Edinger, and his nerve "consumption theory" of brain pathology developed into an important interface of perspectives on nerve damage as well as environmental and social factors.[106]

According to Edinger's consumption theory of the nervous system, it was intellectuals who were most likely to contract neurodegenerative diseases. His idea was that they would consume their "nerve material" through performance of strenuous mental exercises in thinking, long research hours, or manuscript-writing deep into the night. Hereditary factors were considered to be another source of influence on patients' nervous systems and their disposition to attract different kinds of nervous disorders. Edinger proposed one scenario in *The Contribution of Function to the Development of Nervous Diseases* (1908): "When functioning, the nerve cell consumes different substances which have to be permanently replaced. But if the functional process proves to be greater than the capacity of the brain to regenerate [*Ersatzmoeglichkeit*] ... deterioration of nerve fibre tracts takes place."[107] For most neuromorphologists, this process could be detected only by looking through the microscope and comparing normal with pathological brain slices. Yet it is necessary to keep in mind that major social factors of the conceived aetiology were also quite influential beyond the academic confines of the laboratory walls. Edinger may have seen persons born with a "weak" nervous system and individuals exposed to continuing intellectual work as being more likely to attract neurodegenerative diseases, but he also anticipated some rehabilitative potential through changes of environment, such as he had used in physical therapy and early rehabilitation approaches as part of his private medical practice in Frankfurt.

SOCIOTECHNICAL CONCEPTS AND PRACTICES: BRAIN RESEARCH DURING THE WEIMAR REPUBLIC

Contemporary discourse on neurodegeneration also developed into an explanatory concept of military and preventive medicine. It is most strikingly seen, for example, in the case of neurohistologist Max Bielschowsky, who worked at the KWI for Brain Research in Berlin-Buch from 1927 forward. In this particular case, where the concept of "traumatic regeneration" was transferred from a military hospital setting to the hygienic, quiet, and well-equipped KWI laboratory, Bielschowsky situated the question of regeneration in the new epistemic context of "degeneration and exhaustion" discourses in the Weimar Republic. As a reflection of, and in answer to, social demands, Bielschowsky and other Weimar neurohistologists (e.g. Walther Spielmeyer, Karl Stern [1906–1975], and Hans Altenburger [1902–1938]) offered to microscopically discern degenerative occurrences. They started this undertaking with the new histological staining techniques of the contemporary "*silver image*" (Bielschowsky).[108] It revealed the abundance of "nerve fibers in the sclerotic area, which are as dense as those in areas filled with nerves which have myelin sheets."[109] Whereas the former military researcher Bielschowsky had been confident about the existence of nervous regenerative phenomena, as the head of the KWI division of neuropathology he became less optimistic as to the functional potential of regeneration, especially with regard to heredodegenerative diseases. With his laboratory investigations – now placed in the "Weimar degeneration context" – Bielschowsky began to understand axonal growth phenomena and referred to repair mechanisms as types of "healing with defect."[110]

Neurodegeneration and neuroregeneration figured as integrative *sociotechnical concepts and practices* in a variety of experimental and neurosurgical applications. This transformation, together with the general reception of the problem in contemporary morphological laboratories, characterizes many of the changes that took place in the experimental neurosciences in the German-speaking countries. They became further driven and enhanced by the advent of new technologies – such as the electronic microtome, new gold- and aniline-staining derivatives, and pneumencephalographic approaches for the analysis of brain tumours.[111] Bielschowsky and his co-workers at the KWI for Brain Research were no exception in this respect. Rather, the undercurrent of technological change in recent neuroregenerative research endeavours had become embedded in the differentiation of Edinger's and Kurt Goldstein's (1878–1965) Neurological Institute in Frankfurt am Main (see figure 1.2). The Frankfurt institute now combined its departments for clinical psychiatry and neurology with basic neurological laboratory work in comparative microscopical anatomy and pathology.[112]

The laboratory pursuit of "de- and regeneration" in German brain science was also significantly influenced by the succession of various societal contexts from the late Wilhelminian epoch to the Nazi regime. The historical time period in question saw an *assortment of neurocultures* in anatomical and pathological university laboratories, which slowly but steadily reflected cultural changes in an expanded and thus broadening contemporary perspective.[113] These sociotechnical approaches were not simply products of recent advances in the scientific differentiation of somatic neurology and brain psychiatry; they also had a role in the emergence of important interdisciplinary attempts through great collaborative work by anatomists, pathologists, and neuropsychiatrists.

Applying current historiographical methodology may provide more appropriate answers as to how such phenomena as those described here for the field of German-speaking neuromorphology can be looked at as analogous to *sociotechnical experiments*.[114] If one takes into consideration earlier innovative works and methodological advances in the historiography of science generated, for instance, by Frederic Lawrence Holmes (1932–2003) on Hans Adolf Krebs's (1900–1981) experimentation in physiological chemistry, and recent accounts by Daniel Todes of Ivan Petrovitch Pavlov's (1849–1936) physiological factory, or Hans-Joerg Rheinberger's analysis of Paul F. Zamecnik's (1912–2009) protein synthesis, their divergence from what could be called the earlier *laborocentric view* becomes strikingly apparent:[115] All these scholars advocate for the position that it is insufficient to consider scientific achievements of clinicians and experimental research teams in isolation from their technological, economic, and cultural environments. Instead, they demand an analysis of such experimental systems as being intertwined with political discourses and technological innovations during different historical epochs. The fruitful sociotechnical research conditions of the 1920s and 1930s also attracted many international neuroscientists – like the neurophysiologist Henry Head (1861–1940) from London,[116] the Boston neurosurgeon Harvey Cushing, and the Montreal neurologist Wilder Penfield – who flocked to Austria, Switzerland, and Germany for parts of their

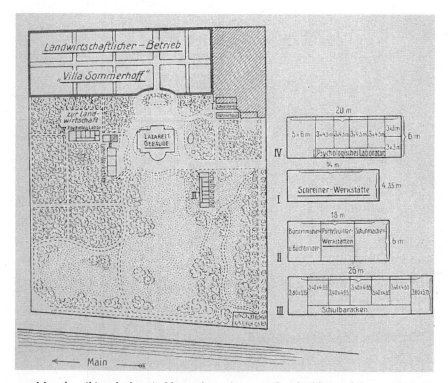

1.2 Map describing the hospital barracks and surrounding buildings of the agrarian colony ("Villa Sommerhoff"), Edinger Institute in Frankfurt am Main, 1919, from Kurt Goldstein, *Die Behandlung, Fuersorge und Begutachtung der Hirnverletzten: zugleich ein Beitrag zur Verwendung psychologischer Methoden in der Klinik.* Leipzig, Germany: F.C.W. Vogel, 1919, Fig. s.n., n.p. Coll. Frank W. Stahnisch. © 2010 Frank W. Stahnisch, Calgary, Alberta.

postgraduate training.[117] With the Rockefeller Foundation's financial support of the Deutsche Forschungsanstalt for Psychiatry, for example, North American students, fellows, and visiting professors travelled again to Munich and other centres of their interest.[118] The Rockefeller Foundation's individual funding program, in return, enabled numerous German neuroscientists to work on the other side of the Atlantic. There, they introduced scientific practices, which were subsequently "enriched" with utilitarian ideals as well as the neurological and psychiatric eugenic perspectives that loomed large in the American and Canadian medical communities.[119]

As alluded to earlier in the preface, if one follows the standard "self-image" of contemporary neuroscientists, one often finds a reluctance that hindered the explicit inclusion in the standard histories of neurology and

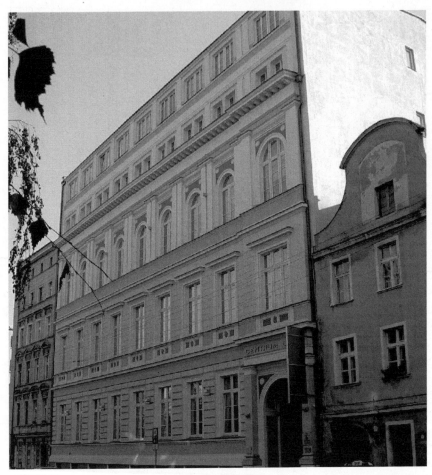

1.3 Otfrid Foerster's first "Neurobiological Laboratory," at the University of Breslau (in the basement of the earlier Department of Dentistry), which was associated with the Friedrich Wilhelms University. Coll. Frank W. Stahnisch. © 2008 Frank W. Stahnisch, Calgary, Alberta.

psychiatry of such individuals as Edinger, Goldstein, or the Breslau neuro-surgeon Foerster (see figure 1.3) among the forebears of an interdisciplin-ary tradition (see also chapters 2 and 3).[120]

If one looks at the writings of contemporary brain researchers since the beginning of the twentieth century, however, and reads administrative as well as organizational materials in the relevant archives in Germany, Austria, Poland, Switzerland, and France, then a very different picture emerges. One instructive historical example can be placed up front here:

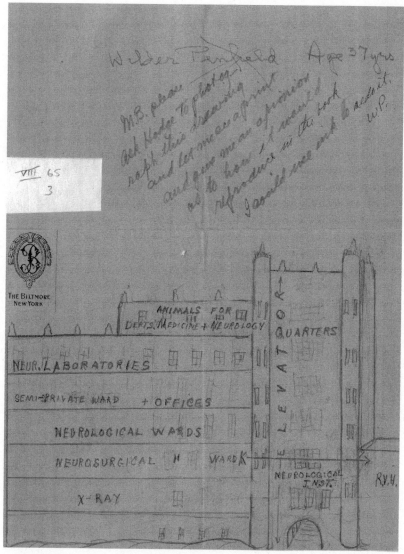

1.4 Sketch of a proposed diagram of the Montreal Neurological Institute, diagram [Online image]. It was drawn by Wilder Penfield in 1929 on letterhead from the Biltmore Hotel in New York. The sketch shows a seven-storey building with floors for an x-ray department, patients, laboratories, and the housing of laboratory animals. The proposed institute is shown as being directly next to the Royal Victoria Hospital (RVH), rather than at its eventual location, across University Avenue from the RVH. Wilder Penfield Digital Collection Wilder Penfield Fonds P142 – Series A (Administration) – Sub-Series A/N (Administration, Neuro; Call Number: A/N 14-2/1). © Reproduction by permission of the Osler Library of the History of Medicine, McGill University, Montreal, PQ.

Canadian neurologist and neurological surgeon Wilder Penfield learned
his operative methods and neurostimulation technique with Foerster during two quite lengthy research periods at the Breslau clinical department
for nervous and psychiatric diseases in 1928 and 1931.[121] He later pointed
out how transformative this research experience had been in his 1932
report to the Rockefeller Foundation and McGill University, in which he
commented on the research set-up and the functioning of Foerster's
Neurological Institute in Breslau:

> Foerster's clinic is above all a clinic in which therapy takes first place.
> Syphilis of the central nervous system is treated energetically by the
> [Homer Fordyce] Swift [1881–1953]-[Arthur W.] Ellis [1907–1935]
> endolumbar method in addition to the other usual procedures.
> Intracarotid injections of salvarsanized serum are likewise freely
> used. Physio- and hydrotherapy are carried out vigorously in the
> special rooms which are well equipped for that purpose. The wards
> are pleasant but the nursing is not of the highest order and decubitus
> is too frequently seen ... *Above all, here Neurology is accompanied
> by therapy.*[122]

After returning from his European tour, Penfield began the successful
development of a structurally similar and very modern treatment and
neuroscience centre (see figure 1.4) that incorporated new forms of thorough diagnostics, encephalographic visualizations, and clinical physiological procedures with electrical measurements in the treatment advances
for epilepsy at the Montreal Neurological Institute.[123]

At the Montreal Neurological Institute (see figure 1.5), Penfield and
his associates developed a vast and detailed research program on the
cortical localization of brain functions, which they investigated by electrically stimulating patients in neurosurgical intraoperative settings.[124] He
closely monitored the movement effects, sensory perceptions, and psychological results in his patients, findings that led to his famous cortical
cartographic map of the homunculus of motor and sensory cortical areas
of the human brain.[125]

From that point forward, theoretical, methodological, and pragmatic
factors were merged in clinical neuroscientific investigation in order to
create groundbreaking forms of research organization:[126]

> In Montreal, the growth of neurosurgical and neurological work has
> been spontaneous and easy because of the universal hospitality here,

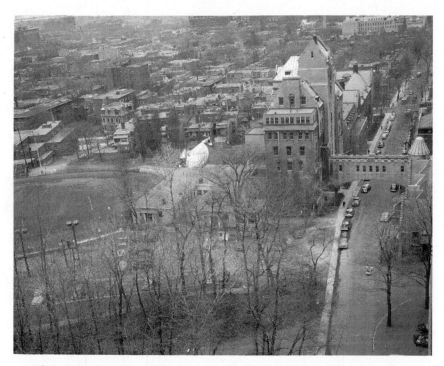

1.5 The Montreal Neurological Institute, with Military Annex and McGill football stadium on the left, 1945 (Archive number: MNI image #9–1099) / Courtesy of the Montreal Neurological Institute, McGill University © Montreal Neurological Institute, Montreal, Quebec.

the generous co-operation from the start by the Royal Victoria and the Montreal General Hospitals, and the kindness of Professor [Jonathan Campell] Meakins [1882–1959] in throwing open his laboratories to us, grasping amateur neuropathologists and neuro-physiologists that we are. The whole undertaking [was facilitated] by Dean [Charles F.] Martin [1868–1953], who was able to interest the Rockefeller Foundation, the Province of Quebec and the City of Montreal in this Institute at a time when the present project seemed doomed to failure.[127]

The methodological differentiation of the program was also reflected in the architecture,[128] organization, and function of neuroscientific inquiry in centres that were built to reflect the new interdisciplinary setting of neuroscientific research.[129] It was a consequence of a division of labour necessary to engage in group sesearch activities so as to respond to greater social demands – in Montreal, Breslau, and elsewhere in America and Europe – to produce results in areas that could no longer be mastered by one individual alone.[130]

By explaining the epistemological meanings of contemporary concepts of interdisciplinarity, I hope to provide answers as to the place, time, and culture in which these transformations occurred in the neuromorphological community from 1882 to 1962. When applying a cultural picture to this early period of neuroscience, interdisciplinary research into neuro-degeneration, brain psychiatry, and holist neurology – perhaps with the exception of a few enclaves, such as the Heidelberg clinic of Viktor von Weizsaecker (1886–1957) – ceased to exist for around three decades after the death, murder, and the forced migration of many of the protagonists during the Nazi period.[131] These disastrous developments, to which the Third Reich had given rise, destroyed the societal and institutional basis for the growth of the interdisciplinary field and forced major neurological and psychiatric leaders to seek refuge in North America, Britain, the Soviet Union, and Turkey, among other destinations of exile, from which many never returned to their home countries. The great disruptions in the neurosciences are even more striking when one takes into consideration the broader influence of many of its protagonists – including Foerster, the Munich neuropathologist and cancer specialist Walther Spielmeyer, Goldstein, and the Vogts – and their followers into account. By their ability to relate to interdisciplinary scholars from various areas and through their impact as academic teachers – neuroscientists such as Foerster, Spielmeyer, Goldstein, and the Vogts – seemed to have influenced entirely new generations of biomedical students, and not only in a reductionist histological study of the brain.

With the application of the concept of interdisciplinarity, I contest scholarly views that argue for a "sudden switch in the ethical framework," the "ideology-ladenness, particularly of German science," or even the "unscientific impetus" of Nazi science and medicine.[132] By addressing the changing societal and cultural contexts in which various patterns of research practice of Nazi medicine pre-emerged, I shall draw a broader picture here of one of the most crucial phases in modern science and medicine at the beginning of the twentieth century. My argument is based on two earlier analyses: the first thesis emanates from the book *Racial Hygiene: Medicine under the Nazis* (1988) by Stanford historian of science Robert Proctor and his argument concerning the political ideologization and "corruption or abuse" of medical science in Nazi Germany.[133] For instance, Proctor proposed "that science [and medicine] thrive only under democracy and that democracy in turn benefits from values implicit in the free pursuit of science," whereas social forces hostile to democracy would lead more or less directly to a decrease of good science. Nazi medicine, however, presents a rather special case – to say the least – of the embeddedness of science in culture and scientific exchanges, which calls for a more substantial and subtle investigation rather than being merely characterized as "pure ideology."[134] I therefore want to pursue an investigation of the general foundations of neuroscience since the German Empire (as particularly addressed in chapters 2 and 3), which enabled medical investigators to conduct military-related research or later unethical human experimentation (chapters 5 and 6). In the hopes of identifying the more international effects of Nazi science and medicine, a scrutiny of the marginalization of patients and people with disabilities as well as the forced migration of Jewish and oppositional researchers and physicians is needed, since these formed important contexts for the emergence of neuroscience as a research field by themselves. It would be inadequate, however, if the medical and scientific activities in Nazi Germany were equated only with "pseudoscience."[135] The claim must rather be made that racial hygiene and anthropology, along with the field of medical genetics, were highly international in their scope at the time, and that qualitative differences between these fields in Germany, Scandinavia, Britain, and the United States were rather insignificant.[136]

It is most pertinent – as historian Fritz Fischer (1908–1999) discussed decades ago – not to overlook the political influences on science and learning during the times of the German Empire, under the conditions of World War I, the Weimar Republic, and the Nazi regime.[137] As such, the research motives, economic factors, and the striving for power will all be analyzed in further detail. Historiographical analysis during the past two decades has somewhat over-focused on the "pseudoscience character of National Socialist research," by addressing important myths about Nazi medicine and health care.[138] We are now entering a period of an ever-deeper understanding of the health policies in Nazi Germany and the motives and actions of Nazi physicians. Depictions of their participation range from reluctant enforcement of early discrimination measures by the German government (e.g. the Civil Service Act of 1933 and the Nuremberg Laws of 1935), to full endorsement of Nazi medical philosophies, such as in the case of Munich psychiatrist Ernst Ruedin or the Wuerzburg neurologist Georges Schaltenbrand (1897–1979).[139]

The political and biological contexts of "eugenics" had an important complementary influence on the field of neuroscience, as many of the diseases of the brain were understood to be inherited. It is interesting to see that a great number of the physicians in the German eugenics movements had previously worked in social medicine and psychiatry as well.[140] For them, neurology and psychiatry became, "in the true sense of the word, a healing medical discipline," because the therapeutic repertoire – electrotherapy, surgery, pharmacotherapy, and physical therapy – was still very limited at the time.[141] These social and technological trends merged into a multidisciplinary, albeit murderous, field in the context of Nazi medicine, where the healing of the sick and the extinction of the weak coincided with barbarous endeavours of health professionals, medical, and neuroscientific researchers. Hence, the state and development of medicine and public health in the Third Reich cannot be regarded as mere contingencies. Moreover, the idea that medical knowledge was intrinsically in conflict with ethical values may also not be regarded as unique to this period alone.[142] The narrative here will serve to answer some of the questions that arise through the conundrums posed by the Nuremberg Trials from 1945 to 1947; namely the impact of *prima facie* absent ethical rules for scientific and medical aberrations during the first decades of the twentieth century. It was this lack of ethical standards that eventually made it necessary to treat Nazi atrocities under the law as "war crimes" rather than as medical misconduct.[143]

There are many more adherents to the thesis that "science thrives only under democracy and that democracy in turn benefits from values implicit in the free pursuit of science," and one could even see it as a well-entrenched view in the anglophone research literature.[144] In my narrative, I shall relate this to Proctor's second thesis,[145] with which I am in principle in agreement, while trying to adjust some of its respective consequences. The conception of medicine following Proctor's exposé is very timely, both with regard to recent developments in the biomedical sciences along with respective scholarship in science and technology studies.[146] If we look at the general history of the field of biomedicine after World War II, the development of new technologies from sophisticated laboratory endeavours is particularly evident. This is the case, for example, in the area of antibiotics, microsurgical techniques, reproduction, and the advent of intensive care medicine since the time of the Korean War.[147] These groundbreaking developments have certainly transformed medicine on a global scale. Moreover, Proctor's observations reflect important elements of medicine today, in that they call attention to the need to recognize "that science-based technologies also serve to maintain social order and to facilitate the policing of society."[148] It is important to address these issues here from a *science-in-context perspective*, because it will shed a fresh light on neuroscientific work of the period under study. Since the 1960s, however – inspired by the foregoing publications of Thomas S. Kuhn (1922–1996) and a renaissance of Ludwik Fleck's (1896–1961) medical philosophy – there have been growing concerns that science cannot be applied only for the improvement of modern societies but likewise can be abused politically and economically. It has further been realized that individual scientists have to be held socially and culturally responsible for their research contributions and forms of investigation.[149] That science generally was not independent of society led to the recognition in the scholarship that the respective forms of science, which society creates, had something to do with the changing cultural contexts themselves. This was shown, for example, in the works of Everett Mendelsohn for biology, Mitchell Ash for social psychology, Ted Brown for psychosomatics, and Barry Barnes for physical technologies.[150]

The realization that science and society are tightly interwoven in modern societies pertains particularly to the issue of medicine throughout the National Socialist period. By looking at the more long-term developments and the international relations of the research fields under scrutiny, my discussion departs significantly from the received view in English-speaking historiography.[151] Until recently, much historical and sociological work has focused on what was seen as the Nazi destruction of science through the expulsion of Jewish researchers from German-speaking universities and the corruption of intellectual values which sealed the fate of contemporary science in Central Europe. As German philosopher Walter Benjamin (1892–1940) once put it, in order to come to grips with the cultural bedrock of artistic, intellectual, and scientific endeavours, it is essential to dare "to brush history against the grain."[152] When trying to disentangle the complex interrelationship of social contexts, scientific progress, and technological occurrences that have taken place in the eighty-year history of German-speaking neuromorphology analyzed here, important inferences can be drawn for the contemporary development of the history of science on the one hand and the meaning of modernity, internationalization, and globalization on the other.

Relating this general issue to Proctor's foregoing analysis allows us to see scientific and medical trends as having continued from the Weimar Republic to Nazi Germany, even though international exchanges were markedly reduced toward the end of the 1930s due to mounting political antagonisms, territorial occupations, and the eventual outbreak of war.[153] In examining these underlying political and cultural influences on major university institutions and extra-university centres in Frankfurt, Berlin, Strasburg, Leipzig, and elsewhere in the following chapters of the book, I will study several crucial methodological processes and foundations relating to neuroanatomy, neurology, and neuropathology. By paying particular attention to the cultural dimension in the historiographical investigation of this emerging research field of the German-speaking brain sciences, I map not only the institutional patterns but also the specific interplay of conceptual, personal, and research relations which provided fruitful breeding grounds for neuromorphology to become a burgeoning *interdisciplinary problem field* in the biomedical and scientific arena of the twentieth century.

THE INDIVIDUAL CHAPTERS OF THE BOOK

In this chapter, I have outlined my historiographical narrative, as it is in itself a particular form of interdisciplinarism, blending sociological and ethnographic approaches from science and technology studies with methodologies from historical epistemology. The restrictions as well as the epistemic reach of the modern concept of "interdisciplinarity" for understanding contemporary forms of research organization have been compared with the historical notions and they have been positioned in the international context that fostered diverse *fields of knowledge* between the 1880s and the 1960s.[154]

In chapter 2, in exploring the disciplinary makeup of clinical and basic research in late Imperial Germany, I focus on two leading research universities of the time, Strasburg and Leipzig. Both universities still displayed a traditional nineteenth-century form of academic organization, in which neuroscientific research took place in autonomous institutes of anatomy and physiology, along with neurological and psychiatric clinics. The third chapter considers the shortfalls of individualized research projects of the time *vis-à-vis* the emergence of specialized neurological clinical departments. This discussion is further situated in a general contextualization of modern life, as it so drastically impinged on the research environment in the younger "reform" universities and extra-university research centres. Heinrich Obersteiner's preceding institute in Vienna serves as an important model for the analysis of interdisciplinarity in German-speaking neuroscience, while the Edinger Institute in Frankfurt am Main and its precursor laboratories at the KWI for Brain Research in Berlin are likewise investigated and compared.

In the fourth chapter, I discuss the impact of war, trauma, and regeneration, since they posed extreme external demands on contemporary neuromorphological research endeavours. Developments in field hospitals and veterans' clinics during and after World War I led to the sociopolitical dimension of *Grossforschung* ("big science") already in the early years of the Weimar Republic. This process was facilitated by three national and international foundations: the Deutsche Forschungsgemeinschaft ("German Research Council"), the American Rockefeller Foundation, and the Kaiser Wilhelm Gesellschaft ("Kaiser Wilhelm Society").

Chapters 5 and 6 follow these examples of prolonged continuity into the National Socialist period, while looking specifically at German-speaking neuromorphologists from the old guard and those biomedical researchers who entered the system after the 1930s, when the unifying alignment (*Gleichschaltung*) of German academia had almost been completed.[155] In the fifth chapter, I trace the changing societal emphases on research, along with the new concepts in neurology and psychiatry, during the final years of the Weimar period. Political conflicts, the increasing popularity of the eugenics movement and racial hygiene, as well as pressing economic influences reframed interdisciplinary neuromorphological work within the context of social medicine, *Volksgesundheit* ("public health"), and tighter political control mechanisms.[156] These become increasingly apparent when focusing on international relationships between Germany, Switzerland, and the United States.

Moving beyond the Weimar period – in chapter 6 – I examine the impact of the National Socialist German Workers Party's *Machtergreifung* (seizure of political power) and its effects on German neuroscience and psychiatry. Already in 1933, the newly inaugurated anti-Semitic laws and the oppression of socialist and democratic movements led to the first wave of forced migration of large numbers of neurologists and psychiatrists, the majority of whom had been ousted from their universities and state-affiliated positions. They fled, in particular, to the neighbouring Netherlands, the United Kingdom, and North America; this exodus is illustrated by examining the local contexts of Amsterdam, London, and New York City, where many of the émigrés arrived.

In the seventh chapter, I propose a theoretical analysis of various "unintended" theory-changes in the neurosciences that were due in large part to the forced migration processes. I explore particularly the interactions between pathology and psychiatry, neurology, and public mental health, as well as the transformations in new neuroscientific agendas.

Historiographically, the focus is placed in this chapter on neuroscientific institutions in New York, Bethesda, and Brooklyn in the United States, taking into account the biographical fate of quite successful "normal scientists." Also, I provide a comparison between the fate of émigré neuroscientists from preceding German-speaking research communities and their new host countries, Canada and the United States.[157] Previous research on émigré neuroscientists – Herbert A. Strauss and Werner Roeder (1983), for example, or Mitchell Ash and Alfons Soellner (1993) – has focused mainly on individual biographies and the interrelation of political changes with the rejection of the persons concerned.[158] Here, rather than focusing again on specific biographies of individual émigré neuroscientists, I explore various organizational patterns, technical skills, and neuroscientific know-how, as it crossed the Atlantic with the academic refugees from their German-speaking countries of origin.[159]

Chapter 7 addresses the historical development of interdisciplinary work, while summarizing the theoretical considerations. In this chapter I provide an outlook on the influences of early interdisciplinary centres in the German-speaking scientific community on the establishment of modern-day neuroscientific research institutions through the analysis of medium-sized working groups at Dalhousie University (Halifax) and McGill (Montreal) in Canada, along with the University of Pennsylvania in the United States. Likewise, some of the consequences of World War I, such as the massive exodus of German-speaking neurologists and psychiatrists, as well as the slow restitution of transatlantic relations between the Federal Republic of Germany and the United States, are described at length. Some views are provided there too on the altered context of the steady reanimation of the German-American research relations in the early postwar period.

After World War II, however, the broader outlook on neuroscience (or in its German original *Hirnforschung*) as a new interdisciplinary enterprise (with the integration of morphological, functional, behavioural, and cognitive perspectives) was scarcely represented in West Germany for almost twenty years, a period in which disciplinary formations and paradigms tended to lead scientific research.[160] The 1940s to the 1960s particularly witnessed the emergence of the connections and integrative knowledge field of the "neurosciences" as a new and comprehensive entity on the international level, with an enormous reach into the social and behavioural sciences, cross-over areas to information and computer science, and the new and emerging fields of molecular biology and human genetics.[161] Since the 1960s these cutting-edge trends have tended to be overshadowed by subsequent mainstream developments in the neurosciences.[162] It needs to be pointed out, however, that on the margins of the then-dominating disciplines of neuromorphology and neurophysiology, the 1940s and 1950s also saw considerable advances in research groups and subdisciplines "on the edge" of brain research, examples being neurotoxin investigations (in medical research), neurobehavioural research (in ethology contexts), and synapse research (with the help of electron microscopy).[163]

As chapter 8 on the postwar consequences and developments in neuromorphology will show, when we place these occurrences in the wider context of twentieth-century biomedical science[164] it should be mentioned that the specifically "interdisciplinary" endeavour, which the "Neuroscience Study Program" of St Louis–trained neurophysiologist Frank Schmitt represented at the Massachusetts Institute of Technology in Boston, was a major ignition point for the expansion of the neuroscience landscape in the early 1960s.[165] With its integrative approach to the neurosciences, as stated above, Schmitt managed to bring together an international group of eminent researchers from various disciplines and stimulate their productive interaction in the study of the nervous system.[166] However, thus far, there exists no adequate historical account on the origins of such interdisciplinary research programs in the neurosciences as we know them today. In focusing on the theme of interdisciplinarity in structural research activities in German-speaking neuroscience from the 1880s to the early 1960s, the impact that three different political and cultural systems – German Imperialism, the experiment of Weimar Democracy, and later the National Socialist period (the immediate postwar period in West and East Germany consecutively struggled with the infamous heritage and burden that the Third Reich had left for the sciences in the FRG and the GDR alike)[167] – had on the emergence and transformation of this new research field become more discernible and comprehensible. The historical narrative can thus furnish us with new, augmented insights into how important interdisciplinary work was perceived to be in neuroscience and its research organization.

Although the following chapters are primarily organized in chronological order, each one also has its own thematic and epistemological topics of interest, as can be gleaned from the main chapter titles or section titles. A thematic discussion left incomplete in one of the earlier chapters is thus sometimes resumed in later ones related to a distinctive topical interest, and I provide signposting on how the chapters interlink with one another. In each chapter, I trace both the chronological and systematic changes in neuroscientific research in the specific period under discussion. This historiographical narrative touches on pre-existing accounts within the scholarship – accounts, for example, of changing institutional histories, transformation in transatlantic relationships, and exchanges between researchers and neuroscience trainees during the pre-1950s-neurosciences. The concluding perspective will contribute to our current understanding of general issues of knowledge-transfer, positive and negative receptions in American neuroscience, as well as the cultural matching of divergent "national research styles."[168]

Looking at émigré neuroscientists who escaped the Nazi terror regime, and examining their work profiles, allows for additional insights into the biographical and institutional settings that were essential for the formation of various *topoi* of modern historical epistemology.[169] These subjects include the interrelation of practice and theory, the organization of mutual research actions, and cultural differences in scientific hypotheses-generation.[170] It is interesting to note that one of the consequences of the reintegration of differing communities of neuroscientists into pre-existing American scientific cultures was the gradual though effective transformation of this field into one of most prolific areas of knowledge production in postwar medicine, a process that I compare with the earlier traditions in the German-speaking neuroscientific communities before World War II.

The Disciplinary Makeup of Clinical and Basic Research in Imperial Germany

The Case Examples of Strasburg and Leipzig

I believe that the time has come when the localization of brain functions can no longer be investigated simply with clinical or experimental approaches. Instead, brain anatomy itself claims to be received in all related questions and I will hence base my observations today exclusively on the relevant anatomical facts.

Paul Flechsig[1]

The period of the Wilhelminian Empire (*Deutsches Kaiserreich*) is known for being one of the most politically charged phases of Western science and medicine, especially, as historian Wolfgang Mommsen (1930–2004) reminds us, in regard to its implications for German history in the first half of the twentieth century.[2] In this chapter I consider some of the underlying and intricate developments in the research organization and historical structure of medicine and science of German imperialism up to the final years of World War I. Two case examples in particular will help us to identify and trace the succession of cultural and political contexts in relation to the emergence of different research traditions in brain science. By considering the changing patterns of academic self-understanding from the Wilhelminian Empire to the outbreak of the Great War, I have gained insights into the process of state-administered institutionalization of scientific pursuits along with the effect of the hierarchies and knowledge differentials that shaped and constrained the historical development of German medicine until 1945.[3] In consideration of German historian Fritz Fischer's seminal work *From Kaiserreich to Third Reich* (1986), I extend the analysis from the final years of the German Empire to the end of World War II:[4]

After 1866 and 1871, Germany came to experience a more recent line of continuity – that of monarchial-bureaucratic Prussia – which incorporated its military-state tradition into its founding of the German Empire or *Kaiserreich* of 1871. Transcending all political changes, this new continuity retained its dominance, despite modifications and varieties in intensity, until 1945, as may be seen from the example of the two world wars.[5]

The specific reasons for such an approach here lie in an understanding of the respective contexts of science and medicine in the century's first decade, rather than in the political developments with which historians Fischer and Mommsen were concerned when they examined Germany's role in the events leading to the outbreak of World War I.

THE MORAL ECONOMY OF THE SCIENTIFIC PURSUIT

When focusing on the continuities and breaks in the system of science and medicine from the late Wilhelmine period to World War I, transformed patterns of morality, medical science, and applications in health care can also be effectively traced. These include, for example, changes brought about by authoritarianism and social obedience toward hierarchies, military applications, and political influences on the pursuit of higher learning, as these related to the field of neuromorphology.[6] Such contextual academic patterns have been intriguingly analyzed by Fritz Ringer among what he described as a "besieged caste" of scientific mandarins in the German university system:

> [*The Decline of the German Mandarins*] deals with the opinions of German university professors from about 1890 to 1933, particularly with their reaction to Germany's sudden transformation into a highly industrialized nation. About 1890, the impact of an abrupt economic expansion began to be felt in Germany … To German academics, the whole period … seemed a continuous upheaval, a particularly unpleasant *introduction to the problems of technological civilization.*[7]

By examining some of the continuities and discontinuities in the scientific approaches from the Wilhelmine Empire to the Weimar Republic, my narrative will show how contextual and practical meanings of interdisciplinarity already existed in the early field of German neuromorphology.[8] In its etymological meaning, "neuromorphology" (Greek: *neuro-* for "nerves" and *morphé* for "form") is the study of the gross anatomical and histological structures of the brain and spinal cord. The research field of neuromorphology is seen here to include neuroanatomy, neuropathology, and aspects from neuroimmunology, neuroradiology, and neurosurgery. I take this research perspective to also encompass important allied sciences, as well as their clinical applications in neurology and psychiatry.[9] Even in the practice of neurology, basic methods of post-mortem analysis, histopathological staining techniques, and topological diagnostics counted among the leading-edge trends and showed the importance of neuroanatomy for clinical research.[10] Illnesses of the central nervous system were diagnosed primarily on a somatic and thus neuroanatomical basis, before electrophysiology further encroached on the field and, in certain respects, came increasingly to dominate neurology and psychiatry.[11] Altogether, my goal is to trace the formative stages toward an interdisciplinary neuromorphological tradition in early twentieth-century German medical history in its formative, institutional, and interactive paths.[12]

Yet I am jumping ahead in my historical narrative; let me begin by describing what I mean by *moral economy* specifically in the field of early neuroscience and brain psychiatry. In this, I follow the interpretation of American-German historian of science Lorraine Daston in her analysis of the cultural assumptions in contemporary forms of science. For Daston, a moral economy in relation to science refers not to financial, market, labour, and production elements in the pursuit of scientific research alone but rather to an organized system that displays certain explicable but unpredictable regularities in research and education. It further describes the intricate ties to scientific activities such as inscriptions, measurement, or methodical interpretations that imbue the pursuit of *moral economies of modern scientific and medical knowledge generation.*[13]

Looking at the neurologists and brain psychiatrists who engaged in neuromorphological research in the latter decades of the nineteenth century, my object here could be interpreted as an analysis of the causes and effects of degeneration phenomena of physical bodies and minds through the scientific disciplines involved.[14] I have chosen to take the formation of the clinical departments of psychiatry and neurology (*Kliniken fuer Psychiatrie und Neurologie*) in Strasburg and Leipzig as a starting point, since they later emerged as leading institutions in the contemporary clinical fields.[15] Their experimental pathomorphological laboratories, which had already opened by the turn of the century, offered ample opportunities for brain research to take place in the vicinity of clinical surroundings. Accordingly, pathological organ materials, clinical observations and measurements, and cadavers for post-mortem dissections were available for sophisticated laboratory work. Brain anatomists, neuropathologists, and neurological clinicians viewed the inauguration of such laboratories as supporting a focused way of investigating the brain's structure and function. Yet clinical departments soon tried to incorporate such innovative research facilities into university medical schools and, for a brief period afterward, clinicians had even found themselves losing ground against their basic science competitors – a professionally challenging situation that they quickly aimed to reverse.[16]

On the basis of Canadian historian of medicine George Weisz's analysis of continental hierarchies in academic medicine, I shall describe the first phase of historical developments up until the outbreak of World War I as the period of the "Wilhelminian institute mandarins."[17] This was a period when eminent institute directors held complete sovereignty over decisions and policies, running their own specialized institutes as "little kingdoms." These institutions closely represented the hierarchical structure and arbitrariness of the Wilhelminian Empire within the limited confines of the scientific institutes and clinical departments at the level of individual German research universities. Subtle tendencies for change only emerged with the end of World War I, as is intricately described in John Craig's analyses "The German University and Alsatian Society" and "From *Universitaet* to *Université*," in which he used the University of Strasburg as his case example. The German-French interwar period is discussed here at length as an important political context in which national research styles dissolved into international research programs.[18] I should mention two analytical constraints at the outset, however: I will limit my discussion to the development of the morphological neurosciences and focus particularly on German-speaking brain researchers, since the development toward interdisciplinary cooperating groups, research programs, and neuroscientific centres was most prominent in Germany, Austria, and Switzerland during this period, which will also serve as a connecting thread to the narrative of the following chapters.

THE PERIOD OF THE WILHELMINIAN INSTITUTE MANDARINS IN STRASBURG

The medical professors at Strasburg from the late Wilhelminian period to the 1920s adopted influential and almost omnipotent roles in the biomedical sciences as institute "mandarins." The German *Ordinarius* professors among them, who moved to Strasburg immediately after the Franco-Prussian War (1870–71), had been explicitly hired in a political attempt to showcase the capacity of German research and higher education in the recently annexed Alsace and Lorraine, with its French-speaking Université de Strasbourg, prominent since the Napoleonic wars.[19] The incoming academics settled into palatial institute buildings, which were financed largely through reparation payments by the French government, as stipulated in the peace treaty of Frankfurt of 10 May 1871. However, these German professors came to Alsace-Lorraine at a time when the majority of the population rejected the new rulers as envoys of the dominating Prussian government and, even worse, of militaristic oppression.[20]

As with the founding of the Faculté (Libre) de Médecine à Nancy in 1793 under Napoléon Bonaparte (1769–1821), the inauguration of the University of Strasburg in 1872 by the new government of the German Empire was pursued as a step in a larger political plan. The inaugurated Kaiser Wilhelms Universitaet Strassburg[21] had been the only new research university in Germany after the creation of the Friedrich Wilhelms University in Bonn (1818) more than half a century earlier. If it is true that "science goes where the money is,"[22] then the founding of the Kaiser Wilhelms University can be seen as an excellent example. It was highly unusual for a German-speaking university at the time to have three-quarters of its faculty offered positions in the highest rank of full professors, with large groups of subordinate research staffs. These *Ordinarien* received a salary nearly double that of their academic peers in the Prussian capital of Berlin. It comes as no surprise, then, that the Kaiser Wilhelms University emerged as one of the important centres of German-speaking neuroscience – similar to other fields of the natural sciences and advanced scholarship in the humanities at Strasburg.[23]

One of the most prominent new hires at the Kaiser Wilhelms University was the neuroanatomist Wilhelm Waldeyer (later, Von Waldeyer-Hartz [1836–1921]), who came from the Friedrich Wilhelms University of Breslau, where he had led one of the large anatomical institutes in Prussia. Waldeyer was well known for his pioneering work in comparative anatomy on the gyration of the cortex in humans and animals, as well as for his publications on the cell theory of nerve tissue.[24] Among his pupils were the Frankfurt neurologist Ludwig Edinger (1855–1918), the neurohistologist Carl Weigert (1845–1905), and the neuroserologist Paul Ehrlich (1854–1915).[25] Furthermore, Christian Friedrich Wilhelm Roller (1802–1878), a prominent clinical psychiatrist and founder of the State Psychiatric

Asylum of Illenau, became a *Privatdozent* in the anatomy institute, where he worked on the structure of the neuronal ganglia (a now obsolete term for large agglomerations of nerve cells) in the vestibular organ. His research program on the nervous innervation of the inner ear became so successful that one of the nerve colliculi, which receives afferent nerve axons from the sacculus structure of the labyrinth (important for the balancing function of posture and gait in humans and animals), still bears his name: the nucleus vestibularis inferior (Roller). During the 1870s, Roller further developed an important collection of histological slides on the network of the tracts of the spinal marrow in humans and primates.[26] After Waldeyer's retirement, an accomplished successor for the chair of anatomy was found in the neuroanatomist Gustav Schwalbe (1844–1916), who came to the Kaiser Wilhelms University from the University of Koenigsberg in East Prussia.[27] In Strasburg, Schwalbe continued the neuroanatomical tradition with his own work, which eventually led to the identification of the nucleus vestibularis inferior.

The institute of experimental physiology, only a few buildings away from the architectural quad that housed the anatomical and pathological institutes (see figure 2.1), was chaired by Friedrich Goltz (1834–1902). His research on functional localization of the cortical areas of the brain became one of the landmark findings in nineteenth-century neuroscience. Edinger commended Goltz's neurophysiological work in his autobiographical account: "He determined that many actions of the so-called 'higher life of the soul' [*als hoeherseelische Handlungen gedeutete Verrichtungen*] were merely the expression of isolated parts of the nervous system."[28] An important pupil of Goltz was the experimental physiologist Albrecht Bethe, who between the 1910s and 1930s became one of the German pioneers in clinical neurorehabilitation and functional plasticity.[29]

Although the psychiatrist Richard Freiherr von Krafft-Ebing (1840–1902) may be seen as marginally important in the development of German-speaking neuromorphology, he nevertheless deserves mention here. Krafft-Ebing complemented other star members of Kaiser Wilhelms University's founding faculty (1872–73) in the wider field of neuroscience and contributed substantially to the climate of the research-minded medical faculty. Later becoming one of the most prominent of European psychiatrists, it was in Strasburg that Krafft-Ebing consolidated his psychiatric program on the classification of mental illness based on the differentiation of various "psychoses" as psychological and degenerative forms. With the arrival of his successor, Friedrich Jolly (1844–1904) in 1873, the morphological perspective gained further momentum in the neurosciences.[30]

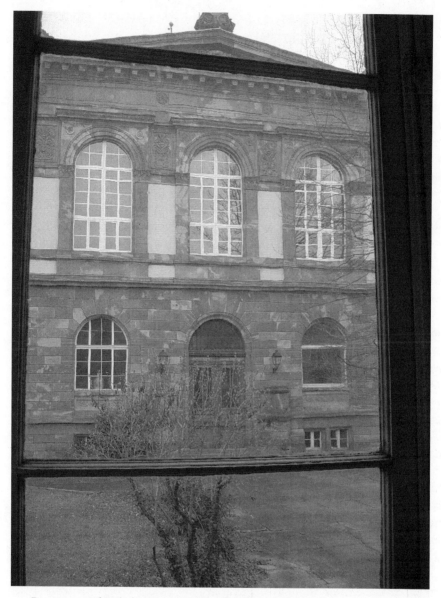

2.1 Department of Pathology at the University of Strasburg (built in 1872). Coll. Frank W. Stahnisch. © 2008 Frank W. Stahnisch, Calgary, Alberta.

Parallel to his clinical research, Jolly pursued intensive investigations on the ganglia cells of the spinal marrow in traumatic diseases and neuro-syphilitic conditions – a program into which he integrated various experimental studies by his clinical assistants as well. Jolly also pioneered innovative steps in the Strasburg community care system, in that he convinced the municipality to build a clinical department of psychiatry in 1876 (see figure 2.2). It served the mentally ill of the city and the Alsatian region, and became a partly autonomous research institution in which various perspectives of psychiatry found an interdisciplinary integration.[31]

The founding of the clinical department of psychiatry in Strasburg marked a new developmental phase during which a greater number of clinical wards and research divisions were opened (see figure 2.2). Initially, as German science historian Beatrix Baeumer has pointed out in comparing the chemical and medical laboratories at German research universities, the creation of scientific institutes had been the main priority for ongoing building activities.[32]

The two-stage development could certainly be related back to a scientific orientation that the earlier French concept of a *faculté-hôpital* had envisaged. This concept of the *faculté-hôpital* foresaw a tight interrelationship of medical institutes with the demands of the hospital for which these units should cater.[33] Yet, in addition to such innovative developments in biomedical research in the context of a growing city, the arrival of another influential faculty member on 20 April 1872 should also not go unnoticed. The anatomical pathologist Friedrich Daniel von Recklinghausen (1833–1910), probably more than any other Strasburg professor, personified the leading basic science ideal of the time, and he became one of the most highly regarded teachers of the Kaiser Wilhelms University. Von Recklinghausen was a pupil of the eminent pathologist Rudolf Virchow and, as dean of the new medical faculty and administrative curator to the university, he determined the course of the new research university for a full decade to come. A further substantial to the field of clinical neuroscience was his pathological analysis of the phenomenology of generalized neurofibromatosis in the 1880s, which has since come to bear his name internationally as *Morbus von Recklinghausen*.[34] Von Recklinghausen's science-mindedness was all-encompassing, and the development of medicine at the Kaiser Wilhelms University flourished under his leadership. He strongly supported the diversification of the institution by hiring innovative clinicians, securing freedom in research directions, and initiating major exchange programs for postgraduate students. Strasburg during this period developed strong ties particularly with universities in the United States (Madison-Wisconsin and Columbia), France (Paris), and Japan (Tokyo), which led to a continued influx of international researchers until the dawn of World War I.[35]

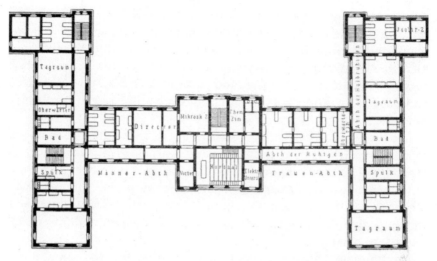

2.2 Architectural plan of the University of Strasburg's clinical department of neurology and psychiatry (Klinik fuer Neurologie und Psychiatrie der Kaiser Wilhelms Universitaet Strassburg), ca 1880 – 103 AL 1157. © Courtesy of the Archives départementales du Bas-Rhin (103 AL 1157) à Strasbourg, France.

THE STRASBURG NEUROSCIENTISTS IN THEIR "RESEARCH TEMPLES"

Even though the Strasburg *Ordinarien* ruled their institutes in an autocratic fashion, like glorified Chinese mandarins, the overall influence of von Recklinghausen as the university curator was still felt on all levels.[36] I would go so far as to call the communications structures he created the "system von Recklinghausen," since they endured even until the Great War; it was a successful organizational system that subsequent university curator Christian Riele (1841–1922?) acknowledged publicly at the fiftieth anniversary of von Recklinghausen's graduation:

> Immediately after the opening of our university, it was essential to organize the development and completion of all areas, especially those in the Medical Faculty. All the individual parts had to be aligned in a harmonious way, so that they could actively and freely move, *just as the little wheels in a clockwork, which relate to one another without constraining or breaking each other.*[37]

Important elements in the smooth running of the mechanics of the Strasburg clockwork were the central units of the medical sciences, in which participating researchers complemented each other's work, to the extent that laboratory investigations at the University of Strasburg surpassed those of most other comparable faculties in the German-speaking countries until the late 1880s. Besides being evident in the significant role that physiological chemistry played as "an integrative science and an interdisciplinary research direction," a teamwork approach to neuroscience investigations could be found also in the broader area of oncological research. This field thrived not only in the Kaiser Wilhelms University but also in other leading research institutions of the time such as the Deutsche Forschungsanstalt for Psychiatry in Munich, the Friedrich Wilhelms University of Breslau, and the Friedrich Wilhelms University of Berlin (see also the map in the frontmatter to this book). Particular examples in neuromorphological research were studies of brain tumours, cerebrospinal fluid transport and infections, as well as spinal marrow structures.[38]

Despite official affirmations of the innovative organization and the quality of the research output from the Kaiser Wilhelms University,[39] some deep-rooted nineteenth-century academic traditions nevertheless still prevailed, having a significant effect on early Strasburg neuroscience. Career paths within the field of neuromorphology, for instance, had been all but predictable at the time, since the new researcher elite had been subjected to contingent contracts, limited term placements (*Rotationserlasse*), and autocratic direction of their own research by the hovering directors. The hierarchical structure of the institutional relationships was felt right through to the subordinate levels of research assistants (*Hilfsassistenten*), assistant professors (*Institutsassistenten*), and associate professors (*Extraordinarien*). Consequently, even prominent brain researchers such as Ludwig Edinger were threatened with an early end to their academic careers.[40] Even though Edinger had been keenly promoted by his influential mentor, the clinician and internist Adolf Kussmaul (1822–1902), and maintained excellent contacts at the anatomical institute of the Kaiser Wilhelms University, he nevertheless found himself in a position where he had to leave the Alsatian capital. By the turn of the century, the system of frequent job rotations had become the rule rather than the exception for most basic medical researchers.[41]

With such a lack of institutional stability, the Kaiser Wilhelms University experienced severe constraints on the growth of established research programs – and in some ways the very existence of its neuroscience programs became endangered. As French medical historian Christian Bonah has shown, a noticeable process of the "aging of the full professors in

Strasburg" continued until the outbreak of World War I, resulting in crowded career paths for young *Privatdozenten*, for whom vacant positions became extremely rare.[42] Yet most of these researchers held medical degrees and, like Edinger, were obliged to seek positions as medical practitioners or choose jobs in the public health sector. Despite the affirmative rhetoric of university administrators at the time, a huge contingent of promising researchers was thus irretrievably lost. This process was visible not only in Strasburg but in many other German and Austrian universities as well.[43]

Toward the end of the century, the very hopeful atmosphere of the Kaiser Wilhelms University's founding years had been dissipated, even though the intensity of its academic work remained comparatively high on every level of research.[44] Excellent senior researchers such as Waldeyer and Jolly were subsequently lured away from Strasburg to Friedrich Wilhelms University of Berlin. By means of a successful political move through which Prussia tried to regain former academic terrain, the Strasburg researchers were offered exceptionally attractive research infrastructures in Berlin. Many of the vacated positions at the Strasburg Kaiser Wilhelms University would never again be filled, thereby setting in motion a process that lowered the institute's ability to attract the brightest and the best among contemporary researchers. Another result was the overburdening of the faculty members who stayed in the capital of Alsace-Lorraine, as the excellent instructor-student ratio of the founding years was substantially diminished.[45] Contrary to the intensive decade after Kaiser Wilhelms University's exciting founding years, which had been characterized by strong personal relationships among the chairs of the departments and their co-workers, research circumstances became less collegial and the atmosphere increasingly gruff. Witness a letter of complaint written by the embryologist Dr Franz Keibel (1861–1929), *Ordinarius* professor and director of the anatomical institute, to his dean on 3 December 1915:

I would like to express my strong concerns over the recent complaints that my colleague *Herr Hofrat Professor [Arnold] Chiari* [1851–1915] has raised, because he felt irritated that inventory numbers had been fixed to objects in our shared lecture hall. If he had ever addressed this issue to me in a single word, I would have known how to take care of this – in the way that he himself requested. Since *we are all forced to remain under the same roof*, it appears to me the simplest thing that we accommodate each other.[46]

Personal frictions, decreasing willingness to cooperate, and a pervasive new mindset among *Ordinarius* professors to take their whole research groups (comprising laboratory scientists, house officers, and research assistants, etc.) along with them to the new Kaiser Wilhelm University from their former university, from which they were hired – thereby marginalizing and excluding Strasburg's own young researchers – came to dominate. The earlier atmosphere of mutual understanding (*gemeinsame Geisteshaltung*) of the founding decade gradually faded away when the second generation of exclusively German professors assumed university leadership roles.

WORLD WAR I AND CHANGES DURING THE GERMAN-FRENCH INTERWAR YEARS (1914–1933)

The prolonged period of prosperity, social innovation, and optimistic nation-building that had prevailed since 1871–72 ended abruptly with the outbreak of war on 3 August 1914, quickly initiating years of violent national clashes. The Great War was devastating in its disruption of the trend toward modernity and democracy in Europe. German historian Thomas Nipperdy intriguingly summarized the impact of the war in the following way, emphasizing that for Europeans it was not only a disruptive break in the history of their continent, but prefigured a multi-decade process of major social upheaval to come:

> Everyone had believed that they were on the defensive, and everyone had been ready for war. Most, however, overrated the threats to their own existence, while all underrated the violence and the epochal character of the coming war. The war came, not because all or many were exasperated by the peace, nor because of their eagerness to actually begin a war. If one looks at the amount of freedom for each individual decision-making of the historical actors, then everyone had their share in seeing the crisis come to a head.[47]

The outbreak of war was the result of many underlying social, scientific, and technological developments that had begun accumulating in the final years of the nineteenth century.[48] Military command structures, for example, asserted increasing influence over the civil administration system in Wilhelminian universities, affecting particularly the background training of researchers in clinical neurology and psychiatry. The growing influence of such command structures (*Kommandierungsregeln*) in the medical service of the army (*Heeressanitaetswesen*) – which included hundreds of physicians as officers of the reserve – became more and more palpable after the early 1890s. Particularly after the mobilization of faculty, clinicians, and researchers into the German army medical corps in the 1910s, the demands of technological warfare, convalescent needs for the war injured, and sanitation provisions for the German people emerged as predominant themes. These trends are reflected, for instance, in the scope of many dissertations supervised at the Kaiser Wilhelms University between 1912 and 1919. In the area of neuroscience, dissertation topics now dealt with problems of peripheral nerve traumata, wound healing, neuropsychological assessments for the military service, and the prevalence of mental illness, along with therapeutic options for treating veterans with neurasthenia and shellshock (*Neurastheniker* and *Kriegszitterer*).[49]

The process of warfare did more than provide a natural impulse for medical research at the universities' clinical departments, however. One year into the war, the negative effects of economic austerity also became apparent. The absence of conscripted personnel was now felt on the research assistant level – in areas such as preparing collections of microscopic objects and the day-to-day practical needs in clinical wards. And, since male physicians had been ordered to the fronts or military hospitals, vacancies were more often filled with the women who remained behind. Many women took over the roles of the absent assistants and increasingly assumed medical and scientific functions that were formerly deemed "completely unsuitable" for them. Working tasks included the preparation of bodies for pathological purposes; assistance in *post-mortem* dissections; cleaning, repairing, and adjustment of microscopic equipment; care for laboratory animals; bloodletting and intravenous injections in the clinic; neuropsychological testing; or simply necessary repair work in the offices of the institutes and clinics. As an example, the director of the Strasburg institute for anatomy, Franz Keibel, wrote a fast-track application to the university curator:

> Your Excellency,
> Allow me to please submit to you the following request to be permitted to advertise for another female microtomist. We would like to hire Fraeulein [Maria] Hinburg as the microtomist in our institute of pathology, since she has already worked in our institute during the morning hours. She would be paid for the whole duration of the war 60 M[arks] ... with your agreement, from the salary allocation for the vacant research assistant.[50]

On the basic research side, departments of anatomy and pathology during the times of the war economy had to manage with only the annual, benchmarked funds for their regular routine work (in teaching, specimen preparations, and *post mortem* services for the university clinics and city hospitals), while at the same time the clinical field of neurology experienced an unexpected increase in military interest. Under the leadership of neurologist and psychiatrist Robert Wollenberg (1862–1942), the neurosciences at the Kaiser Wilhelms University created new fields of activity, an example being the clinical description of nerve lesions or investigations of glial scar tissue in the peripheral nervous system and the central nervous system. The scope of these endeavours remained fairly limited, however, due to the lack of human resources. This situation became an embarrassment for researchers, since they now sat on sackfuls of money never seen before. Yet technological equipment (fine mechanics and optics for microscopes) was hardly available on the market, as most supplies of that nature were of prime interest to the military, particularly the artillery.[51] Although clinical neurosciences effectively had more financial support than ever, the situation was a Pyrrhic victory, since the money could not be used to transform allocated infrastructure into effective research programs. At Strasburg, Wollenberg and his collaborators nevertheless struggled along and tried to compensate for the lack of supplies through relentless laboratory investigations with the limited means available.

After the war, though, Wollenberg was ousted from his position as a full professor by the new French government. Like most of the German, non-Alsatian faculty members, he took all his protocols, object slides, laboratory notebooks, and data archives with him, and for a period of two years became a neuropathology professor at Marburg University in Hesse. Having received a subsequent job offer from the University of Breslau, he moved to the Silesian capital and continued as the chair of its prominent clinical neurology department.[52] The embryologist Franz Kleber (1899–1975), another offspring of the Strasburg neurosciences in the 1910s, continued his training as a visiting scholar at a number of American institutions and after his return to Germany received an offer from the University of Freiburg, where he continued a research program on neurogenesis from a comparative perspective.[53]

When the new dean of the medical faculty, the Alsatian internist Georges Weiss (1861–1929), took office after the war in 1919, he actively promoted an equal-opportunity policy to avoid nationalist splits among the professors. Despite such efforts, however, most German-speaking academics left

Strasburg for universities in Germany, Austria, Switzerland, and elsewhere. During the transformation years of the early 1920s, the new French government changed its policies, since most of the organizational elites were eager to hold on to the existing – and often younger – scientists and clinicians, many of whom were still versatile researchers.[54] Adding to the problem faced by the new government due to the exodus of the German-speaking staff, it proved impossible to attract an acceptable number of ordinary scientists, least of all highly renowned professors, to the new French university.[55] In this sense, it was fortunate for administrators that many of the Alsatian *Privatdozenten* and former assistants had remained in the province due to their family ties, and were eager to continue in their positions or to seek faculty promotions. The exodus of high-profile academics back to the "right side of the Rhine" thus became a major opportunity for Alsatians to acquire vacant chairs at their regional university.

It should not be overlooked that, from a cultural perspective, the new Alsatian professors also played an important role in the re-establishment of French-German scientific relationships in the postwar period. In this respect, histologist Claude L. Pierre Masson (1880–1959) can probably be seen as the most active and prolific researcher of the French faculty during these years. He joined the University of Strasburg after leaving the Pasteur Institute in Paris and transformed his department into a leading brain tumour institution. Following a research period in North America, to which he had been invited, and having personally witnessed the early rise of Fascism and Nazism in Europe, he eventually decided to return to Canada as a professor of pathology at the Université de Montréal in 1927.[56]

Apart from star researcher Pierre Masson, it was the Alsatian professors, including anatomist Andreas Forster (1873–1960) and the psychiatrist and neurologist Jacques Felix Pfersdorff (b. 1878), who built and nurtured the new French-speaking faculty. It is interesting to note the enthusiasm of the founding professors in re-establishing a veritable research university in Alsace, which was very similar to the creation of the Kaiser Wilhelms University yet with much less outside financial support.[57] For the neurosciences this proved to be particularly valuable, since an interdepartmental program in neuropathology had crystallized around Masson's chairmanship. The research pursued at the university became centred on questions of cerebral sclerosis and neurofibromatosis. However, due to the insufficient research funds from the Strasburg General Hospital (the former *Buergerhospital*), clinical neuroscience did not experience the same *élan scientifique* that it had at the turn of the century.[58]

When compared with other leading-edge centres in German-speaking neuromorphology between 1910 and the interwar period – centres such as Berlin, Leipzig, Munich, and Breslau – the development of neuroscientific research at the University of Strasburg can only be described as a history of continuous decline throughout the first half of the twentieth century. While American educator and university researcher Abraham Flexner (1866–1959) emphasized in his influential "Report on Medical Education in Europe" (1912) for the Carnegie Foundation for the Advancement of Teaching, that "productive scientists in Germany had not long or consistently been connected with universities, but have labored as individuals," it became obvious that not only individuals but also general social contexts had dramatically changed the framework of biomedical research at Strasburg University (the link to the build-up of the early Nazi Period in Alsace-Lorraine is described and discussed later in this chapter).[59] This historical case of morphological brain research at the University of Strasburg is highly instructive, since it demonstrates the making, rise, and fall of interdisciplinary programs as *neuroscience in context*.[60] This narrative also provides important perspectives on the involvement of the neuroscientific endeavour with spheres of government, military, and industrial interests, which gradually expanded the horizon of inquiry and knowledge production after the Wilhelminian period.[61]

THE EARLY SITUATION IN LEIPZIG

The development of scientific medicine at the University of Leipzig is strongly associated with the physiologist Carl Ludwig (1816–1895), who not only introduced the paradigm of "physical physiology" to the local research environment but was also instrumental in creating the largest department of physiology in the world in the latter half of the nineteenth century.[62] Ludwig and the Leipzig school of physiologists introduced important experimental approaches in neurophysiological research through a quantifying methodology of self-inscribing kymographs and original vivisectional techniques. This was shown, for example, in the assumption of the Leipzig experimental practices in the subsequent demonstration of the electrical excitability of the motor cortex by Gustav Fritsch (1838–1927) in Berlin and Eduard Hitzig (1838–1907) at the University of Halle.[63] Another famous researcher, who became the doyen of behavioural neuroscience at Leipzig, was the psychophysiologist Wilhelm Maximilian Wundt (1832–1920) – "the founding father of experimental psychology."[64] Although he was not a neuromophologist, the analysis of the principle of "Psychophysiological Parallelism" from his Leipzig colleague, the philosopher and physicist Gustav Theodor Fechner (1801–1887), became an important heuristic principle for experimental applications in laboratory neuroscience.[65] Wundt and Fechner helped to create an interdisciplinary mindset for research in contemporary neuroscience, which expanded the confines of the local medical faculty to include collaborations with philosophers, psychologists, and physicists at the university, as well as doctors in the city of Leipzig.[66]

Leipzig's claim to fame in morphological brain research began to emerge in 1877 with the return of the neuroanatomist Paul Flechsig (1847–1929) from Vienna, where he had stayed and collaborated with Heinrich Obersteiner. Flechsig had been offered an associate professorship (*Extraordinariat*) in neurology and psychiatry along with the promise that he would be made the director of the new clinical department of neurology and psychiatry.[67] However, it was more than five years before the new department was finally opened on 2 May 1882. The creation of this institution can be seen as an architectural and organizational merger of three major traditions at the end of the nineteenth century: In Flechsig, who was himself a pupil of the eminent Leipzig experimental physiologist Ludwig, a neuromorphologist had been hired to support the somatic approach in psychiatry following the philosophy of Wilhelm Griesinger, according to whom "*all mental diseases are in fact diseases of the brain.*"[68] While training with Ludwig, Flechsig had risen to prominence as he advocated for the construction of a "city asylum" in Leipzig-Doesen for the public health community (see figure 2.3), essentially a compromise of Griesinger's own concept of acute psychiatry in Heidelberg with later Berlin developments.

In Berlin, Griesinger had likewise advocated for pavilion-style psychiatric buildings attached to the university hospital for research purposes and acute psychiatric cases. Chronically ill patients, on the other hand, had to be transferred to agrarian colonies outside the city confines.[69] A third influence on Flechsig came from the research impetus (*Wissenschaftsideal*) that had captured German-speaking medical science since the second half of the nineteenth century.[70] Flechsig immediately seized the opportunity when the department of neurology and psychiatry opened:

When the Ministry of Cultural Affairs and Public Education of the Kingdom of Saxony approached the *rapporteur* [Flechsig] in the spring of 1878 to organize an autonomous clinical department for the insane, which had to incorporate all necessary auxiliary means

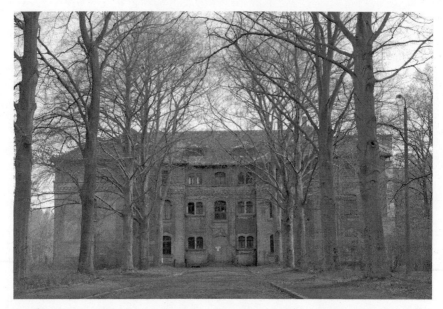

2.3 The main entrance area and building of the clinical department for psychiatry and neurology (inaugurated in 1882) at the University of Leipzig, as it appeared in 2005. Coll. Frank W. Stahnisch. © 2008 Frank W. Stahnisch, Calgary, Alberta.

for the care of the mentally ill, no institution of this kind was in existence – neither in Germany nor elsewhere – which could have served as a model. Although there had been a variety of psychiatric clinical departments, they differed greatly in the way they were organized from what was envisaged at Leipzig.[71]

In the same year that the Leipzig clinical department of psychiatry was opened with the intention of being "used for psychiatric teaching purposes," Obersteiner inaugurated his multi-disciplinary brain research institute at Vienna University.[72] Flechsig's rhetorical announcement about the uniqueness of his department must of course be taken with a grain of salt, since it disregarded Obersteiner's parallel academic program. Yet, in truth, a stunning number of ten other institutions in the German-speaking countries were unable to fulfill Flechsig's expectations as a model for a complete institute for neurological and psychiatric research and care, even though they had their own local properties and advantages for different types of research programs.[73] The dedication of his book *The Clinical Department for the Insane* of 1888 (*Irrenklinik der Universitaet*

Leipzig und ihre Wirksamkeit in den Jahren 1882–1886) to the "Ministry of Cultural Affairs and Public Education in the Kingdom of Saxony" certainly explains the superlatives that were used in the political language of the new *Extraordinarius* professor.

The continuing development of early neuroscience endeavours in Leipzig resulted in part from the specific location of the clinical department for neurology and psychiatry, since it had been built in close proximity to the other research institutes in the "medical district" (*Klinisches Viertel*). Yet beyond what Flechsig had stated, the research impetus did not become embedded in the architectural arrangement with adjacent medical science institutions. The whole area was far away from the inner city of Leipzig and could not be reached with public transportation. The complex itself, however, consisted of a three-storey main building and two aisles on each side for male and female wards, while an isolation ward for infectious diseases was later added in the park-like quad. The main building accommodated the offices of the physicians and researchers, and housed the central brain research laboratory. Forty years later, in 1927, however, the laboratory facilities became independent from the hospital, yet continued their work on the same hospital grounds until the end of World War II.[74] The number of patients treated by the clinical department during the first years of its existence, from 1878 to 1886, totalled 1,894, the highest number for any clinical department in Germany at the time; and about a quarter of these patients had been *Nervenkranke* (neurological patients with somatic forms of illness).[75] While the hospital had forty staff members (wardens, nurses, and technicians, and so forth), the doctorial staff consisted only of a chief physician – Paul Flechsig at the time – and two assistant physicians: the illustrious Emil Kraepelin, who in 1917 became the founding director of the Deutsche Forschungsanstalt for Psychiatry in Munich – which only later in 1924 became incorporated into the Kaiser Wilhelm Society – and Georg Lehmann (1855–1918). The latter had studied in Leipzig and then continued his postgraduate training under Jolly in Strasburg. Socialized in the morphological tradition in psychiatry, Lehmann had been considered *secundo loco* during the job search for the associate professorship, which Flechsig then received. His lifelong friend Flechsig later recommended him as director of the clinical department of psychiatry at the University of Munich, after Bernhard von Gudden (1824–1886) had tragically drowned during the suicide act of King Ludwig II (1845–1886) of Bavaria.[76] Even though the professorship went to Oswald Bumke, who became von Gudden's successor in Munich, Lehmann stayed on as a consultant and staff-attending physician.[77]

During Flechsig's headship, the Leipzig clinical department of psychiatry and neurology continued as a morphologically oriented research institution. This orientation was soon represented in its name change to the "clinical department for mental and nervous diseases" (*Psychiatrische und Nervenklinik*) in 1888, at which point its designation as a "hospital for the insane" disappeared. During his more than forty years of service, Flechsig kept the morphological tradition of the department alive until he retired in 1920, at which time other psychiatric traditions were incorporated into the clinical environment. This development is exemplified in the work of two of his pupils: as a psychiatrist, Erwin Niessl von Meyendorff (1873–1943) published extensively on neuroanatomical problems of the organization of the human cortex, the interdependence of higher cortical functions *vis-à-vis* their localizational organization, and generally on the anatomical principles of the brain's functional mechanics (*Prinzipien der Gehirnmechanik*).[78] Also, Friedrich Wilhelm Quensel (1873–1957) conducted neurological and anatomical studies on the brain before he left the hospital to become chief of service in specialized union hospitals for miners near Leipzig.[79]

Although it has been argued that the morphological tradition had its difficulties in altering clinical perspectives at the beginning of the twentieth century, Flechsig and his collaborators maintained important relationships with basic researchers in the department of anatomy and pathology. These contacts included frequent exchanges of elective students and summer interns as well. For these trainees a stay at the unit proved a worthwhile research experience before assuming assistant positions in other neuroscientific institutes.[80] These collaborations came to fruition through personal continuities over the four decades that Flechsig was the chair of psychiatry and neurology, as well as an independent director of the brain research institute.[81] Important in this respect are the interchanges with the director of the Leipzig department of anatomy, Wilhelm His (1831–1904), who was also interested in neuromorphological research on nerve cells ("neurons") as distinct anatomical and functional elements. For his own comparative research aims, His developed new staining derivatives and a stationary microtome for the automatic slicing of histological objects,[82] methodological advances that brought international researchers and trainees to Leipzig, including the leading Hungarian neurohistologist Michael von Lenhossék (1863–1937) from the University of Budapest.[83]

THE FORMATION OF SUPPORT NETWORKS IN BRAIN
RESEARCH FROM IMPERIAL GERMANY
TO THE BEGINNING OF THE EARLY POSTWAR PERIOD

Wilhelm His had been a supporter of what came to be called the contemporary "neuron doctrine," but other researchers of his group reached different conclusions, supporting instead the syncytial theory of nerve alignments in the brain.[84] Among them, in addition to the prominent neurohistologist Camillo Golgi (1843–1926) in Italy, was the Leipzig anatomist Hans Held (1866–1942), who succeeded His as the chair of anatomy. Held promoted the idea that the neuronal texture in the body displayed a continuous morphology. He interpreted this as a structural similitude to other bodily organs (such as the liver and kidney tissues).[85] Those who agreed with Held argued that the microscopic evidence of the neuronists entailed too many artifacts, leading to controversial results based on the sudden stopping of nerve cell filaments in the microscopic slides. This finding was often seen when the objects had been perpendicularly sectioned during the preparation process of the slides. Meanwhile, Held and his co-workers built a theoretical argument around the findings of Emil Du Bois-Reymond (1818–1896). It showed that the action potential (the *Nervenstrom*) could electrophysiologically follow continuing nerve tracts but would stop at structural discontinuities. Held's argument was that the action potentials could "not hop" over the gaps from one nerve to another.[86]

A striking case is that of one of Held's pupils and main opponents of the succeeding electron microscopic interpretation of the neuronal synapse: German neurohistologist Karl Friedrich Bauer (1904–1985), who later became the head of the institute of anatomy at the Friedrich Alexander University in Erlangen, received numerous international awards and degrees, along with the honour of *Commendatore dell' Ordine al Merito della Repubblica Italiana*.[87] Bauer himself was trained at the Leipzig Flechsig Institute after he had received his medical licence to practise in 1930, and he continued to work as a research associate with Held from 1930 to 1935. When Held became professor emeritus, Bauer went to Berlin to receive his *Habilitation* with the infamous Nazi anatomist Hermann Stieve (1886–1952) at the Charité.[88] Even though research technologies had by then changed from light microscopes to electron microscopes, with the *neuroanatomical community* increasingly accepting the view of the neuron theorists, Bauer kept to the convictions of his teacher, whom he always cited as an *argumentum auctoritatis*.[89] Held had been a fervent opponent of the Spanish histologist Ramón y Cajal (1852–1934) at international medical conferences such as International Brain Commission meetings, and as Bauer's mentor he became quite an influential player in neuromorphology from the 1910s to the 1930s.[90] With his assumption of the Erlangen chair, later in 1947, however, Bauer undertook to create a new school of neurohistologists:[91]

> E[ber]. Landau [1878–1959] (1948) says that the neurohistologists know the difficulty it takes to receive instructive slides ... Whether neuronists or non-neuronists – as he pointed out – we are all seeking to discover the structure of the synapse between the nerve cells in the region of the hypothetical "ultranerve" ([John N. Langley [1852–1925]).[92]

Yet, other than Bauer, postwar Erlangen neuromorphologists had not been trained in these new technologies; nor had they been part of the wider neuroscientific networks involving American researchers. Otherwise, they would have been better able to reconnect with global research trends after the war.[93]

Similarly, the previous academic setting of Flechsig, His, and the other neuromorphologists at Leipzig University was quite different from that of most communities at German and Austrian universities after the Great War. Their common influence was not confined to particular areas of research; together they provided forums for a free exchange of philosophical and scientific ideas, for example in what they called the "Nerve Circle" (*Nervenkraenzchen*), an ongoing gathering of researchers, psychologists, philosophers, and other professors interested in the brain (between 1890 and 1920). For nearly three decades, this early neuroscience interest group met in one of the oldest coffee houses in downtown Leipzig. In addition to His's and Held's associates, neurologist Adolf von Struempell (1853–1925), and psychiatrist Oswald Bumke also took part in these meetings.[94] The participants in the illustrious *Nervenkraentzchen* exchanged opinions on the many questions that might be raised about the brain and mind, from neuromorphological issues to psychiatric cases, epistemological research questions, and the nature of the human soul, in what was a thoroughly humanistic afternoon pastime.[95]

This liberal atmosphere was also highlighted in Edinger's early scientific visit to Leipzig after his 1881 MD graduation from the Kaiser Wilhelms University in Strasburg (see chapter 2). He came for a year of postgraduate training with Carl Weigert to study new staining techniques for nervous tissue, such as aniline dyes for nerve cells and fibrin as well as myelin stains for nerve sheaths identification.[96] At that time, Weigert was assistant professor in the institute of pathology, to which he had followed his mentor, Julius Friedrich Cohnheim (1839–1884) from Breslau.[97] While collaborating primarily with Weigert, Edinger also sought research input and advice from Flechsig in the clinical department of neurology and psychiatry, as well as from Wilhelm Heinrich Erb (1840–1921) in neuropathology. Soon afterward, however, Erb received an offer from the University of Heidelberg, where he founded one of the first specialized neurology departments.[98] Even if a number of these brain researchers worked only transiently in Leipzig before continuing on to an academic niche in the German university system, the sheer concentration of investigators represents the vibrant situation that existed between the 1880s and 1910s and demonstrates Leipzig's influence as one of the foremost centres in the German-speaking neurosciences. It is pertinent to note how Edinger tried to combine the different aspects of neuroscientific research that he had in mind as a new, comprehensive form of research organization of the type he had experienced in Strasburg, Paris, and above all in Leipzig during his academic *Wanderjahre* in Central Europe. In accordance with his strong appreciation of the free collaborative exchanges and overtly stimulating *Nervenkraentzchen* at the University of Leipzig, Edinger pushed strongly for Weigert to be with him in Frankfurt am Main. To that end, he successfully managed to garner a large salary for the latter in 1884 out of the endowment of the Senckenberg Foundation, and thereafter he invited Weigert to join him.[99]

With regard to the influences of researchers in Leipzig, Flechsig was the unquestionable centre of gravity for neuroscientific research in Saxony, while also maintaining deep personal relationships with the versatile neuroanatomist His. Together, they became interested in elucidating the structural conditions of the nerve tracts in the brain and sense organs, in a collaboration that famously culminated in Flechsig's work on the auditory pathway (*Gehoerwindung*). His, in addition, ventured into comparative studies of the autonomic nervous system, which allowed him to identify the "Bundle of His" of the autonomic innervation toward the atrioventricular node of the heart muscle.[100] The research progress made in Leipzig and so many other institutions also attracted a large number of postgraduate students and visiting researchers to the Saxon metropolis for parts of their training. Among them were Michael Foster (1836–1907) and Woodrow Wilson (1856–1924) from the United States, along with

Henry Head from the United Kingdom. To further these visits, the nerve and brain research departments at the University of Leipzig received even larger amounts of financial support from the Rockefeller Foundation.[101] This support had been planned as a long-term financial investment from the American side, in order to recreate and sustain the international science exchanges.[102]

Of course, non-American international researchers also benefited from the infrastructures and training opportunities in the leading research programs. An instructive example is Michael von Lenhossék, who arrived from the Hungarian University of Budapest to work with Wilhelm His on experiments about regeneration phenomena in nerve endings.[103] Von Lenhossék's contribution to the "neuron doctrine" and his discovery of the "growth cone" is indicative of the fruitfulness of interchanges at the University of Leipzig up until the 1930s. The university and its institutions built a legacy in neuroscientific research not only for this Hungarian histologist but likewise for a considerable number of contemporary brain researchers.[104]

The impact of the strong neuromorphological tradition at Leipzig was much more visible in somatic neurology than in the area of clinical psychiatry, however. Even though Oskar Vogt – who was an assistant physician with Flechsig in Leipzig from 1894 to 1895 – would later open up toward clinical hypnotic therapy of the nervously ill; he came to be better known for his histoarchitectonic work at the KWI for Brain Research in Berlin. The brain psychiatrist Siegfried Walter Loewe (1884–1963) also deserves mention here, since it was he who first tested the drug *Luminal* in 1916 on his Leipzig hospital patients. What was intended as a sleeping drug for the mentally ill came to be one of the first successful introductions of a pharmacological treatment for epileptic patients. Among the clinicians were Heinrich Klien (1875–1941), who worked on diagnostics of psychiatric and nervous diseases, and Carl Schneider (1891–1946), who pursued research on the psychopathology of schizophrenia.[105] With the Nazi *Machtergreifung*, however, Schneider assumed the directorship of the department of psychiatry at the University of Heidelberg and later became infamously known for his advisory work in the *Aktion T4* euthanasia program of the Nazi government.[106]

With Flechsig's final retirement in 1927, a qualified successor was needed to continue the morphological tradition in brain psychiatry. It proved to be difficult, however, for the search committee to find good candidates from the psychiatric side, although not the neurological one. Their first choice had been for the application of the doubly trained psychiatrist and psychologist Richard Arwed Pfeifer (1877–1957). Pfeifer began his studies in philosophy, in which he became a research assistant of Wilhelm Wundt at the University of Leipzig, before he changed to medical studies in Leipzig and Munich between 1912 and 1915. During the first year of the war, Pfeifer was conscripted as a staff-attending physician in a military hospital on the Eastern front in Russia. Beginning in 1918 he worked in the barracks of the Lazarett Regiment in Leipzig-Connewitz, before entering the clinical department of psychiatry and neurology at the university. In 1920, he became a consultant physician and earned his *Habilitation* with a study that used new intravascular dies and a comparative radiological approach on the angiotechtonics of the brain. Subsequently, at the end of 1924, he rose to the rank of full professor.[107] Pfeifer was respected as "the only person who knows the whole collection of brain preparations and histological slides," a collection that was perceived as unique in the world and which Flechsig had curated for over four decades. Pfeifer was now identified as "the only person who could preserve and sustain it" as an intellectually rich and scientifically usable neuroanatomical and neuropathological collection. Despite finally receiving the job offer on 1 June 1927 as the chair of brain research and Flechsig's successor, the committee still held some reservations about his application, since his research was deemed quite narrow and "extremely occupied with anatomical and brain pathological questions."[108] Furthermore, it was pointed out that his neuroscientific knowledge was clearly "not in the area of clinical psychiatry," as some of the clinical professors had hoped for in Flechsig's successor.[109]

Pfeifer was further personally antagonized by the director of the clinical department of psychiatry and neurology, Paul Schroeder (1873–1941), who had joined the faculty from the Northern German Ernst Moritz University of Greifswald. Schroeder became grossly irritated by the fact that an autonomous brain research chair had been created in what he considered to be "his own" department. From Schroeder's letters sent to the medical faculty and the search committee it becomes clear that he did not have an adequate understanding of the historical development of the unique research organization at the University of Leipzig. Instead, he made constant complaints: "Herr Professor Pfeifer is like a foreign particle (*Fremdkoerper*) in the institute which is subordinated to me;" or "I (Schroeder) only heard by chance a few days ago, when chitchatting in our laboratory that a foreign visiting professor had been pursuing experimental research in it for several weeks. Pfeifer did not notify me about this visitor, yet instead only sent a letter to the Principal of the

University." Schroeder was clearly anxious that he could not personally control the communication, research, and educational activities of Pfeifer, working in what he perceived as "his own institute."[110]

Despite these frequent attempts to threaten Pfeifer personally, Pfeifer remained in his position. His superiors ignored Schroeder's complaints, appreciating the international benefit in the continuation of the tradition at their university. Flechsig's highly visible landmark institute continued to attract large numbers of international researchers to Leipzig, and it was seen as a major research unit of the university for both scientific reasons and public outreach relations. The complexity of the situation nevertheless displayed many of the problems inherent in organizing an interdisciplinary system of collaboration and research in the contexts of the time. Literally, the brain research institute was a "foreign body" that resisted what American interdisciplinarity scholar Thompson Klein has called the "incorporation" by the larger and thus encompassing system in the attempt to create interdisciplinary surroundings.[111]

Flechsig's immediate, though short-term, successor as the director of the clinical department of psychiatry and neurology was Oswald Bumke, who became well known internationally through the publication of his *Handbook of Neurology* (1935–37) with Otfrid Foerster.[112] Oswald Conrad Edouard Bumke had studied medicine in Freiburg, Leipzig, Munich, Halle, and Kiel, from which he graduated in 1901, and he subsequently worked at several psychiatric and neurological institutions at the universities of Freiburg, Rostock, Breslau, and Leipzig between 1910 and 1924. Bumke published his influential *Textbook on Psychiatry* (*Lehrbuch der Geisteskrankheiten*) in 1919, and – in 1923 – was included among the group of illustrious physicians to visit Lenin, after the Russian leader had suffered a severe stroke. Other German-trained consultants to Lenin included: Foerster from Breslau, who led the team, Adolf von Struempell (1853–1925), a neurologist from Leipzig, Max Nonne (1861–1959) from Hamburg, and Salomon Henschen (1847–1930) from Uppsala in Sweden, along with two surgeons and one internist from the United Kingdom.[113] In 1924, after his training period in psychiatry at the University of Leipzig had ended, Bumke became Kraepelin's successor in the psychiatry chair at the University of Munich. There, he became fully engaged in large-scale investigations and epidemiological research on "nervous degeneration" disorders. From 1928 to 1930 Bumke edited the eleven-volume *Handbook of Mental Diseases* (*Handbuch der Geisteskrankheiten*), which, like its predecessor, was published by Springer Press.[114] Following the celebrations surrounding the eightieth birthday of Paul Flechsig in 1927, the Brain Research Institute at the University of Leipzig became autonomous, since Flechsig had continued the somatic tradition of brain research and psychiatry on the basis of his strong conviction that all mental diseases are in fact diseases of the brain.

In this chapter, I have examined the disciplinary makeup of clinical and basic research in the late Wilhelminian period in Germany, while concentrating on two leading universities of the time, Strasburg and Leipzig, as a distinct case comparison. Both universities displayed a traditional nineteenth-century form of academic organization, before the outbreak of World War I, a structure in which neuroscientific research took place in specialized institutes of anatomy and physiology, as well as neurological and psychiatric clinics. In this sense, they present us with the *status quo* of brain research at the outset of the twentieth century, which came to be transformed in the decades after the end of the Great War during the interwar period. These considerations further set the stage for this book to guide the analysis of the emergence of interdisciplinary thinking and early clinical neuroscience research centres in the German-speaking countries from the later decades of the nineteenth century to the early interwar period. This chapter has provided constructive insights into the close collaborations between Strasburg and Leipzig, as representative examples of an ever-growing network between leading researchers and clinicians in early German neuromorphology from the very beginning of the twentieth century.

3

Shortfalls of Individualized Research, the Emergence of Clinical Neurology, and the Demands of Modern Life,

1910s to 1930s

Frankfurt am Main and Berlin

The ideal goal of the study of brain anatomy is a very ambitious one. We desire so thoroughly to understand the organ with which mental processes are associated that we shall be able to predict its functions ... To be sure, we are still very far from this goal. When we consider what we know about the human brain, its overwhelming complexity seems even simple compared to what we have observed of its activities.

Ludwig Edinger[1]

During the interwar period, in an otherwise disjointed discipline based on individualized research endeavours, a new type of interchange between neuroanatomy, experimental neurology, and clinical psychiatry emerged through connected research cultures. Such *experimental neurocultures* served as a stellar feature for early regenerative projects in the area of neurology and psychiatry (see also the Introduction).[2] Vitally intertwined with societal developments such as discourses on human degeneration and neurasthenia, as well as the experiences of brain-injured Great War veterans, events in the realm of brain research and clinical neurology could no longer be regarded as isolated.[3] Each of these cultural developments influenced researchers' conceptualization, scientific ideas, and even their research orientation. This process is mirrored, among other places, in reports and grant proposals that actively addressed societal concerns in general or the needs of funding institutions in particular.[4] Using the concept of *sociotechnical approaches*,[5] this chapter demonstrates that methodologies of neuronal de- and regeneration studies in German-speaking neuromorphology were more than simply products of recent differentiations of neurology or psychiatry. The consecutive changes were brought about by interdisciplinary efforts that derived from great collaborative work among contemporary brain researchers from various areas of investigation in the basic and clinical spheres.

In looking at these methodological interrelationships it proves valuable, from a history of medicine perspective, to consider the dimension of trauma research between 1910 and 1930, particularly if we want to understand the newly configured research culture in German neuromorphology.[6] As a "seductive hypothesis," this perspective helps in appreciating the forms of use, the historical connotations, and the modifications of notions of trauma and degeneration employed by clinical researchers at the time.[7] Instructive cases for the interwar period are those of the Heidelberg psychiatrist Viktor von Weizsaecker and Berlin neuropathologist Max Bielschowsky (see also the discussion in chapter 1). For von Weizsaecker, the notion of trauma was integrated with an anthropological approach of the "healing of the social body," whereas for Bielschowsky it rose to prominent neuromorphological meaning. For Bielschowsky, the individual experience of trauma was bound to an inherited disposition in what was seen as "degenerate patients"; at the same time, he acknowledged that morphological changes of the brain could also be brought about through physical and psychological wounds.[8]

Disciplinary transformations toward larger-scale working groups and programs in contemporary German-speaking neuroscience therefore followed individual technological advances as well as societal concerns. Researchers such as von Weizsaecker and Bielschowsky embraced the pursuit of de- and regeneration early and in a way that Karin Knorr-Cetina has described as a "condensation of society in the experiment."[9] This amalgamation between the scientific and cultural sphere – the condensation of society in brain research – is followed here on the basis of *laboratories in context* in neuromorphological centres from the 1910s to the 1930s. Earlier discourses on the "mental and physical degeneration" of modern man had already risen to notoriety under the societal conditions following World War I and during the Weimar Republic.[10]

THE "AGE OF NERVOUSNESS" AND RESEARCH EXCHANGES IN NEUROMORPHOLOGY

In building psychiatric and neurological theory, "degenerative views" underpinned widespread cultural beliefs about what Joachim Radkau has intriguingly called the "age of nervousness," describing neurasthenia as emerging from the practical needs of "the medical consultation room" rather than any from specific theoretical psychopathology.[11] Radkau's perspective on such social requirements of medical diagnostics in neuropsychiatry really puts the narrative in the right place. It strongly emphasizes the practical necessities of the time – the need to deal with a perceived increase in nervous diseases deemed to have arisen with the demands of urbanization, mechanization, and a highly competitive society.[12] Contemporary living conditions brought a soaring number of bourgeois, male, and high-performing individuals into the clinics and asylums of *fin de siècle* neurologists and psychiatrists. Trauma research therefore became an emerging field of interdisciplinary research during the first decades of the last century.[13] Shared experiences of war – physical and mental exhaustion, hunger, and frequent impressions of despair – had become deeply embedded in German and Austrian society.[14]

Yet even the ubiquitous phenomenon of "nervousness" in the busy Wilhelminian society was rendered obsolete overnight by the traumas of the "war to end all wars."[15] With the outbreak of war, traumas of the brains and minds of soldiers and affected civilians took hold in the collective consciousness of the public and physicians alike. The shell-shocked *Kriegszitterer*, with their visible limb-shaking after enduring periods of stalemate in the trenches, became a pan-European phenomenon, assuming the status of a real neurological epidemic. Already by September of 1914, this scourge had flared up, and by the end of the war almost two hundred thousand German veterans had experienced shell-shock disorders.[16] In addition to psychologically traumatized soldiers, there was also a group of another two hundred and fifty to three hundred thousand physically injured veterans who returned from the front with injuries of their nervous systems. During the interwar period, these "brain-injured warriors" (*Hirnverletzte Krieger*) crowded the asylums and neurological rehabilitation units to the extent that adequate therapy could often no longer be provided.[17]

After a review of how laboratory technologies became fused with views on nervous degeneration at the end of the war, we will be better able to determine the role of social pathologies (such as alcoholism, social deviance, and crime) in the transformation of brain anatomy, neuropathology, and clinical psychiatry. The final discussion of this chapter follows common perspectives on German society further into the experimental laboratories of the 1930s. It provides an integrative account of how societal representations and experimental research influenced each other at the end of the Weimar Republic's political torment. The decades between 1910 and 1930 were increasingly taken up with investigations into de- and regeneration in German brain science.[18] During this period, there emerged a transformed concept of "trauma" that brought together hybrid notions and research practices from various disciplines.[19] These develop-ments not only left their legacy in modern psychological and psychiatric occupations but they also integrated narrative components, neurological theories, and psychoanalytical treatment forms.[20]

Conceptual and methodological frameworks of psychological trauma research frequently overlapped with neuroanatomical interests. They even became embedded in efforts to find the microstructural lesions that trau-matic episodes left imprinted on the structure of the brain and spinal cord.[21] This research direction is particularly evident in laboratory experi-ments on nerve fibre regeneration by Albrecht Bethe at the University of Frankfurt and Max Bielschowsky's research into the regeneration of central nerve axons. Bielschowsky in particular pursued these analyses in Oskar and Cécile Vogt's brain research laboratory in downtown Berlin, and since the 1920s at the new KWI for Brain Research in Berlin-Buch on the northeast outskirts of the Prussian metropolis. While Canadian neurosurgeon Wilder Penfield had collaborated closely with other research-ers in that laboratory and institute during his 1928 visit to Germany, he had described personal relationships as rather difficult. Oskar Vogt, he wrote, had a tendency to intellectually retreat and focus exclusively on his work with his wife, Cécile:

Oskar Vogt was all-alone in one sense. He had every facility that he could use. He had associates, like his wife and the neurocytologist Max Bielschowsky, but no one to compete with him. When one is alone, it is too easy to go off on a tangent.[22]

In the laboratories of individuals, the research impetus was oriented around the internal demands of researchers' specific field of study, such as the functional anatomy of the human nervous system. The results were then applied with comparative intentions to different animal models, such as pigeons, goldfish, hamsters, and rabbits.[23] When neuromorphological regeneration work began to be pursued in leading neuroscientific labo-ratories, however, the findings became of pivotal importance to contem-porary debates in the *public sphere*, which were determined by the conflicts in major political arenas.[24]

BRAIN PSYCHIATRISTS' VIEWS ON HEREDITARY
NERVOUS DISEASES

For psychiatrists who had been predominantly engaged with issues of
moral (psychological) and cerebral degeneration at the time, the methodological boundaries between the medical and scientific disciplines they
drew upon were not clear-cut.[25] Junior researchers often developed their
particular brain research agendas, whether as a consequence of their setting in highly acclaimed centres for brain research or simply for reasons
contingent on their earlier studies in anatomy, biology, or psychology.
This tendency is apparent, for example, among many of the *Privatdozenten*
in the field of neuroanatomy, neuropathology, and brain psychiatry, of
whom about one third had a personal Jewish background. Like the adjunct
professors of neurology Alfred Goldscheider (1858–1935) and Max
Bielschowsky at the University of Berlin, they often ran productive laboratories along with innovative private clinics at the same time.[26] This
pattern may be presented as a general feature of the generation of young
brain researchers who became particularly instrumental for the interdisciplinary field of de- and regeneration in German neuromorphology at
the beginning of the twentieth century. Up-and-coming academics carved
out for themselves the places they wanted to be in or the specific laboratory methods they sought to learn. This strikingly innovative but institutionally unstable culture in Berlin was in fact comparable to those of other
medical research fields – such as dermatology and venerology, paediatrics,
and urology – alongside well-established disciplines around this time. As
Timothy Lenoir has pointed out:

> The notion of the lifeworlds as the precondition for objective science
> is a valuable additional resource for thinking about linking pragma-
> tism with our concerns about instrumentation, skill, practice, and the
> material embodiment of dispositions, taste and other cultural forms
> that do crucial mediating work between disparate domains … The
> focus on practice shifts our gaze to the mundane, to the construction
> of instruments, the manipulation of experimental apparatus in the
> time and space of the laboratory, and the relationship of these practical
> activities both to the "object" and to its theoretical representation.[27]

It should not go unmentioned, however, that, apart from *the cultural
forms of the lifeworlds* of their laboratories, clinics, scientific associations,

and other professional habitats of the Berlin *Privatdozenten*, well-established chairs clung to more traditional types of research production.[28] Full professors in normal anatomy and morphologically oriented pathologists were regarded as addressing basic research questions incommensurable with those raised by their colleagues in clinical psychiatry and neurology. This was particularly so since most worked explicitly with animal models or human dissection material, and the transferability of their findings to the human organism was not that simple to establish. The methodological divergences in fact resulted in a puzzling persistence of large-scale morphological research programs at the beginning of the twentieth century. In this ambivalent context, established programs that addressed issues in neuronal regeneration were likely to be paired with innovative developments only at the fringes of the field. Notable, for instance, were research activities on the attracting and repelling factors of nerve growth, acute-phase and late-onset neural sprouting, and the relationship between training effects (of both animals in their experimental settings and human patients in their clinical wards) and neuroplastic phenomena. All of these, however, lacked accepted labels and offered few career opportunities for young investigators.[29]

If one takes a closer look at de- and regenerative endeavours in contemporary brain science and leaves aside the fact that neuropsychiatry could not draw on the same "cultural capital" as was aligned with the laboratory sciences, it becomes palpable that after the turn of the century broad psychiatric concepts came to infiltrate basic and clinical research.[30] An influential aspect of such knowledge transfer "from bedside to bench" can be seen in Wilhelm Griesinger's notion of *neuropathy* (*neuropathische Schwaeche*). It subsumed disorders that displayed transient signs of agitation. It is instructive to note here that Griesinger, in his book *Mental Pathology and Therapeutics* of 1867 (*Pathologie und Therapie der psychischen Krankheiten*), saw the respective phenomena as an interlacing of hereditary and environmental causes:

The cases are proportionately rare, but cannot be questioned, where such mental anomalies, after being developed, pass slowly and gradually without further appreciable injurious influence into actual insanity. Much more commonly the nervous constitution is but a predisposing circumstance, besides which something else is necessary [in order that] the moderate mental aberration may pass into profound insanity, may become an actual cerebral disease.[31]

The assumed interplay between hereditary factors and environmental causes among constitutional neuropathies was further explained in a handbook contribution written by one of Griesinger's followers, the Munich internist Hugo Wilhelm von Ziemssen (1829–1902), in 1877:

> We venture to assume that catalepsy [forms of psychological fits with stupor] belongs to the large group of disease conditions designated by Griesinger [as] constitutional neuropathies ... and also that a predisposition dependent on congenital preformation of certain portions of the central nervous system generally precedes the appearance of the cataleptic attack. This supposition is yet further supported by the fact that we often observe catalepsy in families in which certain members are disposed to other disturbances.[32]

With his pathogenic notion of "irritable weakness," seen as describing congenital nervous diseases, Griesinger alluded back to French-Austrian psychiatrist Bénédict-Augustin Morel's (1809–1873) concepts of *dégénérescence*, which the latter had published in his *Treatise on Physical, Intellectual and Moral Degeneration of the Human Race*, in which he postulated that an original healthy and moral state of human society had existed in the past and diagnosed subsequent deteriorations from this state as a consequence of alterations in people's germ material.[33] Morel had in 1857–58 published his infamous though highly successful book, which was fully dedicated to the social problem of "degeneration" and its psychiatric and neurological underpinnings (see also my discussion in chapter 5). It was well received by the emerging field of clinical and brain psychiatry, as its protagonists believed it would help prove that psychiatric diseases had an identifiable (and thus in principle curable) somatic basis.[34] However, it is interesting to note that, in addition to clinical psychiatrists, a number of related approaches were also influenced by the broader scientific context of degeneration theories (*théories de dégénérescence*) – and even early eugenics thought within academic European psychiatry, especially among scientists and clinicians who worked with psychiatric patients at the same time.[35]

Morel's ideas became widely attractive to European psychiatrists, neurologists, and pathologists during the latter half of the nineteenth century. Among them was the eminent Swiss psychiatrist Auguste Forel (1848–1931) and the equally acclaimed neuroanatomist Constantin von Monakow (1853–1930) at the University of Zurich. Both medical researchers integrated Morel's approach into their neuropsychiatric theories about the pathological afflictions of the mind and increasingly began to search for somatic and morphological alterations in the human brain due to hereditary and "degenerative" influences.[36] Another scholar who sought somatic and morphological alterations in the human brain was the versatile pupil of Rudolph Virchow, Wuerzburg-based neuropathologist Georg Eduard von Rindfleisch (1836–1908).[37] In his *Lehrbuch der pathologischen Gewebelehre* (1867–69), he applied a Morelian interpretation of physical, intellectual, and moral degeneration to the human brain and spinal cord, which can be seen as a starting point of research into a new clinico-pathological view of the somatic foundations of psychiatric illness and mental disease. German medical historian Volker Roelcke has intriguingly shown that when Morel's publications appeared in Wilhelm Griesinger's influential clinical textbook, *Mental Pathology and Therapeutics*, Morel's notion had been received as a strict neuropsychiatric concept "stripped of its socio-*dégénérescence* political, moral, and collectivist aspects."[38] Griesinger effectively applied the concept of nervous degeneration in a much narrower sense than Morel, relating it to a hereditary aetiology of individual diseases of the mind and brain. For the Berlin brain psychiatrist and many of his followers, degenerative pathologies were thus basically associated with somatic correlates:[39]

If anywhere, here we are entitled to speak of *degeneration*. This is why this group of states has been grouped under the name of degenerative psychoses proper. In a wider sense, however, this term still includes a series of other mental disorders arising from pathological predispositions, in particular general neuroses, manic-depressive insanity, certain forms of feeble-mindedness[,] and perhaps also paranoia.[40]

In his famous article "On Degeneration" ("*Zur Entartungsfrage*"), published in the *Zentralblatt fuer Nervenheilkunde und Psychiatrie* (*zblNP*) in 1908 and thus long before the beginning of World War I, Emil Kraepelin likewise had argued that the aetiology of neurasthenia resulted from the general technological and urban conditions of modern life.[41] These views about nervous degeneration by the doyen of German psychiatry became so powerful that they even affected later approaches in social medicine and psychoanalysis in the Weimar Republic. Kraepelin's clearly stated view was that the war-traumatized had not become ill because of the conditions of industrialized warfare, but because of the inherited and physiological nature of their bodies, which these individuals had had since their birth – which gave rise to their nervous diseases under the straining conditions of warfare:[42]

> War involves a great number of mental causes of insanity. [Robert] Sommer [1864–1930] proved that active service in peacetime only renders psychopathically predisposed persons ill and causes no more cases of mental disorders than those observed in the civil population, but years of war are usually accompanied by a considerable increase in mental diseases ... Hence, the clinical pictures are, on the one hand, severe neurasthenic states and fright psychoses, on the other, concussion psychoses, exhaustion psychoses, epilepsy, and, above all, paralysis which appears essentially as a consequence of syphilis so frequently contracted during a campaign.[43]

In the following decade, positivistically oriented brain psychiatry came to reject many of the above-mentioned psychological symptoms associated with "traumatic neurosis." This could be seen as a reflection of a sternly nationalistic self-understanding, which many clinical neurologists and psychiatrists held at the time, having been socialized in the military or held positions in the army reserve. Conversely, shell shock symptoms and depressive states came to be interpreted as intentional behaviours of veterans to change the social insurance system of the Weimar Republic in a pathologic struggle for pensions (as *Rentenbegehren*).[44]

This attitude is similarly evident in Kraepelin's own notions of the pathology of war neuroses. He increasingly reduced his earlier assumptions of a somatic aetiology of injury-related neuroses in war and industrial contexts. In fact, he saw war neurotics as displaying a "premorbid and inferior" constitution, with their "tendentious wish- or purpose reaction to receive advantages" in times of war in order to achieve the desired result of being liberated from service at the front.[45] Kraepelin's tendentious concept became the predominant position in German-speaking psychiatry, neurology, and insurance medicine right up until the 1930s:

> If one interprets traumatic neurosis as an effect of the insurance system on psychopathic and weak-headed people, who became paralyzed by this process, then the essence of the diseases manifests as an inability to cope with disadvantageous external conditions. The oppression of drive and mood, because of his fixation on the compensation question, along with the exaggeration of the whole situation can only be understood as a sign of the patient's helpless submission to the struggles for autonomy of his personality.[46]

"Trench neuroses" and "pension neuroses" now became coined as defence diagnoses. They rose up as psychiatric fighting words used by many German-speaking *Nervenaerzte* whose purpose was to protect not only the public health system against what they saw as illegitimate claims of their patients, but also their psychoanalytical colleagues.[47] Only a very small number of neurologists continued with research projects that sought structural correlates of traumatic neuroses.[48] These discussions about the aetiological place of psychotherapy were furthermore reflected in the social discourses of the Weimar Republic, and the demands of modern life were interpreted as inducing aspects that exacerbated the pathological dispositions of "bad hereditary stock." The performance of the nervous system was viewed as impaired as a consequence of nutritional problems and genetic conditions. This position lent additional support to the assumption that biomechanical changes on the fine structural level rendered "degeneration" phenomena observable only through microscopic investigations of nervous tissue.[49]

Moreover, the term "neuropathic dispositions" came to represent developments in the sociocultural context in many passionate social debates about the consequences of urbanization, industrialization, and the medical implications of the labour question.[50] Such health issues were reflected by prominent psychiatrists who focused on "nervous degeneration" as a rhetorical means for promoting their own research agendas as scientific champions of an increasingly politicized health care field.[51]

STAINING METHODS, REGENERATIVE PHENOMENA, AND "NEUROCULTURES" IN CONTEXT

With the advent of the war and subsequently during the Weimar Republic, neuroanatomical and histopathological methods rose to the level of standard methodologies in research programs on nervous de- and regeneration.[52] Contemporary experimental methodologies aimed particularly at: (1) analyzing growth forms of nervous tissue, (2) discerning structural origins of axonal sprouting, and (3) investigating the relationship of the histological nerve structures in reticular networks.[53] Analyses of regenerative phenomena in the brain and spinal cord were thus included in diverse methodological perspectives. These among others had their origins in cell theory, embryological morphogenesis, or crossover programs between embryology and pathology.[54] In the first decades of the twentieth century, nerve cell theory enjoyed a growing interest that laid out a particular context for de- and regeneration studies. Innovative histological techniques such as haematoxylin, chromic acid, and methylene blue stains were introduced as by-products of late nineteenth-century chemistry. These techniques lent high currency to research programs on the nervous system, while they became progressively used for the microscopical identification of complex neurocellular architectures – most prominently reflected in the histological research program of Cécile and Oskar Vogt in Berlin.[55]

One does not need to be a neuromorphologist to quickly appreciate the potential that microscopical tissue studies offered for contemporary research directions on nervous de- and regeneration. The staining of tissue slices enabled researchers from a variety of disciplines to pursue projects in respective laboratories or clinical wards. Neurohistologists could now investigate the material as long as they wished and, with the introduction of tissue fixation methods such as changed paraffin protocols, silver damp impregnations, and cryo-drying of the nervous textures, new ways of demonstrating de- and regeneration phenomena could be found.[56]

Psychiatrists, neurologists, and clinical pathologists used the new staining methods in a multitude of laboratory animals – from frogs and dogs to monkeys, and so on.[57] Investigations were taken one step further by relating clinical phenomena to laboratory models and *post-mortem* findings. The new preparation methods supported a transformation of the results from various morphological disease forms (such as regeneration in nerve injuries, hereditary diseases, and tumour growth).[58] Scientific discourses on what counted as de- and regeneration phenomena became deferred to a privileged place in medical knowledge production: the experimental laboratory in neuromorphology. As described in Spain, in Ramón y Cajal's influential book *On De- and Regeneration in the Nervous System* (1928), refined argentum stains were thereby rendered as the "gold standard" for visualization studies of neuronal growth behaviours. Here, Cajal summarized the deep conundrum of the field:

> No histologist has been able to demonstrate with absolute certainty the reality of regenerative phenomena in the white matter of [the motor cortex]. For our part, by dint only of persistent explorations were we able, finally, to discover unquestionably active production of nerve fibers, although ephemeral and, therefore, frustrated.[59]

Similar statements directed at colleagues in the neuromorphological community resonated well with the intensely dynamic atmosphere in contemporary brain research.[60] However, the extraordinary increase in staining methodologies for microscopic purposes and the investigation of in vitro tissue cultures can only be understood within the embracing context of the anatomico-mechanistic tradition.[61] Standard approaches perceived the central and peripheral nervous systems as a delicate framework, which was seen as composed of nerve fibre tracts and nerve sheaths, which acted as the substrates for higher central nervous system functions.[62] For its fundamental physiological actions, the brain was thought to further depend on nutritional factors from outside sources, a theoretical interpretation that crystallized in the views of the Frankfurt neurologist and neuroanatomist Ludwig Edinger (figure 3.1), whose "consumption theory" (*Aufbrauchtheorie*) of brain pathology developed as a *trading zone*[63] of perspectives from nerve injuries, regeneration, and social factors. Edinger's brother-in-law, the neurosurgeon Siegmund Auerbach (1860–1923), described this intriguingly in 1915:

> According to Edinger, all diseases of the nervous system were divided into nerve lesions, toxic effects, and consumptive processes. The latter have their origin (1) in extraordinary demands on the normal tracts, and (2) on normal regenerative processes … Many individual fibre tracts are, by their very nature, endowed with sufficient physical strength to cope with the normal functional demands. Types: the hereditary nervous diseases; most of the combined dorsal tract pathologies; spastic paralyses; amyotrophic diseases.[64]

URBANIZATION, BOURGEOIS CULTURE, AND THE LOCAL CONTEXT IN FRANKFURT AM MAIN

Research institutes are thoroughly intertwined with the social developments, economic dynamics, and technological infrastructures of their specific locations. That is the case whether the confines of mental asylums are situated far from urban centres, on university grounds, or amid the buzzing life of metropolitan areas. Modern cities have emerged not only as lively cultural sites but also as centres of the construction of new knowledge as Sven Dierig, Jens Lachmund, and Andrew Mendelsohn have pointed out in their specialized *OSIRIS* volume *Science and the City*. "Science and scientific knowledge have shaped the urban way of life from the rise of transport and communication systems to the reordering of social, geographic, and architectural space."[65] The interrelationship of the urban economy and scientific work in brain research is most evident in the case of the founding of Edinger's Neurological Institute in Frankfurt am Main.[66] The process of its organization was forced by external circumstances toward a unique research position. It took place in the context of a dynamic and far-reaching transformation of the city's culture and its social and scientific networks, which gradually changed the life of the Hessian metropolis after the turn of the century.[67] Edinger's institute was formally established as an affiliated unit of the University of Frankfurt when it was founded as a *Buergeruniversitaet* in 1914.

This is perhaps a good moment to present some biographical details about Ludwig Edinger and some of his colleagues. Edinger was born in 1855 into a Jewish family in Worms, near Frankfurt, as the fifth child of clothing entrepreneur and member of the Parliament of Hesse-Darmstadt Marcus Edinger (1820–1872). The major shift in Edinger's career can certainly be identified as occurring at the moment when he turned to the rich cultural milieu of Frankfurt. In 1909, in his newly opened Neurological Institute (*Neurologisches Institut*), he began to develop many facets of a modern, team-based centre of the neurosciences. A closer look at Edinger's career reveals heuristic insights as to how interdisciplinary work was initiated and sustained in the new organizational setting of his institute.[68]

Edinger had settled in Frankfurt am Main in 1883 as one of the city's first clinical neurologists (*Nervenaerzte*) and soon opened a successful private clinic along with an outpatient department in Sachsenhausen, a larger city hospital. The development of this agglomeration into a thriving research institution was exceptional, since the growth of Edinger's institute took place in a mercantile city that had not previously had any higher learning institution. Its ongoing research nevertheless depended on a tradition of civic pride, individual ingenuity, and public sponsorship. The role of the city, its bourgeois culture, and its scientific developments during the Weimar period have been interpreted in terms of what German historian Gunther Mann (1924–1992) has called the "medical republic of Frankfurt."[69] This assessment of the scientific urban context within which Edinger worked as a neurological scientist substantiates many facets of the way interdisciplinary work became organized in the 1910s and the way that contingent factors played into its successful development for many decades to come. We must certainly acknowledge that this process took place despite the given sociocultural context, which did not always favour the movers and shakers of the early field of neuromorphology.

As we can gather from Edinger's personal history, the academic situation at the end of the nineteenth century repeatedly proved to be a hindrance to the intellectual accomplishments particularly of Jewish researchers, who tried to find their place among the diverse specialties in

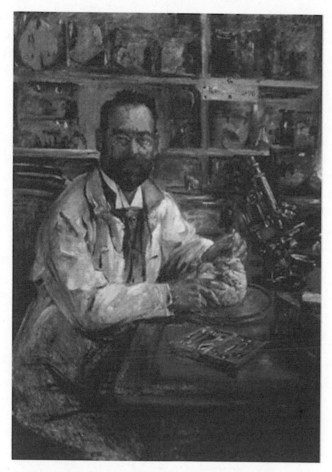

3.1 Portrait (B.1956.01) by Lovis Corinth of Ludwig Edinger, professor of medicine, Frankfurt am Main, 1909 (oil on canvas, 145 x 110 cm). (Edinger, Tafelbild, Portrait, Frankfurt am Main, 1909, Öl auf Leinwand). © Copyright: Historisches Museum, Frankfurt am Main, Germany (Horst Ziegenfusz).

academic medicine that were increasingly established alongside the traditional disciplines of surgery, gynaecology, and medicine.[70] In reflecting on the interdisciplinary endeavours in German-speaking neuroscience, it seems necessary to look for what later MIT Neuroscience Research Program director Frank Schmitt called the emergence of "hybrid fields," which brought people together from different research areas.[71] The notion of a hybrid field is also valuable when characterizing Edinger's own conceptual work, through which he undercut rigid nineteenth-century organizational styles in his laboratory at the Senckenberg Institution and later the Neurological Institute.

Edinger studied medicine in Heidelberg between 1872 and 1874, where comparative morphologist Carl Gegenbauer (1826–1903) was his teacher; and at the University of Strasburg from 1874 to 1877, where his MD thesis of 1877, "On the Histology of the Mucosa of Fish and Some Remarks on the Phylogenesis of the Glands of the Small Intestine" ("Ueber die Schleimhaut des Fischdarmes nebst Bemerkungen zur Phylogenese der Druesen"), was supervised by influential anatomist Wilhelm Waldeyer.[72] While at Strasburg, Edinger had the best introduction to the methodology of microscopic research when working in Waldeyer's tower laboratory overlooking the entrance of the *Buergerhospital*.[73] His medical training also brought him into close working relationship with the neuropathologist Friedrich Daniel von Recklinghausen, who had described the histopathological signs of neurofibromatosis for the first time. Intellectually, after he had been hired as a professor of medicine in 1876, Edinger was even more influenced by the new head of the medical service, Adolf Kussmaul. Immediately after his military service in Worms and Strasburg, Edinger began a clinic internship with Kussmaul, whom he admired for his broad knowledge of differential diagnoses. Yet most decisive for Edinger's later interests was his work as an assistant in neurohistology. In Kussmaul's clinical department, Edinger was given the opportunity to investigate the pathological material of all the brain tissues derived from patients who had succumbed to their illnesses.[74] Without no external supervision, he began to study neuropathology independently in a field that he perceived to be relying on simple microscopical technology, because, as he wrote, "histological dyes are still inadequate and slides are not prepared more anterior than the frontal end of the pons, because 'any understanding of the normal' ends at this point" in the brain.[75]

What had been a personal dissatisfaction during his Strasburg years later served as an inspiration for Edinger to change the course of neuroanatomical research. After three years he was obliged to rotate his internship. He now went to work with the internist Franz Riegel (1843–1904) at the University of Giessen in Hesse, where he completed his *Habilitation* thesis, entitled "Inquiries into the Physiology and Pathology of the Stomach" (1881).[76] Immediately thereafter, he used his first release from duties to participate in meetings of major societies such as the German Association of Natural Historians and Physicians (Gesellschaft Deutscher Naturforscher und Aerzte), and to make pilgrimages to major academic centres in Europe, which put him into contact with many luminaries in the brain sciences. In 1882, for example, Edinger went to London to visit English neurologist William Richard Gowers (1845–1915) at the National Hospital for the Paralysed and Epileptic, and then to Berlin to work with microbiologist Robert Koch (1843–1910) and psychiatrist Carl Westphal (1833–1890). He later visited the University of Leipzig, where he stayed with neuroanatomist Carl Weigert and psychiatrist Paul Flechsig, along with neurologist Wilhelm Heinrich Erb. Moreover, in 1883, Edinger went to Paris to spend some time of his *Wanderjahre* in Jean-Martin Charcot's (1825–1893) illustrious clinic at the Salpêtrière, before eventually returning to Frankfurt am Main.[77]

Until this point, nothing extraordinary had really happened in Edinger's peripatetic career. It could even be speculated at this point whether we would be as interested in his biography today, if his travels had not brought him to the cultural milieu of Frankfurt, which came to serve his intellectual needs so well (see chapter 1 for the specific reasons). Needless to say, his career was far from being planned and should rather be seen as a biographical accident. Since Edinger had been born into a Jewish family, his plans to work as a medical practitioner and give student lectures at the University of Giessen were suddenly interrupted when the principal of that university prevented him from teaching and thereby exercising his *Venia legendi* privileges. Since the end of the 1870s, German sectarian universities had experienced some opening toward students of different faiths – with Protestant students being accepted at Catholic universities (such as Wuerzburg and Munich) or Catholic students at Protestant universities (such as Halle or Erlangen).[78] Yet it was not uncommon, especially in the smaller universities, for Jewish academics to be officially denied their academic rights, even though they might be promoted to adjunct and assistant faculty status. Within medicine itself, widespread anti-Semitism could be particularly found in the traditional fields of surgery, medicine, and gynaecology. Anti-Semitic behaviours were also noticeable, however, in nineteenth-century specialties such as dermatology, urology, paediatrics, and neurology, which many assimilated Jews entered.[79]

Consequently, twenty-eight-year-old Edinger was barred from an academic career in the University of Giessen and it was thus that he settled as one of the first clinical neurologists in the city of Frankfurt. With this move, genuinely, he made a virtue out of a necessity, finding liberal urban surroundings that fostered his brain research needs. Edinger's first neurology practice was in the Frankfurt neighbourhood of Sachsenhausen at 30, Schifferstrasse, in a medically underserved community where a number of private philanthropic hospitals had been built. The practice at Schifferstrasse later developed into the outpatient department of Sachsenhausen's city hospital when it was founded in 1895. This coincidence brought hundreds of new patients into a care relationship with Edinger. His important clinical and pathological observations serve as evidence of his thorough interest in neuromorphological studies. It was with this good fortune that he was eventually able to build a brain research unit with the Senckenberg Foundation, a philanthropic foundation, inaugurated on an endowment basis by the natural historian Johann Christian Senckenberg (1707–1772).[80] Edinger was approved as a scientific member of the society in 1883 and two years later became a member of the local physicians' organization and the Senckenberg Society of Natural Scientists.[81]

Writing later about the Senckenberg Institute, Edinger recollected with pleasure that "never before and never again did [he] find a society of people of such a pure spirit and goal-directedness."[82] This harmonious working relationship can be perceived as an important stimulus for the creation of his own department in 1903.[83] Although it was initially set up in the cramped environs of a single room of the Senckenberg Institute of Anatomy, Edinger's department became entirely devoted to the study of neurology and neuroanatomy. Here, he tried to integrate the different aspects of neuroscientific research that he had experienced in major centres such as Strasburg, Berlin, Leipzig, and Paris. In his autobiographical notes, Edinger frequently mentioned the work of others in relation to his own: comparisons to Flechsig's application of Weigert's myelin nerve stain or Charcot's clinical observations, for instance.[84] Since he had to set up private practice and many necessary instruments, office stationery, and storage items were hard to obtain, his first years in Frankfurt were quite difficult. However, he managed to establish himself as an accepted researcher in the field of comparative neuroanatomy (see figure 3.2), and the whole process subsequently proved far from unsuccessful:

Everything that I needed was not very easy to get ... Old saucers, glasses, and whatever I could find in my mother's household to serve my needs was taken away and reinstalled in the new home. Further, I wrote to Professor [Johann Friedrich] Ahlfeld [1843–1923] the director of the Marburg University department of obstetrics, [to ask] whether he could send all kinds of aborted embryos (Fruechte) ... It had always been a secret hustle and bustle when another box arrived by post and when I had to smuggle it into my flat without the knowledge of my landlord.[85]

Such were the dire circumstances under which Edinger – with the help of his assistants – managed to produce his highly successful textbook *Lectures on the Structure of the Nervous Central Organs* of 1885 (*Vorlesungen ueber den Bau der nervoesen Zentralorgane*).[86] It was due to the fame of this textbook that he was invited to be an associate professor at the Senckenberg Institute in 1896. It can certainly be said that Edinger's activities were successful not only because he managed to bring researchers from different disciplinary areas – such as anatomy, pathology, and clinical neurology – together into one neuroscientific institution, but also because of his personal efforts to forge active interdisciplinary knowledge exchanges. He asked useful research questions, organized regular journal clubs, and further planned meetings with other medical researchers in the Senckenberg Society.[87] Edinger and his group were engaged, for example, in creating new instruments such as refined microtomes for histological analyses and developing psychological measuring apparatuses to improve the testing capacities of the institute's program to investigate the brain injuries of war veterans. Likewise, Edinger sought additional, non-medical co-workers to provide technical assistance as well as administrative help. For these activities to take shape, the institutional surroundings of the bourgeois city of Frankfurt proved indispensable.[88] Edinger's institute thus became established in a rather commercial and entrepreneurial city that depended largely on learned societies and colleges to provide material and financial resources. In a way, this *niche* was both constraining and enabling for Edinger's work – and for the work of his Frankfurt group composed of Weigert, a neuropathologist, and neurologist Adolf Wallenberg (1862–1949) – since he could now realize his plans with the Senckenberg Natural Science Foundation. In 1885 Edinger also became a member of the local medical association.[89]

Relying on Edinger's academic recognition and his solid relations with members of the medical community, Weigert had also come to Frankfurt – in 1885 – as the new director of the Senckenberg Institute of Anatomy. Edinger's astonishment, as a Jewish scientist, at encountering such a supportive academic setting also speaks to the cultural liberalism and entrepreneurial spirit of this central German city. Frankfurt's bourgeois milieu served as an important vantage point for the continuation of neurophysiological, neuropsychological, and neuroanatomical research, which made a vital contribution to the creation of his prototypical neurological institute.[90] Edinger's endeavours to create an interdisciplinary community of researchers interested in the brain were further encouraged by personal contacts among the members of local learned societies and by the freedom of thought possible at the creative fringes of the rather inflexible and controlling hierarchical structures of German universities.[91]

As Dutch experimental neurologist Paul Glees (1909–1999) wrote in his biographical article on Edinger in the *Journal of Neurophysiology* in 1964 – astutely informed by Edinger's daughter, the Harvard neuropalaeontologist Tilly Edinger (1897–1967), along with his own firsthand experience – "Goldstein and Edinger invited their young collaborators regularly to their homes for discussions on a variety of neurological problems."[92] And Edinger had participated in other informal meetings in Frankfurt institutions. Prior to Weigert's unfortunate early death in 1904, the institute had already established collaborations with outside researchers and proven its capacity in the clinical field. In this respect, Edinger and Weigert had worked with the notable psychiatrist Heinrich Hoffmann (1809–1894) and the pathologist Carl Friedlaender (1847–1887) in Frankfurt, along with the neuroanatomist Adolf Wallenberg in the city of Danzig in Pommerania.[93]

At this stage, many students and visiting researchers from America, England, Belgium, The Netherlands, and France came to work at the Frankfurt institute. One was prominent neurologist Friedrich Heinrich Lewy (1885–1950) from Berlin, who stayed with Edinger for four months, later needing to emigrate to the United States during the National Socialist period. Paul Glees himself had visited Edinger's Institute during the interwar period and later joined neurologist Cornelius Ubbo Ariëns Kappers (1877–1946) in the comparative anatomical department of the Central Netherlands Brain Research Institute (Nederlands Instituut voor Hersenonderzoek) after it was founded in 1909. Glees later moved to the University of Oxford, where he had an illustrious research career and contributed a new silver-staining method, winning several scientific prizes in neuroanatomy.[94] Edinger's international correspondence kept him in close contact with the American zoologist Charles Judson Herrick (1866–1960), who had been one of the founding members of Clark University together with his elder brother, the psychologist Clarence Luther Herrick (1858–1904).[95] Herrick was not only a pioneer in comparative neuroanatomy but also brought the psychoanalyst Freud from Vienna for a lecture tour and Ramón y Cajal for demonstrations on his new staining technique to America.[96] In 1904, Clarence Luther Herrick wrote about Edinger and his brother in the *Journal of Comparative Neurology* that "these two men [Ludwig Edinger and Charles Judson Herrick] were generally regarded as the founders of comparative neurology as an organized scientific discipline (figure 3.2), the one in Germany the other in the United States."[97]

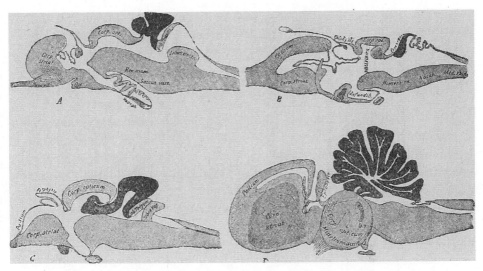

3.2 Depiction of semi-diagrammatic sagittal sections through different vertebrate brains: A, Brain of Ray; B, of an Amphibian; C, of a trout embryo; D, of a Bird (1899) © Courtesy of the US National Library of Medicine, Bethesda, Maryland, USA.

It was another eight years, however, before Edinger could exchange his private apartment laboratory for a one-room laboratory in the Senckenberg anatomy building in 1903. This coincided with his designation as the inaugural director of the Neurological Institute. When the new Senckenberg Pathology institute (then at 225, Gartenstrasse) also became available to him in 1907, these institutional surroundings became merged into a full-fledged brain research institute. It was in its department of pathology that the foundation was laid for the shaping of the new unit that eventually became known as the Frankfurt "Neurological Institute." By then it had become an interdisciplinary workplace for various perspectives on the study of the nervous system: the comparative, morphological, experimental, and clinical. Being conceptually influenced by the Austrian neuromorphologist Obersteiner and his earlier foundation of the "Neurological Institute" in Vienna, as well as by Vogt's "Neurologische Centralstation" in Berlin (see also chapter 1), Edinger went further by establishing new forms of institutional organization that also paved the way for innovative collaborative brain science.[98]

In the first phase of its development, the Edinger Institute became one of the contributing bodies that in 1912 declared support for inaugurating the new university as a philanthropic institution.[99] Consequently, with the opening of a university in Frankfurt, Edinger was also made a full professor of neurology and had two departments under his aegis: the department of anatomy and the department of pathology. They both fulfilled service tasks for the adjacent city hospitals, such as *post-mortem* dissections of patients with difficult clinical symptoms, as well as gross anatomical analyses of tumours or the study of aborted embryos. He could furthermore rely on his practice in the outpatient department for nervous diseases (*Frankfurter Poliklinik fuer Nervenkranke*). Edinger was also successful in luring to Frankfurt the Heidelberg neurologist Georg Dreyfus (1879–1957), who joined him in his clinical efforts during World War I. Dreyfus was a pupil of the neurologist Wilhelm Erb, who had been his MD supervisor at Heidelberg. After two years of military service on the Western Front, Dreyfus came to Frankfurt, where he was awarded his *Habilitation* and became an honorary professor with strong interests in neuropathology investigations.[100] Edinger also soon collaborated with the clinic of Villa Sommerhoff, the nursing home that had been run by internist August Knoblauch (1863–1919) since 1900, as well as with Goldstein's affiliated Institute for Research into the Effects of Brain Injuries.[101]

The war effort necessitated decisive cuts in funding for the university, however, and the incorporation of the outpatient clinic within the grounds of the university's medical school could not be realized. The outpatient unit had to await the end of the war. It was then managed by Dreyfus, Edinger's successor as the head of the clinical department, who continued the clinical neurological work, engaged in growth of the outpatient department, and assumed new rolès in the vicinity of other health care facilities. This success story came to a tragic end with the rise of Nazism and the loss of Dreyfus's position, after the latter was obliged to flee to Zurich to continue his work as a neurologist in private practice.[102]

After his death in 1918, Edinger's legacy in clinical psychology was continued by Kurt Goldstein. Goldstein had attended the Friedrich Wilhelms University of Breslau, where he studied medicine and, in 1903, graduated with his MD also on the basis of a morphological thesis. "On the Structure of the Posterior Columns [of the Spinal Marrow]: Anatomical Contributions and a Critical Revision" had been supervised by the psychiatrist and aphasiologist Karl Wernicke in the clinical department of psychiatry. Goldstein's philosophical thoughts, especially on the replacement of higher functions lost after brain injuries, were further influenced by his cousin, the Hamburg cultural philosopher Ernst Cassirer (1874–1945), and his conceptual views on the interplay of form and function in biology and art.[103] Between 1906 and the outbreak of war,

Goldstein completed his residency in neurology and psychiatry at the University of Koenigsberg in East Prussia (today Kaliningrad in Russia), after which Edinger was offered the directorship of the Frankfurt Institut zur Erforschung der Folgeerscheinungen von Hirnverletzungen (Institute for Research into the Effects of Brain Injuries) (see also figure 1.2).[104] There, he joined the experimental neuropsychologist Adhémar Gelb (1887–1936), who was already active in the Frankfurt institute and directed the neuropsychological service until 1930, when both men left the city for Berlin.[105] As one of his American friends, the Harvard neuropsychologist Hans-Lukas Teuber (1916–1977) put it in a later biographical essay, the group of people who joined Goldstein was heterogeneous. Yet their working relations, the conceptual enrichment, and long-term exchanges revealed that this interaction was the crystallization of fruitful interdisciplinary work, which essentially built on the friendship with Gelb in the Frankfurt Institute. While Goldstein had a much more philosophical attitude and greater clinical neurological interest, it was Gelb who contributed the technicalities for succinct and analytic laboratory experimentation on human subjects. Their collaboration led to a remarkable friendship relation as well as breathtaking scientific productivity.[106]

Having introduced Edinger and Goldstein as early examples of interdisciplinary neuroscientists at the beginning of the twentieth century, it now seems appropriate to mention some important qualities that characterized this group of contemporary brain scientists, a classification that will help analytically in the descriptions of the subsequent chapters. Because neurology was not yet fully independent from medicine and psychiatry, major research advances frequently took place at only the fringes of the medical establishment.[107] Also, it must be remembered that neurology and brain psychiatry were not well-paid disciplines at the time and that most of the protagonists in this field were often therefore very young and striving individuals. A considerable number were among the medical professionals of Jewish descent who happened to concentrate in the most cosmopolitan German cities, such as Berlin, Munich, Frankfurt, and Breslau, all of which had sizable Jewish communities.[108] In these particular urban intellectual milieux – as German historians Till van Rahden and Ulrich Sieg have pointed out – the number of Jewish physicians could reach 50 percent in the related clinical and research fields.[109] In general, these early brain scientists were well educated, often in both the humanities and the natural sciences in the German *Gymnasium* high school tradition, experimentally and clinically apt, and highly innovative.

However, these unique qualities can hardly be attributed to them simply because they were such a "homogenous group."[110]

The division by the university administrators of the clinical department of the Edinger Institute consecutively into an outpatient department and a rehabilitation department under Goldstein's leadership notably resembled the split between neurology and psychiatry. The previous twinning of the two clinical sciences in Germany had gradually entered into a process of separation. German neurologists, in particular, were not entirely supportive of this development, which, in any case, was not completed in Germany at the university level until after World War II. The institutional separation under Goldstein hence reflects less a difference of philosophy than a difference of *scientific* methodology. On a political level, the plan was to further subdivide the clinical department into a neurological and psychiatric division, when the psychopathologist Karl Kleist (1879–1960) arrived in Frankfurt in 1920.[111]

The external institute of Villa Sommerhoff (figure 1.2) had been approved by the university's board of regents as a specialized academic unit for neuropsychology and -pathology. Its directorship was given to Goldstein, a holistic neurologist; and Walther Riese (1890–1974), an assistant professor, became its deputy director, joining Goldstein's experimental program on the physical constitution of the brain from Berlin at the end of World War I. The Institute for Research into the Effects of Brain Injuries, where Goldstein now worked, had been independent since February of 1916. The inauguration of Villa Sommerhoff as a research institute stood in the context of the provision of dozens of new military hospitals for the nearly quarter million war-injured soldiers that Verdun had cost the German military.[112] According to Goldstein's own descriptions:

> It consisted of a ward for medical and physiotherapeutic treatment, a physiological and psychological laboratory for special examination of the patients, and theoretical interpretation of the observed phenomena, a school of retraining on the basis of the results of this research, and finally workshops in which the patient's aptitude for special occupations was tested and where he was taught an occupation in line with his ability.[113]

Additional neuropsychological collaborators of Goldstein and Riese in Frankfurt included the psychiatrist Favel Friedrich Kino (b. 1882) and the psychologist Hans Max Cohn (1886–1933), who was later killed by Nazi perpetrators as one of the early inmates of the political concentration camp Dachau. Throughout his whole time in Frankfurt and Berlin, Goldstein relied on the collaboration with his friend and co-worker, the experimental psychologist Adhémar Gelb. The latter was a pioneer in the development of psychological patient testing, which he advanced by building on Wilhelm Wundt's Leipzig foundations and using research apparatuses received from Gestalt psychologists.[114]

It is particularly interesting that after Edinger's death the search commission of the medical faculty became much more occupied with the organizational complexity of the interdisciplinary tradition than with the fate of neuropathology. Their minutes reflect this difficulty well and show how challenging it was for them to determine the scope of the institute and its level of collaboration within the university and also with outside hospitals, societies, and city bodies.[115] They could hardly inventory the scientific output and methodologies of Edinger's collaborators, since they fell into categories as diverse as medicine, anatomy, public health, clinical psychology, experimental psychology, and even psychoanalysis. This picture motivated some commission members to propose that the units related to the pre-existing university departments be dismantled.[116] Fortunately, the majority of the members rejected this proposal on the grounds of Edinger's astounding scientific reputation. Had this new interdisciplinary organization not been so successful since the 1910s, it is highly likely that the institute's legacy would have been destroyed by the discipline-oriented normal scientists even before the Nazis arrived. Yet the achievements of the Neurological Institute's members were so evident that major damage was prevented. Certainly, this centre was important for the new university; it was helpful that it could be recognized as a private postsecondary institution.[117]

Eventually, the Edinger Commission endorsed the continuation of a brain research centre in Frankfurt and favoured the application of Walther Spielmeyer, the director of the neuropathology department at the Deutsche Forschungsanstalt for Psychiatry in Munich, as an excellent successor (see also chapter 1). Spielmeyer's experiences with the network of the various Munich institutions – separate clinical departments for psychiatry and neurology, emerging laboratories for psychiatry, discussions about a KWI institute for laboratory research[118] – all spoke to his ability as a problem-solver, one who could pull the Frankfurt chestnuts out of the fire. Disappointingly, however, Spielmeyer rejected the offer when it became clear that the Rockefeller Foundation would engage in the creation of a new research institute for brain psychiatry in Munich under the umbrella of the KWG, which eventually became established in 1924.[119]

The directorship of the Frankfurt institute was eventually given to Goldstein – in 1918–19, since Wallenberg, the primary contender for the chair, had decided not to accept the job offer but remained chief of service at the Municipal Hospital of Danzig. The major limitations were the inferior financial means offered by philanthropic endowments, which had taken a serious hit in the war economy. In direct comparison, state-funded research institutes at traditional universities were in much better financial shape. Outside contenders such as Wallenberg, who worked in well-paid positions in the public hospital system, simply did not wish to risk receiving low-paid, contingent jobs within a volatile academic research context that were completely dependent on the availability of philanthropic funds, as in the situation of Frankfurt's Senckenberg institutes.

The second phase in the development of the Frankfurt Neurological Institute ended with the negotiations of the directorship search committee in 1918. These occurred after the majority of the faculty members had favoured the continuance of the institute with six divisions, amounting to an increase by two from the former clinical department and morphological departments, which included a psychological and neurological department. In addition to such internal differentiation in the institute itself, the external exchanges that Goldstein arranged with members of the Frankfurt psychoanalytic society had been very valuable for the ongoing program. For instance, he ran mutual colloquia with Karl Landauer (1887–1945) from the Frankfurt Psychoanalytic Institute, which allowed Goldstein to engage in advanced discussions of clinical psychiatric research, theoretical issues, and changes in group therapy.[120] In the Frankfurt colloquia, they discussed questions related to the pathological course of speech in neurological patients, the latest research in functional localization, and behavioural changes in war-injured soldiers. Landauer had himself been a pupil of Kraepelin and Freud before, a perfect background that aligned well with Goldstein's orientation toward holistic neurology. Like Goldstein, however, Landauer also had to flee Nazi Germany and seek refuge nearby in Amsterdam. When the Wehrmacht occupied the Netherlands, he was brought to Bergen-Belsen, the concentration camp where he tragically died shortly before the camp's liberation by British forces.[121]

Despite the bold vision of the university's committee and Goldstein's agreement to become the successor to Edinger's chair, the austere circumstances of the Weimar period annihilated these plans. Ongoing research became further concentrated and was reduced to only three serviceable divisions: neuropathology, neuroanatomy, and psychological research.

An associated palaeoneurology unit, led by Edinger's daughter Tilly at the Senckenberg Museum of Natural History, complemented these. What was basically a one-woman unit continued fruitful research on the reconstruction of brain morphologies in dinosaurs, molded from plaster casts, comparative studies with living reptiles, and approximate brain size measurements. Immediately before war broke out again in 1939, Tilly Edinger fled to Cambridge, Massachusetts, where she successfully continued her research for many decades at Harvard's Museum of Natural History.[122]

Plans to extend the institute had to be dropped in the late 1920s, mainly because of financial factors related to Weimar hyperinflation and the Great Depression, but also because Karl Kleist was given the vacant chair for psychiatry with all its clinical responsibilities. He likewise advocated an altered conception of neuronal degeneration – essentially modifying Edinger's earlier consumption premise of nerve morphology (see also chapter 1).[123] When Kleist began to investigate brain-injured veterans in his clinical department, he stressed the case for societal issues being of fundamental neuromorphological interest. This view was clearly reflected in a 1924 address to the German Psychiatric Association and the Society for German Neurologists (Sitzung des Deutschen Vereins fuer Psychiatrie und der Gesellschaft Deutscher Nervenaerzte) in Innsbruck:

The restoration of the neurological research tradition in psychiatry has quite different origins other than being a mere resumption of philosophical and psychological traditions … We see a steady development instigated through a massive influx from brain-pathological war experiences, additionally fostered by numerous observations on the encephalitis epidemic.[124]

As a result of Kleist's integration of all the clinical divisions from the former Edinger Institute into his own department of psychiatry, Goldstein was left with only three serviceable research divisions for himself and his collaborators. The new director of the neuroanatomical department was the zoologist Victor Franz (1883–1950) from the University of Halle;[125] and the director of the neuropathological department was the neurologist Heinrich Vogt (1875–1936) (investigating special forms of tuberous sclerosis), joining the institute from the Deutsche Forschungsanstalt for Psychiatry in Munich. Both researchers continued their work during the National Socialist period and, while Vogt died early, Franz left Frankfurt for the University of Jena after Goldstein's move to Berlin. These developments constituted a major setback for

Edinger's legacy, since most of the members had left Frankfurt when the interdisciplinary institute was reduced to an academic torso. Franz assumed the position of a professor of zoology at the Ernst Haeckel House in Jena, and only after the postwar Soviet administration placed him under examination did it resurface that he had been a member of various Nazi party organizations.[126] This could also explain why he refrained from following Goldstein's group to Berlin. After Goldstein, Gelb, and Riese had departed from the Edinger Institute in 1930, it became fully incorporated into the psychiatric clinical department, which was led by the ardent eugenicist Arnold Lauche (1890–1959) from 1937 to 1945. Only after the war did the institute become re-inaugurated under Spielmeyer's pupil Willibald Scholz (1889–1970), who led it back into the MPG in 1954 and who was later succeeded in the directorship by the neuropathologist Gerd Peters (1906–1987) in 1961 (see also chapters 8 and 9).[127] Following a short period at the Moabit Hospital in Berlin, Goldstein, along with Tilly Edinger, had to emigrate for good to the United States, where they both recommenced their research careers.[128]

THE GROUND LEVEL OF RESEARCH IN THE FRANKFURT NEUROLOGICAL INSTITUTE

When looking at the forms of research organization in the Edinger Institute, the descriptions of its postwar director, Wilhelm Kruecke (1911–1988), are useful; they point to the high level of investigations conducted at this centre.[129] First, there had been Edinger's attempts to apply Weigert's histological staining methods of in a variety of neuroanatomical fields. These research activities led to the discovery of the tractus spinothalamicus (1895) as a sensory pathway from the sense organs of the skin to the thalamus in the diencephalon, proving that it connected with the thalamus rather than the cerebellum. Moreover, they resulted in the discovery of the Edinger and Westphal nucleus, which has remained a neuroanatomical eponym to this day. The related discovery of the parasympathetic nucleus of the third cranial nerve (the nucleus accessorius nervi oculomotorii) between 1885 and 1887 in pathological studies with human specimens was only made possible by these new staining techniques.[130] The basic advances of histological technologies had subsequently given rise to innovative comparative studies regarding neencephalization, which culminated in the pathological autopsies of neuroanatomist Heinrich Vogt (1875–1936), that is, on a person without a cerebrum (*Mensch ohne Grosshirn*).[131] Edinger's own interests had extended beyond neuroanatomy and

-pathology alone; he was likewise engaged with issues of psychology and psychoanalysis, while including neuroanatomical research with clinical and psychological observations.[132] This was a very innovative approach, as is evident from other practitioners such as Vienna psychiatrist Sigmund Freud, Zurich psychiatrist Auguste Forel, and Berlin brain researchers Oskar and Cécile Vogt as well. They were all engaged in similar forms of interdisciplinary work, creating large research groups and circles, along with undertaking publishing activities in a wide spectrum, from anatomy to psychology – and even philosophy.[133]

Edinger himself had a high regard for clinical work, which often served as a vantage point for his laboratory investigations, one instance being when he gave Goldstein a job in the neuropathology department in 1914 to study the impact of brain injuries and tumours. However, the medical situation of World War I soon took over and Goldstein was offered the directorship of two military hospitals (*Reservelazarette*). It is quite significant that Edinger, who clearly thought that Goldstein would be his research associate, allowed him to freely decide: "Your work with patients is of a much higher importance than my theoretical work in the laboratory."[134] Edinger and Goldstein carried on their close collaboration, and their work was reflected in a number of Edinger's publications on regenerative processes. Goldstein, in his Institute for Research into the Effects of Brain Injuries, continued his work not only on scientific diagnoses but also on rehabilitation schemes for the brain-injured. Most promising was his project of early patient rehabilitation, soon followed by brain surgery and wound closure as described in his important 1919 report, "The Treatment, Care, and Evaluation of the Brain Damaged." Here, Goldstein stated that 73 percent of the patients had been able to return to their prewar positions, 17 percent could still start a new job, and only 10 percent remained unemployed, while another 10 percent had to be hospitalized.[135] Villa Sommerhoff already possessed what Edinger had in mind for the future direction of his institute: a clinical ward for physiotherapeutic treatment, a psychophysiological diagnostics laboratory, a training school and, further, working places for the patients. In particular, Goldstein attempted to integrate brain psychiatry and neurology to complement his holistic approach:

At that time [mental diseases] were considered the expression of abnormal brain conditions. The study of the nervous system was taken for granted, and I became attracted by professors who were occupied with studies in this field: the anatomist, Professor [Alfred]

Schaper [1863–1905], who was interested in the embryonic development of the nervous system; the famous psychiatrist, Professor Carl
Wernicke, who tried to understand the symptoms of the patients psychologically and to combine this understanding with the findings on
their brains; and Professor Ludwig Edinger, who laid the foundations
of comparative anatomy of the nervous system.[136]

The interrelation of the institute with the other medical, psychiatric,
and biological research units in Frankfurt was accordingly developed to
serve the need for an analogical knowledge transfer from research animals
and comparative studies, to the morphological understanding of the
human brain. This endeavour was supported by a *new model of a division
of labour* between neuropathological, clinical-neurological, and psychological research.[137] The resulting circle of knowledge generation and
application likewise fed into earlier observations that the group at the
Edinger Institute had made (such as detailed analyses of parts of the
corticothalamic nerve tracts and insightful comparisons of embryological
brain development in diverse mammals and other higher animals, as
well as the application of structural findings to a reconceptualization of
cortical function and localization). It appears very unsurprising to us
today, but at that time in history it was a *revolutionary model of organizing brain science*, since it broke with the strict specialization of the nineteenth century, particularly at contemporary faculties of medicine.[138]
      When these organizational transfers at Edinger's Frankfurt Neurological
Institute are related to the conceptual side of brain research at this centre,
we may realize that cerebral function served here as a heuristic hypothesis. It meandered freely between investigations made on the morphological side and those brought about by traditional physiological
approaches "to realize the importance of interrelating structure and
function" as a biological problem.[139] However, it was not a new conceptual idea; such a correlative approach between brain structures and
physiology can be traced back to the functional anatomists. It was already
present in the French veterinarian Félix Vicq-d'Azyr (1746–1794) and
pathologist Marie François Xavier Bichat (1771–1802) at the end of the
eighteenth century, or in localizational neuropathologists of the nineteenth
century from Paul Broca (1824–1880) in Paris to Friedrich Leopold Goltz
(1834–1902) at Strasburg.[140] Most intriguingly, however, it became a
regulative idea that bundled the research activities on the cerebral cortex
around a generalized understanding of localization.[141] In this respect,
Edinger's regulative idea itself worked on both the intellectual and

management level, when he built the organization of the Frankfurt Neurological Institute. The interrelationship of form and function was further reflected in his "consumption theory" (*Aufbrauchtheorie*) of nervous diseases, interpreted as a wasting and degenerative process of central nervous tissue.[142] In his autobiographical account, posthumously published in 1919, Edinger expressed:

> Toxic agents do not cause this process [of regeneration], as neurologists had thought earlier on, but it is based on brain damage, with the nerve function being responsible for ensuing nervous degeneration.[143]

As with other degeneration theories, Edinger assumed a crucial incongruence between the genetic set-up of the nervous system and its physiological conditions, particularly visible, it was thought, in the processes of modernization with their increasing demands through both work life and the constraints on human behaviour. If an individual could not cope with the "minimal nervous tissue pathologies" such as neuritis after strenuous work or noxious influences due to cold temperatures, then the normal brain morphology went into partial tissue degeneration.

Edinger's *Aufbrauchtheorie* thus served as a model for what he and others understood as an increase in degenerative nervous disorders, by combining clinical and psychological observations with neuroanatomical or neuropathological analyses. Like many other contemporary brain researchers, Edinger also integrated large-scale cultural pessimist views with psychiatric concepts about degeneration. These became based on the constraints of modernist tendencies, as is visible in his psychological studies of consciousness during this "Age of Nervousness":[144]

> We will reach a point where the assumption of consciousness will be necessary, but doubtless this point is pushed further away, even if the question is gradually answered in more appropriate forms. When we are able to explain certain actions without the basic assumption of consciousness, then the time will have come when scientists can explain the unknown or the mythical (*das Mythische*) of today.[145]

To use a modern philosophical term, Edinger's position on the functions of the mind could be described as that of an eliminative materialist.[146] He thought that consciousness could in principle be reduced to brain processes, but that the techniques of the time were inadequately sensitive to perceive them. As a result, he acknowledged that there remained a fundamental level of explanation beyond the scope of contemporary neuroanatomy. However, Edinger and other early neuroscientists offered no criteria for what such a reduction would comprise, or if it could ever be achieved. In his own words, "the mythical phenomena in science can only be solved when the methods are available."[147]

Although one frequently finds such reductionist views in Edinger's thinking, it is also possible to discern a complementary position in his work: the supposition that, for the practical neurologist and psychiatrist, human consciousness would forever remain inexplicable:

> We have no clue how it comes about that the activity of a single part of the Nervous System can be rendered conscious of the whole human person. The endeavor to fill the remaining gap in the mind-body-dualism *must* be seen as doomed to failure.[148]

This view is reflected practically in his own research with Goldstein on the neurological consequences of the brain lesions they saw in veterans with gunshot wounds that destroyed circumscribed areas of the cortex, the midbrain, or the cerebellum. Edinger sometimes even ridiculed their mutual research program as the intent to map out the *anatomische Generalstabskarte* of the brain (ordnance map of the brain). With cerebral maps of this sort, morphological findings could serve as vantage points for later neurophysiological and neuropsychological research. This plan was also based on Edinger's belief that neuroanatomical data would never become obsolete; patient records and histories, dissection and histology reports, as well as brain collections should be painstakingly archived.[149]

Having laid out the structure of the Neurological Institute and the complexity of its research projects, we can turn to the cognitive basis of the institute. It is probably best summarized by Goldstein's description in his 1919 obituary of Edinger for the Senckenberg Society as an interdisciplinary parallelism of approaches in his mentor's work: "In Edinger I found an excellent interpreter of the great variations in the relationship of the structure of the nervous system to the behaviour of animals; thus he created a new field of science, 'the comparative anatomy of the nervous system.'"[150] So, what were the broader contours of the interdisciplinary methods used in Edinger's institute? Its research program of comparative neurology of the human psychological faculties originated in the earlier influences of Gegenbauer's "genetic method," which included hereditary and evolutionary perspectives, as well as comparative zoological methodology. Edinger had furthermore been interested in Goltz's cortical ablation studies on dogs, as both of these early neuroscientists had been Edinger's mentors at Strasburg. Once again, they stimulated him to draw comparisons between animal and human brains, with the experiences that Goldstein later recognized from his brain-injured patients, as Edinger described and explained in his autobiography *Mein Lebensgang*.[151]

Edinger's institute had often been described in the biographical notes of neuromorphology research contemporaries such as Adolf Wallenberg, Paul Glees, and Munich neuropathologist Hugo Spatz (1888–1969) as an example of functional neuroanatomy along traditional lines of microscopical research.[152] If we look more closely at the conceptual perspectives that the Frankfurt Neurological Institute presented, however, it is clear that Edinger's career lay fully at the cutting edge of a multi-versed neuroscientific pursuit. In fact, from his practices we can draw a variety of insights for our discussion of emerging forms of interdisciplinarity in the German-speaking neurosciences. First, despite the fundamental practical dimension of neuromorphology, Edinger's research is important for this historical discussion by virtue of its fundamental break with the hierarchical institutional arrangements of contemporary university institutes. In institutional terms, this development parallels that of the Vogts' Neurobiological Institute in Berlin or the brain research at Breslau and Munich. These decisive events took place in the decades between 1910 and 1930, and it is quite remarkable that the respective institutions, despite their affiliation with local universities, assumed a greater autonomy that could account for their considerable success.[153]

Second, how did Edinger's research relate to the overall organization of the Frankfurt Neurological Institute? It is intriguing to see that his personal convictions, influence, and optimism helped to set up the institute even at a time that did not favour his academic plans. On the one hand, we may see the founding of the institute as Edinger's only way to pursue his academic interests in the face of a largely anti-Semitic medical system. This process could easily have led to professional failure and his withdrawal from research life back to his private practice. On the other hand, we may regard the local context of the pre-university learned societies as the enabling context of the scientific culture of Frankfurt am Main. The founding of neuroscientific programs at the Senckenberg took place in a largely mercantile city, in which wealthy bankers, landowners, and industrialists came to act as benefactors due to the immediate experiences of World War I.

Third, from the standpoint of institutional history, the question often comes up: where does one draw the line for the perimeter of an "institute"? Where do its actions begin and where do they end?[154] Rather than inviting us to view contemporary medical institutions from an *intra muros* perspective, as it were, the example of Edinger's Institute illustrates the importance of contextual factors in the choice of the place of a research centre. In a physical sense, his Neurological Institute was linked with his private neurological practice and later a neurological outpatient clinic. It was largely seconded by the Senckenberg Society, which acted as an institutional bridgehead for its brain research activities. Finally, the interdisciplinary research endeavour was complemented by the inclusion of Goldstein's Institute for Research into the Effects of Brain Injuries. Regardless of the perception that the "institute" appeared to be scattered all over the city, which traditional "disciplinarians" in brain research saw as a major flaw in its organization, "interdisciplinarian" members of the search committee for a successor, along with Edinger's collaborators, identified the communication structures and discussion circles as the institute's major asset. Although this level of organization has been neglected in historiographical scholarship, it was what made possible an integration of the various research localities into *one functional whole*.[155] Facilitating the growth of interdisciplinary research at this early stage of the modern brain sciences was crucial for the accomplishment of Edinger's institute.[156]

CHANGING SOCIETAL CONCERNS AND INSTITUTIONAL SETTINGS IN THE PURSUIT OF NEURONAL DE- AND REGENERATION

When taking the medical situation immediately before and after World War I into account and examining the changes in the sociopolitical context of the Weimar Republic, it becomes clear that in this period even specialist discourse on neurodegeneration had shifted.[157] The focus of study moved from traditional problems of clinical rehabilitation in traumatized workers and care for the war-injured, to an emphasis on the investigations of neuronutritional processes.[158] The quest for "hygiene of the nerves and mind" became increasingly intertwined with new industrialized environments and life experiences.[159] Neurodegeneration was seen as a biological constituent of nervous patients, the war-disabled, and trauma victims. It had thus grown into *a hinge concept* onto which both social and scientific meanings could be interchangeably appended. It could accommodate soldiers' responses to severe war conditions such as shell shock, exhaustion, and brain injuries, along with various nervous pathologies that developed during the postwar deprivation and starvation of large parts of the Central European civilian population.[160]

Discourse on neurodegeneration emerged on the one hand as a concept of preventive and military medicine, as can be inferred, for example, from Edinger's work *The Role of Function in the Development of Nervous Diseases (Der Anteil der Funktion an der Entstehung von Nervenkrankheiten)* of 1908.[161] It is necessary to keep in mind that several factors of the envisaged aetiology were social in nature. To Edinger persons born with a "weak" nervous system were those most likely to contract neurodegenerative diseases.[162] Another striking example in this respect comes from the prominent neuropathologist Max Bielschowsky at the KWI for Brain Research (see also chapter 1).[163] In the essential later transfer of the neuroscientific concept of traumatic regeneration from the military hospital setting to the KWI laboratory, Bielschowsky's positioning of the normal *versus* the pathological distinction gave rise to a new epistemic discourse on exhaustion and regeneration. Through the macroscopic research programs of Emil Kraepelin and Oswald Bumke, psychiatric and nervous degenerative changes became associated with the brain's gross morphology. This tradition was further intensified through the fibre-preparatory approaches of Edinger, Bielschowsky, Paul Flechsig in Leipzig, and Theodor Meynert in Vienna, who had begun to search for underlying neurohistological processes during the Weimar period.[164] These researchers interpreted the histological changes of neurodegeneration as pathological responses of the brain to specific injuries, psychological trauma, and inherited diseases, while offering expertise for analyzing degenerative occurrences with their microscopes:[165]

> When observing the preparation with the naked eye, one is quite astonished at the impossibility of finding a distinct border between normal and sclerotic tissue ... The diameter has a homogenous grey or black appearance; under the microscope one can see abundant nerve fibers in the sclerotic area ... Eventually, a long-standing clinical desideratum could thus be solved.[166]

It was quite clear to Bielschowsky that this observation had important implications for questions of nervous de- and regeneration. Whereas "Captain" Bielschowsky, the former military researcher, was convinced about the existence of positive nervous regenerative phenomena, after he had left the front and assumed the directorship of the Berlin KWI Division of Neuropathology he became less and less optimistic about his research findings. The relocation of his program also contributed to this change of direction in assessing the functional potential of regenerative phenomena in heredodegenerative diseases. With his laboratory investigations, Bielschowsky now interpreted growth phenomena, glia cell invasion, and repair mechanisms as forms of an "early expression of necrobiosis."[167]

On the other hand, neurodegeneration and neuroregeneration were seen as integrative sociotechnical concepts in a variety of neuroexperimental applications of the time.[168] This transformation, together with the general reception of neuroregenerative problems in contemporary morphology, characterizes some of the profound changes that took place in the experimental laboratories of the German-speaking neurosciences. Such altered views about neuroregeneration were furthered through the integration of new technologies such as the electronic microtome, staining derivatives, and encephalography.[169] The underlying direction of transformation in neuromorphology became reflected in a more optimistic mood *vis-à-vis* the diagnostic procedures of neuropsychiatry and the development of contemporary therapy. This optimism was rooted in the assumption that the effects of modern social pressures on the brain would be more successfully treatable once a better understanding of the microscopic architectures of nervous tissue was reached. Experimental corroboration of regenerative phenomena, however, still lay in the hands of neurohistologists, who could precisely "see" the effects of nerve-weakness and trauma when they were scrutinized with specific staining techniques. If we were to take an observation by French medical philosopher George Canguilhem (1904–1995) – that "there is no fact that is normal or pathological in itself"[170] – and apply it to the neuromorphological practices of the time, we would realize that societal concerns about nervous degeneration, exhaustion metaphors, and shifts in the research context from traumatology to socio-rehabilitation had already been deeply inscribed in the larger-scale socio-technical experiments of Weimar Germany.[171]

The laboratory pursuit of de- and regeneration phenomena in the German brain sciences was crucially influenced by successive societal transformations. The historical period from the late Wilhelminian Era to the Weimar Republic saw a rapidly changing sequence of differing neurocultures in university laboratories. Social contexts had been extraordinarily altered from the general public discourse about degeneration (*dégénérescence*) in late Wilhelminian Germany to the more modern concern with the reintegration of disabled soldiers into society. Advances in neuroscientific research helped to identify disease processes and offered new treatment options. As we have seen, Griesinger, Kraepelin, Edinger, Goldstein, and Bielschowsky – all of whom worked at separate and geographically distinct research institutions in Germany – tightly integrated current representations from the public sphere into their own neurological and psychiatric work.

Some of them, like Edinger in his neuromorphological program, were quite outspoken about the need to provide responses from both basic and clinical endeavours to the urgent medical demands of German society at the time. By integrating such interdisciplinary efforts into current neuropathological, clinical, and psychological research on nervous de- and regeneration, Edinger, in conjunction with his collaborator Goldstein, managed to transform pre-existing research approaches and treatment options. He emphasized, for example, the plastic reactions of patients' behaviour after injuries, applying early rehabilitation programs or developing individually tailored prosthetic devices for his patients. In so doing, Goldstein's group continued an important tradition that Griesinger and Kraepelin had begun, when re-orienting brain research from the bedside to the experimental bench.[172] In the application of a modern cultural view to methodological advances, laboratory actions, and scientific reinterpretations in neuroregenerative research, the imprint of wider societal concerns became noticeable in the development of new micro-optic technology and encompassing neuromorphological concepts.[173] This was also true for the description of axonal outgrowth phenomena, surgical nerve recombination, and the experimental acceleration of fibre-sprouting processes.

Through his ongoing preoccupation with problems of hereditary development, Bielschowsky in Berlin was well aware of the potential that neuromorphological work had acquired for answering questions on nervous de- and regeneration. Having worked in the context of trauma surgery and military medicine, Bielschowsky was now increasingly guided toward topics related to nerve degeneration by societal concern for understanding the morphological substrate of nerve injuries. Societal concerns also influenced the way he and other neuromorphologists came to view regenerative process in the brain in a predominantly positive light from the late 1900s to the end of World War I. While working in the institutional confines of the experimental neurohistological laboratory at the Berlin KWI for Brain Research, however, Bielschowsky became increasingly less optimistic about the existence of adaptive phenomena. He began to understand them as aberrant processes of axonal growth, glia invasion, or forms of healing with defect.[174] Although plenty of ink has been spilled in the literature over the role of de- and regenerative concepts in psychiatry, psychogenetics, and racial hygiene, little attention has been paid to the undercurrent of transformation in regeneration research strategies between

applied and basic fields of German-speaking neuroscience. These inter-
dependencies between structural anatomical interests and clinical
works were also significantly interwoven in the cultural discourses of
"nervous exhaustion," even in Goldstein's fairly unknown monograph
On Racial Hygiene of 1913 (*Ueber Rassenhygiene*).[175] It is revealing
of late Wilhelminian culture, in which it appeared, and it continued to
be well received during the early years of the Weimar Republic. Goldstein's
On Racial Hygiene contextualizes neurological practices, even though
the state of contemporary knowledge remained underdeveloped:

> The reality of intellect, of self-determination, which even in its most
> primitive form represents essential characteristics of man, dooms any
> breeding experiment of the usual type to failure. However, if the rela-
> tion of hereditary conditions does not aim at specific characteristics
> but aspires to ameliorate the human race by eliminating unfit indi-
> viduals, such an endeavour presupposes a thorough knowledge of
> the significance of individual variances for human natures.[176]

This statement further shows that even the recognized holistic neurologist harboured degeneration and eugenics views consistent with the public
demands of the cultural discourses of the time. Far from being limited to
transformation in the neuromorphological laboratories, the integrative
character of sociotechnical concepts of "neurodegeneration," "neuroregeneration," and "hereditary nervous diseases" were strongly reflected
in brain researchers' discourses of the time. Their *hinge character*,[177]
comprising researchers' assumptions about societal issues as well as deliberate strategies to meet broader public demand, was current in the 1916
war meeting between the Gesellschaft Deutscher Nervenaerzte and the
Deutscher Verein fuer Psychiatrie. In the middle of the war, members of
both societies emphasized that the problem of degenerative psychiatric
and neurological conditions was simply a reflection of the phenomena of
modern cultural degeneration. Interestingly, as the war dragged on, clinical neurologists diagnosed fewer instances of "civil" degenerative diseases.
These developments were all part of a transformation of the research field
of German neuromorphology, which led to altered views about clinical
neurodegenerative and neuroregenerative disorders.[178]

During the latter years of the war, as well as throughout the period
of the Weimar Republic, the increasing prevalence of neuromorphological disease entities gave rise to changing conceptions in the neuroscientific
and psychiatric community. Karl Kleist's address to the combined

meeting of the Gesellschaft Deutscher Nervenaerzte and the Deutscher Verein fuer Psychiatrie in 1924, for instance, reflected more than the undercurrents in neurodegenerative and neuroregenerative investigations. It was also seen as an expression of the influences that the neuroscientific community had exerted on the perception of social pathologies such as alcoholism, venereal diseases, and malnutrition. Kleist's emphasis on a restored "neurological research tradition" was largely the product of such societal concerns. The specific view that modern social life effectively influenced brain health could be understood through an investigation of the microscopic architectures of nervous tissue. Other representatives of the neuromorphological tradition held even stronger environmental views in neuropathological theorizing. Alfred Hoche (1865–1943) in Freiburg and Oswald Bumke in Munich, for example, regarded development-associated psychiatric disorders in their patients as cases of detailed organ-centred substrates:

Many of the hereditary diseases will only become observable in the life of the adult, and then often lead to a considerable disease process. It appears that the ambiguous meaning of the term "hereditary disposition" had led to considerable confusion. On the one hand, it means a "genetic disposition," on the other hand a developmental step of the embryo, which implies something particularly phenotypical. The term "hereditary disposition" naturally depicts something very different in these two cases.[179]

Both Hoche and Bumke later adopted a decisive eugenics framework for their aetiological views, along with their therapeutic and research proposals, under the again-changed public concerns of the National Socialist period in Germany.

CENTRAL STATIONS AND CENTRAL LABORATORIES: THE EXAMPLE OF OSKAR AND CÉCILE VOGT

An analysis of the permeability, interchanges, and parallel developments in modern biomedical science makes it clear that the relationship between psychiatry and brain research in the cultural laboratory of Berlin cannot be presented from within the university system alone. On the contrary, some very important advances in the framing of this interdisciplinary research took place outside the system of Berlin University. The necessary, fertile ground for this endeavour was the network of relationships among psychiatry, neurology, and experimental research that can be compared to the interstitial areas in the urban science spaces of the Prussian metropolis. These intersections among laboratories, private clinics, and academic departments can be observed in the intricate working relationships of neuroanatomist Oskar Vogt, morphologically oriented neurophysiologist Korbinian Brodmann, and clinical neurologist Kurt Goldstein after his move from Frankfurt to Berlin. In this prosopographical initiative, I map out some constellations that were constitutive of the field of brain research and psychiatry in Berlin until the 1930s. My analysis also envisions traffic lines, shortcuts, and blockades in a geographical and intellectual sense, to illuminate the interrelationship between psychiatry and brain research in the Berlin example:

> Electrical No. 68 travels to Rosenthal Place, Wittenau, the *Northern Railway Station, the Mental Asylum*, Wedding Place, Stettin Railway Station, Rosenthal Place, Alexander Place, Straussberg Place, Railway Station Frankfurt Avenue, Lichtenberg and the *Lunatic Asylum of Herzberge*. The three public transport companies in Berlin – the City Trains, the Underground Lines and the Omnibus Lines – *build one public transport network* ... Children under the age of fourteen years can use public transport at a reduced rate, as can apprentices, poor high school and university students, war veterans and disabled people with a certificate from the district city halls.[180]

Interstitium comes to us through the Latin as *inter-stare*: "that which stands in between, while demarcating two different sides and putting these in contact."[181] If one juxtaposes the history of science argument with the metaphor of interstitial space described above, one could exchange "interstitium" with "intersections;" for "traffic lines" one might insert "hospitals and asylums," "physicians' practices," "living room laboratories," or "short and long distances"' and one could understand the status of research as that of a "specific organ function."[182] It then becomes apparent how productive the organs of the extra-university science spaces of Berlin had actually been.[183] The functional whole of contemporary brain research can only be captured historiographically if the geopolitical dimensions of the municipality of Greater Berlin are taken into account.[184] While focusing on the biographies of individual who constituted the working groups in contemporary brain research, this historical narrative also reflects the individual fates, strokes of luck, and human tragedies inherent in the field. For these reasons, in the narrative of this chapter, I avoid concentrating overly on the academic psychiatrists and neurologists of the Charité medical school. On the contrary, the Charité often presented major obstacles to the scientific creativity that emerged at the fringes of the pre-established academic borderlines of faculties, departments, and working units. The burgeoning of the brain sciences in Berlin was strongly aligned with the booming development of the city itself, and particularly with the fruitful intersections between science, art, and public life.[185]

Another important element of brain research in this period was the organizational structure of the "experimental laboratory." In the years from 1910 to 1930, work places, dissection tables, and private cellars became major intersections for clinical departments of psychiatry and neurology (see figure 1.2). The spatial arrangement of studies in the early neurosciences depended on many contingencies in the urban settings.[186] From the middle of the nineteenth century, laboratories in brain research had become closely linked to the process of knowledge generation and had evolved to play important roles in the biomedical research pursuit. However, the definition that the influential French physiologist Claude Bernard (1813–1878) once gave of a "laboratory experiment" appears much too narrow to encompass the variety of venues for contemporary brain research that were active at the beginning of the twentieth century:

> Every experimental science needs a laboratory. The laboratory is the place to which the researcher retreats, in order to derive a new understanding of observed natural phenomena with the help of the experimental analysis.[187]

The situation at the beginning of the twentieth century was different from Bernard's description in two substantial ways. The first may sound trivial, but it was a major concern for the brain researchers involved: neither Cécile and Oskar Vogt, Brodmann, nor Goldstein had actually enjoyed a laboratory "to which they could retreat" in order to pursue their investigations.[188] In its early stages the field was characterized, rather, by perpetual complaints and petitions for acknowledgment and academic respect. The actual acquisition of a formal scientific laboratory only became a reality twenty-six years – and thus a whole scientific generation – later, after the beginning of their respective research activities, as the example of the professional couple of the Vogts shows.[189] Others could not work at the university of their choice, as in the case of Brodmann; or their research had to be carried out beyond established clinical departments, as shown by the example of Goldstein in Frankfurt and Berlin.[190]

And this description does not even mention the rise of Nazism in Germany, which first constrained and later erased many research and career plans such as those of Goldstein and the Vogts, with their respective groups of neuroscientists.[191]

Oskar Vogt, born in 1870 on the island of Husum on the North Sea coast, came to Berlin when he was twenty-nine years old. He studied medicine from 1888 to 1894 at the University of Kiel and spent his final year at the University of Jena, from which he graduated. Vogt then travelled to Switzerland for postgraduate clinical training with Auguste Forel at the psychiatric hospital *Burghoelzli* in Zurich. From 1897 to 1898, he continued his training at the clinical department of psychiatry and neurology at Leipzig University, while collaborating with the brain psychiatrist Paul Flechsig. From Saxony, Vogt headed to Paris to gain first-hand knowledge in neurological operations with the versatile surgeon Pierre Marie (1858–1940). It was here at the Bicêtre that he met his wife-to-be, Cécile Mugnier, in 1898. She had been an associate in neurology in Marie's service. The love affair between the countryside physician and the unconventional scholar from Paris soon led to their marriage in Berlin the following year.

In reviewing their research program, it would be inaccurate to reduce the neuroscientific investigations of this professional couple solely to the activities of Oskar Vogt, since important impulses – the application of deep psychology (*Tiefenpsychologie*), for instance, or their early studies on the basal ganglia, or support for the division of labour in their private Neurological Laboratory – had been initiated mostly by Cécile (see figure 3.3).[192] Their partnership is nicely depicted in Santiago Ramón y Cajal's recollections of his second research visit to Berlin in 1905:[193]

> The married couple Cécile and Oskar Vogt can be found in the Neurological Institute in Berlin, where they both work on a detailed mapping project of the brain, similar to the astronomers who share their whole life with the photographic representations and the cataloguing of the celestial elements and the spatial nebulas ... Until very late at night, the couple still sits on their paired writing desk, where they face each other during their work ... This is where their *Manuscripts on the Disorders of the Soul, and the Anatomy of the Brain and their Mutual Interrelationships* are written.[194]

Oskar and Cécile began to work together in private neurological practice during their first year in Berlin (in 1902), while they also assembled and

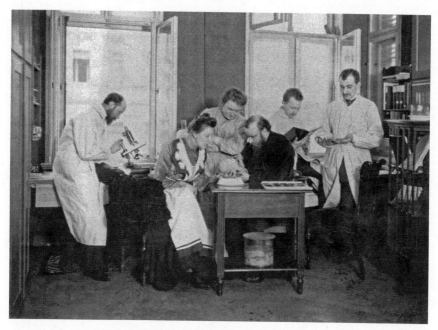

3.3 Oskar and Cécile Vogt at the dissection table in their private living room in Berlin, ca 1903. © Courtesy of C. and O. Vogt Institute for Brain Research, Medical Faculty, Heinrich Heine University Duesseldorf, Germany.

developed a "laboratory" in their own living room for their multidimensional studies of the brain. They charmingly called their apartment laboratory a "neurological Central Station" (*Neurologische Centralstation*), a description much in line with the physical location of their private practice – near the Northern Railway Station of the Prussian capital. Yet it bore no resemblance to the Vienna Neurological Institute, which Obersteiner had "centrally" inaugurated in 1882 – both in geographical respects and in its historical exclusivity. Despite the Vogts' rhetorical claims that the National Hospital for the Paralysed and Epileptic at *Queen Square* in London (founded in 1859)[195] had, together with Obersteiner's institute, served them as a model, their laboratories were by no means comparable. The couple literally had to start their own brain research program from scratch in isolation, "at home."[196] The beginnings of the *Neurologische Centralstation* were humble, but by spring 1898 the Vogts had managed to rent the whole three-storey apartment building of 12, Magdeburger Strasse – to which later the adjacent buildings could also be added – a short five-minute walk from the campus of the Charité. At this time, the philanthropic support of the steel magnates of the Krupp family came into effect for their neuroscientific ventures.[197] The funds received from Friedrich Alfred Krupp covered the rent for the entire building and paid for augmented reconstructions for their animal research (see also chapter 1). This expansion is wittily described in the autobiographical recollections of Thea Luers, the female research assistant of neuropathologist Hugo Spatz at the KWI for Brain Research:

> What may the neighbours have thought or known about the apartment building at the corner of Magdeburgerstrasse [12–]16 in the middle of downtown Berlin W? ... The Vogts had asked that a cage and safety net should be attached, so that their monkeys could very soon swing and rock over the rooftops of Berlin ... While the monkeys performed their gymnastics training on the balcony (which was important for [the Vogts'] work on the localized functional areas of the brain), human brains ... in disguised bags were carried into the house. This happened at the very same time that the high society of Berlin, politicians, writers, poets, actors, and *grandes dames*, were sitting downstairs in their patient waiting room.[198]

In 1910 the anatomist Wilhelm Waldeyer – who had just returned to Berlin from the Kaiser Wilhelms University in Strasburg – supported the Vogts' idea for the creation of a brain research institute and sent letters of support to the Charité. The same was done by eminent neuroanatomist Paul Flechsig from Leipzig, who wrote supporting references to the faculty of medicine in Berlin as well. They pleaded for the creation of such an institute in the new extra-university unit of the *Centralstation* and recommended as its academic director the brain psychiatrist Franz Nissl (1860–1919) of Munich, thinking he would bring both psychiatric knowledge and versatility in neurohistological techniques to the new position. Illustrating the wide political influence of the Krupp family of industrialists, however, the University of Berlin eventually chose Vogt as the director of the planned institute, at a point in time when a new division of brain pathology had just been staffed by one of the most prominent neuropathologists of the time, Max Bielschowsky. Bielschowsky "roomed in" at 12, Magdeburger Strasse, joining the Vogts from Emanuel Mendel's (1839–1907) private neurological laboratory, which was another important research hub in downtown Berlin. He supported the Vogts' microscopical research program in histopathology at what had now by been named the Berlin Neurobiological Laboratory.[199] Although neither Vogt nor Bielschowsky had officially received their formal *Habilitation* allowing them to assume a professorship, they were both appointed adjunct professors to the Friedrich Wilhelms University in 1913. In the following year, the laboratory became affiliated with the university and was incorporated into the Kaiser Wilhelm Society as the new institute for brain research.[200] The construction of the building in Berlin-Buch could only be started in 1930, however, since the funds promised by the Krupp family had just vanished in the Great Depression. This loss triggered a laborious process of finding other international funds. Fortunately, these monies were provided by the American Rockefeller Foundation on the basis of contributions shared among Berlin, the German State of Prussia, and the Kaiser Wilhelm Society. The agreement paralleled a similar funding model chosen for the earlier establishment of the Deutsche Forschungsanstalt for Psychiatry in Munich so that, even under the economic constraints of the time, the construction work could go ahead.[201] Yet, if we review the notes of Rockefeller Foundation Officer Alan Gregg, who visited the Munich institution on 6 November 1928, it becomes apparent that Rockefeller Foundation funds had not been sufficient to actually guarantee its much-needed construction:

> We then went to Vogt's Institute which consists of 3 floors in a cheap apartment house. A surprising show. The Vogts have been working for 17 years with poor equipment and inadequate space, but with a comprehensiveness and persistence which is both admirable and impressive ... (1) The architectonic of the brain as a whole; (2) the localization of both physiological experiment and evidence of several cases of different functions of the brain; (3) the further study of some phases of genetics which may be of special importance in the hereditary determination of brain structure.[202]

With the continued engagement by the Rockefeller Foundation in German biomedicine and especially in the field of brain research, the Berlin municipal government was eventually persuaded to find a piece of land where the new KWI for Brain Research could be built. The project was rescued at the last moment when Alfred Krupp von Bohlen und Halbach (1870–1950) joined these efforts and resumed his father's undertaking for Vogt's central laboratory (*Centrallabor*).[203]

The Vogts were now compelled to leave their apartment in Magdeburger Strasse. All the neighbouring houses had been rented out and considerable dispute had arisen with the other tenants. There had been growing numbers of complaints about the animals on the façades, the awkward research activities, and the suspicious packages from the nearby cemeteries that were spirited into the building by Charité attendants. It was clear to everyone that the institute could not stay in that location.[204] The American officers of the Rockefeller Foundation in Germany continuously gathered information on the Vogts' laboratory and cabled those to the Rockefeller Foundation headquarters in New York. News soon arrived that Oskar Vogt was toying with the idea of applying for the directorship of the Deutsche Forschungsanstalt in Munich. The Rockefeller Foundation became nervous, since this meant that a promising position in Germany would be vacated and that Vogt might leave Berlin altogether. All these developments led to the acceleration of the planning process. The choice for the new institute was a site in Berlin-Buch that the city physician (*Stadtmedizinalrat*) Von Drigalski had identified. Von Drigalski was the leader of the Berlin public health service and in that role supervised the care ratios of the hospitals and asylums. The community of Buch, north of Berlin, had traditionally been the location of many large mental asylums and care facilities. Adjacent to the new location were the so-called Third City Lunatic Asylum (Hufeland Krankenhaus), which guaranteed "a large number of mental patients as study material" for the purposes of the KWI.[205] Vogt was also given charge of a psychiatric department with forty beds, which he "should be able to fill to meet his own research demands."[206] It would be added to the basic research divisions of the institute.

Two other fortunate circumstances then made the creation of the KWI for Brain Research possible:

Another part of this general scheme has ... been realized by the Kaiser-Wilhelm-Society in promoting science in the field of physiology, and this has made it possible to open the Kaiser-Wilhelm-Institute in Berlin, for the study of the brain. Here are engaged: Oskar Vogt, Cécile Vogt, [Maximilian] Rose [1883–1939?] and [Max] Bielschowsky. The first of the above are working on the extension of the teaching on the localization of brain cells, the psychology of the "Neurosen," and the special characteristics connected with the problem of heredity.[207]

Central to the Vogts' research program was the innovative concept of a techtonical analysis of cerebral histological cell layers (*Pathoklisen-architektur*) (see also figure 3.4), designed to elucidate the histology of psychiatric and neurological diseases such as schizophrenia, Morbus Parkinson, and apoplectic strokes.

Sitzungsberichte
der Heidelberger Akademie der Wissenschaften
Stiftung Heinrich Lanz
Mathematisch-naturwissenschaftliche Klasse
Abteilung B. Biologische Wissenschaften
================ Jahrgang 1919. 14. Abhandlung ================

Zur Kenntnis
der pathologischen Veränderungen des
Striatum und des Pallidum und zur
Pathophysiologie der dabei auftretenden
Krankheitserscheinungen

Von

CÉCILE und OSKAR VOGT
in Berlin

Mit 1 Figur

Eingegangen am 21. Oktober 1919

Vorgelegt von H. BRAUS

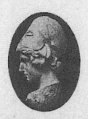

Heidelberg 1919
Carl Winters Universitätsbuchhandlung

Verlags-Nr. 1528.

3.4 Cover page of Cécile and Oskar Vogt, *Zur Kenntnis der pathologischen Veraenderungen des Striatum und des Pallidum und zur Pathophysiologie der dabei auftretenden Krankheitserscheinungen*. Heidelberg, Germany: Carl Winters Universitaetsbuchhandlung, 1919, frontpage / Book courtesy of the Heidelberger Akademie der Wissenschaften, Heidelberg, Baden-Wuerttemberg, Germany (HAdw Digital: https://digi.hadw-bw.de/view/sbhadwmnkl_b_1919_14/0001).

The Berlin brain researchers were well aware that "a new form of pathoarchitectural surveillance of the brains of mental and neurological patients with the help of histological brain slide series had thus far not been undertaken."[208] The grounds on which the KWI for Brain Research was ultimately built were ideal for future expansion. The land had origi-nally been singled out for a new cemetery, and the chapel had already been built with public funding. But that undertaking had to be abandoned because of high ground water levels – the public even humorously dubbed it a "sailors' cemetery." (It remains at this location in the institute park of the Buch campus still today.)[209] The adjacent residential building, which had been intended for the gardeners and wardens of the cemetery, was appropriated for the staff of the KWI, one of whom was Russian geneticist Timoféeff-Ressovsky.[210] Soon after Nazi Party seized power, however, the inaugural institute director, Oskar Vogt, came under attack by local Nazi groups because he was regarded as left-leaning and subversive; and his relatively autonomous position made him more difficult to control. Furthermore, Vogt had been one of the international experts invited to Russia to investigate the brain of communist leader Vladimir Ilyich Lenin[211] and was under suspicion as well for having a French wife.

As early as 1933, the institute was the site of a conspiracy led by faculty member Max Heinrich Fischer (1892–1938), head of the human physiol-ogy department. Fischer betrayed Vogt to the Nazi authorities for the latter's political disloyalties and internationalist leanings. He further enraged a local group of SA members ("Brownshirts") to march against Vogt and threaten the scientists and workers in his Kaiser Wilhelm Institute. On 30 January a troop of local SA members from Buch stormed the institute, ostensibly because the many foreign researchers there were suspected of hosting an Eastern European spy. Not only was the PhD manuscript of Marguerite (1913–2007) – the Vogts' daughter – stolen, but two staff members with foreign passports were taken into custody: the Dutch engineer Jan F. Toennies (1902–1970) and the American geneti-cist and later Nobel prize laureate Hermann J. Muller (1890–1967). These illustrious guests were driven to the Buch police prison.[212] Even though they were soon released, the event gave rise to major international irrita-tion. As Alan Gregg reported:

> Vogt sent car to hotel. Went out to Buch and spent all day there. Vogt has had a good deal of trouble. House surrounded and researched by Nazis. Suspected of communism ... A long and thorough visit to the lab and to the clinic with demonstration of all the kinds of work

going on. Thennis [Toennies] impressed me as much as many of the juniors. Also got first rate impression of the atmosphere of the small observation hosp[ital]. – Patients as happy as under the circumstances they could be.[213]

A tangible threat since the Nazis took control, Vogt was ousted as the director of the KWI for Brain Research in 1936 by means of a signed resignation certificate from the new *Reichsfuehrer*, Adolf Hitler (1889–1945). This was grossly unusual, since it violated the KWG tradition of granting its institute directors lifelong tenure; and it ignored the academic independence of the KWG.[214] Half a year later, in spring of 1937, Vogt was obliged to hand over the directorship to the neuropathologist Hugo Spatz, who had been called from Munich to take up the vacant Berlin position.[215] The Krupp family, who had supported the Vogts since the 1910s along with the American Rockefeller Foundation, thereupon decided to finance the construction of a brain research institute for the Vogts as far away from Berlin as possible. In the later 1930s, the institute was rebuilt in Neustadt, Titisee, in the Black Forest, 660 kilometres from the ruling Nazi ministries. Here, the Vogts managed to continue their research program with a few co-workers until the early postwar period, although they now shifted their focus to the nervous systems of insects (Vogt's *Hummelsammlung*).[216]

MAPPING THE BRAIN IN BERLIN AND TUEBINGEN: THE CASE OF KORBINIAN BRODMANN

In their investigations on the organization of the cerebral cortex, the Vogts were particularly supported by the experienced histologist Korbinian Brodmann, who arrived in Berlin from Frankfurt am Main in 1898. The neurological clinicians Max Lewandowsky (1876–1918) and Max Borchert (1879–1918) soon joined this group in the Berlin Neurobiological Laboratory as well.[217] Brodmann was the son of a farmer in Swabia, where he attended public school (*Volksschule*) in Liggersdorf bei Hohenfels. He then moved to the junior high school at Ueberlingen and graduated from *Gymnasium* college in Sigmaringen and Konstanz.[218] Between 1889 and 1895, Brodmann studied medicine in Munich, Wuerzburg, Berlin, and finally in Freiburg im Breisgau, where he finished his studies in 1895. After receiving his licence to practise medicine, Brodmann went to the University of Lausanne in Switzerland and then came back to Germany to Emil Kraepelin's clinical department of psychiatry in Munich. In 1898

Brodmann received his doctorate from the University of Leipzig with a thesis on ependymal sclerosis, under the supervision of the pathologist Felix Victor Birch-Hirschfeld (1842–1899).[219] His doctoral research consolidated his interests in brain research, as he now took a position as a physician in the department of psychiatry at the University of Jena. He later went to the City Mental Asylum in Frankfurt, where he came into close contact with psychiatrist Alois Alzheimer (1864–1915) (see figure 7.3). In 1901 Alzheimer encouraged Brodmann to continue a career in neurohistology, a path that Brodmann then successfully followed with the Vogts for the next ten years.[220]

Brodmann had known Oskar Vogt for a long time, having worked with him clinically in the Psychiatric Sanatorium of Alexanderbad in the Fichtelgebirge, where Vogt had been chief physician in his early years before leaving for Switzerland and Paris.[221] Now, in 1902, Brodmann joined Vogt again as senior research associate and worked closely together with thirty-five-year-old Max Bielschowsky in the Berlin laboratory.[222] Brodmann undertook prolific publication activities that centred on the cortical architecture of the brain and predestined him to collaborate with the Vogts on the architectonical organization of the human cortex (see also the cover image of this book):

> Brodmann started work with the greatest enthusiasm [and] a sheer untiring work ethic and fulfilled all the tasks that were given to him … The new cell preparations in particular, which were produced with the many augmented staining methods, led to rich results right from our first mutual orientation experiments. On the basis of these observations, I [the technical assistant of the KWI for Brain Research Thea Luers] proposed to him that he could develop the first draft edition of the volume on cortical architecture. Today, Brodmann's cortical maps and his differentiation of the cortical areas can be found in every clinical university department and in every anatomical institute.[223]

Brodmann carried out intensive histological investigations of the correlation of the cyto- and myeloarchitectonic cortical areas between 1901 and 1910. This research was driven by the availability of myelin stains and Nissl stains for various cell layers in the brain, as well as their connectivities. Brodmann's central book on the localization of the cell layers, *Comparative Localization of the Human Cortex* (*Vergleichende*

Lokalisationslehre der Grosshirnrinde), summarized this important work in 1909. "Brodmann's areas," as they are still known, have since then become the recognized functional cell layer mapping of the human cortex.[224] This immense contribution has widely influenced practices in neuroanatomy, neurophysiology, and neurosurgery for a century. And it established the foundation for the ensuing programs of such luminaries as Otfrid Foerster in Breslau, Wilder Penfield in Montreal, Fedor Krause (1857–1937) in Berlin, and Edgar Douglas Adrian (1889–1977) in Cambridge, England.

In particular, the work of Penfield, who as a neurosurgeon studied the neurophysiological properties of Brodmann's areas in his epileptic patients, confirmed Brodmann's microanatomical mapping. It led ultimately to the refinement of the sensory and motor homunculus regarding the functional localization of the human cortex:[225]

The prospect of operating, under local anaesthesia, on a long series of patients who might be cured of their epilepsy had another exciting aspect. The electrical stimulation that must be used to guide the neurosurgeon in his removal of the cause would perhaps tell the thoughtful surgeon many secrets about the living, functioning brain. He could learn what the conscious patient might tell him.[226]

Vogt himself transferred Brodmann's findings onto a variety of stimulation experiments in mammals and subjected these to ongoing histological analyses. He hoped to confirm in humans the earlier stimulation experiments that Foerster, a neurological surgeon, had pursued with his group (including Ludwig Guttmann, 1899–1980, Klaus Joachim Zuelch, 1910–1988, Georg Merrem, 1908–1971, and Fedor Krause) at Breslau University.[227] In fact, Foerster had previously found a correlation between individual patterns of functional organization, as Penfield noted:

Professor Foerster had operated on twelve patients who were sufferers from epilepsy. The fits were caused in some of the cases by war wounds to the brain. In others, the brain injury had been received at the time of a difficult birth. The patients were alive and grateful after operation. I studied the scars he had removed, using the methods I knew so well by that time. It was a golden opportunity. We published those cases together and I have continued such operations with new studies since coming to Montreal.[228]

The German neuroanatomist Karl Zilles (b. 1944) at Duesseldorf University's Cécile and Oskar Vogt Institute has continued their scientific research work since the time of the Vogts' institute in Neustadt.[229] Zilles himself applauded Brodmann's pioneering work on the fine structure of the cortical localization in his biographical entry to the seminal historical dictionary *Founders of Neurology*:

· Brodmann's broad comparative-anatomic approach, his recognition that the cortex is organized anatomically along the same basic principles in all mammals, and his idea of utilizing the morphogenesis of the cortex as a basis for the classification of cortical types and for the nomenclature of the layers, were all instrumental in dispelling the almost hopeless confusion which existed before Brodmann entered the field. *His studies culminated in his famous book,* Vergleichende Lokalisationslehre der Grosshirnrinde ... *which remains the only comprehensive work ever published on this subject.*[230]

Brodmann's scientific career was, however, tragically constrained by the hostile attitude with which the Berlin medical faculty rejected his *Habilitation* and his previous research work, deeming them unsatisfactory.[231] This decision was based on power struggles between the contemporary medical mandarins. Brodmann's thesis was rejected in 1910 because of an unfavourable report written by Theodor Ziehen (1862–1950), who headed the clinical department of psychiatry and neurology. Ziehen's damning report on Vogt's collaborator at the Neurobiological Laboratory could be interpreted as a harsh personal act that harked back to the longer story of how Vogt had become a member of the medical faculty.[232] As noted above, Vogt had begun his neuroscience career outside the Charité medical school in the urban spaces of Berlin. His affiliation with his former *Centralstation* as the university's Neurobiological Laboratory was made possible only through the personal intervention of the minister of the Prussian Ministry of Science, Arts, and Culture in 1902.

And it was clear to everyone involved that the recommendation for this affiliation had been seconded by the Krupp family, together with the local support of the neurophysiologist Theodor Wilhelm Engelmann (1843–1909). Engelmann had supported Vogt all along, since he saw the great potential of the work undertaken at 12, Magdeburger Strasse and sought for himself interdisciplinary collaborations that the rigid university system barely allowed. Administratively, Vogt's laboratory came to be identified as a "special division" of the institute of physiology, even though neurologist Friedrich Jolly and anatomist Wilhelm Waldeyer objected to that move when the petition was submitted to the faculty. They all feared losing some of their own academic turf. More significantly, it appeared likely that they would receive decreasing financial support for their own institutions, should the faculty accept another basic science institute under its jurisdiction.[233] This unhappy situation of intra-faculty politics could not keep the Neurobiological Laboratory from becoming incorporated into the university as per ministerial decree of the Prussian Ministry of Science, Arts, and Culture. But the all-powerful academic mandarins had never forgotten this reduction of their influence. So when the opportunity for retaliation came and Brodmann submitted his thesis for faculty approval, he and his scientific career were sacrificed in their personal revenge against Oskar Vogt.[234]

Following the rejection of his 1908 *Habilitation*, entitled "The Cytoarchitectonic Structure of the Simian Cortex" ("Die cytoarchitektonische Kortexgliederung der Halbaffen"), Brodmann was obliged to leave both the Vogts and Berlin, since his access to the academic community had been formally blocked. However, Brodmann was already well known and scientifically accomplished, and had many personal contacts with senior medical scientists in Germany and abroad. Soon after the shocking Berlin incident, he decided to join the Tuebingen clinical department of psychiatry in 1910, where the psychiatrist Otto Binswanger became his mentor. His *Habilitation* at Tuebingen was speedily approved without any further foul play. Brodmann then quickly rose through the ranks in three years from assistant to full professor at the University of Tuebingen's psychiatry department. After a brief period as a practising pathologist during the war, he finally received a job offer in 1917 from the Deutsche Forschungsanstalt for Psychiatry in Munich.[235] His life had a tragic ending, however – not unlike those of two former colleagues in the Vogts' Neurobiological Laboratory – Max Lewandowsky (1876–1916), who died of typhoid fever in 1916, and Max Borchert, who as a fervent royalist committed suicide at war's end. Shortly after Brodmann took up the Munich position and married Margarete Franke (1896–1918), and just as the young couple was expecting their first child, he passed away. Like many pathologists in the pre-antibiotic era, he had contracted a sepsis as a result of cadaver dissections and died on 22 August 1918 at the age of only forty-nine years.[236]

THE "RED WEDDING" AND THE "BROWN CITY":
ON AN "ABORTIVE CLINICAL TRIAL"
BY KURT GOLDSTEIN

Another important neurologist who entered the urban Berlin academic context of the 1930s was Kurt Goldstein. Born in 1878 into a Jewish family as the seventh of nine children, he was jokingly referred to as "the professor" at a young age by his brothers and sisters. They particularly ridiculed his love of books and philosophy. Goldstein found his schooling at the *Gymnasium* college in Breslau rather boring and lacking sufficient stimulation. Hoping to receive an inspiring education, he moved to Heidelberg to begin philosophical studies, which he indeed found extremely enriching. However, his father – a well-to-do owner of a Silesian logging company – pressured him into studying a profession, rather than pursue what his father saw as "unprofitable studies" in the humanities.[237] Goldstein's early philosophical interests nevertheless remained a vital influence. This is clear even in his succeeding work on holistic neurology, in which he was additionally influenced by his cousin, the Hamburg cultural philosopher Ernst Cassirer. Like Goldstein himself – who always tried to keep in touch with his former collaborators and associates (see figure 3.5) – Cassirer later had to flee during the era of Nazism and emigrated to the United States via England and Sweden. Until Cassirer's death in 1945, the cousins carried on a rich correspondence about matters of philosophy and the holistic interpretation of neurology.[238]

Between 1906 and the outbreak of war, Goldstein continued his clinical training in neurology and psychiatry at the University of Koenigsberg in East Prussia, where he received his *Habilitation*. By this time, renowned Frankfurt neuroanatomist Ludwig Edinger had become interested in Goldstein's work and offered him the directorship of the clinical neurological division in his institute (see also chapter 1).[239] The Frankfurt institute also offered fertile ground for a long-lasting collaboration between Goldstein and Adhémar Gelb, the experimental psychologist who headed the neuropsychological division until 1930. Goldstein's own work would have been impossible without Gelb's tremendous help, since Gelb initially designed the tests for war-injured soldiers and assisted him in developing his research program on speech disorders and complex rehabilitative tasks. Goldstein's experiments with Gelb and Walther Riese on the behaviour and improvement of young brain-injured soldiers in the institute led to many questions about the process of regeneration in the human nervous system.[240] As they did with many of their patients,

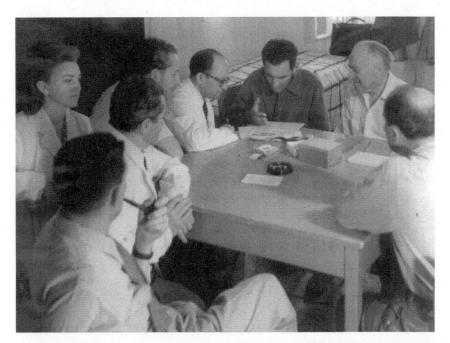

3.5 Kurt Goldstein (second from right) during his visit to Israel in 1958. © Courtesy of Dr Moshe Feinsod, Collection of Moshe Feinsod, Haifa, Israel.

they examined a twenty-four-year-old veteran, Schneider, who had two lesions in the posterior visual cortex, and concluded that other parts of the brain must have taken over the functions that had been lost. The fact that these were thought to reside in destroyed areas led them to postulate that the brain possessed adaptive capacities. The experimenters noted, however, that Schneider was able to read any text through "a series of minute head and hand movements – he 'wrote' with his hands what his eyes saw ... If prevented from moving his head or body, the patient could read nothing whatsoever."[241]

Through these experiments, it was gradually understood that the physical constitution of the brain was part of the process of compensating for functional losses – but that this could not be the full pathophysiological story. When investigating cognitive disorders and their interrelation with practical skills and the reconditioning of patients with shaking limbs, Goldstein and his collaborators realized that the effects of such "catastrophic reactions" could rule out instances of complete destruction of delineated cortical areas. Moreover, Goldstein was convinced that more was to be learned about the regeneration, adaptability, and structure-function relationships than was available at that time. There was certainly some element related to the Weimar cultural context of the "Goldstein group"[242] that brought together such a variety of social meanings in an original and innovative way – shock, *Angst*, paralysis, speech variations, art, craft practices, memory, and hope were all ubiquitous study phenomena well reflected in written exchanges between Binswanger, Freud, Bethe, Gelb, and Georg Klemperer (1865–1946), among their laboratory assistants, war comrades, and Goldstein's humanistic friends. In the case of this group, the dialectic of Weimar as simultaneously a social catastrophe and an unimaginable cultural laboratory for the creation of newly amalgamated scientific and community lifeforms becomes tangible. In fact, Villa Sommerhoff was all in one. It was a study institute, a hospital, a long-term sanatorium, a working colony, a residence hall, and an intellectual salon.[243] The fact that Goldstein was unable to obtain a separate ward for clinical psychiatry to integrate it into his institute could be seen, however, as a further indication of the difficult relationship between academic psychiatry and the emerging field of brain research.[244]

It did not come as a great surprise that Goldstein left Frankfurt in 1930 when he received an offer to head the department of neurology at Berlin's Moabit Hospital. The offer included the opportunity to bring a number of his former collaborators with him and add other brain scientists to complement this neurological research unit. He was fortunate that many of his former collaborators followed him to the capital city, where he soon assembled an illustrious group of physicians and researchers. Between 1931 and 1932, Goldstein was joined by the Jewish neurologist Karl Stern from Bavaria, who had worked with him in Frankfurt and whose thesis he had supervised. After his three years of postgraduate training in neuropathology with Spielmeyer, the world-renowned tumour specialist at the Deutsche Forschungsanstalt for Psychiatry in Munich, Stern agreed to join Goldstein in Moabit, where he founded a division of clinical neuropathology within the department. The brain research facilities at Moabit became further diversified and the cohort of Goldstein's collaborators formed an amazing interdisciplinary group. In Moritz Borchardt (1868–1949), a pupil of Ernst von Bergmann (1833–1907), he attracted one of the first specialized neurosurgeons. Adhémar Gelb, as a major proponent of clinical experimental psychology in Germany, joined him from Frankfurt as well.[245] For a short period the renowned neuropathologist Ludwig Pick (1868–1944) (co-discoverer of "Niemann Pick" disease) headed the neuropathology division in the hospital's basement,[246] but after two years he left for a directorship position in one of Berlin's district pathology departments in Lichtenberg, continuing as a consultant for the Moabit group.[247]

In contrast to Goldstein's work situation in Frankfurt, Pick's new service lay outside the core faculty of the Charité. Moabit Hospital was nevertheless one of the few academic institutions in the city that offered a high degree of organizational differentiation. It also served as a teaching institution, with Goldstein giving guest lectures at the medical school. The hospital consisted of complementary departments of neurology, psychiatry, internal medicine, and pathology. It offered similar working conditions to those that Goldstein's group had appreciated earlier in Frankfurt, and the researchers were now given access as well to acute neurological and psychiatric patients through the curative mandate of the hospital. In this sense, Goldstein had moved into an ideal position to further build on the pre-existing infrastructure, while aligning it with his holistic approach to neurology and psychiatry.[248] Yet at the very moment when the ground had been prepared to position Moabit Hospital as a leading research institute for clinical neuroscience, the advent of Nazism destroyed all promising plans. The director of this city hospital, internist Georg Klemperer (brother of the notable Berlin diarist Victor Klemperer, 1881–1960, and also personal physician to Vladmir I. Lenin), was convinced that their "Jewish" hospital with its social care roles for the nearby proletarian communities of the "Red Wedding" would soon become a target for political oppression.[249]

Klemperer became greatly concerned about an offensive news article dated 21 March 1933 in the Nazi propaganda paper *Der Stuermer* (*The Attacker*), in which Goldstein was personally criticized for being a Jewish physician in a high social position, and a psychoanalyst whose prime interest was to care for mentally disabled patients, rather than to eradicate "this burden" from the public health system.[250] Such negative views on eugenics had widely infiltrated the German-speaking medical community on all levels, as evidenced for instance by Max Nonne's successor in the chair of neurology in Hamburg, Heinrich Pette (1887–1964). In his inaugural lecture to the students and faculty, Pette stated: "It is one of the main tasks of a clinical department of neurology to organize programs in social hygiene that are based on selection."[251] Disguised as a rational approach to public health in an underfunded social system, similar rhetoric from contemporary neurological peers targeted the way Goldstein and others approached brain-injured and psychiatric patients – all the more so because holistic neurology was quite labour-intensive and involved intuitive acts of understanding and care seemingly transcending natural science:

> In accordance with the spirit of the times in medicine, I was attracted
> to the idea that sickness should not be considered something that
> befalls the individual from the outside, but that one should rather
> treat the sick personality, a concept which had gained wide consideration in Germany already at the beginning of the century.[252]

And Klemperer's concerns were warranted: the very fact that approximately 70 percent of the physicians in the Moabit Hospital had Jewish backgrounds and about 10 percent of the nurses were organized in left-wing unions made it a suspicious institution in the eyes of Nazi officials.[253]

Klemperer warned Goldstein that the situation was dire and that he should leave the country immediately to save his life. Unfortunately for both, Klemperer's clairvoyance was accurate. On 1 April 1933, while seeing patients in his practice, Goldstein was taken into custody. According to the recollections of his assistant, Edith Thurm (1892–1964?), Goldstein had even pleaded with the SA men to wait until he could see all his patients. Yet he was handcuffed and taken outside, while the Brownshirts shouted: "Everyone can be replaced – and this includes you as well!" As a prominent member of the "Socialist Physicians Union," Goldstein was taken to one of the most brutal prisons at General-Pape-Strasse in Berlin, where he was also tortured. After a few weeks, however, a former student of his, Eva Rothmann (1878–1960), used her acquaintance with Nazi psychoanalyst Matthias H. Goering (1879–1945) – the cousin of the Luftwaffe high commander and Reichsminister without specific portfolio Hermann Goering (1893–1946) – to request that Goldstein be protected. Immediately after Goldstein had been set free, he fled to Switzerland and from there found refuge in the Netherlands.[254] Although he at first experienced Dutch exile as a safe haven, his working context in Amsterdam was quite dissociated from psychiatry and neurology, despite having been made possible through a connection with Dutch neurologist Bernard Brouwer (1881–1949). The latter arranged for Goldstein to be given office space in the institute of pharmacology at Amsterdam University. Yet, despite their German certificates, neither he nor his fiancée could receive medical relicensing, and they were barred from practising medicine.

In order to make the best of this situation, Goldstein continued to work on a major theoretical treatise, *The Organism* (*Der Aufbau des Organismus* – see figure 3.6), for which he became internationally renowned. During

DER AUFBAU DES
ORGANISMUS

Einführung in die Biologie unter besonderer
Berücksichtigung der Erfahrungen am
kranken Menschen

VON

Dr. KURT GOLDSTEIN

FRÜHER HONORAR-PROFESSOR AN DER UNIVERSITÄT BERLIN

HAAG

MARTINUS NIJHOFF

1934

3.6 Front cover of Kurt Goldstein's *Der Aufbau des Organismus. Einfuehrung in die
Biologie unter besonderer Beruecksichtigung der Erfahrungen am kranken Menschen.*
Amsterdam, The Netherlands: Martinus Nijhoff, 1934. © Title page of Goldstein, Kurt,
Der Aufbau des Organismus, Berlin 1934; Courtesy of Zone Books, Brooklyn, New
York, USA.

this time, he was supported by a two-year fellowship from the American Rockefeller Foundation, which enabled him to finish the book, subsequently published by Martin Nijhoff in The Hague in 1935:

> His stipend (2,000 guilders) during the past year was provided jointly by the Dutch Academic Assistance Council and the Rockefeller Foundation. His Dutch colleagues were anxious that he remain in Amsterdam for at least another year under the same terms, but being convinced that there was no future for him in Holland either in a university post or in practice ... Prof. Goldstein has been offered facilities for research at the Psychiatric Institute, Columbia Medical Center, and the Foundation and Emergency Committee in Aid of Displaced Foreign Physicians have been asked to supply the necessary stipend.[255]

With no possibility of remaining in Amsterdam, Goldstein and his now soon-to-be wife, Eva Rothmann-Goldstein – daughter of the Berlin neuroanatomist Max Rothmann (1868–1915) and sister of the neuroanatomist Hans Rothmann (1899–1970), who emigrated to San Francisco to continue a successful career at the University of California, San Francisco – now decided to leave the Netherlands. Upon their arrival in New York in 1935, Goldstein tried for a third time to resume his career, while seeking a collaboration with the immigrant German psychologist Martin Scheerer (1900–1961), with whom he founded a laboratory at Columbia University. The lab provided a working place in which Goldstein could pursue his research work in parallel with a demanding neurological practice in New York City. From 1937 to 1938 he also lectured on neurological theory at Harvard University and on neuropathology at Columbia University. Together with other luminary émigrés in New York – such as the philosophers Max Horkheimer (1895–1973) and Erich Fromm (1900–1980), who had come to the United States from the University of Frankfurt – Goldstein conducted further studies in social psychiatry. His research project on the "authoritarian character" at New York's New School of . Social Research had clearly been informed by the experiences of the large group of exiled scholars who joined this research centre. The structure of the New School included many academics, economists, and non-professional supporting members.[256] Until Goldstein's death in 1965, the New School of Social Research remained an intellectual refuge for him.[257]

Goldstein's loss of his physical affiliation with the neurological and psychiatric research communities in Frankfurt and Berlin had many negative effects on the development of his research program on addressing problems in neurology and the phenomenology of brain injuries. His research never reached the level of prominence he had achieved previously at the two centres in Germany. For the institutional and personal reasons given above, it could not be replicated in other international venues such as Amsterdam or New York. This was even the case at Columbia University and at the academic Montefiore Hospital with its research facilities in Brooklyn. Goldstein's peer researchers considered his approach to neurology as alien, undisciplined – not even "neurology" at all. Arriving only a few years before his retirement age, Goldstein needed to cope with many difficulties in his new start in North America. This third attempt to establish himself in an urban context, with different academic communities, proved too difficult to accomplish.[258] Even though his collaborative earlier publications with Gelb in Frankfurt had been well received in the American communities of psychology and rehabilitation medicine, his more psychiatric and holistic publications soon fell into oblivion – culturally, they seemed like products of quite foreign "Germanic" scholarship.[259]

The relationships between early brain research, psychiatry, and neurology in the German-speaking countries show that developments toward an interdisciplinary neuroscience field were not pure "success stories." Looking at the examples of Frankfurt University and the KWI for Brain Research in Berlin-Buch, as well as the extra-university laboratories of the Vogts and Goldstein in downtown Berlin, it becomes clear that it was impulses originating from the outer edges of the field that led to the emergence of this interdisciplinary area of neuroscience. The analysis of the interstitial transitions within the urban science spaces in the Berlin metropolis shows that *important accomplishments and contributions were produced outside the established university system*, with its rigid structures, strict hierarchies, and inflexible traditions. This change speaks as well to the intensity of the personal energy and creativity that individuals such as Edinger, the Vogts, Brodmann, and Goldstein must have been able to summon. Only with such commitment could they have established their early interdisciplinary research institutes and centres despite the lack of support from established medical and scientific faculties.

As we have seen, these researchers were operating largely outside mainstream institutions. The narrative of this chapter has shown that any description of intramural laboratories would offer too narrow a representation of the research surroundings of the early German-speaking neuroscientists. As intersections of open research methods, respective experiments, and laboratories, the extra-university settings of these early brain researchers and psychiatrists became a showcase for a variety of processes of modernization in the early years of the twentieth century. In this exploration of the contingencies of this early episode of brain research in Frankfurt and Berlin, even though their local histories were very different, this observation is particularly relevant. The interstitial segments of the urban science spaces in Berlin literally arose as "laboratories of real life,"[260] with transformations, disputes, and influences that could hardly be planned for. Furthermore, the denial of a psychiatric clinic in Frankfurt to Goldstein, the rejection of Brodmann's *Habilitation* Charité dissertation, the antagonism of the contemporary neuromorphological context, and the imposition of Nazi power posed huge challenges for the burgeoning innovative research field of interdisciplinary brain sciences.

4

War, Trauma, Regeneration

External Influences and Cultural Nervousness Considered in Neuromorphological Research

There can be no doubt that political, social, and cultural circumstances, and anything else that may here be included, have an extraordinary influence on the human nervous system. Nervousness has indeed increased to an enormous degree at the end of our nineteenth century ... Its causes can easily be found in the spirit of our day, in the modern way of life, in the progress and the sophistication of our culture, in the new creations of modern being, and indeed in social intercourse.

Wilhelm Erb[1]

It may well be that this quotation, which I refer to as a *Zeitdiagnose* in the full sense of the term as a "medical diagnosis" of contemporary culture, was known to the neurologist Wilhelm Erb's peers, colleagues, and students. It was popularized by Erb in his academic convocation address at the University of Heidelberg, "On the Growing Nervousness of Our Time" in 1893 ("Ueber die wachsende Nervositaet unserer Zeit") at the height of the Wilhelminian restoration in the early 1890s. Even if Erb is not personally credited in the literature, the cultural diagnosis of "increasing nervousness" had by then clearly become a popular trope, as historian Joachim Radkau has shown in his seminal book, *The Age of Nervousness: Germany between Bismarck and Hitler* (1998). Although this diagnosis has become a fairly accepted view in historical scholarship, it is intriguing to note that the decades of increased nervousness have indeed been predominantly associated with the more psychiatric or psychological aspect of German *Nervenheilkunde*.[2] It is hard, if not impossible, to find a good translation for this specialty. While "neuro – logy" since the nineteenth century would convey the meaning – "nerves" and the Greek work *logos*, which adds the connotation of knowledge as well as healing – this etymology still does not cover the semantic field sufficiently. In Germany, clinical neurology and psychiatry in the context of basic research and health care organization were very different from those of comparable communities in other European countries and America. Whereas in Britain, neurology and psychiatry had separated into two specialties in 1894,[3] for instance, *Nervenheilkunde* in Germany continued to include most psychiatrists and a number of doctors in internal medicine even throughout the period of the Weimar Republic.[4]

It is evident that, as the chief of the clinical department of internal medicine at the University of Heidelberg, Erb was definitely not the type of professor his contemporaries would have associated simply with the custodial professions of the alienists or mental hygienists. Quite the contrary. Erb had made important neuroanatomical discoveries (such as nerve fibre and cell degeneration phenomena following syphilis infections).[5] He also introduced diagnostic measures into medicine such as methods for electropuncture ("Erb's reflex hammer") and a number of diagnostic clinical signs ("Erb's Points" – the points of the emergence of peripheral nerve branches). He was certainly an exemplary representative of a psychosomatic doctor *avant la lettre*.[6] At the same time, the Heidelberg neurologist's accounts of the adverse influences of society at large were shared by many of the colleagues he addressed at the Ruperto Carolae Dies Academicus in the overcrowded *Aula* of the university on 22 December 1893. Erb's views of the general world picture (*Weltbilder*) serve as a guiding theme throughout this chapter, especially as we search for associations of somatic neurology with psychiatric and even psychoanalytical explanations *for* and treatment *of* the cultural phenomena of the time. The primary question for me is how social and political tropes became so effectively associated with somatic explanations of the functioning of the human body? Not only were researchers themselves influenced by the broader cultural developments of their time, but they coined new theories about the structure and function of the brain to account for the effects of such external, social and political influences on their research work. Some neuroanatomists even went so far as to look for the morphological changes related to the phenomena that they observed in both their patients and society at large. The heterogeneous field of *Nervenheilkunde* in interwar Germany instructively reveals to historians how these soft "external factors" became hard "research subjects" for the cutting-edge neuroscientists of that time.[7]

In this chapter, I address this *problématique* by structuring the narrative in two parts. In the first, I briefly map three specific manifestations of "modernity" that represented major long-term problems in Weimar Germany. These were not addressed exclusively by contemporary neurologists but posed social challenges to the considerably nervous Weimar Republic: There was widespread concern among bourgeois Germans that the cultural process of "degeneration" had intensified since the turn of the century, a perception that was also prominent in England, France, and elsewhere. In the context of Germany, it was interpreted as being precisely the social condition that had led Wilhelm II (1859–1941) – with his visibly "crippled" and "nervous" arm – to embrace militarism and push for war.[8] The development of World War I was seen to have accelerated the process of cultural degeneration by "killing society's best men in action," while leaving large groups of "crippled and weak individuals" behind.[9] There was a strong perception among contemporary professional elites that the German and Austrian people were physically and mentally "exhausted" from the strain of warfare, and that this influence would endure for decades:[10]

> For professional reasons we are obliged to support the terrible negative selection of this war in the interests of justice … The sick and the weak, the psychically inadequate are not suited to the strains and horrors of this war, and must … sooner or later be withdrawn from the front. But the more this happens, the more terribly the burden of fighting and the necessity of death fall on the healthy and vigorous part of Germany's male population.[11]

Medical patients were accordingly diagnosed both on grounds of physical exhaustion and significant loss of bodily strength, and on psychological grounds of depletion of their mental vigour. Veterans and war-injured were described by their neurological and psychiatric doctors as being left behind "tired" and with no incentive to work "in these hard times" immediately after the Great War (see figure 4.1).[12] Corresponding to the way the physical constitution of Weimar Germans was seen to have suffered from the war experience, "the physical constitution of the brain" now presented a medical concern that needed study to understand the devastation in which society as a whole found itself. "Negative selection," "traumatic injuries," and "exhaustive states" gradually assumed a material basis, even though they were invisible to the naked eye. Since most practitioners did not have high-end microscopes at their disposal, they needed to rely on support from the brain research laboratories of anatomists, pathologists, and serologists.[13]

After introducing these topics, I address the intellectual working contexts of two major representatives of the field of *Nervenheilkunde*: Viktor von Weizsaecker, a psychosomatically oriented psychiatrist at the universities of Breslau and Heidelberg; and then Max Bielschowsky, a highly prominent neuroanatomist and head of the division of neurohistology at the KWI for Brain Research in Berlin-Buch (see figure 4.2). When analyzing their research into the new human repair work needed after the war, I examine the ways in which these neuroscientists incorporated particular questions from the Weimar period into their academic research and private writings, as well as their social behaviour as members of the professional German elite. In addressing these questions, I map out the ways in which Weimar neuroscientists helped reshape current discourses about the perceived "pathologies of modern life," which had led to the catastrophe of the war, as well as the subsequent revolutions and economic downturns.[14] From whichever angle these medical experts approached the constitution of the mind-brain relation, they immediately faced the *malaise de la modernité*, which Canadian philosopher Charles Taylor (b. 1931) has defined as "certain characteristics of the contemporary culture and society, which many people perceive as a form of cultural regress or decadence, rather than a progress of our civilization."[15]

DEGENERATION

With its two million German dead and nearly 2,700,000 physically and psychologically mutilated soldiers, the end of World War I inevitably gave rise to overwhelming social concerns. Foremost among them were the health of the population and the treatment of war-injured soldiers.[16] To compound those concerns, the devastating social situation faced by the Weimar Republic – founded on 11 August 1919 – led to widespread reconfigurations within the medical system. These were particularly tangible in the emergence of left-wing Weimar governments after the war, with their emphasis on addressing such social demands as public health, which was of key importance to the middle- and lower-class populations. This shake-up in the provision of health care also translated into a differentiation between the military hospital system and institutions for veterans' health care, along with new cultural conceptions of illness in a more holistic understanding.[17] Irrespective of where, on the spectrum from somatic to psychological, physicians and early neuroscientists sat

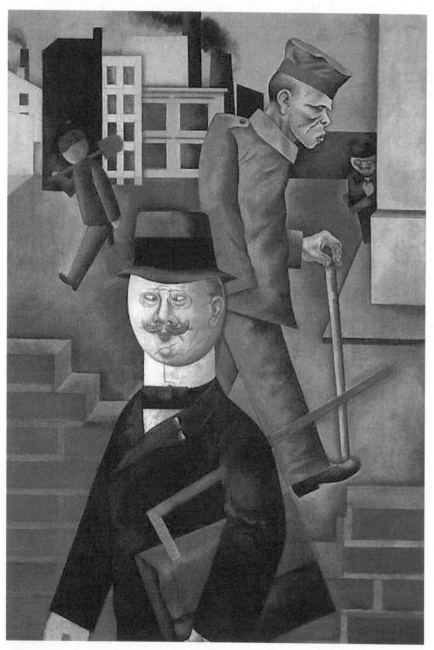

4.1 George Grosz, *Grey Day* (1921) (oil on canvas, 80 x 115 cm) (ART 564363 – 2088171) / 1921 Courtesy of Nationalgalerie, Staatliche Museen zu Berlin, Preussischer Kulturbesitz, Berlin, Germany © Permissions received from Art Resource, Inc., New York, USA and from the Estate of George Grosz / SOCAN (2019).

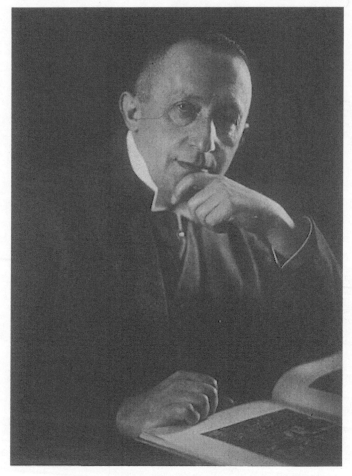

4.2 Portrait photograph of Max Bielschowsky (ca 1930) © Courtesy of the US National Library of Medicine, Bethesda, Maryland, USA.

in their views of the causes of the illnesses of individual Germans, the underlying reconfigurations were worked into the framework of "bodily and mental degeneration."[18] This dichotomy was also the subject of ongoing professional debates among psychiatrists and neurologists in the Weimar period. Different protagonists of the Deutscher Verein fuer Psychiatrie, such as the psychiatrists Emil Kraepelin, Ernst Ruedin, and Alfred Hoche, or the neurologist Oswald Bumke, had developed often-conflicting socio-, psycho-, and neuropathological concepts to account for the apparent increase in functional nervous disorders seemingly related to the impact of urban life conditions on modern civilization. Bumke's view was clear:

It is a most decisive fact that every generation before us would have been as healthy or as diseased, if they had had to live under the very same conditions as our life. This makes it less urgent to ask whether we have become a sicker [generation] or whether the specific nervous diseases of our times are more severe than those of our ancestors ... That *all* the phenomena of degeneration we are able to discern could be attributed to *external* and *social* causes is much more important than the dispute about whether nervous degeneration has increased.[19]

Following on the ideas of the Swiss psychiatrist Bénédict-Augustin Morel, the aforementioned protagonists further posited the existence of an originally healthy and moral state that had subsequently deteriorated as a result of an alteration of people's germ material. The important step now was that Morel's views became closely linked to the *mental and physical degeneration* of modern man and the alteration of germ material became attributed to the effects of modernization in general as well as to the economic working conditions of the 1920s and 1930s. In the ongoing debates in neurology and psychiatry, "nerve weakness" and "neurasthenia" even became a symbol for modern culture and found their direct expression in the bodies of the soldiers who had suffered mass deaths and severe mutilation "*vor Verdun,*" in the words of novelist Arnold Zweig (1887–1968).[20] Weimar-era discussions focused on the acceleration of the "neurasthenic" character, which American neurologist George Miller Beard (1839–1883) had presented in his monograph *American Nervousness: Its Causes and Consequences* (1881). Beard described the neurasthenic patient as having "fine, soft hair, delicate skin [and] nicely chiseled features," which distinguished this population of "sufferers of the better sort" as the "indoor classes."[21] What must be kept in mind, however, is that in this scrupulous study of neurasthenic identity, Beard manifested his own bourgeois self-identity along with the class of patients he treated in his private practice in New York City: white, wealthy, urban citizens, primarily men of the brain-working class, men of the "desk, the pulpit, and ... the counting room," responsible for keeping the engines of modern civilization running.[22] The medical conditions rife among such individuals were the inevitable effect of a new disease that was caused primarily by "modern civilization" and in return "paid for by nervousness":

Our civilization hangs by a thread; the activity and force of the very
few make us what we are as a nation; and if, *through degeneracy*,
the descendants of these few revert to the condition of their not very
remote ancestors, all our haughty civilization would be wiped away
... The lower must minister to the higher ... For every brain-worker
there must be ten muscle-workers ... The America of the future, as
the America of the present, must be a nation where riches and culture
are restricted to the few.[23]

By 1919 Beard's views had reached Germany at the height of its postwar
turmoil. They fell on fertile soil in the social experiment of the Weimar
Republic, as new forms of modern living were being introduced under
the prevailing conditions of austerity that saw the postwar hunger blockades and soon the massive effects of the Great Depression. Professional
and scientific elites were definitely thinking they had lost out completely,
as exemplified by the ongoing protestations about the high number of
injured war veterans. This is reflected, for instance, in Hamburg neurologist's Max Nonne's account of nervous degeneration in the immediate
aftermath of the German Revolution of 9 November 1918. In a similar
vein, Heidelberg professor Wilhelm Erb wrote a pessimistic letter on
2 February 1919 to neurologist Adolf von Struempell (1853–1925) at the
University of Leipzig:

I am not a philosopher or enough of an optimist to look confidently
into the future[, because] we have to envisage a complete downfall!
And this mainly due to the particular moral comportment of our
so-called "people," in all its degeneration, laziness, abstinence from
work, and craving for pleasure – with all its consequences for the
privation of coal, nutrition, and the state and order of the Reich. At
its top, the Reich is now run by a group of jackasses and weak idiots,
who only think about *discussing* political matters without energetic
decision and *action*.[24]

Arch-conservative Wilhelm Erb used his neurological training to frame
a social perspective on Germany's downfall. He saw the conditions of
modern life as factors that induced nervous diseases predicated on predisposing conditions caused by "bad hereditary stock." To Weimar psychiatrists and neurologists, the pathological cause of neurasthenia and its
related disorders was a matter of the quantity of exogenous noxae and
widespread pressures in the cultural conceptions of mental and physical

health.[25] In his letter to Von Struempell, Erb also used his professional background to diagnose the downfall of Kaiser Wilhelm's *Angst Neurasthenia* by painting a full neurasthenic world picture to his colleague. The circumstances of modern life, he wrote, were inducing factors on top of a variety of predisposing conditions such as poverty, immorality, and an ever-weakening general work ethic among the people. If it was a moral failing of the neurasthenic Kaiser for having led the German people into war, it was now a failing of the lower classes that they did not minister to the higher ones: society's best had died in action, and Erb's view was that Germany would therefore fall into the hands of the lower classes, leading to the ultimate decay of its society.[26]

This concept that a social causation could account for neurasthenia had been formulated in an influential 1908 article by Munich psychiatrist Emil Kraepelin entitled "On Degeneration" ("Zur Entartungsfrage"). It thus appeared only three years after the Deutsche Gesellschaft fuer Rassenhygiene was founded in Munich.[27] Kraepelin's discussions of social degeneration in this *ZfNP* article in fact implied a major shift of concern – away from seeing the social origins of disease as affecting the individual toward an understanding that saw the "collective culture" or "folk body" as endangered through somatic degeneration.[28] In "On Degeneration," Kraepelin identified a number of relevant phenomena in modern society that his psychiatry colleagues should more directly address. Among these he included the increased frequency of insanity, higher suicide rates, and greater numbers of epileptics and drug addicts, along with the decline in the general birth rate. Epidemiological data, however, were available only for some of these crude assumptions, and most of these views had been based on a preselected patient *clientèle* in the department of psychiatry and neurology at the University of Munich.[29] Furthermore, since this account was written during peacetime, Kraepelin emphasized the role played by alcohol and syphilis as agents toxic to the "germ plasma," which to him signified the moral degeneration of modern German society at large.[30]

In this respect, what could have been more devastating than the war, with its millions of casualties "negatively selected" from the germ line of the body of the people, as his contemporary psychiatric colleagues Ruedin and Hoche repeatedly and rhetorically asked?[31] Both had later taken up Kraepelin's legacy in institutionalized contexts and spread Kraepelin's views. Ruedin became the inaugural director of the Demographic Study Unit (Demographische Abteilung) at the Deutsche Forschungsanstalt for Psychiatry in Munich, after it was founded on 13 February 1917.[32] As for Hoche, he had always advocated for a clinically oriented form of psychopathology to accompany the promotion of neurology-based social degeneration theory. Before 1919 there had been considerable debate about the real increase in epidemiological numbers for degenerative diseases; after the war with its enormous casualties and disabled veterans, there was no longer any debate.

Earlier, in 1909, in his review of Kraepelin's work in the *Archive for Racial and Social Biology* (*Archiv fuer Rassen- und Gesellschaftsbiologie*), Ruedin had agreed with Hoche's skepticism about the value of available data on the putative increase of "nervous disorders" at the beginning of the twentieth century. With the end of the war, however, and with nearly three million wounded soldiers returning from the front – among them five hundred thousand with neurological and psychiatric conditions – this epidemic of neurological disease could not be denied. Likewise, the continuing discourse on biological degeneration was bolstered by an increase in the numbers of syphilitics, who became conceptually associated with the return of the war veterans to their homeland – as were individuals who suffered from alcoholism, which became a particularly worrisome condition among veterans as well.[33] Vacant work places and social roles were, according to Kraepelin, further filled with "below-average material which the weakened process of natural selection left behind in the arena of humanitarian activity."[34]

Since they believed that the process of "natural selection" as advocated by Charles Darwin (1809–1889) had been slowed down in postwar Germany,[35] Ruedin and Hoche launched severe polemics against social welfare programs during the Weimar Republic. In a Kraepelinian vein, welfare programs to them represented unwarranted expenditures because they lengthened the lives of individuals "of low value" and thus contributed to the deterioration of "germ plasma."[36] These psychiatrists also launched their negative agenda against another postwar development, although this volley had instantaneous social repercussions. They turned against the enactment of the Nationaler Rentenplan, designed to meet the needs of war-injured veterans. The creation of this program had been a considerable task. Basic numerical facts highlight the financial burden of this endeavour, since the Weimar government now had to cater financially for another 525,000 widows, and 1,100,000 orphans.[37] To accomplish this Herculean task, the Ministry of Finance set aside one billion, two hundred million Reichsmark, an amount that later had to be raised to four billion Reichsmark. This gigantic sum amounted to one third of the new republic's budget before the international stock markets crashed on Black Friday, 25 October 1929.[38] Under the Weimar government, care for war victims had been transferred from military to civic responsibilities under a three-pronged national system that was locally organized: the Labour Ministry's pension offices administered pensions, the National Insurance System facilitated medical care, and pension courts reviewed complaints and made decisions regarding the claims of individual cases. Supporters of the Nationaler Rentenplan had certain ideas about how the living conditions of disabled war veterans, widows, and orphans could be improved. Providing work in the general job market as well as in rehabilitation settings was seen as the most urgent step to help with the reintegration process of each individual back into society.[39]

And, while bodily mutilations could be compensated for – with wheelchairs, crutches, or arm-prostheses, for example – to assist reintegration into the industrial labour market, such accommodations proved vastly problematic for those with psychiatric and neurological conditions. Bumke had specifically addressed this problem in his book *On Nervous Degeneration* from the perspective of the Leipzig school of brain psychiatry and neuroanatomy (see also chapter 2).[40] However, the only criterion of value that he saw in social programs dedicated to caring for the conditions of "nervous degeneration" was that this group of patients would be brought again to the level of economic subsistence. He particularly emphasized that it was the strenuous occupations in the modern administration, communication, and service industries that needed the greatest attention from psychiatrists and neurologists:

It has not really been confirmed that the intellectually most demanding and exhausting professions, such as those of the lawyers, physicians, and financial tradesmen, would predispose individuals to functional nervous diseases, as many psychiatrists and neurologists have thought. Rather, it appears to be ordinary office work, which can be hardly reconciled with the earlier views.[41]

This claim had, of course, been around as a cultural thesis in the *Age of Nervousness* before World War I, but with Weimar it became the battle credo of the far right and early Nazi physicians. They repeatedly tried to marginalize psychiatric and neurological patients, along with the clinical researchers who actually tried to improve their living conditions.[42] It was the view of traditional right-wing psychiatrists that the social medicine agenda of the Weimar Republic had put the cart before the horse, in that it supported the majority of "degenerate patients" – alcoholics, syphilitics, and patients with neurodegenerative diseases – in its campaign against the postulated dysfunctionality of the social and political system. As champions of a highly politicized form of medicine, Hoche in Freiburg, Ruedin in Munich, and Max De Crinis (1889–1945) in Berlin scientifically spearheaded many of the Nazi social reforms regarding the implementation of racial hygiene means, spoke out in support for the segregation and forced sterilization of psychiatric and neurological patients, and seconded coercive psychiatric treatments in their patients.[43]

EXHAUSTION

For years and years this superior power [modern living conditions] had been active, and when strong exhaustion eventually set in, this was not because of the work itself, but because of the unhealthy conditions.

Rainer Maria Rilke[44]

Related to the central trope of degeneration was the discourse about the various forms that "exhaustion" could assume. Who could better speak to this than the director of the Kreuzlingen sanatorium and doyen of *Daseinsanalyse* ("analysis of being"), Otto Binswanger? He had also acted as clinical mentor to Carl Gustav Jung (1875–1961); and in his own 1922 *Handbook on Medical Experiences in the World War 1914–1918*, Binswanger wrote about the formation of psychiatric and neurological conditions:

When I found myself faced with the task of presenting our experiences of war hysteria within a narrow framework, I soon realized that with the mass of observational material available, I could only do the subject limited justice. We had never before been confronted by such a quantity of male hysteria.[45]

What Binswanger had in mind by alluding to "war hysteria" is spelled out in the disease categories of the statistical data in the "German Army Medical Services Official Report" to the German Reichstag for the years 1914–18.[46] These revealed that about 613,000 members of the field and reserve armies were being treated in military hospitals for "diseases of the nervous system" – head injuries, gunshot wounds, cramps, attacks of war hysteric, shell shock, and trembling, war neuroses, or nervous exhaustion.[47] Two major cultural issues were represented in the statistical picture of the most horrible circumstances of the time: first, the vast number of nervous system diseases could be seen as "a logical and necessary outcome of the realities of modern combat," as American historian Eric Leed has argued in No Man's Land: Combat and Identity in World War I (1979); especially the disempowering of human soldiers in the face of military materiel.[48] This was manifest during continuous artillery and machine gun fire, which rarely allowed for human decision-making or prior anticipation of the horrific attacks. Frontline soldiers felt they had no agency in their own fate, obliged to resign themselves to their almost complete exposure to "higher non-human" factors. Immobilized, they were consigned to passivity "before the forces of mechanized slaughter."[49] To conceptualize, research, and treat these conditions, both psychiatry and neurology adopted interdisciplinary practices from industrial management; one such concept with its respective responses was exhaustion.[50]

An ardent advocate of the aetiological position that organic changes in the nervous system were due to the insurmountable strains of warfare was the Berlin neurologist Hermann Oppenheim (1858–1919).[51] In his writings and political statements, Oppenheim drew attention to the fact that the Great War had been the first time in the history of all belligerent societies that a clinical diagnosis of "mass traumatization" had been made. Several of his colleagues concurred, including the dynamic psychiatrist Pierre Janet (1859–1947) in France, neurologist William Halse Rivers Rivers (1864–1922) in England, and the dynamic psychiatrists Sigmund Freud and Josef Breuer (1842–1925) in Vienna.[52] Freud himself formulated the change of perspective in 1920:

> The war that has just ended has created a vast number of injured patients and presented them for medical observation. This has also led to a decision in the old debate about the causation made in agreement with the functional psychological interpretation. By far the majority of medical doctors today do not believe any longer that war neurotics suffer due to organic lesions in their nervous system. The most sensible among them have now decided to exchange the term "functional deteriorations" for the non-ambivalent notion of "mental deteriorations."[53]

For Oppenheim, the mental deteriorations that the neurologists and psychiatrists observed during the war were an expression of the concept that he had already introduced in 1889 – the concept of "traumatic neurosis."[54] Throughout the war, this notion experienced a renaissance; in German and Austrian societies it now represented a mass phenomenon.[55]

Thirty years earlier, Oppenheim had already interpreted "traumatic neurosis" as a psychophysical reaction to severe forms of trauma, while the
disease itself led to manifest organic changes in the central nervous system
of patients:

> For the causation of the illness, the physical trauma cannot alone be
> held responsible. A much more important role is here taken by the
> mental situation of the individual itself, the shock and the concussion
> of the soul.[56]

However, Freud always discriminated between "traumatic neuroses"
and traumatic experiences that were influenced by a specific "mental
reality" presented through external factors such as injuries or war neuroses, which "scattered the former foundations of an individual life."[57]
Freud's aetiological interpretation in his psychopathology of neuroses
saw patients confronted with forms of deep suffering that led them to a
"psychological fixation" on elements of their individual past. He also
tried to exclude the neurological concept of microtrauma in nervous
systems, along with other assumptions of a "non-psychical reality" of
human traumatology.[58] As an important cultural trope since 1900, the
notion of "trauma" had grown to be an intellectual leitmotif in many
European societies and it emerged at the same moment that Freud was
introducing it as a psychoanalytical concept of what could be seen as
"modernity"; or, more correctly, the "other side of modernity," including
its vast social, psychological, and medical pathologies.[59] The trauma of
war, flight, forced migration, hunger, and economic depression became
deeply embedded in the memories of an entire generation. This collective
experience has been emphasized in historiographical perspectives on the
Weimar Republic and the rise of Nazism in Central Europe.[60] "Nervous
Trauma" – like its sister concept of "neurodegeneration" – became a
dominant theme in neurology, psychiatry, and psychotherapy, spreading
sentiments of healing and wholeness to other contexts and broadening
the various medical interpretations of trauma.[61]

In addition, the problem of the "objectivity" of trauma became of
particular concern to a number of disciplines, each of which intended to
solve it in its respective albeit limited way. Throughout his career, Freud
remained somewhat ambivalent *vis-à-vis* his psychopathological views:
"I do not believe in my Neurotica any longer," he wrote in a letter on
21 September 1897 from Vienna to otolaryngologist Wilhelm Fliess
(1858–1928) in Berlin.[62] By this time, Freud had abandoned his earlier

"seduction theory," which assumed that sexual abuse was a major source of hysteric illnesses such as traumatic neuroses; yet he now theorized that the genesis of neuroses was triggered by childhood "fantasies" about sexual experiences in the past. Thus, Freud's abandonment of his earlier psychological aetiology, which he had developed between 1885 and 1887, subsequently led to disagreements in contemporary communities of neurologists and psychiatrists. It is interesting to note that Freud held onto the concept of a triggering instance only in his theory of neuroses and saw a drive to repeat earlier traumatic behaviours in his clinical patients. In his psychoanalytical theory, this aetiology was doubtless seen to have had a real experience at its source.[63] In a similar way, Oppenheim fervently defended the supposition that the influences of war could have left enduring traces in human body architecture. Most notably, he defended his views at the 1916 "joint War Conference" of the Deutscher Verein fuer Psychiatrie and the Gesellschaft Deutscher Nervenaerzte, while manoeuvring himself into a stalemate of critique from his colleagues, many of whom had active military careers paired with strong nationalistic convictions.[64] For Oppenheim, however, who had been an accepted expert in neurology and keenly served as field medical advisor to the German army:

[It was] inconceivable that doctors trained in neurology and psychiatry, to such an extent, could disregard the effects of the war's violent mental and psychical traumas, and assume that they left only a fleeting impression on the nervous system.[65]

Oppenheim's view aligned well with Weimar's public health initiatives and social welfare programs, which envisioned mutually beneficial interactions to heal Germany's open social and political wounds. However, it is important to be aware of the dialectical nature of these arguments as well: as one contemporary doctor from a Nuremberg military hospital, the orthopaedic surgeon Hermann Gocht (1869–1938), pointed out, the war had created a new set of conditions for disabled veterans as well as German society at large. Disabled soldiers needed to be capable of performing the same tasks and skills as their able-bodied and mentally healthy comrades, so that they would once again receive commensurate social acknowledgment as "productive members of human society:"[66]

It is the restoration of function, i.e., the ability to work again and to accomplish something, that is of the greatest importance. This holds true not simply with respect to the limbs of the severely injured and their will to work, but also for the general public, the entire nation, and the state.[67]

As Gocht saw it, veterans should become re-attached to their work machines as soon as possible in order to regain their full social value through reintegration into the industrialized production process. With the economic crises following 1923 and 1929, however the postwar economy exerted its own antagonizing influences on social reconstruction. As acclaimed writer Erich Maria Remarque (1898–1970) later put it in his novel *The Road Back* (1931): "'It's my idea that we're sick, Georg. We have the war in our bones still.' Rahe nods. 'Yes, and we'll never get it out again!'"[68]

In such times of austerity the contemporary diagnosis of exhaustion was certainly not limited to war veterans, widows, or orphans. Exhaustion, in the sense of degeneration, became a widespread trope and cultural phenomenon in German postwar society, and it was frequently believed that Germans had given everything they could for the war effort. In addition to the millions of lives snuffed out on the battlefields, they had lost their hopes, aspirations for the future, and their physical health. Many felt profoundly fatigued and had no incentive to contribute to society.[69] "Nutrition" was likewise a physical and metaphorical concept that became associated with physical exhaustion too, particularly after the "hunger winter" of 1918–19. The Freiburg neurologist Alfred Hauptmann (1881–1948) summed up the situation in a letter to Hamburg neurologist Max Nonne during what he found to be a most depressive holiday season:

> I think it is the only way out that we now work on the creation of our new political life [because] the thoughts that those ganglion cells secrete, which are only nourished through dry bread, beet roots, or dumplings, are themselves very pale and smelly. I sincerely hope that the New Year does *give rise to some beefsteak- and lobster-thoughts again*![70]

The "healing of the war-injured" likewise came to represent the healing of a whole nation – a nation that in the early years of the Weimar Republic was on the threshold of losing faith in cooperative work and cultural community. War-injured soldiers exhibited exhaustion, laziness, and a general inability to meet the demands that the peacetime administration called for in the postwar reconstruction phase (see also figure 4.1). The prevalence of "pension neurotics" troubled the Labour Ministry's larger project to convince German employers that war veterans were generally capable of working in industry again, while also making employers aware of their patriotic duties to bring injured veterans back into their civil positions. During this process, neurologists and psychiatrists came to play an active role in perpetuating the dominant negative picture: Already during the war, they had been seen as symbols of authority in the *triage*-like distinction between those diagnosed as actually wounded and those seen as "malingerers" trying to avoid military service. Further, wrote Nonne, the soldiers themselves could tell the difference:

> Despite their severe mental and somatic wounds, I have only seen a few soldiers, who showed symptoms immediately after they had been wounded (up to three hours, before they were brought behind the lines), which could really be grouped with the "traumatic neuroses" ... That there are fewer cases of "tr[aumatic] neur[osis]" than during peace times is an effect of the whole situation itself: the other soldiers understand very soon that they have a coward in their group and will treat him miserably.[71]

The occupational practices of the German military command, during the war and the postwar period relied almost exclusively on civilian-trained doctors. The most prominent examples were the Tuebingen psychiatry professor Robert Gaupp (1870–1953), the Berlin psychiatrist Karl Bonhoeffer (1868–1848), and Max Nonne in Hamburg – who could only apply their prewar diagnostic repertoire to the new population of soldiers and veterans. Even though a number of these counselling physicians were themselves conscripted into the German army, they had received no special training in military psychiatry or traumatology before entering the battle-fields, military hospitals, and rehabilitation sanatoria. The German situation of clinical neurology and basic trauma research differed from parallel histories of shell shock and trauma care in Britain, Canada, and France.[72] In Germany it was the neurologists and psychiatrists who assumed the vital roles as decision-makers between life (for soldiers who could be transported to hospitals behind the front) and death (for soldiers who were sent directly back to the battlefields).[73] For many veterans, these physicians represented Wilhelminian oppression and were held responsible for much of the physical and mental suffering inflicted on ordinary trench soldiers. Veterans' perennial question, "Where are your wounds, *Herr General*?" was thus also turned against their practising and treating doctors in the polyclinics, asylums, and military hospitals during and after World War I.

The depth of these resentments against neurologists and psychiatrists co-opted into the military is captured in the anecdote that Prof. Nonne needed to escape from his clinical ward at Hamburg-Eppendorf hospital, since "the mob was out to raid it" in revenge. Similarly, the patient August Grundmann attacked and tried to suffocate Vienna psychiatrist and later Nobel-prize–laureate Julius Wagner-Jauregg (1857–1940) in the spring of 1920 in Austria, during a state of hypnosis. In a therapeutic session with Prof. Wagner-Jauregg, Grundmann had relived bad memories from battlefield hospitals and mistook his psychiatrist for the medical front officer.[74] Such violent experiences were not surprising, given the right-wing attitudes that neurologists and psychiatrists often proudly and publicly proclaimed against pension-neurotics, as occupational counsellor Adolf Becker (b. 1871) wrote:

The fight against the fear of work is a question of conscience of the highest order. The occupational counselor must act as the nation's guardian and educator in enforcing his program and, like a father, simultaneously use sternness ... and thus restore the mutual love and trust as well as strictness and seriousness that were once present in close family circles as well as in the family life of community and civil households.[75]

Irrespective of the medical and social roles of many German *Nervenaerzte*, the patriotic desire to heal the wounds of the war, diminish mutual guilt, and contribute to the growth of the Weimar economy was seriously threatened by the fact that the restoration of health and productivity in postwar Germany drained more than a third of the national budget.[76] During the subsequent period of inflation in the 1920s, Germany required a drastic expansion of its welfare and public health systems. Not to mention the burden that the budding democracy faced as a result of provisions in the Treaty of Versailles requiring Germany to pay the astronomical sum of 269 billion gold marks in war reparations. The gist of these developments is well outlined in Detlev Peukert's formative book *The Weimar Republic: The Crisis of Classical Modernity* (1989), in which Peukert shows how the costs of the expansion of the welfare programs hobbled Weimar's governments from its humble beginnings.[77] Exhaustion from the physical and psychological toll of the war was reflected in the bureaucratic and depersonalized circumstances of the hospitals and doctor-patient relationships. After visiting the metropolitan hospitals in Berlin, journalist and former World War I officer Willi Meyer (1858–1932) described these circumstances in a series of shocking articles in the *Berliner Tageblatt*:

The bitter struggle of the war continued ... behind hospital walls, where real life tragedies played themselves out, behind the barred windows of insane asylums, [among men] whose faces were now only deep holes or folds of scars ... men who lost limbs and succumbed to deepest despair.[78]

Not only do the examples of "exhausted" and "nervously degenerate" patients show what bad shape the welfare system was in, but they also are indicative of Germany's profound social crisis. In the Prussian State Assembly, for example, Herman Beyer (1876–1931), the representative of the Social Democratic Party of Germany on the committee for the public investigation of war neuroses – and former military doctor – argued that physicians who denied the status of "being war disabled" to psychologically traumatized veterans acted against the common-sense beliefs of most Germans.[79] In making the case for the effects of psychological war traumas, he attacked the biologically minded brain psychiatrists and neurologists who wanted to take war neurotics off the Nationaler Rentenplan because they could find no neuromorphological lesions or other organic phenomena that would account for the damage to patients' nervous systems. For morphological reductionists such as Gaupp in Tuebingen, Bonhoeffer in Berlin, and Nonne in Hamburg, the absence of clear microscopic lesions justified the view that "shivering limbs" were caused by predispositions, which they emphasized to greater or lesser degrees. At the same time, different authors ruled out direct war interferences such as grenade explosions, machine gun fire, or compression sickness due to collapsing trenches and bunkers.

As some neurologists and psychiatrists viewed it, the war had confronted clinicians with an "otherwise unprecedented spatial and temporal concentration of case studies," and most of these turned out to be psychological in nature and not an object of neurological treatment. West Prussian social hygienist and member of German parliament, Hermann Beyer attacked the somaticists in the hearings of the Prussian State Assembly, eliciting the following response:

The rejection of the status of war disabled made by Professor [Ernst] Meyer [1871–1931] of Koenigsberg and other doctors employed by the state is in the majority of cases unfounded and it runs against the sentiment of the entire nation. In addition, under no circumstances should purely economic considerations, as described by Dr Meyer, be made the sole basis for granting pensions to these sick individuals ... Our society should provide a feeling of justice for all those whose injuries are the responsibility of the state.[80]

Clearly, more than the social sense for compensation was at stake in these political debates, since Weimar Germany invigorated a *quasi* ergothera-peutic sense of trust, action, and recovery through the equation of health with work. Health care administrator Hermann Hartmann (1863–1923), who inaugurated the first meeting of the combined German Medical Association in Leipzig in 1900, wrote an instructive manual for evaluating doctors, providing detailed advice about health care, which all disabled veterans and their families should receive.[81] Hartmann clearly emphasized national healing through mutual work efforts:

The war-wounded and their dependents have suffered exceptionally under the nerve-shattering effects of the world war: their speech, their movements, their ability to feel, their inner being was funda-mentally changed through today's murderous torments to the body and spirit ... It is crucial to convince the individual war-wounded and widows to trust themselves again, to awaken in them the will to act, the desire to live and the self-confidence that they are useful limbs of the national community.[82]

In Hartmann's publication war victims were depicted as being deeply alienated from the social democratic view that their physical and mental suffering had social meaning and that they must be fully reintegrated into German society. But this view of political reintegration through mutual work was idealistic; it was also undercut by the turmoil of the never-seen unemployment rates which the Weimar Republic had to face. It amounted to 15–20 percent, or six million people, who were out of the work force by 1933, an unemployment rate that shattered the young republic to the core.[83] The impact was felt even in high military ranks. Representatives of the German and the Habsburg armies who went to the Fifth International Psycho-Analytical Congress in Budapest in 1918 discussed setting up a large number of psychoanalytically oriented hospitals for war veterans, but their defeats in the Great War and the subsequent economic crises in these two countries annihilated all these medical and public health plans.[84]

Already before the outbreak of war, extended research activities on all questions of trauma causation had taken root in the vicinity of Freud's clinical psychoanalytical group in Vienna and increasingly also in Berlin. These centred on an understanding of the different types of psychological reaction to traumatization, and their psychoanalytic occupation with the aetiology and pathology of traumas was soon received in broader medical and psychological circles.[85] Protagonists of psychiatric and neurological stimulant treatments (such as cold and hot water treatments, forms of sleep deprivation, and therapeutic electropuncture) became increasingly interested in the psychoanalytic treatment options of "traumatic neuroses." And some even started training in psychoanalysis to add this perspective to their clinical work.[86] Berlin neurologist and psychiatrist Karl Abraham (1877–1925), Budapest psychoanalyst Sándor Ferenczi (1873–1933), and Berlin social medicine physician Ernst Simmel (1882–1947) – who was later forced into exile in Los Angeles – became particularly active in treating war-related nervous diseases and traumatic neuroses. At the Fifth International Psycho-Analytical Congress in Budapest, these clinical researchers presented their profound experiences: "On the Psychoanalysis of the War Neuroses" ("Zur Psychoanalyse der Kriegsneurosen," International Psychoanalytic Press, 1919). The themes and general structure of the congress had been planned so as to mimic yet critique the 1916 "war congress" of German psychiatrists and neurologists in the Deutscher Verein fuer Psychiatrie and Deutsche Neurologische Gesellschaft – which had previously emphasized the malingering nature of the war neurotics.[87]

Conceptually, Freud understood many war-related illnesses as the result of a personal conflict on the psychological level of the "I" in his threefold model of the human mind,[88] which he presented in Budapest as a cultural tension between the moral and social values of the "I in peace times" (*Friedens-Ich*) and the martial "ego of the soldiers" (*Kriegs-Ich*).[89] For Freud, the psychological conflict began in the minds of soldiers, when their "I in peace times" realized how much they had been corrupted by the new "parasitic alter ego" that took possession of them. Freud's examples were frontline soldiers who avoided killing their enemies in the trenches ("since they were much like them"), but had to operate machine guns, heavy artillery, and grenade throwers, knowing that these would kill human beings.[90] While clinical neurologists and psychiatrists had substantial reservations about the psychoanalytical idea of a "flight into disease" as a psychological defense among war neurotics, it was nevertheless quickly received in the medical community. For contemporary psychoanalysts present at the congress in 1918, the treatment of the mass phenomenon of war neurotics represented an opportunity for the new discipline of psychoanalysis to work toward a broader acceptance of psychoanalysis in the public as well.[91]

However, as Freud later resignedly stated during the aftermath of Budapest, this could no longer be realized since World War I was soon to end with the victory of the Triple Entente. Acute forms of diagnostics and therapies for war neurotics were now no longer needed.[92] As a consequence of the exchanges between the neurologically and the psychoanalytically trained military doctors, many war physicians behaved like the field officers at the end of the war. For them, war neurotics were nothing but "scrimshankers," and physicians avoided prescribing any legitimate psychological or somatic treatment form to these shirkers.[93] While Freud had lamented in October 1920, during the Wagner-Jauregg law case concerning his being victimized by being violently pounded by a patient in a therapeutic setting, that "doctors acted like machine guns behind the trenches," it now became evident to some that neurologists and psychiatrists were becoming the very foremen in the industrial assembly lines of Weimar German society.[94]

THE PHYSICAL CONSTITUTION OF THE BRAIN

What does the brain do? What should it do? You know the brain ... The brain cannot do anything. They seem to understand: How can this heavy mass think? ... They have seen a human brain. It is a wet, heavy, and sponge–like substance of whitish-grayish color.

Alfred Doeblin[95]

The treatment of the war neurotics – "the degenerate psychopaths" (Kraepelin) or the "brain cripples" (as the Wiesbaden psychiatrist Ewald Hecker, 1843–1909, called the chronically ill) – by the German and Austrian social welfare systems was continuously traumatic. Their adverse experiences virtually mirrored the state of economic distress inherent in the new republic's health care programs. At each regular medical evaluation, which determined the pension status of the patients, most doctors told the war-disabled that they were malingerers.[96] Only grudgingly, for example, did neurologists and psychiatrists comply with German law in giving war veterans the pensions to which they were legally entitled. In fact, "war neurotic" patients became symbols of victimhood, who critically invoked that this was the "thanks of the fatherland" for enduring all the suffering in the war theatres of the Great War. As a consequence of the deep antagonism between war-injured soldiers and the medical community, physically disabled veterans began separately to organize themselves against war neurotics. They believed they would otherwise jeopardize their own struggles to secure pensions during these tight economic times. Veterans suffering from physical brain injuries – such as gunshot wounds, grenade splinters, or bayonet stings – feared that with their visible palsies, uncontrollable shaking, and broken speech, they would become similarly stigmatized as "hysterics" or "whiners." A schism emerged in doctors' psychiatric and neurological perspectives as well as on the level of patient advocacy.

In 1927 the Association of "Warriors with Brain Injuries" (Bund der hirnverletzten Krieger) was founded as a national advocatory organization. During their first pan-German meeting in 1927, the chairman of the Munich branch, the medical doctor and politician Willy Boehm (1875–1938) – a reserve officer, instructor, and survivor of a physical head injury – submitted a twenty-three-page brochure that outlined the types of occupational therapies needed to treat blindness, deafness, paralyses, and gait problems. Boehm went into great detail to reassure his audience that brain-injured veterans were special cases:

> To put it briefly, the subjective complaints made by brain-injured disabled veterans are the expression of severe alterations in the brain itself; they must be seen as completely different from perhaps similar sounding words that are produced by neurotics and hysterics. These complaints are often so severe that the disabled veterans who are experiencing these issues will never [in their entire lives] be able to overcome their difficulties.[97]

Boehm's booklet on official state medicine policies as well as later works offered ready solutions to the medical problems faced by many pension courts, as they tried to assign different rates to a variety of neurological wounds along with the appropriate compensation for individual treatment and rehabilitation forms. The specific demands of men suffering from "head wounds," rather than from "nerve injuries" or "nerve shock," were thus based on socioeconomic interests and necessities according to a general middle class work ethic.[98] Former officers such as Boehm and those veterans who organized themselves against the psychologically traumatized in the work houses (Arbeitshaeuser) for war-wounded soldiers made a strong case for the social acceptance of disabled men.

By 1927 they no longer stood alone because neuromorphological research had progressed and focused more directly on microstructural changes of memory-related brain areas such as the hippocampus, speech-related changes (as in the areas that Wernicke in Breslau and Paul Broca, 1824–1880, in Paris had discovered), or regenerative phenomena in the visual cortex. These advances seemingly added credibility to the claims of veterans and the group of benevolent neurologists and psychiatrists. Oppenheim had for a long time been the only prominent advocate of structural changes after war-related traumas, but soon many up and coming neurologists hopped on the bandwagon as well and helped create a morphological research program in the field of neurotraumatology throughout Germany. Researchers such as the Berlin internist Alfred Goldscheider, the holistic neurologist Kurt Goldstein in Frankfurt, the neurohistologist Max Bielschowsky (see figure 4.2) in Berlin, Frankfurt neurophysiologist Albrecht Bethe, and the young neurosurgeon Wilhelm Toennis (1898–1978) in Wuerzburg particularly addressed the regenerative phenomena of the brain in their laboratory investigations. At the same time, the search for a "psychopathic constitution" or psychiatrically relevant "degenerative dispositions" of the brain continued. During the postwar period it was clear to nearly everyone that the neurological and psychiatric conditions of war-injured veterans were of an often-changing nature, which made it necessary to find new concepts and expressions that could accommodate the dramatic differences between soldiers who had experienced psychopathic episodes, and others who had returned home nearly unaffected by any medical conditions.[99]

As Cologne psychiatrist Gustav Aschaffenburg (1866–1944), head of the military clinical department of psychiatry, stated in his *Constitutional Psychopathology* (1923), the "psychopathic condition" had to be seen as an "innate degenerative inferiority of the nervous system with abnormally deep and enduring reaction" to emotional excitement.[100] And this was clearly not a concern for clinical psychiatrists alone, since Hamburg neurologist Max Nonne had earlier pointed out at the 1916 war conference that this diagnosis would indicate an "individual disposition" (*einen persoenlichen Zustand*) to abnormal operations of existing psychological functions. With the end of the war, there were new rehabilitation institutions and laboratory capacities, along with sufficient human resources through the returning doctors, researchers, and laboratory assistants (see chapter 2 regarding the constraints of World War I on medical research), who again ventured into detailed pathological and microanatomical studies of brain trauma. Conversely, neurologists in the trenches had only had a short moment for the physical examination of the wounded, in order to exclude a possible "brain concussion:"

The soldiers ... who dug their comrades up from the destroyed trenches often spoke of their unconscious condition and sometimes [they] even had retrograde amnesia. In very few cases did I find hysteric monoplegia, hysteric sensibility disorders, mutism, or tremor, *et cetera*. It will be interesting for you to know that people with these conditions had earlier on (yet not always) been seen as softies (*schlappe Leute*) by their platoon comrades.[101]

Although the military hospitals behind the lines were quite different and usually allowed time for the physical examination of the patients and their full medical history, they were badly equipped with diagnostic apparatuses. Moreover, they lacked the necessary higher-quality laboratories and sufficient dissection rooms, as Paul Weil (1874–1932), a former lecturer of the Strasburg Kaiser Wilhelms University institute for anatomy, complained during a vacation visit from the western front in October of 1914. Weil wrote that he had seen so many patient cases that it gave him ample opportunity to build a large collection of wartime brain specimens. Nevertheless, he had too many clinical obligations, no technical assistants to help him, and neither a microscope nor sufficient time to pursue this project as a full-scale research program.

Weil's Strasburg institute director, Franz Keibel, therefore offered to help by setting up a military courier service. The service guaranteed that from time to time a few of Weil's pathological specimens from the front hospitals were secured for the anatomy collection at the Kaiser Wilhelms University. Yet once this material arrived, it could not be studied scientifically, as there were no research assistants left to support Keibel in his home institute. A plan was soon formed to preserve the collection until the end of the war, when physicians and research assistants could return and begin a large-scale postwar research program on the vast medical "field experiment" that the war had offered physicians. The working conditions at the Strasburg institute, however, put a spoke in Weil's and Keibel's research wheel; the institute heating needed to be cut back in the war winters. Only a few offices and the living rooms of the institute assistant and secretary in this huge research palace could be kept warm – and only by drastic means. The inventory of all wooden shelves, dissection tables, books, and journal articles was burned. Delicate neuroanatomical specimens soon decayed, while military pathologist Weil was left presuming they were in a secure space 300 kilometres away from the combat front.[102]

The very idea that traumatic injuries incurred through the effects of explosion pressure, bullet ricochets, and even head bleeding after hand-to-hand combat changed "the physical constitution of the brain" by now had become a subject that fascinated morphologically minded neurologists and neuroanatomists. Yet research was not possible. Wilhelm Erb put this succinctly in a letter from Heidelberg to Adolf von Struempell in Leipzig on 21 October 1921:

[Research] practice is almost put on complete hold. Although I could still work on this and that, as I have a lot of nearly finalized things flying around, I find neither the time nor the leisure for such work. The misery of our Fatherland, the sorrows about living accommodation and federal taxes, the incompetence of our state officials, and the abysmal meanness (*bodenlose Gemeinheit*) of our enemies are a heavy burden to me![103]

The scientific debate on whether such traumatic experiences had been "inscribed" in the somatic substrate of the brain had to await the further investigation and analysis that would only be possible in peacetime – during the Weimar Republic. Following the discussions about "degeneration" and "exhaustion" above, one of the key proponents of the somatic approach to mental and nervous disease, Munich psychiatrist Oswald Bumke, undertook a full-scale analysis of the notion of the "physical constitution of the brain," which he reported on in his address to the Gesellschaft Deutscher Naturforscher und Aerzte in September 1911. It was subsequently published as the chapter on "Culture and Degeneration" in his book *On Nervous Degeneration* of 1912 (*Ueber Nervoese Entartung*), in which he drew close associations between the mental and neurological pathologies influencing modern life.[104] Referring explicitly to the earlier contributions of Kraepelin, Hoche, and Ruedin, Bumke first surveyed the conceptual and empirical features that underlay the condition of "nervous degeneration." He interpreted the condition in terms of a biological deterioration of the species or at least the social collective of human beings. Like many other psychiatrists and neurologists of this period, Bumke posited a consequent accumulating deterioration of the genetic pool of the people.[105] In his letters to the Deutsche Forschungsgemeinschaft, he therefore requested further support for research on the underlying morphological conditions in the nervous system as they were changed by the immediate influences of the war on mental and nerve pathologies.

Another Weimar doctor who deserves our attention is the prominent psychiatrist Viktor von Weizsaecker. He is of particular interest for his efforts to integrate philosophy, social psychiatry, and neuroscientific innovations in his encompassing program of psychosomatically oriented neurology. Von Weizsaecker's high degree of cultivation in the arts and humanities served him well for his theoretical projects in neurology and psychiatry, which were embedded in a broader approach to medical anthropology toward his patients with speech disorders.[106] This paradigm now allows for a closer study of the cultural exchanges and interrelations between neurology and Weimar society.[107]

THE CASE OF BRAIN PSYCHIATRY: VIKTOR VON WEIZSAECKER IN BRESLAU AND HEIDELBERG

Already the unlearned mind can teach us that real help – and not repair – that a humanistic – and not a technological – approach creates the core value of medical practice. In the brain-injured patient, we encounter changes of structure. In each medical action, not the provision for any purpose but the human encounter is the centre-piece of real therapy.

Viktor von Weizsaecker [108]

The influences of the Great War and the Weimar Republic on contemporary therapeutic practices are quite evident in the case of the Heidelberg psychiatrist Von Weizsaecker, one of the most prominent and internationally acclaimed German neuropsychiatrists of the first half of the twentieth-century. Von Weizsaecker was born in Stuttgart and had studied medicine in Tuebingen, Freiburg, Berlin, and Heidelberg, where he also became an assistant clinical physician to the psychosomatics-minded internist Ludolf von Krehl (1861–1937). All throughout the war – from August 1914 to November 1918 – he served as a captain in the military corps and worked in various first aid hospitals on the Western Front. Certainly, one of his most vivid impressions had been his involvement in field trauma care during the gruesome almost year-long battle of Verdun in France. Weizsaecker and his physician colleagues were confronted by mass casualties and by unimaginably horrible injuries that they had never before seen. As a commanding captain-physician, Weizsaecker was responsible for the first aid *triage* program in his section of the frontline. He was obliged to decide which of the injured soldiers should be taken behind the lines for care and which ones left to die, since it was impossible to provide medical treatment for them under such dreadful circumstances.[109] As with many of his contemporary neurologists and psychiatrists, the experiences of war became a determining leitmotif in von Weizsaecker's subsequent work.

After the war had ended, the trauma model emerging from Pierre Janet's research in Paris became a most influential one also in the German-speaking field of *Nervenheilkunde*. Janet's trauma model was based on a cognitive dissociation of the influences of negative memory and the intention to emphasize specific positive recollections, following the trauma model of Sigmund Freud and Josef Breuer. Freud and Breuer had deferred the psychological defence strategies to the domain of the "unconscious," while Janet in return perceived the faculty of memory as a conscious psychological element:

> Memory is defined through consciousness and it is thus everything other than pathological. Conversely, it really forms the basis of the adaptation of man to his environment. When experiences are only perceived but not integrated into a personal narration, a narration that is both – a recollection and an action – but remains dissociated, then this is the absolute contrary of memory, namely amnesia: the complete loss of any coherence.[110]

In this definition, memory is complemented by actions and particularly patients' ability to recount and tell a story. Janet saw that psychological traumas would stop the narration of histories as well as the continuity of a particular personal character. Accordingly, in his view, severe traumatic experiences (whether psychological or physical) were those that could no longer be integrated into the earlier self-picture that patients had of themselves, and it was this inability to integrate them that influenced and fractured the patient's consciousness.

Whereas Freud had understood "a model of repression and unacceptable longing, and accordingly only found diverse hysteric aggregate states in his patients,"[111] Janet now diagnosed "multiple personalities."[112] In the planning of their therapeutic procedures, Freud and Janet also followed quite different paths. In their early practice and research, both dynamic psychiatrists tried to liberate traumatic memories in their patients under hypnosis, in order to gain access to the original trauma and make it available for their patients' biographical narration. Janet, however, less of a rationalist than Freud had been in his therapeutic practice, saw amnesia as exemplifying a vital healing faculty of the traumatized mind. Where Freud tried to identify the original trauma in "free associations" or the analysis of dreams, Janet went in a therapeutically opposite direction, actively trying to influence his patients under hypnosis that the real trauma had never existed and could thus be "forgotten." This therapeutic practice came to be known as Janet's "psychological amputation method."[113]

At the end of World War I, von Weizsaecker had himself become a prisoner of war with the American troops and, since he held the rank of captain, he was only released in 1920. Between 1920 and 1941 he assumed the headship of the non-autonomous neurological division in the department of internal medicine at the University of Heidelberg, where he inaugurated a specialized unit for psycho- and ergotherapeutic treatment of "war neurotics."[114]

Following his promotion to associate professor for clinical medicine at the University of Heidelberg, in 1922, Weizsaecker continued to apply for numerous chair positions throughout Germany, yet even as a veteran medical officer from the front lines he encountered a lot of resistance, since strictly right-wing candidates, and later members of the National Socialist German Workers' Party (NSDAP), were always preferred over him. Quite revealing in this regard are the letters exchanged between von Weizsaecker and the Hamburg neurologist Max Nonne, after von Weizsaecker had been rejected as the latter's successor in the chair of neurology. Hereafter, external reviewers, such as the Bonn professor of internal medicine Friedrich Schultze (1848–1934), for instance, might so subtly mention that Weizsaecker's influence was questionable: "I cannot understand his writings anymore. His stupidity (*Dummheit*) is too strong. But *clinically* [Weizsaecker's work is] still very important."[115] The psychiatrist Carl Schneider from the University of Heidelberg more pointedly complained about Weizsaecker in a letter to the Munich epidemiologist and racial hygienist Ruedin, dated 2 January 1935:

He [von Weizsaecker] remains very cool regarding our new movement [the Nazis], but remains certainly loyal to it. Emotionally, however, he is really not attuned to it. This has obviously contributed to the situation that despite his scholarly accomplishment, he has yet not received an offer for another position at an outside university.[116]

Von Weizsaecker finally received a job offer from a peer institution some years later. The neurological surgeon Otfrid Foerster in Breslau had died in 1941 and a national search had been on for a prolonged period of several months in which no suitable academic successors could be found. The local search committee from the Neurological Clinic at Breslau University continued its work incessantly to try to select an "outstanding and decent scholar being nearly as broad and renowned as Foerster," in order to keep the interdisciplinary activities of the Neurological Institute and those in the psychiatric clinic sustained and intact. After Weizsaecker had again taken part in the war offensives of Eastern and South-Eastern Europe between 1939 and 1941 – and thus proven his "loyalty to the movement" – his application was eventually accepted. He received the offer to occupy Foerster's vacant chair and was made an *Ordinarius* professor in Breslau. This position was short-lived, however; the Neurological Institute and medical school of the Silesian capital, like most of the city, was completely destroyed in the Battle of Breslau between January and March 1945.[117]

In Weizsaecker's biography as well as his psychiatric work, the nature of the postwar Weimar period, perspectives on the military, and a philosophical investigation of the meaning of the pathologies of modernity all came together. Most important were Weizsaecker's analyses of the shortcomings of modernity and the new forms of treatment that he developed in his "anthropological medicine." In this approach, he saw doctors and patients jointly as the subject of medical practice, and their mutual rapport became crucial to his interpretation of *Nervenheilkunde*, a position that he developed especially from his own experiences as a military physician on the Western front. He dismissed the objectification of "patient material" of the sort found in traditional medical research – which he saw as an ambivalent, yet complementary foundation of the prevailing healing enterprise. Weizsaecker also fashioned interdisciplinary methods from a range of approaches, received from Freud's psychoanalytical practice, from new psychopathological developments since Kraepelin, and from the neurophysiological findings by Foerster and others that he integrated into his concept of the "Gestalt cycle" (*Gestaltkreis*). According to the Gestalt cycle concept, modern medicine would have to be reoriented – while following the interconnectedness of organismic physiology, sense impression, bodily movements, and the adaptation to external influences – and its perspectives integrated in encompassing interdisciplinary ways.

Just as the Weimar Republic aimed generally at reunifying its defragmented society, Weizsaecker thought to transcend individual perspectives on the body and mind by forging on with the social dimension of medicine. This is most evident in his widely received work of 1930, *Social Disease and Social Healing (Soziale Krankheit und soziale Gesundung)*. The book addressed question related to the adaptation of war neurotics, the return of social neuroses in the postwar period, and the general interplay between societal changes through individualism and the devastating economic downturns of the period. Weizsaecker thus aimed to transform the concept of "mental pathologies," as introduced by American psychologist Granville Stanley Hall (1844–1924), into the notion of a "social disease."[118] Just as Weimar social politics and public health depended on concepts of reintegration of individuals into the labour market, and healing of the "public organism" through medical reconstruction endeavours (e.g. neuro-rehabilitation, technological innovations in prosthetics, and long-term care options for chronically ill war veterans), Weizsaecker's therapeutic work centred predominantly on the notion of the "ability to work" (*Arbeitstauglichkeit*), as he wrote in 1933:

A person is ill when he is unable to aspire for work, what he socially needs to do … Nervous incapacity to work basically means that the spiritual community with society has been disrupted for the individual person; and this case is politically, ethically, and religiously the most prominent of all.[119]

Weizsaecker's "anthropological medicine" was the foundation of his theorizing in all his writings about the hermeneutic dimension of "the meaning of illness" and the "ways of adaptation" of each psychiatric and neurological patient. In historiographical research, Weizsaecker is often understood as a "conservative revolutionary,"[120] an important concept that in research literature is still underrated as to its implications for the group of medical doctors, neurologists, and psychiatrists that had been trained in Wilhelminian times and made their first steps into medical practice during World War I and the Weimar Republic.[121] It is certainly revealing to see medical protagonists of his time strongly clinging to their professional ideals from the earlier prewar Imperial times. Yet, other than the apathetic characters in the famous novel *Man without Qualities* of 1930 (*Der Mann ohne Eigenschaften*) by the Austrian writer Robert Musil (1880–1917), neurologists and psychiatrists of the time proactively experimented with innovative answers to "mental pathologies." As in contemporary right- and left-wing theories, these medical recommendations – similar to Weizsaecker's "anthropological medicine" – were couched in a reformatory project aimed at "society" and "the people" at large, often still in militaristic language:

It can easily be demonstrated in many cases that the social community itself has been destroyed, i.e., its organic action-relations are
harmed, and it is this disruption which has to be seen as a major
cause for the development of individual disease ... We all know how
much faster this aim can be reached if the state decides to fight
unemployment and foster the rational organization of a civil work
force and an army, because this does away with all therapeutic
patchwork.[122]

For Weizsaecker, the early 1920s, characterized by the vast context of
war neurotics and physically injured veterans, had become a threat to the
"health of the nation." Medicine, according to him, needed to provide
ready answers to such large social problems; alcoholism, psychological
depression, and the effects of growing aggression were frequently encountered by contemporary psychiatrists and neurologists. His "anthropological
medicine" supplied a partial answer in psychiatric wards, sanatoria, and
institutes for the brain-injured, where it aimed at rebuilding the personal
self-esteem and autonomy needed for patients to become a part of the life
of a community again in war-scarred German society.[123] *Interdisciplinarity*
in this sense was not limited only to a new form of research organization
in central institutes, as I have already explored them above in the cases
of the Vienna, Strasburg, Leipzig, Frankfurt, and Berlin brain research
centres (see also chapters 2 and 3). Interdisciplinarity, as practised by the
Heidelberg brain psychiatrist von Weizsaecker as well as the Berlin laboratory neurohistologist Bielschowsky, meant an increasing use of conceptual
advances from outside the specialized and confined fields of their respective
disciplines. These became closely interwoven with the ongoing clinical
and basic neuroscientific activities. In this sense, the approaches of Weimar
brain researchers bore fruitful results in the *hybrid theories and practices
of contemporary socio-technical therapies and approaches.*

THE CASE OF NEUROHISTOLOGY:
MAX BIELSCHOWSKY IN BERLIN

The biologically most interesting part of the problem of regeneration is the
restoration of function in the innervated parts of the mixed nerves, which had
been destroyed through the breaking of their continuity ... Experimental research has shown that, in reality, there will never be a reunification of identical
fibres, and it has been thought that the key for solving this riddle would lie in
the extraordinary adaptability of the Central Nervous System.

Max Bielschowsky and Gerhard Unger[124]

As already mentioned, it has been quite common to place practising physicians such as the brain psychiatrist Weizsaecker in a framework of culture and exchanges with non-medical spheres of social life (such as philosophy, social theories, and political discourse). However, the circumstance that medical figures such as Weizsaecker were also visible public intellectuals during the Weimar Republic led, rather, to their clinical and research work being analyzed amply in research literature.[125] Major interdisciplinary developments in neurology, psychiatry, psychoanalysis, and other brain research fields, on the other hand, have often not received the necessary attention to be given their due as important processes in the emergence of the early field of neuroscience. In this respect, it is not a major challenge to place such important early neuroscientists as Adolf Wallenberg in San Francisco, Otto Loewi (1873–1961) in New York, or Sigmund Freud in London, who were later forced to emigrate under the Nazis, into the context of the social developments of their time as well. Their significant contribution to theoretical works in psychiatry and neurology was also profound for the cultural context of the time, through their intensive research on "nervous trauma" and "nerve regeneration." In addition, it appears imperative from a historiographical perspective to take brain histologists and neurologists such as Bielschowsky in Berlin and Goldstein in Frankfurt and Berlin into account as well.[126] How did they develop and change their working theories of the mind-brain relationship? How was the process of trauma and degeneration research reconfigured at the working desks of their laboratories, in the clinical wards, and in their neuropsychiatric practices?

It is a much more demanding task, in fact, to investigate how less prominent and more scientifically oriented laboratory neuromorphologists addressed nervous disease and the mind-body relation at the time. Since 1927, this context led, for example, to psychoanalytical trauma researchers no longer being alone in their research intentions since some researchers strove to find somatic correlates for psychopathological phenomena as well. Neurohistologists, in particular, attempted to analyze microstructural changes in the memory areas of the brain, via cell-structure investigations of the hippocampus (Bielschowsky's and Held's histological analyses), looked for structural changes in the language system (particularly Wernicke's and Broca's areas), and sought regenerative phenomena in the visual cortex of brain-injured patients (Goldstein's and Bethe's experimental observations).[127] While Oppenheim had long been the most visible protagonist of a somatic theory of the "traumatic neuroses," a group of younger and interdisciplinary-minded neurologists now began to take a similar position. They influenced an early research program of neurotraumatology *avant la lettre*, which strove to analyze plastic reactions in the central nervous system following the external and internal destructions of its parts.[128]

However, individual disciplinary projects had at first demonstrated rather loosely associated forms of cooperation (e.g. sending microscope equipment, slides, or laboratory animals and organ specimens to other departments), while exchange relationships with psychoanalytical and neurological research projects were often of a purely local nature (see also chapter 3). Anatomists and neurohistologists were often hidden away at their workbenches in respective departments or brain research laboratories – independent of whether these were small, such as the Frankfurt Edinger Institute, or large-scale institutions such as the KWI for Brain Research in Berlin-Buch. The discrepancy between public awareness of major figures on the one hand and early neuroscientists' contributions to societal discussions on the other hand was intriguingly pondered by Leipzig brain psychiatrist Paul Flechsig. In a letter dated 13 August 1915 to Ludwig Edinger he wrote:

When looking at the enormous tragedy of our days one does not feel interested in anything else anymore except the daily news and events … What is brain anatomy at a time when empires are falling to pieces and the practical necessities become overwhelming? I am strongly concerned that after the war has ended, no civilized nation will spend any money any longer on such a foolish problem.[129]

One neuroscientist whose research I want to describe in more detail, for whom brain research was not just "a neurology of disaster," is the Berlin neurohistologist Max Bielschowsky. For his predecessors – such as Oskar Vogt or the Zurich neuropathologist Constantin von Monakow – neuromorphology needed to be engaged in broader cultural and political discussions. Von Monakow had once said that the debate about "nervous degenerates" in the public health system was a "fight that has to be, it helps us to exist, strengthens us, and gives us superiority." His position was that somatic and morphological alterations in the human brain were due to hereditary, "degenerative" influences.[130] For Bielschowsky, at first, neuroscientific work in the laboratory was much more unequivocal and offered an intellectual "escape from worldly problems"; or, as he had stated, anatomical research became a "*Weltflucht*."[131] However, even for him, broader societal issues could not be completely avoided, since *Weimar's concerns poured through the interstitial walls of his* KWI*'s department of neuropathology.* In fact, during this time dozens of publications from Bielschowsky's neuropathology department at the KWI appeared in leading medical journals. They had been devoted to a penumbra of problems regarding nerve trauma, regeneration, and the surgical and medical treatment of nerve lesions. All this activity underlined Bielschowsky's great anatomical productivity and important contributions to the ongoing discourses in basic medicine and clinical neurology.[132]

In the wider context of the reconstructive and reparative approaches to the war-injured bodies of German military veterans, Bielschowsky, like his peer neurohistologists Walther Spielmeyer (Munich), Karl Stern (Frankfurt), and Hans Altenburger (Breslau), sought to provide specific somatic answers to the pressing question of the diseases of the central and peripheral nervous systems. His research was certainly not limited to neuromorphological research methodologies; in his private neurological practice he went even further to test the effects of rehabilitative and deep psychological therapy:

The biologically most interesting side of the regeneration problem is the restitution of function in those innervated regions, where the functions have become lost due to the traumatic injury of the nerve shaft ... However, experimental laboratory research has instructed us that, in reality, there will never be a complete reunification of exactly the same fibers. It is thought that the key to solving this riddle has been found in an extraordinary capacity for adaptation in the central nervous system.[133]

Max Bielschowsky was born into a Breslau Jewish family on 19 February 1869. Like many influential neurologists and psychiatrists of his time, he was part of a generation that extended the German-speaking field of *Nervenheilkunde* in a variety of directions from neurology and internal medicine, to experimental psychology and beyond. Indeed, his personal socialization into the flourishing Wilhelminian society of 1871 emerges as the major factor for our understanding of his particular relationship with the later political and cultural context of the Weimar Republic. Bielschowsky was educated at the integrative and humanistic Jewish *Gymnasium* college of Breslau, and it is no coincidence that the entrepreneurial milieu of the Silesian capital shines through Bielschowsky's intellectual background on many occasions.[134]

Bielschowsky had also pursued his medical studies in the culturally buzzing cities of Breslau, Berlin, and Munich and wrote his medical dissertation in 1893 on a cerebral "Case of Suppurating Perityphlitis that Led to Septic Blood Poisoning" (Ueber einen Fall von Perityphlitis suppurativa mit Ausgang in Septico-Pyaemie) with the prominent brain psychiatrist Emil Kraepelin as his mentor and Alois Alzheimer as his main supervisor at Ludwig Maximilians University.[135] He then pursued advanced postgraduate training with some of the most renowned brain anatomists of his time, such as Ludwig Edinger and Carl Weigert in Frankfurt between 1893 and 1896. It was also at Edinger's Institute (see chapter 1) that, at the age of twenty-six, he developed the "Bielschowsky silver impregnation method" for nerve cells, which still bears his name today.[136] The new staining technique also allowed for the visualization of structural changes within the nerve cells themselves, a technological advancement that fostered innovative studies of intracellular conditions in degenerative diseases. A particularly good example is of course the well-known disease form that the psychiatrist Alzheimer had identified and described in his famous patient Auguste Deter (1850–1906) in 1906.[137] Bielschowsky and Alzheimer had been in close contact at the University of Munich, the Edinger Institute in Frankfurt, and later at the Deutsche Forschungsanstalt for Psychiatry in Munich. It was therefore no coincidence that Bielschowsky had subsequently become interested in pursuing further research into the disease that Alzheimer had described as a "very obscure pathology of the cerebral cortex."[138] With his innovative research work in neuromorphology, Bielschowsky reached a better description of the pathologies inside nerve cells affected with Alzheimer's disease, which also subsequently gave rise to the international use of the eponym "Bielschowsky bodies."[139]

Although already well known in the emerging community of neuromorphological scientists in Germany, Bielschowsky, being Jewish, could not receive a full academic position in the university system at that time. He decided, therefore, to go into private practice in Berlin and to continue teaching neurohistology as an instructor at Friedrich Wilhelms University. This was also the period that featured some of his main clinical discoveries in medicine, such as the symptomatology of "Scholz-Bielschowsky-Henneberg diffuse brain sclerosis" or "Dollinger-Bielschowsky syndrome," with which he contributed to the advancement of neurology.[140]

In 1904 Berlin neurologist Mendel enticed Bielschowsky to become the neuropathologist of his private neurological clinic and laboratory, a very prominent venue in the urban science spaces of Berlin. In the nineteenth century it had served for training most of the specialized neurologists and internists who worked at the general city hospitals outside of the capital's university system. Mendel's clinic had raised the profile of clinical neurology in Berlin to a world-class standard and continued its activities until Mendel died in 1907.[141] With the creation of the KWI for Brain Research in 1910, however, Bielschowsky went to work with the Vogts and became the first head of the institute's neuropathology division.[142] It was one of the few differentiated departments that contributed directly to the overall research program of Oskar and Cécile Vogt later at the KWI (see figure 4.3). When joining the Vogts, Bielschowsky increasingly developed his neuro-morphological staining approaches toward an integrative research program of neurotraumatology. Many impulses for this endeavour may have come from his own therapeutic work with brain-injured soldiers from his private practice. Also, the exchanges with Oskar Vogt about the latter's therapies in hypnosis seemed to have played an important role in this respect, after he had used the method widely in different forms of psychiatric diseases. The research program of the Vogts on the development of the cytoarchitecture of the cortex (*Pathoklisenarchitektur*) under different environments and social conditions became further involved with exceptional elite brains. This involvement was most prominently represented in the histological analysis of Lenin's brain in the Soviet Union, into which Bielschowsky's investigations had been integrated as well (see chapter 1).[143]

Despite Bielschowsky's outstanding productivity, his laboratory conditions were quite modest in relation to the tasks he had to pursue to keep his research program going. These other tasks included the many forms of cooperation and duties necessitated by his private clinical practice. In order to facilitate his research work, Bielschowsky even needed to pay out of his own pocket for his two laboratory assistants in this "one-man department," which he likewise supported from the revenues of his extra-clinical activities. He continued nevertheless to work in parallel with his private neurological practice, while pursuing his neuropathological research at the KWI at the same time, before he was ousted from this position by the Nazis in 1937 on account of his Jewish origins.[144] The development of Bielschowsky's laboratory can also be seen as a reflection of the changing cultural concerns in various periods from the Wilhelminian period to the Weimar Republic. His main research interest at the beginning of the century had been the aetiology of growth processes of brain tumours, certainly strongly influenced by the fact that Spielmeyer, his mentor (see figure 4.4), was one of the most distinguished neuro-oncologists of that time.[145]

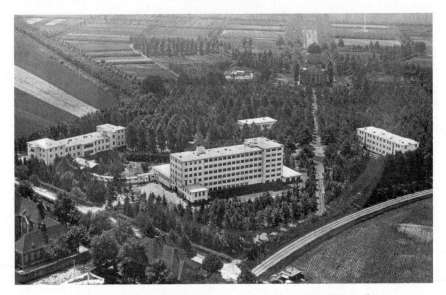

4.3 The Kaiser Wilhelm Institute for Brain Research, No. I/3 in Berlin-Buch, ca. 1930
(c) Courtesy of the Archives of the Max Planck Society, Berlin, Germany.

As recent scholarship on the KWG has shown, because biomedical research in Imperial Germany was so concerned about the insufficient knowledge of cancer – the "number one enemy of the state" and a burden on its aging population – additional funding was made politically available to foster wider approaches to oncology research – including the brain.[146] This concern about rising cancer rates and insufficient research knowledge into its pathologies became tangible as well in the "social organism" of the German Empire, which had extended its reach into the colonies of South-West Africa, Shanghai, and the Bismarck Archipelago, seeking a unified identity for early nationhood. This broadened social context subsequently included the health of all German people, now geographically dispersed, and defences against cancer and the tropical diseases, such as malaria, bilharziosis, and sleeping sickness, encountered in the colonial context.[147] Certainly, there was a lot of support both academically and financially for research work on cancer, even though non-surgical treatment options had to be deferred to the distant future.[148] These concerns and influences are prominent in Bielschowsky's *The Behaviour of Axis Cylinders in Tumours* (1906) and can be seen as characteristic of his own work along with that of many of his peers in neuro-oncology. Above all else, an adequate phenomenological description for

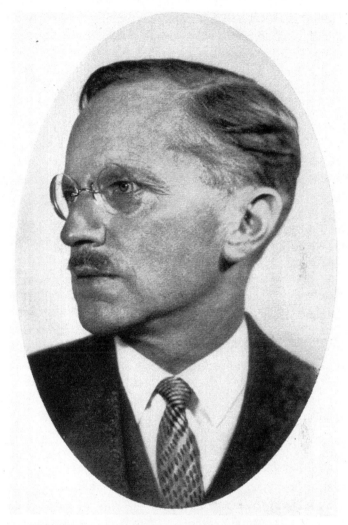

4.4 Walther Spielmeyer at the Deutsche Forschungsanstalt fuer Psychiatrie in Munich, ca 1926 © Courtesy of the US National Library of Medicine, Bethesda, Maryland, USA.

the differentiation between "normal" and "pathological" growth phenomena needed to be found, so as to guarantee better diagnoses between the morphologies of "good nerves" and "enemy tumour tissue."[149]

When Bielschowsky was conscripted into the Eastern German Army in the course of preparations for war against Russia in 1914, his research concerns changed. Together with Ernst Unger (1875–1938) – a pupil of the first Berlin neurosurgeon Ernst von Bergmann – and the orthopaedist Bruno Valentin (1885–1969), Bielschowsky began to publish on peripheral nerve lesions and treatment options in cases with microtraumas. Until World War I broke out, knowledge about traumatic nerve lesions had been largely limited to investigations from animal experiments. Yet many uncertainties remained as to the transferability of this heuristic knowledge to applications in the human body. The group newly formed around Bielschowsky began to establish standards for surgical treatment practices, with recommendations for when it was advisable to operate, when to interpose the injured nerves, and how to manage rehabilitation protocols. This program led to numerous surgical and neurological publications, which appeared between 1917 and 1925.

Many of Bielschowsky's more detailed neuromorphological insights furthered our understanding of secondary degenerative phenomena due to peripheral nerve lesions following injury. These observations had only become possible on the basis of Bielschowsky's staining approaches with ammonia silver salt solutions.[150] It could even be argued that Bielschowsky was still to some extent interested in the same kinds of problems as before the war, yet he now applied this practical knowledge to the social concerns of military medicine, such as the treatment of gunshot wounds and grenade splinter injuries. At the same time, it was clear that the general outlook of his research changed under the influence of the new context, where an emphasis on neuro-oncology (Imperial Germany) was replaced by traumatology (during World War I).[151] Here, we can see an important practical and philosophical shift away from the methodological concerns of an *Imperial neuro-epistemology* – concern with nutrition, metabolism, and cancer – toward a *World War I epistemology*, which mainly faced the practical problems of injury prevention, wound healing, and the restoration of function in the wake of the traumatic effects of war. Bielschowsky still continued his experimental work in the latter context, when he was relieved from his duties in the army's medical corps in 1917 and returned to Berlin.

Oskar Vogt had originally given the headship of the neuropathological division in his laboratory to Bielschowsky, with the idea that the latter would support his group-collaborative efforts. Vogt's purpose was to create wider interdisciplinary knowledge about the cytoarchitecture of the brain at his institute, and Bielschowsky now extended that mandate in the Weimar years to pursue cutting-edge research on nervous de- and re-generation.[152] Later, as a full scientific member of the KWG between 1925 and 1934 and secured by that tenured role, Bielschowsky discarded many of the duties he had carried out for Vogt, and continued working mainly on his independent agenda until 1933. Threatened by the Nazi government, Vogt himself now began to blackmail Bielschowsky in a letter dated 6 July 1933 to physicist Max Planck (1858–1947) on the leadership board of the KWG. This intervention eventually accelerated Bielschowsky's exile to The Netherlands. Vogt had been hostile to Bielschowsky quite early on, since he personally perceived that his division head did not follow through with his assigned research duties and align with the overarching program of the KWI for Brain Research.[153] In retrospect, however, one would have to affirm that Bielschowsky's research program did, in fact, tie in nicely with the scientific "pathoclitic idea" of the Vogts, since Bielschowsky investigated the basic submicroscopic changes in nervous tissue as representing changing functional demands on the brain and spinal cord. The methodological differences between Bielschowsky and the Vogts were in fact based more on differences in perspective than on lack of communication and differences of a visibly qualitative nature.[154]

In consequence, Bielschowsky transferred his research on "traumatic regeneration" from the military hospital setting, in the epistemological context of the Weimar Republic, to address "degeneration and exhaustion" in his exile in the Netherlands again. After such changes had become associated with the phenomenological observations of clinicians in the past, Bielschowsky and his collaborators offered the possibility of microscopically discerning how degenerative occurrences were rendered visible.[155] Bielschowsky's own investigations of cortical gyration during the development of the cerebral cortex seemed an excellent verification of a condition that the Rumanian pupil of Charcot, George Marinesco (1863–1938), had recently described as "pathogénie de l'idiotie amaurotique" in 1936.[156] Most evident in the identification of this new disease was the intersection of psychopathological phenomena, neurohistological changes, and the "physical constitution of the brain" – a paradigm for Bielschowsky's foundational concerns about the psychophysical interrelations with neurological diseases that he emphasized in the "heredodegenerations":

There can be no doubt, however, that in the question of what chiefly determines such diseases, the abnormal germ-line of the individual has to be closely observed. It is legitimate to subsume even those forms under the notion of heredodegenerations, which are without similar hereditary background.[157]

It was quite clear to Bielschowsky, in his ongoing preoccupation with the development of brain morphology, that this line of enquiry had important implications for nervous de- and regeneration as well. The rather pessimistic assumption about restitution after nerve lesions may also be seen as a corrective stance *vis-à-vis* Kraepelin's clinical school, since it embodied some pessimistic cultural assumptions of the neurologists, psychiatrists, and psychoanalysts active during the Weimar Republic.[158] With his laboratory investigations now placed in the context of "Weimar degeneration discourses," Bielschowsky began to understand axonal growth, neuroglia invasion, and continuous repair to be forms of "healing with defect." He shared this attitude with a chorus of neuroanatomists, who were as pessimistic about this research direction as they were about the outlook of Weimar society in general. A striking example is provided by the right-wing neuropathologist Julius Hallervorden (1882–1965), who later so drastically profited from the Nazi regime, after he had become the head of the department of neuropathology in the KWI for Brain Research and began to use this position to procure himself organ specimens from prisoners as well as later also through the T4 euthanasia action on psychiatric patients and people with disabilities.[159] Hallervorden wrote on 18 December 1931 from the Brandenburg state asylum to Spielmeyer in Munich:

> A visit in Bielschowsky's home and in our own institution in Berlin [the KWG's Harnack House]. Everybody is very depressed. And they all have the feeling that we are floating into a new chaos with increasing velocity.[160]

When trying to characterize the development of histopathological investigations in Bielschowsky's program, the particular context of Weimar culture appears crucial, since the culture of this leading brain science centre had been inscribed in parallel into neurology, clinical practices, and laboratory research. Bielschowsky held onto his KWI post until 1933. When the "Law of the Restoration of a Professional Civil Service" forced him out of that position, he fled Germany first to exile in the Netherlands and then, with the German occupation, further afield to London, where he tragically died in 1940. Bielschowsky's former position remained vacant for about five years, certainly because of Vogt's personal quarrels with local Nazi groups and his loss of the directorship of the KWI for Brain Research in 1937.[161] Eventually, in 1938, Hallervorden became Bielschowsky's successor as the head of the

Neuropathology Division. Here, some of the most questionable research activities were undertaken, such as the use of brain material of approximately seven hundred patients from nearby Brandenburg psychiatric asylums who were murdered in the so-called euthanasia programs.[162] Thus it was that concepts explored prior to 1933 contributed to the prevailing atmosphere of the 1933–45 period that enabled the realization of brain investigations. These investigations would not have been sanctioned before the Nazis' rise to power, yet they nonetheless built upon pre-1933 theoretical concepts, as in the case of Hallervorden's drastic eugenics and racial anthropology studies. Overall, then, cultural influences did not stop at the doors of contemporary research laboratories, as Vienna-born theatre director Max Reinhardt (1873–1943) so strikingly captured in his ambivalent *aperçu*: "What I love – is the taste of transience on the tongue – every year might be the last."[163]

Of course, the historical narrative of this chapter has come a long way; developments in neuromorphology were not confined to occurrences in science and medicine but were part of the highly complex circumstances of Weimar cultural life as well.[164] This makes it difficult to fully capture the tumultuous, agonistically creative, and in the end politically disastrous fourteen years – under sixteen different national governments – of German history. Most Germans had not favoured the early-postwar Weimar period at first, in which an external, victor-enforced derivative of British parliamentarism was mandated onto the remaining pre-war aristocratic and imperialist structures, belief systems, and prevailing public behaviours. Eventually, however, the Weimar experiment was accepted *faute de mieux*, being perceived as a generator of new answers to the problems of an increasingly modernized society and level of cultural life.[165] Given these antagonisms within large parts of Weimar society, it is astonishing to see the enormous national and international impact that Weimar Germany had socially, in the arts, and in the sciences, as many scholars – quite prominently historian Eric Hobsbawm in *The Age of Extremes* (1994) – have emphasized. It became a "centre of modernity" with its sharpened, bitter kind of creativity, paired with an intelligence unrestricted by convention that "hit the nerve of the time."[166]

I have described above how the welfare state and the health care system of the new German republic took shape around the *problématique* of "degeneration," within the specialized discourse of *Nervenheilkunde* after the turn of the century. It intruded forcefully into society with the public perception of the devastating causes of World War I and the returning "war-nervous" veterans. Our focus on the physical constitution of the brain has made it clear that those "pathologies of modernity" and "catastrophic effects of war" were seen by contemporary neurologists and psychiatrists as being based in the brain and nervous system. These structural and formative origins needed to be examined with new clinical, psychological, and even microscopical means. When looking at conspicuous proponents of the Weimar brain sciences – such as Viktor von Weizsaecker and Max Bielschowsky – the interdisciplinary merger of concepts, theories, and practices among neurology, psychiatry, and neuroanatomy becomes noticeable in the context of the larger social project of forming a group of experts for sociomedical repair of the human body after the Great War.

In a time fuelled by patriotic desire, medical doctors and patients alike had been expected to contribute to the common good of the German people. Neurology thereby became part of an entire system designed for social re-integration (*Wiedereingliederung* – the re-incorporation of constitutive parts) of individual members into postwar Weimar society. As such, in the medical areas of neurology and psychiatry, pre-existing concepts, approaches, and technologies from the Wilhelminian period became re-inscribed into the Weimar landscape. Disabled veterans, themselves quite reflective, both emphasized and criticized such continuities in the early neurosciences in the transition from Imperial to Weimar Germany, based as they were on the pre-existing status hierarchies, militaristic mentalities, and political roles of their physicians and therapists. Subjected to what they believed were forms of violence similar to what they had experienced in the trenches in France, and Russia before, war veterans in particular were concerned about the situation in the health care clinics of a capricious economy in Berlin, Munich, and Hamburg. They claimed that the state had persisted in brutalizing the physically and mentally scarred by relying on the very same physicians as had been active in the latter years of the Wilhelminian Empire.

Cultural influences exerted through the Weimar Republic had thereby no longer been confined to the "catastrophic reactions" of war injuries and their treatment. Nor were they limited to the peculiar *national style of Nervenheilkunde* that paved the way for various sorts of psychosomatic and holist approaches – as in Weizsaecker's anthropological medicine.[167] Nevertheless, substantial influences from the cultural leitmotifs of the Weimar period found their way into the neurological theories, clinical practices, and methods of leading German-speaking brain research centres.[168] Cultural changes brought about by the altered political contexts affected the work of experimental laboratories and made an intellectual "escape from world problems" (Bielschowsky) impossible.

During World War I special funding and resource support was given to experiments in regeneration, oncological research, and investigations of neuronal rehabilitation, while with the beginning years of the Weimar Republic neuropathologists had increasingly begun to occupy this research area from a "nervous trauma" perspective.[169] Of course, the parallels between the concepts of "racial degeneration" and "neural degeneration" should not be overdrawn, since investigations of neural degeneration and associated cultural metaphors from contemporary political discussions were noticeably linked with the programs of individual brain researchers, neurologists, and psychiatrists. Nevertheless, in looking more closely at the intersecting fields of neurology, psychiatry, and neuroanatomy, one may notice an ever-closer "culturization" of such discourse. Though known in principle to social and cultural historians of medicine, that discourse penetrated equally deeply into the fields of somatic neurology and the psychiatric segment of *Nervenheilkunde*, as seen in the most materialistic research discipline of them all: human brain anatomy!

5

The Later Weimar Period

Political Conflicts, the Rise of Eugenic Concepts, and International Influences on Interdisciplinary Work in German Neuroscience

The war not only exhausted us. It also tremendously exhausted our opponents. And from this feeling of exhaustion come their efforts to recover their losses from the German people and to bring the idea of exploitation into the work of peace. These revenge and rape plans require the strongest protest ... The German people are determined to hold responsible those who can be proven to have committed any intentional wrongs or violations. Yet one should not punish those who were themselves victims, victims of the war, and victims of our previous lack of freedom.

Friedrich Ebert[1]

IN THE LATE WEIMAR PERIOD

By 1857 Bénédict Augustin Morel had written his well-known and infamous *Traité des dégénérescences physiques, intellectuelles et morales de l'espèce humaine* (*Treatise on Degeneration and Physiology*), which was dedicated entirely to the social problem of "degeneration" and its psychiatric and neurological underpinnings. European psychiatrists, neurologists, and pathologists enthusiastically received Morel's ideas into their neuropsychiatric theories and for the latter half of the nineteenth century searched for the somatic and morphological alterations in the human brain. Swiss psychiatrist Auguste Forel and German-Swiss neuroanatomist Constantin Von Monakow, for instance, integrated Morel's approach into their views and began to search for the morphological alterations in the brain that they theorized were due to hereditary influences (see figure 5.1).

In this chapter I investigate some of the continuities and contrasts in the early eugenics tradition in German-speaking countries, where that social movement gained many followers among psychiatrists and neurologists. During the Weimar Republic, this particular community made the eugenics discourse their own program and integrated it into their clinical and research work, as the German Nobel laureate Gerhart Hauptmann (1862–1946) wittily parodied in his novels: "She answered him: Degenerate or not degenerate! Who could live free and easy, if we listened to you doctors and your diagnoses?"[2] Eugenics discourse at the beginning of the twentieth century was remarkably attractive not only to physicians and biological or social scientists.[3] Eugenics programs promised to redefine human morality and especially the modern soul. This prospect accounted for the fact that professional psychiatrists and neurologists were open to the implications of eugenics thinking for questions of diagnosis, psychiatric treatment, and the academic standing of their discipline.[4]

Eugenics originated from various sources in the life sciences and likewise addressed mental illness from a variety of angles: it was not confined to theories of heredity, but extended to physiological experimentation on human embryonic development, and to psychiatry and neurology, preventive medicine, sociology, and the population sciences. The individual case studies discussed in this chapter nevertheless follow a common perception of eugenics (or *Rassenhygiene* in German parlance) as a late-nineteenth and early-twentieth-century phenomenon. This is not simply for historiographical reasons but has the methodological purpose of mapping out the important academic trends in the emergence of the interdisciplinary field of early neuroscience.[5]

Quite frankly, biological scientists, psychiatrists, and social philosophers were not the only ones to have been influenced by ideas envisioning the "breeding of social elites." On the contrary, eugenic thinking was highly popular with many public intellectuals who specifically embraced the modernist critique inherent in its applied programs and their redefinition of the modern soul.[6] Berlin literary scholar Eberhard Hilscher, for example, has gone so far as to diagnose Hauptmann's writings as an instance of "the encyclopaedic approach of the Late-Bourgeois Epoch" of the nineteenth century.[7] Indeed, several of Hauptmann's works deal with the popular scientific discourse of eugenics. *Before Sunrise* (1889) (*Vor Sonnenaufgang*), Hauptmann's first major literary success, offers a critical

Zur Frage der B R A I N C O M M I S S I O N (Internationale Hirnkommission)

Die wichtigste Aufgabe, welche der Braincommission von der internationalen Akademienassoziation zugewiesen wurde, war , abgesehen vom
Austausch der Berichte, literarischer Arbeiten, Gründung von Hirninstitu-
ten und - Museen etc - gegenseitige wissenschaftliche Hilfeleistung und
Cooperation und womöglich planmässige Organisation der Hirnforschung.
Seit Jahrzehnten und bis heute herrscht nämlich auf diesem Gebiete eine grosse Verwirrung, ja ein Chaos. Das Forschen und Untersuchen war hier
lange eine Art Liebhaberssache und die Autoren - darunter Berufene und
bes. Unberufene begannen ihre Studien häufig ohne genügende physiologische und anatomische Vorbereitung, ohne festeren wohlorganisierten
Plan, oft auch ohne leitende, das gesamte Forschungsgebiet (auch der Psychologie) berücksichtigende Gedanken. Die Mehrzahl der Arbeiten war per-
sönlichen Zwecken, wissenschaftlichen Ausweisen gewidmet. Die Autoren gin-
gen von ihren Sondergebieten, von ihrer bisherigen vorwiegend allgemein-
medizinischen Vorbildung aus (Klinik, anatomische & physiologische Institute, Irrenanstalten), sie schöpften ihre Anregung von ihren oft nur
einseitig orientierten Lehrern oder aus der in der ganzen Welt zerstreu-
ten, von den mannigfaltigsten Gesichtspunkten (meist praktisch) und nur
Spezialinteressen literarischen Bruchstücken, und suchten so tastend
und ohne festen Plan weiter zu bauen, verlegten sich oft mehr auf tech-
nische Methoden und gelangten selten in ihren Beiträgen und einseitigen
fragmentarischen Darstellungen, die sich in fruchtbarrer Weise in grös-
sere biologisch zusammenhängende Fragenkomplexe eingliedern liessen.

5.1 Conceptual paper by Constantin von Monakow on the International Brain
Commission and the discussion regarding inclusion of a continuous committee
on neurology and eugenics, 1921. © Courtesy of the Archive for Medical History
of the University of Zurich; Monakow, Constantin von, Correspondence, Box 2;
PN 097.01.444 (Monakow).

representation of a dogmatic eugenicist arriving in a small Silesian coal-mining town where he witnessed the destruction of family relations by alcohol-dependent relatives.[8] Hauptmann scholars have acknowledged that the literary figure of the eugenicist in Hauptmann's 1889 drama was modelled in part on the German physician and eugenicist Alfred Ploetz (1860–1940), a friend of the dramatist from his student days at the University of Breslau.[9] What is less well known, however, is that this champion of the German racial hygiene movement and protagonist of extreme eugenics measures provided the model for a minor character in Hauptmann's later work, the 1913 novel *Atlantis*, which developed out of his initial visit to the United States in 1892.[10]

In comparison to the negative portrayal of the dogmatic eugenicist in *Before Sunrise*, the framing of eugenics in *Atlantis* strikes an ambivalent note, displaying a noticeable measure of tentative endorsement.[11] Common topics include the "tiredness of Europe" (*Europamuedigkeit*), the "ship of fools," and the dilemmas of modernity – also widely inherent in the discourse of neurologists, psychiatrists, and psychoanalysts at that time. Furthermore, *Atlantis* incorporates biographical realities such as Hauptmann's marital difficulties and his later sojourn in the United States in 1894. The diagnostic-utopian dimension of eugenics is reflected in the characters of *Atlantis* who try to find their place between the Old and New World, with Hauptmann covering more generally the present conditions of society and humanity. It is possible to see in Hauptmann's dramatic focus a positive reception of the dogmatism of American eugenics, as represented by American birth control activist Margaret Sanger (1879–1966). For Sanger, whom Hauptmann had not met but whose work he eagerly followed, the incentive for making contraception generously available to women was a eugenic one: "More children from the fit, less from the unfit – that is the chief issue of birth control."[12] And Sanger's double aim certainly paralleled a division of eugenics reform into positive and negative eugenics in the United States, a division that not only Hauptmann but also the German *Nervenaerzte* were to find appealing for their eugenics-oriented programs.[13]

Given these considerations, it would be completely artificial to analyze only the scientific versions of eugenics discourse in the German-speaking context, while discussions of psychiatric, geneticist, and medical issues took place in sometimes secret intellectual circles and networks that also spanned the Atlantic.[14] This is pertinent in Hauptmann's example from the arts, and it helps us identify some of the relationships that linked actors from disparate societal and cultural groups with one another.

Through his brother Carl (1858–1921), Gerhart Hauptmann became acquainted with the Munich racial hygienist Alfred Ploetz, as both went to *Gymnasium* college together – in the 1880s – in the Silesian metropolis of Breslau.[15] Ploetz, along with Carl and Gerhart Hauptmann and other Breslau students, formed an intellectual circle around common eugenic interests, which came to be known as "The Pacific" (Der Pacific). This acquaintance grew into a friendship and strong intellectual bond that lasted until Ploetz's death at the beginning of World War II. Soon after its founding in 1883, Ploetz's club aroused the suspicions of the Wilhelminian Imperial police as it was assumed that this new group – like many political associations (*Vereine*) of the late Bismarckian Era – was providing a source of socialist agitation against the leading classes of the new German Empire.[16]

In 1886 the Pacific association became the subject of legal action in the so-called Breslau Anti-Socialist Law Case (Breslauer Sozialistenprozess). A year later, Hauptmann himself was called to court to testify about the nature of his relationship to Ploetz, who had just left for Switzerland to escape his antisocialist pursuers.[17] Ploetz followed another Pacific club member, Ferdinand Simon (1861–1912) – who had become a medical student in Jena and now studied medicine in his exile in Switzerland, under the controversial brain psychiatrist, insect anatomist, and public health expert Auguste Forel.[18] A fervent opponent of alcoholism, in line with the temperance behaviour movement, and an early supporter of women's rights activists, Forel had gained a wide following among progressive students. By that time, he was in fact one of the most renowned European psychiatrists and he remained the longtime director of the University Mental Institution Burghoelzli in Zurich. As early as 1892, Forel had justified the sterilization of the mentally ill as a "national sacrifice" similar to "that of the soldier in times of war."[19] In fact, as an influential racial hygienist he publicly voiced support for racist and eugenicist policies in 1907:

> I was always of the opinion that there are too many feeble-minded, degenerate, and bad people, whereas there are not enough healthy, intelligent, striving, good, and socially acceptable ones. I am an opponent of quantity Malthusianism but a friend of quality Malthusianism, i.e., a disciple of a conscious and reasonable eugenics as it was advocated by F[rancis] Galton [1822–1911].[20]

In the early 1890s, Forel had inaugurated a discussion circle on issues of eugenics that attracted large numbers of anti-establishment thinkers from the faculty and the student body, most of whom were refugees or foreign students from Germany, Austria, Hungary, and Russia. It is interesting to note that, in addition to Ploetz, this group also included Carl Hauptmann, as well as, later, his brother Gerhart Hauptmann, the Munich writer Frank Wedekind (1864–1918),[21] the Basel physiologist Gustav von Bunge (1844–1920) in Switzerland, and the anthropologist Rudolf Poech (1870–1921) from Innsbruck in Austria.[22] Reminiscing about his experiences in Forel's circle, Gerhard Hauptmann noted that "at that time, questions of heredity had already been discussed widely in medicine and beyond in many other fields. Under the leadership of Forel and Ploetz, this was also the case in our circle."[23]

ALFRED PLOETZ: NORTH AMERICAN IMPRESSIONS AND EARLY GERMAN APPLICATIONS

In 1890 physician Alfred Ploetz graduated with his MD from the University of Zurich. He soon married Pauline Ruedin (1866–1942) – the sister of the later geneticist Ernst Ruedin (1874–1952), who was likewise trained as a medical doctor in Switzerland. During the same year and in a state of professional uncertainty, Ploetz and his wife emigrated to Springfield, Massachusetts, on the American East Coast. Here, the couple lived in a predominantly German-speaking community for four years, and Ploetz used the time to search for ways to realize his ideas for political reform. Cultivating his eugenic ideals, Ploetz was caught up in ongoing post–Civil War debates about creating better American citizens as a means of healing the wounds of the devastating intra-American conflict. To this end, he attended the University of Chicago for a time, studying leading American philosophers and utopian thinkers such as Lester F. Ward (1841–1913), John Coulter (1851–1928), and Charles Davenport (1866–1944).[24] From his new family home in Springfield, he set out on various exploratory journeys to investigate political reform movements in Western Canada and the Northern United States. One of these took him on a four-month field trip to the obscure Icarian Colony in the northern part of Iowa. However, the Icarian political experiment in egalitarianism proved to be a disappointment for him and, foreshadowing his friend Gerhard Hauptmann's criticisms of American society after his first visit to the United States, Ploetz blamed Icarian social "disorganization" on the racial mix within the community.[25]

Having practised as a medical doctor, Ploetz felt a great disillusionment with the limits of both American social reform politics and contemporary medical research practice. He had embarked on medical studies in Zurich to prove that "he could be useful to Mankind" but became disheartened when he realized that "the real gardener takes care of a garden full of healthy trees, but our work is directed towards unhealthy germs and diseased and pathetic vegetation."[26] He was forced to confront the fact that, despite many attempts, social Darwinist and proto-eugenic thought had not – from his perspective – made much practical progress on the North American continent. He came to accept instead a belief common among American eugenicists of the time, that modern society was a sickened entity, attacked from within by "sickly growths." Ploetz later put forward an image of human society as "a body made up of cells" (in 1904) similar to the picture painted earlier by pathologists around Rudolf Virchow (1821–1902) in Berlin, and emphasized that the health of the social organism as a whole relied on the health of its individual members.[27] He now viewed negative eugenics – a medical approach which, at its most drastic, included surgical intervention and forced sterilization in neurological and psychiatric patients and asylum inmates – as the best way of preventing what he saw as such dysgenic developments.[28]

Ploetz wanted to better understand the genetic ways of disease inheritance and means of prevention. After his exploratory journeys on the American continent, he opened a new medical practice in Springfield with his wife. In his free time he started a research project in heredity and began to breed chickens. As this interest in animal breeding and questions of heredity fascinated him, the wandering Ploetz set out anew and moved to Meriden in Connecticut.[29] By 1892 he had already compiled hundreds of family genealogies and, with the help of a secret German lodge, augmented this large data set by gathering family-tree information on the mentally ill, alcoholics, and "social deviants."[30] Ploetz was convinced that this fieldwork in one of the strongholds of the American eugenics movement would be crucially needed for the enactment of a wider social reform program. He envisaged this program as a way of guiding the competition between the races that had built modern American society. One of his followers described Ploetz's attitudes in 1924:

Ploetz understood the danger of a weakening of natural selection, and its counter selective (dysgenic) action. He also had a clear and full realization of the danger of excessive limitation of … the meaning of eugenics, and … *the study of the inheritance of mental disorders.*[31]

The work in eugenics and breeding, which Ploetz pursued as a temporary émigré physician in America was, like that of many of his reformist
colleagues and friends, deeply rooted in late nineteenth-century sanitary
and hygiene movements.[32] Both Ploetz – as the doyen of German eugenic
thinking – and the experimental biologist Charles B. Davenport – the
leader of New York's human breeding movement and later head of the
Eugenics Record Office of Cold Spring Harbor – harboured beliefs in
Nordic superiority, which formed the centrepiece of their ideology.[33]
Davenport developed strong professional relations with German racial
hygienists such as Ploetz and the physician Fritz Lenz (1887–1976),[34]
who was invited by leading American eugenicists to describe the status
of eugenics in Germany for the *Journal of Heredity* in 1924. Here, Lenz
explicitly emphasized common intellectual ground between white Western
Anglo-Saxon and German eugenicists. He referred back to Ploetz, who
had "noted in particular that the Anglo-Saxons of America would be left
behind, unless they developed a policy that would change the relative
proportions of the populations."[35] Germans understood the problem all
too well, since they anticipated soon being in a similar situation – with
respect to what they understood as the detrimental effects of the "Rhineland
bastards" (offspring from African-French occupation troops and German
mothers), the perceived increase of the Jewish population in major cultural
metropolises, and above all the "Slavic takeover" of the eastern German
lands. Moreover, Lenz discussed the devastating effects of World War I:

> A quarter of the young manhood of Germany remained on the bat-
> tlefield; another quarter, although surviving, was badly hurt in mind
> or body. Encouraged and supported by an enemy outside, Bolshevism
> spread inside the commonwealth [*Volkswohl*]. It is not strange alto-
> gether *that a baffled and fatalistic spirit has manifested itself here
> and there.*[36]

Ploetz's major textbook, *Foundations of Racial Hygiene* of 1895
(*Grundlinien einer Rassenhygiene*), which summarized many of his
American experiences from the 1890s, served as an important point of
departure for the eugenics doctrine in twentieth-century medicine in
Germany and abroad. In 1895 his volume was published under the title
*Foundations of a Eugenics: Part I, The Efficiency of Our Race and the
Protection of the Defective* (*Grundlinien einer Rassenhygiene. Band I,
Die Tuechtigkeit unserer Rasse und der Schutz der Schwachen*). It

introduced the term "Racial Hygiene" (*Rassenhygiene*) to the German and increasingly international readership, since Galton's term "eugenics" (the science of good genetic stock) had not yet been adopted into German. In fact, in the German-speaking context, the two terms were used interchangeably. Galton, who had coined the notion of eugenics in his *Inquiries into Human Faculty and Its Development* in 1883 and established the direction of the program in the English-speaking world, pursued pioneering empirical research that focused on the hereditary foundation of mental traits such as "intelligence," "addiction," or "criminal behaviour," before leading psychiatrists – such as Kraepelin in Munich, Alzheimer in Frankfurt, or Robert Sommer (1864–1937) in Giessen – hopped on the eugenics bandwagon to pursue their independent research on the question.[37] But while Galton had focused on rather general social questions, the new eugenic psychiatrists took a notably stronger empirical stance by analyzing the "individual preconditions" of alcoholism, poverty, or prostitution, and sought distinct forms of individual "correction."

As in the case of Ploetz, this difference in early approaches from eugenics to German clinical psychiatry may likely have its explanation in a growing academic interest in agriculture and animal breeding. As a matter of fact, before the term "eugenics" was coined, Galton had long referred to his principles as *viriculture* ("the development of manhood"), and frequently used the agricultural terms "stock," "breeding," or "strains" in his work. Such analogies show that the ideals of health and fitness were less a "return to nature" than a new cultural construct during difficult social circumstances. On the basis of his own field research on chicken heredity in America, and relying on his vast data set from human family genealogies, Alfred Ploetz further developed the opinion that a broadened understanding of general hereditary processes would also help eugenicists, psychiatrists, and public health functionaries to support the "best stock" of the German race in its multiplication. He argued that, "A well understood and thoroughly researched system of racial hygiene forms the basis for the highest super-individual norms for all human action."[38] It is further interesting to note that, although Ploetz focused on "super-individual norms" in a German form of national eugenics and privately held anti-Semitic views, he still included Jews among the leading population groups, and – before 1933 – did not advocate eugenics programs that were associated with anti-Semitic actions.[39]

In a similar manner, Ploetz jumped over his own shadow, by addressing a number of decisions that had tragic repercussions in his private life. Ploetz was so stern to his family that after his return from the United

States – in 1898 – he divorced Pauline Ruedin because the marriage had remained "childless."[40] Ploetz then married Anita Nordenholz (1868–1957?) and moved to the town of Herrsching near Munich, where he found a new sphere of activity. The couple had two sons, Ulrich and Wilfrid, and a daughter, Cordelia – thus bringing the family situation perfectly "in line" with Ploetz's ideas about the need for strong, well-educated families. In the early 1900s, Ploetz began deviating from his long-held socialist ideals and adopted the view that modern society could only be reorganized by following the principles of social Darwinism.[41]

This change is likewise reflected in Ploetz's 1904 launching of the journal *Archive for Racial and Social Biology* (*Archiv fuer Rassen- und Gesellschaftsbiologie*). At the same time, Ploetz became a driving force for the inauguration of the German Society for Racial Hygiene (DGR) in 1905.[42] In 1907, together with the Berlin anthropologist Fritz Lenz and the Munich psychiatrist Arthur Wollny (1889–1976), Ploetz helped to form a secret circle within the Society for Racial Hygiene known as the Circle of the Norda (Ring der Norda). This group was modelled on Forel's circle in Zurich.[43] In 1910 Ploetz, Lenz, and Wollny developed their secret circle into the intellectual and likewise athletic "Archery Club" of Munich (Bogenclub Muenchen), which would become the second most influential private circle in the German eugenics movement until the advent of the "Third Reich." All these secret, lodge-like associations were created around the accepted idea of "saving the Nordic Race" (*"zur Rettung der nordischen Rasse"*) and were formed to promote "Nordic Thought" and often health and gymnastic activities (*Leibesuebungen*) in what was seen as the field of Nordic-Germanic racial hygiene.[44]

The virulent eugenic views of the Archery Club were later integrated into the political "Expert Council for Population- and Racial Politics" (Sachverstaendigenbeirat fuer Bevoelkerungs- und Rassenpolitik), which Wilhelm Frick (1877–1946), as the minister of the interior of the Reich, inaugurated in 1933. Ploetz, Lenz, and the Freiburg anthropologist Hans F.K. Guenther (1891–1968), as well as the Munich psychiatrist Ernst Ruedin, who had by then joined the Deutsche Forschungsanstalt for Psychiatry, were members of the subcommittee of this council, the "Working Group on Racial Hygiene and Racial Politics" (Arbeitsgemeinschaft fuer Rassenhygiene und Rassenpolitik: AG II).[45] It also had the task of scrutinizing proposals for new laws before they were reviewed by political decision-makers in the chambers of the Reich.[46] Ploetz's case and the activities of the Division on Racial Hygiene and Racial Politics demonstrate that by the end of the 1920s, eugenic assumptions had at their core a social diagnostic approach that conceived of the human biological condition as both the principal source of many political problems and the means by which these ills could be medically cured. The materialist analysis of that kind of *scientific socialism* evaluated political struggles mainly in terms of economic relations.

By contrast, the eugenicist critique of modern society – as argued by Forel in Switzerland and Ploetz in Germany – increasingly perceived social ills in terms of the sickly, degenerate, or moribund strains in the "social body" of Western cultures. It sought to formulate medical and therapeutic suggestions as to how the vitality of the national body could be restored irrespective of altered transatlantic transfers. The natural body, as it came to be idealized in eugenic discourse, could only be achieved by undoing civilization's ill effects, an undertaking for which international psychiatrists like Kraepelin, Alzheimer, or Ruedin in Germany, Adolf Meyer (1866–1950) at Johns Hopkins University, and G. Alder Blumer (1857–1940) at the Canton Asylum in South Dakota in the United States, as well as Charles Kirk Clarke (1857–1924)[47] from the Toronto General Hospital in Canada, were eager to come forward with public health solutions.[48] To them, eugenic thinking offered an opportunity to prove the legitimacy of their discipline in its fundamental striving for professional acceptance, especially in its competition with neurology and internal medicine. The related trope of "degeneracy" often referred to the cramped housing conditions in major industrialized cities, poor diet due to the prevalent alcoholism of the urban proletariat, and the aristocratic inbreeding and physical inactivity of the idle rich.[49]

Fundamental to eugenic discourse was the idea that culture, society, and the nation should be regarded as an organism that was subject to mental debilities as well as economic and social decay. The deployment of social-organic models in eugenics discourse and psychiatric applications has already been well documented in the scholarly literature.[50] This reflects a broader tendency of evoking natural and organic models as an idealized corrective to fragmented modern lifeworlds. Eugenicists generally understood their mission as a medical one; that is, the prevention and cure of individual and societal diseases, and psychiatrists as well as neurologists were no exception to that rule.[51] Independent of the political, medical, or psychiatric approaches, eugenic programs came to be viewed not simply as therapeutic measures for individuals but also in terms of Ploetz's *Rassenhygiene*, as holding the solution to the "political responsibility for the causal problem."[52]

EUGENICS, PSYCHIATRY,
AND TRANSATLANTIC TRANSFERS

The years from the 1890s forward were watershed years in the development of neurology and psychiatry in the German-speaking context, a period in which both areas were still seen as one and the same discipline or institutionally belonging to the broadly encompassing field of internal medicine.[53] As a number of German and Austrian medical historians (such as Heinz-Peter Schmiedebach, Wolfgang Eckart, and Hans-Georg Hofer) have pointed out, the cultural diagnosis of "growing nervousness" was a popular trope when explaining the rivalry between psychiatry and neurology in Germany and Austria by the late nineteenth century.[54] Although that has become a fairly accepted view, it is valuable to note that "nervousness" has rather been associated with the psychiatric or even psychological part of the integrative field of *Nervenheilkunde*. While American psychiatry and neurology had already split into two separate fields by 1874, *Nervenheilkunde* in Germany continued right into the Weimar Republic to include most psychiatrists and a great number of doctors and researchers in internal medicine. In Munich, for instance, the teaching and treatment of neurological diseases was later pursued under the direction of Bumke in the psychiatric clinic, which also comprised the representation of neurology from 1924 onward. However, it wasn't until 1925 that the Heckscher Asylum was created as the first neurological hospital in Munich, thanks to a large endowment from a German-American philanthropist in recognition of the needs of brain-injured war veterans.[55] It therefore comes as no surprise that the Heidelberg neurologist Wilhelm Erb, one of the foremost protagonists of his discipline, had earlier used the terms "nervousness" and "nervous degeneration" interchangeably in his central academic address "On the Growing Nervousness of our Time" in 1893.[56]

When Erb gave this lecture as principal (*Rektor*) of Heidelberg University, he addressed the issue of "nervous degeneration" at the height of cultural restoration in the Wilhelminian Empire.[57] Erb's statement can serve as a guiding perspective for the second part of this chapter, in which I examine the postulated material changes in the brain that contemporary psychiatric discourse associated with "nervous degeneration." It must be noted that this view not only reflected psychiatrists' professional assumptions, but a prevalent opinion among bourgeois Germans that "cultural degeneration" had rapidly increased since the turn of the century.[58] In the same context, a stronger concern for the individual body resulted in widespread medical reconfigurations, programs to sustain public health, and new cultural conceptions of psychiatric illness. Irrespective of the somatic or psychological pole of this spectrum, the specific medical reconfigurations took place in a discursive framework about "bodily and mental degeneration."[59]

For neurologists and psychiatrists alike, this was to have a continuing dimension until the first decade of the twentieth century when different proponents of the Deutscher Verein fuer Psychiatrie – such as Kraepelin and Ruedin from Munich, Hoche from Freiburg, or Bumke from Leipzig – entered a debate concerning what they thought to be as an increase in "functional nervous disorders." This proto-eugenic view had been around in the Central European discussion since the time of Bénédict Augustin Morel (see chapter 4).[60] Morel's highly influential volume presented a comprehensive theory of the causes and the aetiology of the variability of social traits, psychological behaviour, and mental illness.[61] His *Traité des dégénérescences physiques, intellectuelles et morales de l'espèce humaine et de ces causes qui produisent ces variétés maladives* (1857–58) widely influenced clinical and brain psychiatrists who believed it would help prove that mental diseases had a somatic basis and that clinical psychiatry would be socially and politically useful.[62] In the German-speaking countries, this argument also contributed to efforts to achieve the goal of professionalizing clinical psychiatry and garnering its full independence from its neighbouring disciplines.[63]

It is interesting to note, however, that not only psychiatrists but also a number of related scientific approaches were influenced by the broader scientific context of degeneration theories (*théories de dégénérescence*).[64] This is striking, for example, in the works of the German-speaking Auguste Forel and the neuroanatomist Constantin Von Monakow from the University of Zurich. Both physicians integrated Morel's approach into their theoretical pathology and increasingly began to search for morphological alterations in the human brain due to hereditary influences. Primary for Monakow, in this regard, was the biological picture of an ongoing struggle for survival "that has to be, it helps us to exist, strengthens us, and gives us superiority" – not the least in regard to what he saw as "nervous degenerates."[65] The contentious issue of "mental and physical degeneration" became more prominent in the first two decades of the twentieth century, during what Radkau has called *The Age of Nervousness* between the times of Bismarck and the National Socialist period.[66]

In a situation similar to that which Ploetz and others encountered in the United States, professional elites were almost obsessed with the idea that they had lost social control – a view that gained widespread currency after Imperial Germany was defeated in 1918.[67] This argument had been prominently formulated in Kraepelin's famous article "On Degeneration," which appeared in 1908, long before the outbreak of war.[68] Until now, few researchers have taken notice that Kraepelin's interest in "nervous degeneration" and possible eugenic solutions actually arose in close communication with the bacteriologist Max Gruber (1853–1927) at the Munich Institute for Hygiene.[69] As with many of the other leading eugenicists in Germany, Gruber was personally connected with American eugenics societies, thanks to his former activities as a Habsburg consul in America. In fact, Gruber and Kraepelin mutually published *Wall Charts on the Alcohol Question* (*Wandtafeln zur Alkoholfrage*, Munich 1911), which went on travelling exhibitions, were used in public health campaigns, and appeared in the popular Hygiene Display of 1911 in Dresden. Gruber had been in close contact with the prominent medical publisher Julius Friedrich Lehmann (1864–1935), the latter being instrumental in the creation of the Munich circle of racial hygienists.[70] Furthermore, he made students acquainted with the development of eugenics in the United States through a well-known textbook, *Reproduction, Heredity, Racial Hygiene* (1911). In the same year, he delivered an influential address to the Deutsche Gesellschaft fuer Rassenhygiene – comprising twenty-one psychiatrists, thirty-one physicians and twelve biologists – in which he examined the falling birthrate in terms of eugenic arguments.[71]

Gruber's views actually implied a major shift in concern away from the social origins of mental disease, as impinging on or affecting the individual, toward a biological perspective that envisaged modern changes in the "folk body" directly altering the population's genetic make-up. Gruber complained especially that racial hygiene was "still so unaccomplished and the general public not willing to accept sterilization as a respective means for the betterment of the race."[72] In his landmark publication "*On Degeneration*" ("*Ueber Entartung*") Kraepelin, the doyen of German clinical psychiatry, identified a number of medically relevant phenomena caused by modern society which, he argued, had to be addressed solely by psychiatrists and neurologists.[73] These included an increased frequency of insanity, a higher suicide rate, rising numbers of drug addicts, and a decline in the general birth rate. In this respect, what could have been more devastating than the 1914–18 war, with its millions of casualties that translated into a negative selection from the *germ line* ("gene pool"), as this became interpreted by his psychiatric colleagues Ruedin and Hoche (see also figure 5.2).

By explicitly formulating a psychopathology- and neurology-based degeneration hypothesis, Ruedin, as the director of the demographic study unit (*Demographische Abteilung*) at the Deutsche Forschungsanstalt for Psychiatry in Munich, and Hoche, as director of the clinical department of psychiatry at the University of Freiburg, continued Kraepelin's legacy.[74] For those still at work in university mental hospitals, there was much frustration with the progress of psychiatric and neurological research and lack of new therapeutic options, while they increasingly sought help and support from "negative eugenics" in conditions of "hereditary or early childhood degeneration of the brain:"

> For the non-physician it must be pointed out that conditions of "mental death" have to be faced in [this] group, in the dementia-associated changes of the brain, in conditions that lay people call the softening of the brain, in dementia paralytica ... juvenile dementia praecox – in which a great number of patients reach most advanced states of imbecility – and in the gross morphological changes of the brain.[75]

SOCIAL PROBLEMS, EXTERNAL RESEARCH SUPPORT, AND THE EMERGENCE OF BRAIN PSYCHIATRY

Whereas before 1919 there had been considerable debate among neurologists, psychiatrists, and other physicians about the increase in the numbers and the diagnoses to be included in the group of so-called "degenerate patients," by the end of the war the widespread phenomenon had now become apparent to society at large. Among the disabled soldiers who returned from the fronts, approximately five hundred thousand displayed specific neurological and psychiatric conditions, a drastic situation beyond any doubt.[76] Since they saw that the Darwinian process of "natural selection" had decelerated in postwar Germany, physicians and anthropologists such as Ploetz came to perceive the health situation of the German people as "badly hurt in mind or body."[77] Ruedin and Hoche, who had launched severe polemics against the social welfare programs before the Weimar Republic, now became even more agitated. In a Kraepelinian vein, both psychiatrists saw such programs as unwarranted expenditures because they would secure the longevity of "low value" populations that negatively

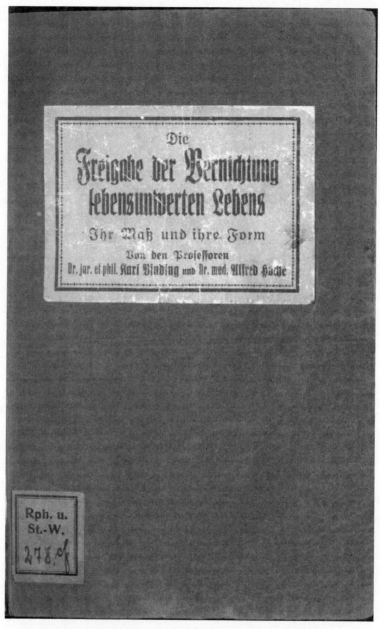

5.2 Karl Binding and Alfred Hoche. *Die Freigabe der Vernichtung lebensunwerten Lebens. Ihr Mass und ihre Form.* Leipzig, Germany: Johann Ambrosius Barth, 1920. © Book cover courtesy of the Saechsische Landesbibliothek, Dresden, Saxony, Germany (s l u b; https://digital.ub.uni-leipzig.de/mirador/index.php#3c290429-cf9b-4ce8-b109-8a38dd7a95dc).

contributed to the "germplasm."[78] The resulting increase in the numbers of the psychiatrically and neurologically ill would, they stated, lead "to an unacceptable burden for the welfare state, especially as so little [was] currently known about the treatment and long-term development of these conditions."[79] Their criticism was also directed at the Nationaler Rentenplan, which had been designed to meet the needs of the vast army of war-injured veterans returning back from the fronts after 1918 (see figure 4.1).[80]

While somatic injuries and bodily mutilations could be compensated with wheelchairs, crutches, and arm prostheses for reintegration into the industrial labour market, this rehabilitation proved to be a great problem with many psychiatric conditions, specifically those addressed as the group of "nervous degeneratives" by clinical psychiatrist Oswald Bumke.[81] He had been trained in the Leipzig school of brain psychiatry and became Kraepelin's successor of in the chair of psychiatry at the University of Munich in 1924. Bumke saw no societal value in public health programs designed to meet the needs of the medical conditions of the "nervous degenerates" (*die nervoes Degenerierten*). Instead he regarded it as the duty of these patient groups – who suffered, for instance, from dementia praecox, hereditary tissue degeneration, or the effects of chronic alcoholism – to guarantee their social existence through their personal means. This claim had, of course, already been made before the war;[82] but with the political conditions of Weimar Germany, it became a battle cry both of rightist psychiatrists, as in Hoche's clinical work (which emphasized individuals' defunct hereditary status) and likewise of left-wing reform psychiatrists, as in the case of early Ruedin's psychiatric genetics. Psychiatrists and neurologists alike focused on "nervous degeneration" as a rhetorical means to strengthen their individual claims as proponents of an increasingly politicized health care field and emphasized the cost-effectiveness of state-run public mental health programs:[83]

> Demographic research into heredity has the central aim of scrutinizing the genetic and biological conditions of the German people, in order to arrive at an adequate knowledge of its mental and physical conditions for general and practical use of the state.[84]

These discipline-building developments occurred in a period when international relations and academic exchanges were becoming increasingly popular, especially between European psychiatrists and young American medical doctors. The resulting interactions brought about significant modifications in the medical and intellectual landscape on either side of the Atlantic.[85] Between the establishment of the Deutsche Forschungsanstalt as an institute of the KWG in 1924 and the declaration of war by Germany on the United States in December 1941, for example, nearly two hundred students and junior researchers from North America had travelled to Munich to work in the laboratories and clinical wards of the institute.[86] Yet, such processes were not limited to the experiences and personal developments of the proponents of the eugenics movement. One of their legacies was to have crucially influenced some of the wide-ranging decisions within major funding institutions in their international and transatlantic engagement, as well as the long-term support of personal, philanthropic, and political projects.

A noteworthy example of an individual deeply enmeshed in transatlantic relations was the Swiss-born psychiatrist Adolf Meyer. He maintained contacts with American colleagues from an earlier research visit, and later became a professor of psychiatry in Baltimore, Maryland, as well as a leading figure in American psychiatry.[87] Meyer represents a "central node" of the American neuroscientific network and was a referee for the Rockefeller Foundation as the major funding institution of biomedical research before World War II.[88] Meyer's engagement and the Rockefeller Foundation's decision-making processes essentially fostered a pre-existing, tightening network in medical science between basic researchers, public health workers, and clinical psychiatrists, that influenced the availability of research funds for psychiatry, while directing support into preventive eugenics and later sterilization programs: "I should like to see a clinic give one half of its beds to intensive work on a limited district and bestow the other half on intensive work on special clinical problems."[89] But what Meyer did not mention was where and how those patients who were not of "research interest" to the contemporary psychiatrist – that is, the chronically ill and those born with hereditary conditions – would be cared for.[90]

The Rockefeller Foundation's financial engagement extended well beyond North America. From the early 1920s onward, the foundation had been one of the first foreign institutions to respond to the devastating effects of World War I on German institutions of higher learning.[91] In fact, the recovery of many major scientific endeavours (*Grossforschungsanstrengungen*) in postwar Germany is inconceivable without taking the Rockefeller Foundation's major financial contributions into account (see also the Introduction).[92] The international funding body supported noteworthy university departments and research units, and during the Weimar

Republic it became a primary stakeholder in the eugenics-related KWI for Brain Research in Berlin-Buch (figure 4.3), the KWI for Anthropology in Berlin-Dahlem, and the Deutsche Forschungsanstalt for Psychiatry in Munich.[93] This support was initially mediated largely through its Paris bureau, which was established in 1919 immediately after the war, to help first to retain crucial French institutions as loci for research training of American postgraduate trainees. The main strategic planner and arbiter of that support was Alan Gregg (see figure 5.3), the executive officer for Rockefeller Foundation's advancement of brain research and psychiatry,[94] about whom scientist J. Robert Oppenheimer (1904–1967) once said, "he probably exerted as much influence on medical education as William Osler [1849–1919] and Abraham Flexner before him."[95]

This international funding body was highly influential in establishing scientific relations between German and American psychiatrists and eugenicists. While the exchanges of American and German psychiatrists had until 1910 been rather personal undertakings, this substantial funding source led to strengthened transatlantic links between Germany and the United States.[96] Throughout the 1930s and into the early 1940s, American money invigorated scholarly research ties in Germany's "Brain Triangle" (see chapter 1), which was formed by Ernst Ruedin's Deutsche Forschungsanstalt in Munich, the KWI for Brain Research in Berlin, headed by the Vogts, and the Neurological Institute in Breslau, which Otfrid Foerster had created (in 1925). Yet, rather than being an altruistic engagement in German neuroscience, the large sums of money for the development of research institutions served transatlantic exchanges between researchers on all levels – basic and clinical, non-experienced and advanced:

> The first most important type of aid is directed to the improvement in the teaching of Psychiatry ... As examples of aid to the teaching of Psychiatry the Rockefeller Foundation is supporting departments of Psychiatry at Yale, Harvard, Washington University in Saint Louis, Chicago, Duke, and Tulane and is largely responsible for their initiation ... Research grants have been numerous and more widely scattered, i.e. including the Maudsley Hospital in London, the University of Edinburgh, and Universities in Germany, Norway, Sweden, Holland, Belgium, Switzerland, Canada, and Australia.[97]

The Rockefeller Foundation's individual funding program also enabled a number of German psychiatric researchers to work on the other side

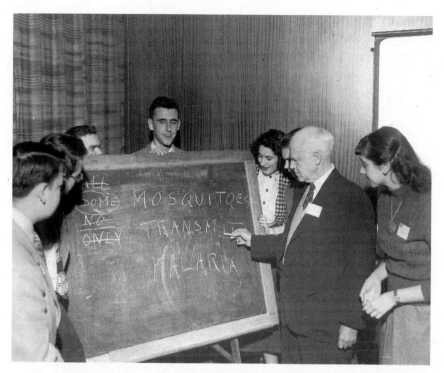

5.3 Alan Gregg (second from right). The head of the Rockefeller Foundation section for psychiatry, psychosomatics, and brain research, illustrates *The Importance of Medical Research* with 1953 finalists of the Society for Science and the Public (STS) © Courtesy of the US National Library of Medicine, Bethesda, Maryland, USA.

of the Atlantic. In both directions, these individuals introduced scientific practices, which became subsequently "enriched" with utilitarian societal ideals (as in the United States) as well as research perspectives on hereditary disease (as in the German-speaking context).[98] Adding to these large-scale commitments for brain research centres, the Rockefeller Foundation's funding programs were particularly active in international exchanges and the support of reciprocal transfers of knowledge. These, in turn, contributed to an atmosphere of receptiveness regarding the emerging Nazi ideology in the 1920s and 1930s. Indeed, the burgeoning fields of eugenics and hereditary diseases proved to be of central interest in the establishment of a racial science, such as Ruedin's intensive epidemiological research program on the inheritance of nervous diseases.[99] Although the Rockefeller Foundation itself did not engage in ideological projects, it continued its funding activities in smaller endeavours even during the 1930s:

The Forschungsanstalt in Munich is a conspicuous example owing to Ruedin, its nominal director, of the racial policy of the Nazi government [!] and on the subject of that policy it is obvious that there are very deep as well as entirely articulate opinions in this country both in the board and out.[100]

To give another example: The particular case of the Deutsche Forschungsanstalt and Rockefeller Foundation's funding of brain research in the Munich area is revealing in respect to the policies of this funding body for integrating eugenic and public health thought in its support of individual neurologists, psychiatrists, and neuropathologists in German research institutions. As planned by its founder, Emil Kraepelin, the Deutsche Forschungsanstalt had been inaugurated as a psychiatric research institute in 1917 and started to function in 1921. It soon became a paradigm institution for neuroscientific research in the Western world under the farsighted leadership of the neuropathologist Walther Spielmeyer and the serologist Felix Plaut (1877–1940), who succeeded Kraepelin in the directorship of the institute and its departments:[101]

> Prof. Kraepelin, who has always been able to attract a very capable body of workers about him, planned a comprehensive institute covering both clinical and laboratory aspects of psychiatry with the object of investigating the causes of insanity and of finding methods of prevention, cure, and alleviation. Of the various activities planned, covered by six headings in his original scheme, four departments were working in 1925 – anatomy, serology, genealogy, and psychology. [Further sections], hoped to be established, are chemistry, physiology, *biological inheritance, and statistics. Plans also include work in industrial problems* and a clinic.[102]

Despite the Rockefeller Foundation's expectation that the Deutsche Forschungsanstalt would further develop into a multidisciplinary research institute, since the end of the 1920s it had shown a tendency in its divisions to focus on areas of racial anthropology, inheritance, and eugenics-related genealogy. Long before the Nazis had come into power, the head of its genealogical research division, Ernst Ruedin, had been made the director of the institute, and – in 1933 – was referred to by German psychiatrists as a "*Fuehrer*" in psychiatry, while also being the permanent director of the Deutsche Forschungsanstalt. This decision was a significant turn away from the rotation principle of the acting director becoming director only for a fixed term of several years before a new director was elected from one of the division heads of this research institute. Yet during the year 1935, when the international monetary exchange rates became increasingly worrisome to German budgets, the Rockefeller Foundation continued to shuffle money in.[103] The Rockefeller Foundation steered quite an ambivalent course of scientific reviews, which, for example, saw the Deutsche Forschungsanstalt receive money even into the war years in 1943. During Ruedin's headship of the Deutsche Forschungsanstalt for Psychiatry, the intricate system of relating research in brain psychiatry with epidemiologic investigations was augmented by considerable research support from the Deutsche Forschungsgemeinschaft and the Ministry of Health.[104] These political alignments resulted in a hiving off of neuroscientific research activities, which then were supplemented with psychopathological, anthropometrical, and genetic counselling programs.[105]

The Rockefeller Foundation defended its continued funding on the basis that Spielmeyer and Plaut were involved as individual recipients of the contributions. Ruedin, however, always found ways to channel part of this financial support into the Deutsche Forschungsanstalt's general endowment, thus securing the foundation's contribution to the demographic division's program on psychiatric eugenics and public mental health.[106] Rockefeller Foundation funding activities frequently added up to quite substantial amounts, due to the concentration of well-supported psychiatrists within the major centres in the big "Reich" cities. As such, the foundation's continuing support of brain research centres and eugenic psychiatric projects can be seen as a direct expression of its own preoccupation with sustaining the research exchanges and training conditions of North American investigators in German laboratories and hospital wards. When, for example, neuropathologist Hugo Spatz succeeded Spielmeyer as the director of the department of neuropathology in Munich in 1935, and after Willibald Scholz was hired from Bonn to follow Spatz in 1937 upon the latter's move to Berlin, they both immediately approached the Rockefeller Foundation's Paris office and received financial assistance for scientific technology and apparatuses for their neurohistological programs. Even after World War II, Scholz was able to impress the foundation with the idea that "the genetic materials collected by Ruedin were really valuable" and could be added to by future eugenic research programs, making it "even more important as a source material."[107] In his working diary kept from the 1910s, Gregg shows the extent to which relations with German psychiatrists had continued throughout the Weimar era, and even in the National Socialist period. This collaborative development

was based particularly on genetics and social epidemiological research
and training programs in psychiatry.[108]

How far this new trend in somatically oriented brain psychiatry had
developed became clear in a report letter to the Rockefeller Foundation
in New York City, written by Spielmeyer in Ruedin's institute on
27 November 1934 – that is, one year after the Nazis had seized power
– in which Spielmeyer informed Gregg about the changes in direction that
contemporary clinical psychiatry had taken:

> In the field of medicine, both practice and scientific research is con-
> cerned primarily with genetics and race hygiene, as you know. You
> convinced yourself of that this summer, during your visit.[109]

I have so far spoken of continuities, differences, and breaks in the eugenics
tradition within the emerging discipline of Brain Psychiatry in Germany
and North America. This inquiry makes it clear that a transatlantic network of leading psychiatrists and neurologists existed long before the
advent of Nazi ideologies, from the latter half of the nineteenth century
forward.[110] Apart from medicine and biological science, many associations and clubs had served as interfaces for the increasing popularity of
eugenics on both sides of the Atlantic: The Berlin Society for Racial
Hygiene, inaugurated in 1905, included a secret circle, the Nordische
Abteilung, founded in 1910.[111] In the same year, Ploetz turned his Nordic
Circle (Ring der Norda) association in Munich into a pre-Fascist "Secret
Nordic Circle," which, in addition to sponsoring racial-hygienic agitation
and programs, attempted to initiate an intellectual reorientation, a return
to "old Indo-Germanic roots" (altindogermanische Wurzeln); similar
anti-modernist forms of social critique could also be found in many
eugenics programs on both sides of the Atlantic.[112]

The findings presented in this chapter further emphasize the strong
currents of cultural influences on the field of psychiatry and its theoretical
advances from bourgeois fears of "nervous degeneration" in Wilhelminian
society to brain psychiatry's concern with conditions of "nervousness,"
the treatment of "war neurotics," and influences of hereditary disease
during the Weimar period. These foci were not just limited to the peculiar
German style of Nervenheilkunde, but cultural forces influenced psychiatric and neurological theory via day-to-day work in hospitals and mental
asylums. This characterization may seem overly medical, but in fact it is
not: we are no longer dealing here simply with a medicalization of the
cultural discourse in Nervenheilkunde as Radkau's Age of Nervousness

suggests (see also chapter 2). When taking a closer look at psychiatry and neurology as emerging scientific disciplines at the beginning of the twentieth century, it is, rather, the "culturization" of medical discourse that becomes apparent.

Although German, American, Canadian, British, and Scandinavian eugenics all contained unique elements, there was significant common ground between the particular "national styles" of eugenic thinking.[113] The British eugenics movement had already been molded in the 1880s and 1890s by Francis Galton and Karl Pearson (1857–1936) before it was transferred to the United States and Canada. In America it was particularly Charles Davenport who kept close contact with Lenz on the other side of the Atlantic, and he was well aware of Ruedin's massive research program on psychiatric genetics in Munich. In Norway, Jon Alfred Mjøen (1860–1939) was deeply influenced by the German movement of "racial hygiene" as put forward by Lenz's colleague Ploetz. Likewise, although succeeding generations of eugenics leaders came from widely diverse political perspectives, they all shared the belief that the human species as a whole was endangered by the tangible effects of modernization, especially through the contexts of armed conflict such as the American Civil War (for the American situation) and the Great War (for the European situation). Nevertheless, eugenics thinkers assumed that these "degenerative conditions and diseases" could be prevented by science along with the ensuing neurological and psychiatric applications. Modern society could be improved, they thought, by the marginalization of the feeble-minded, the physically unfit, and the morally corrupt through planned restrictions on the reproduction of "inferior grades of humanity."[114]

Research-minded German brain psychiatrists of the late nineteenth century, such as the prominent luminary professors Kraepelin and Alzheimer, promoted the view that basic research into "neurodegenerative diseases" should first be advanced before specific action could be taken – but they took eugenic theories as a starting point of much of their own investigations.[115] There were many views on how the direction of human evolution could be controlled, with American psychiatrists calling for hospitalization, anti-miscegenation legislation, and in some cases sterilization of the "brain degenerates."[116] Later, German brain psychiatrists like Hoche and Ruedin saw little advantage in experimental basic research of hereditary conditions. They favoured instead statistical human "phenotype" databases to track the specific biological and psychological traits of the feeble-minded and mentally ill, helping to create state-planned public health actions. In a way, they all admitted that there was no way of precisely knowing the extent of inferiority of the mentally ill, but in the end, their ideology remained remarkably intact.

The engagement of clinical neurologists and psychiatrists in discussions of eugenics measures also developed into a strategy of bolstering professional recognition and the renown of particular disciplines, especially at the turn of the century. Psychiatrists and brain researchers such as Auguste Forel and Constantin von Monakow had been instrumental in this regard as they developed a much broader "holistic" picture of their discipline as an all-encompassing social-medical program.[117] Eugenic thinking of the period, with its strong racial assumptions, thus became an important discursive tool that served clinical psychiatry in establishing its own professional identity *vis-à-vis* biology and medicine. This development was also fostered by conceptual transfers and personal relationships in the German-American context, which went far beyond disciplinary boundaries and included scientists, medical doctors, literary writers, and social philosophers alike, all of whom were intrigued by what they saw as the enormous utopian thrust of this sociopsychiatric enterprise.

6

The *Machtergreifung* of the National Socialists and Its Effects on the German-Speaking Neurosciences

Marginalization – Oppression – Forced Migration

THE EMERGENCE OF THE *BRAUNE BEWEGUNG* AND NAZI THREATS

As [Arnold] Zweig indicated, expressionism, cinema, literature, an explosive theatrical world – they all had their roots in the dual sensibility of the vast destructiveness of war and the powerful creativity of revolution. And they were sustained by the very fragility of Weimar's political order, which *lent a continual sense of edgy nervousness to Weimar society* that imbued the cultural realm.

Eric Weitz[1]

The status of the medical profession in Germany during the National Socialist Era has been the subject of much research, with scholarly consensus being reached on many grounds – regarding, for instance, the central issues of racial anthropology, public health, and the murderous activities of Nazi physicians.[2] The intensive scholarship has given an encompassing picture of the changes in academic societies, along with the development of basic research practices.[3] This holds particularly true for the Nazi seizure of power – the *Machtergreifung* – and its impact on medical disciplines such as neurology and psychiatry, along with the interdisciplinary field of the brain sciences. A more comprehensive account of the history of Nazi medicine – its influence on German society, its medical, scientific, and administrative corps, the infamous human subject experiments, and its involvement in and representation of racial hygiene and euthanasia killing programs – remains, however, to be further developed. Moral and ethical problems are posed not only by the humiliating treatment of patients with mental and neurological problems; the perspective of the prevalent closed-caste mentality (*Corpsgeist*) of the medical establishment also must be taken into account.[4] What strikes today's scholars is that only selected traits of a socio-political nature have been sufficiently explored as to their influence on medicine during the National Socialist period.[5] Accordingly, I focus in this chapter on the cultural context, in order to understand the broader picture behind the ousting of oppositional and Jewish brain researchers, the marginalization of disabled patients, and ultimately the perfidious murder of asylum inmates in the euthanasia programs.[6]

Nazi medicine provides an illuminating case study for newer aspects in the historiography of science – interpreting the evolution of medicine and its aberrations on the very grounds of its interactions and entanglements with culture.[7] This is the theme I want to apply here to the emerging research field of neuromorphology at the beginning of the twentieth century. This field of focus will allow us to unearth more general trends in the history of medicine during the period that later, along with changing transatlantic relations in the early neurosciences, also became the context of the forced migration process. The international dimension of psychiatry, neurology, neuroanatomy, and neuropathology became so important for the growth of biomedical knowledge that it deserves greater scrutiny as well. This is especially true when we consider the hundreds of researchers in neuroscience-related fields who crossed the Atlantic in both directions and follow their trajectory from their working context in the Weimar Republic to their expulsion under the Nazi regime. It was in similar ways that the field of applied eugenics came to influence the development of neurology and psychiatry in the German-speaking countries from the 1930s to the 1940s.

There are also systemic reasons why the neurosciences offer a fruitful case study for considerations about Nazi medicine. The new health programs, as well as cultural and medico-legal views on the neurologically handicapped and mentally ill, saw an unfortunate evolution of eugenics programs into family counselling of parents, marriage laws, and forced sterilization regulations. This trend served as the backdrop for the profound transformations in the public mental health system that made psychiatric and neurological patients the prime targets of applied eugenicists. These developments were additionally empowered by the growing enthusiasm for racial hygiene, forced sterilization, and the later euthanasia programs among the mentally ill. What is crucial for my narrative is the expulsion of what the Nazis saw as "Jewish medicine and science," which included particular areas of psychiatry and neurology along with psychoanalysis, medical sexology, and socialist public health.[8] The normative contexts of medicine and psychiatry had been steadily redefined since the 1920s, a period heavily influenced, as we have seen, by the experiences of World War I and the early years of the Weimar Republic. Furthermore, these developments also caused medical scientists to step out of their normal doctor-patient relationships and discard traditional ethics of mutual respect and support. They began to openly antagonize their Jewish colleagues, particularly socialist and humanist doctors, who themselves resented the increasing radicalism of the medical system.[9] By setting the case of Nazi medicine within the perspective of Stanford historian of science Robert Proctor – who has criticized the positivist view that basic democratic conditions are necessary for scientific development as being unrealistic – we can perhaps better understand neuroscience's embeddedness in culture and international relations. It would be inadequate to limit it by calling it "pseudoscience" or "pure ideology," because in the field of early neuroscience this was simply not the case, even though medical ideology played a significant role in the reshaping of the health care system and framing the context for research programs that had a strong political bias.[10]

I look first at some of the general transformations of scientific institutions that enabled clinicians and medical researchers to link with the eugenics and euthanasia networks emerging at the time of the *Machtergreifung*. These were changes that ultimately led brain scientists to conduct fatal human experiments that took advantage of the political programs of murdering children and patients in psychiatric hospitals. The fact that these developments, in return, became strongly intertwined with the marginalization of Jewish and oppositional neurologists, psychiatrists, and basic researchers makes it necessary for us to dwell on the sociopolitical context of the related transformation of the German medical corps. Finally, in laying the groundwork for my later discussion of its global effects, I discuss the major implications of the exodus of German-speaking medical doctors through a number of illustrative case examples. Since these occurrences are themselves related to the development of German-speaking neuromorphology toward the middle of the twentieth century, they also need to be considered here.

REDEFINITIONS OF HUMAN LIFE AND VALUES
IN NEUROLOGICAL AND BRAIN PSYCHIATRIC
PERSPECTIVES: THE CASES OF GEORGES
SCHALTENBRAND AND ERNST RUEDIN

Two instructive examples related to the field of neuroscience are particularly worthy of mention as I highlight some general elements of the Nazi health care system. They give us evidence that many instances of Nazi medicine cannot be regarded, as some scholars have emphasized in the past, simply as having been determined by top-down political orders (as in the German term *Auftragsforschung*).[11] Quite often, the involvement of physicians and researchers came as a result of strategically planned decisions on the part of individuals who strove for public acknowledgment and an increase in research resources.[12] Furthermore, we need to take into account that the changing normative context of research with human subjects in the Third Reich – which can also be related to neurology, psychiatry, neuroserology, neuropathology, and neuroanatomy – frequently allowed medical scientists to pursue their aims "bottom-up," as it were.

The first example is that of the human experiments of one of the most renowned proponents of clinical neuroscience at the time: the American-trained Wuerzburg neurologist Georges Schaltenbrand. Schaltenbrand completed his medical studies in Munich and continued clinical and research specializations with major international neurologists of the time, including the brain psychiatrist Emil Kraepelin in Munich, the neurologist Max Nonne in Hamburg, and the Dutch neurologist Bernardus Brouwer (1881–1949) in Amsterdam. Moreover, the award of a Rockefeller Foundation research fellowship enabled him to join the neurosurgical research laboratory of Harvey Cushing in Boston from 1926 to 1927. Taking further advantage of the Rockefeller Foundation's commitment to the creation of Western-style medical schools in China during the country's opening phase before the communist revolution, in 1928 Schaltenbrand took a senior position as an associate professor of neurology at the Peking Union College.[13] Until this moment in his career, Schaltenbrand had been an established "normal scientist,"[14] a recognition that subsequently led to a job offer from the University of Hamburg later that year. He accepted this offer and was appointed as a faculty member in Nonne's neurological clinic, assuming also, in 1928, the headship of the neurology department as a full professor with Wuerzburg University.[15]

Schaltenbrand had been a staunchly conservative physician, who himself held onto many social values of the late Wilhelminian Empire. He was, for example, a member of the right-wing *Stahlhelm* organization, the political party branch of the German *Reichswehr* in which he had grown up during his adolescence. However, he was different from many of his other colleagues in that he did not embrace Nazi ideology from the start but appeared to have changed his opinion only in 1936–37. An affiliation with the NSDAP proved beneficial for his promotion in the academic system, opening further doors for research support, for instance, through the Deutsche Forschungsgemeinschaft's increased funding for experimental laboratories. Interestingly, one sees in this change of political opinion, to coincide with his accepting a full professorship of neurology at Wuerzburg University, what can fairly be interpreted as an opportunistic move.[16]

Schaltenbrand initiated his controversial experimental series into the viral hypothesis of multiple sclerosis in 1940, after he had created an extensive brain research laboratory in Wuerzburg. This study was explicitly set up in an interdisciplinary form and built with infrastructure funds from the Deutsche Forschungsgemeinschaft. For his research into the "aetiology of Multiple Sclerosis," Schaltenbrand had first established a "primate farm" on the hospital grounds themselves.[17] When the grant was awarded, 15,500 Reichsmark were planned for the acquisition of apes and primates as necessary experimental models. However, with the outbreak of World War II, as the funding that the Deutsche Forschungsgemeinschaft received for non-military related research was cut back, this amount became substantially reduced. Schaltenbrand's investigations thus had to begin under serious resource limitations; less than half the intended amount was paid out for the ape farm in this conglomerate involving clinical departments, laboratories, and service offices and units. The whole set-up of the experiments was constrained by the lack of sufficient numbers of animals to run the test series required for neurological research into the "infection hypothesis of multiple sclerosis" that Schaltenbrand and Toennis in Wuerzburg, as well as Pette in Hamburg had advocated for.[18]

The pilot studies were based on xenotransfusion experiments in the apes, with the technical assistance of a larger group of collaborating physicians and researchers such as Hans Wolff (1912–1958), Horst Vierheilig (1905–1940), and Josef Schorn (1896–1955?). These physicians had close ties to the general hospital at Regensburg, where Wolff became department head of clinical neurology in the period after World War II.[19] It emerges from historical source material that Schaltenbrand deliberately sent project outlines to the "big science section" (*Grossforschungssektion*) of genetic biology (*Fachausschuss fuer Gemeinschaftsarbeiten zur Erbbiologie* – since 1935, *Anthropologie und Rassenbiologie*), in order to tap into major infrastructure funding for the creation of his interdisciplinary program. This big science section of the Deutsche Forschungsgemeinschaft was headed by professor Hans Conrad Julius Reiter (1881–1969), president of the Reich's ministry of health, while Schaltenbrand repeatedly tried to win the major Deutsche Forschungsgemeinschaft-funding network for explicit support of his multiple sclerosis research. He accordingly emphasized genetic factors in the pathological aetiology of multiple sclerosis and claimed to have successfully produced results that sustained the hypothesis of an inflammatory aetiology of the disease.[20] Later, he even made his experimental findings in humans widely available, choosing to publish his work in two major German-speaking formats – the periodical *Klinische Wochenschrift* (1940) and his so-deemed "classical" monograph *Human Multiple Sclerosis* in 1943 (*Die Multiple Sklerose des Menschen*), with Springer Press.[21] These publications by one of the best internationally known clinical neurologists must have caught the attention of leading German-speaking neurologists, not least because of Schaltenbrand's sensational claims of having cleared a major pathological pathway in one of the most prevalent diseases. Schaltenbrand likewise openly acknowledged that he had used clinical psychiatric patients. He had injected them with blood from apes with multiple sclerosis–like symptoms, along with blood from human patients, while not indicating any consent for these experiments on the part of their relatives or their guardians.[22]

Schaltenbrand's first publication from 1940 contextualized his laboratory experiments within the current theory of a viral genesis of multiple sclerosis. However, a hotly contested debate ensued, in which only a fraction of contemporary neurologists followed Schaltenbrand's complex argumentation. For most, the impact of exogenous toxins, effects of vascular thrombosis, neuroglial overgrowth, and dietary components were just primary pathological factors of the respective aetiology of the disease.[23] Although Schaltenbrand's program thus represented a minority view, his credentials from earlier experimental work in the biomedical centres of New York, Peking, and Hamburg were impeccable and he already had several contributions to clinical neurology to his credit. The Wuerzburg research program and its investigators were working on a cutting-edge endeavour, scientifically on a par with the best clinical research conducted by international groups in Paris, New York, and

Toronto[24] that were also pursuing investigations into the infectious aetiology of multiple sclerosis. It would therefore be a mistake to denigrate Schaltenbrand's contemporary neuromorphological research program as mere "pseudoscience."[25] What made his human experiments so problematic was the way they downgraded ethical values and the fact that Schaltenbrand and his co-workers conducted research on psychiatric patients, for which they actively sought the support from high Nazi officials. According to his own monograph, Schaltenbrand personally believed that he had induced an infectious multiple sclerosis–like illness in monkeys through cisternal injection of cerebrospinal fluid taken from his patients.[26] These investigations were based on xenotransplantational cell suspension experiments, and the outcomes were reproduced in line with clinical behaviours and pathological observations under the microscope.

According to the outline of the research methodologies established between 1935 and 1940, Schaltenbrand's second experimental series consisted of a "control" of the xenotransfusion experiments with monkey cerebrospinal fluid. The fluid was deliberately introduced into human patients by way of high-risk intrathecal injections into the spinal canal just underneath the occipital bone of the skull. To Schaltenbrand and his collaborators, this experimental series performed in dozens of patients appeared medically justifiable. The physicians claimed they had "only used already demented individuals" (*"nur schon verbloedete Menschen"*), as he wrote from the wards of the nearby Werneck psychiatric asylum (Heil- und Pflegeanstalt Werneck) in Lower Franconia. In the wake of these animal-to-man xenotransfusions, two of the patients developed serious physiological complications and died. Hastening to conduct *post mortem* analyses after these fatal outcomes, Schaltenbrand found demyelization signs in the affected central nervous system, as he had expected. These findings appeared to prove his prior hypothesis from animal observations and led him to publish his research in the early 1940s in prominent German-speaking medical journals.[27] What can be interpreted as a natural step for a clinician of the time – wanting to test his animal experiments also in humans to consolidate the hypotheses – constituted in the two fatal cases a murderous shift of the research program.[28] It rendered the experiments unethical even when seen from the underdeveloped pre-1930s ethical standards of the German medical community.[29]

The lack of funds from the Deutsche Forschungsgemeinschaft due to the advent of World War II also led Schaltenbrand "to jump the experimental queue," in keeping with his active pursuit of Nazi officials' continued support. He did not even wait for this to become official, addressing the *Aktion T4* directly, and emphasized in very crass ways that the "idiots," "vegetables," and "demented patients" of the Werneck psychiatric asylum were well suited for the experiments, since they just represented "life not worth living."[30] Within this opportunistic context, it is evident how Schaltenbrand used the new political situation to his advantage, since it allowed the Wuerzburg research program to proceed to active human experimentation. It is telling that he refrained from carrying out the experiments on his own neurological patients at the University of Wuerzburg, apparently recognizing the high-risk character of the research attempt. Instead, he deliberately reached out to the Werneck asylum in its remote location on the assumption that, as part of the patient murder system of *Aktion T4*, those patients would be killed "anyway."[31] What was particularly galling in this context was the moral relapse even to pre-1900 standards within the contemporary overarching medical framework of racial hygiene (*Rassenhygiene*).[32] Rather than being governed by respect for the value of the individual and the best interests of the patient, according to the ethical principle of *salus aegroti suprema lex*, the neurological experimenters defaulted exclusively to the biologistic view of racial fitness.[33]

Schaltenbrand was an example of a high-achieving "normal scientist" – and an opportunistic researcher – using the pretense of National Socialist ideology to further his own aims. In terms of our perspective on interdisciplinary connections, it is significant that Schaltenbrand's department and laboratory at Wuerzburg University had emerged outside of an explicitly Nazi-dominated care system. Yet he tried to build connections with high-profile institutions beyond the confines of the university hospital – the big-science network of researchers funded by the Deutsche Forschungsgemeinschaft, subsequent alliances with the Reichsgesundheitsamt, and further contacts with Nazi officials, as well as administrators from the *Aktion T4* program.[34] At Werneck, humiliating forms of research could be carried out at a "safe" distance from the spotlight of the university medical school. In the urban context of Wuerzburg, on the other hand, patients' relatives and family doctors would likely have asked inquisitory questions, thus endangering the interdisciplinary form of research organization of the Schaltenbrand type in the early 1940s.[35]

Quite striking in this context as well is the case of another, more "revolutionary scientific" figure and leader in the field of biological psychiatry – the Swiss psychiatrist Ernst Ruedin, institute director of the Deutsche Forschungsanstalt for Psychiatry in Munich. At the Deutsche Forschungsanstalt for Psychiatry, every aspect of Nazi medicine came to be tightly connected with neurological and psychiatric clinical practice and research, as can be seen by its focus on genetic brain disorders, the organization of vast statistical field studies in all the German states (*Laender*), and its later use of euthanasia victims for research purposes.[36] Ruedin himself had studied medicine at the universities of Geneva, Naples, Heidelberg, Berlin, and Dublin, and from 1899 on pursued his residency at the psychiatric clinical department (Burghoelzli) of the University of Zurich under the famous psychiatrist and psychoanalyst Eugen Bleuler (1857–1939). During Ruedin's later period as a registrar in the prison medical department of Berlin-Moabit, he even developed left-wing leanings on social public health issues.[37] However, when he received the directorship of the genealogic-demographic department of the Deutsche Forschungsanstalt in 1931, he came under the influence of the racial hygiene program of his brother-in-law Alfred Ploetz (see also chapter 5), which fundamentally changed his medical and political views:

Apart from a brief exploration of the biological races in relation to their cultural values, I will use the word [eugenics] merely as designating a human collective that exists through generations, while being based on its physical and mental qualities. This can be easily pursued, since collective explanations such as the ones mentioned in the previous sentence are likewise validly applied to smaller and larger communities of humans.[38]

In subsequent years at the Munich Deutsche Forschungsanstalt, Ruedin developed his psychiatric approach toward an "empirical genetic prognosis" of mental disorders, through which he could finally align his "socialist intentions." His career was by no means a singular development pertaining to the German-speaking context in brain psychiatry alone; it exemplified events throughout Central Europe in an increasingly internationalized field.[39] Ruedin's widespread reputation is demonstrated by the fact that four years after the Nazis came into power, he was approached to give the keynote lecture to the World Population Conference in Paris. Moreover, in the spring of 1939, the Swedish eugenicist Gunnar Dahlberg (1893–1956) from the Statens institut foer rasbiologi (The State Institute for Racial Biology) in Stockholm invited him to present one of the four plenaries at the Human Genetics Section of the Seventh International Genetics Congress in Edinburgh from 23–30 August 1939.[40] At the Edinburgh congress, in which Ruedin put forward his racial doctrines already infused with anti-Semitic undertones, he stimulated American

eugenicist Clarence G. Campbell (1927–1997) to praise the Nazi government as a political model for the United States:[41]

> It is from a synthesis of the work of all such men that the leader of
> the German nation, Adolf Hitler, ably supported by the Minister of
> the Interior, Dr. [Wilhelm] Frick [1877–1946], and guided by the
> nation's anthropologists, its eugenicists, and its social philosophers,
> has been able to construct a comprehensive race policy of popula-
> tion development and improvement that promises to be epochal
> in racial history.[42]

By using Hitler and his political regime in public addresses as a symbol
for his research aims, Ruedin laid the groundwork for his legendary
machinery for grant money acquisition and pulled out all the stops for
creating a scientific empire of psychiatry, genetics, and brain research in
Germany. From the end of the 1930s, he was credited with numerous
academic awards and recognized as the leading expert in the field of
psychiatry (*Reichsfuehrer der Psychiatrie*) by the Gesellschaft Deutscher
Nervenaerzte. It was little more than a small step in the advancement of
his career, when former socialist Ruedin became immersed in national
socialist views and received full membership in the NSDAP in 1937.[43] A
description of this instructive case can only be complete, however, when
international developments are included in the picture as well. Due to
the scientific renown of its founder, Emil Kraepelin, the Deutsche
Forschungsanstalt for Psychiatry continued to be a heavily subsidized
institution, receiving infrastructure funds, research support, and individual
fellowships from the American Rockefeller Foundation as well.[44] In fact,
the Rockefeller Foundation manoeuvred an ambivalent process of scientific
reviews that saw the Deutsche Forschungsanstalt for Psychiatry still receive
money from that American institution until 1943. Grant payments to
individual researchers continued even until 1945, when the institute was
partially destroyed by an American bomber attack on Munich.[45]

The historical case of Ruedin is thus indicative of the relationship
between the new field of psychiatric genetics and neuropathology and the
contemporary context of anthropology and eugenics. It further speaks to
the direct influence of the Nazi government's involvement in all the medical associations as unifying alignment (*Gleichschaltung*) during the Third
Reich. In the internal processes of the Deutsche Forschungsanstalt for
Psychiatry, which had become a full clinical and research institute of the
KWG in 1924, this alignment resulted in higher intake of patients from

all over Germany for clinical research. Furthermore, brain psychiatric and neuropathological investigations intensified, through the institute's connections with other local hospitals, pathological departments, and mental asylums. Specific analyses of psychopathology, anthropometry, and family relations were included in the records of individual psychiatric hospitals and mental asylums. Ruedin strove to create the largest reference database on psychiatry, pathology, and epidemiology in the world.[46] It soon became even more significant than Davenport's Eugenics Record Office at Cold Spring Harbor, New York, thanks to Munich's concentration and depth of information on psychiatry and public mental health for the German territory.

The cases of Schaltenbrand and Ruedin both offer good examples of the influence of contemporary cultural transformations on the context of early neuroscience. Schaltenbrand and Ruedin used various means to gain official support for their scientific endeavours under the new political constellations, while both worked toward compatible long-term goals. The flow of resources was so generous in the early decade of Nazi Germany, that neither Schaltenbrand nor Ruedin saw any compelling reason to alter their programs, given that their research at the University of Wuerzburg and the Munich Deutsche Forschungsanstalt was so favoured by the new party officials.

TWO DEVELOPMENTS DURING THE THIRD REICH
IN LEADING FORMER NEUROSCIENCE CENTRES:
THE CONTRASTING CASES OF STRASBURG AND LEIPZIG

As I have already indicated earlier (please see chapter 1), it is important for our purposes to assess the institutional reconfigurations brought about by the successive political changes in Germany in the first half of the twentieth century. The University of Strasburg offers a compelling scenario for institutional observations related to the neurosciences in the National Socialist period. It results from the city's exceptional geopolitical position. When Alsace and Lorraine were occupied again by the German *Wehrmacht* after the defeat of the French army on 22 June 1940, the new chief of the Nazi civil government, Robert Wagner (1895–1946), promoted the marginalization of the "French cultural influence of the interwar period." This process had considerable consequences on the science and medical administrations, which French historian Patrick Wechsler has intriguingly mapped in his dissertation, "La Faculté de Médecine de la Reichsuniversitaet Strassburg (1941–1945)."[47] Once again, the Reichsuniversitaet of

Strasburg became a figurehead of German academia in the annexed province, and it was specifically established to demonstrate the "superiority
of German science and culture." Professors were selected not only on
scientific merit but also on the basis of their socialization and role in the
NSDAP and other party bodies. In this respect, ophthalmologist Karl
Schmidt (1899–1980) had joined the University of Strasburg as its new
principal (Rektor) from Berlin and was accorded the autonomous right
to select the academic staff of the Reichsuniversitaet.[48] Such an encompassing political privilege had been unheard of in the seven-hundred-year
history of German universities, with their primary grounding in faculties,
commissions, and other checks and balances.

The leadership role in the neuroscience field was soon taken on by the
new Ordinarius professor August Bostroem (1942/43–44), who had
joined the Reichsuniversitaet from the neurology hot spot of Leipzig
University. He was accepted by the Nazi government as an appropriate
curator to lead the university administration and had been actively
engaged in the NSDAP and NSLB (National Socialist Teachers League)
since 1933. Bostroem was given the organizational task of "restoring"
the clinical departments of psychiatry and neurology into one single entity.
The disciplines had been separated because of the further specialization
and organization of psychiatry during the time of the French University
of Strasburg. In 1942, however, the directorship was passed on to Nikolaus
Jensch (1913–1964) who, as a loyal member of the NSDAP and the SA
(the Brownshirts), was a more uncompromising Nazi than Bostroem had
been. Bostroem, thus politically thwarted by Nazi officials, concentrated
his somatic research on encephalitis, experimental biology, and the pathology of neurosyphilis. Even though Nazi officials had expelled him from
his leadership position as a curator of the Reichsuniversitaet, however,
Bostroem still agreed with the new Nazi medical philosophy, which he
also applied on his clinical service.[49] Among his peers in psychiatry and
neurology, Bostroem had furthermore been known as a supporter of
negative eugenics, and particularly forced sterilizations in families with
an occurrence of physical and mental disabilities.[50] Jensch himself pursued
racial hygiene and anthropological questions more directly, in that he
conducted research on the psychological development of homosexuality
and anthropological craniometry. These activities became funded by the
Deutsche Forschungsgemeinschaft in line with its working group on
human and biological genetics.[51]

An extreme chapter in the history of the medical faculty of the
Reichsuniversitaet Strassburg is associated with the work of the director

of the anatomy department August Hirt (1898–1945). Hirt was a Swiss citizen and took German citizenship after his *Habilitation* at Heidelberg University, a move that can be interpreted as a career-oriented decision. Hereafter he applied for jobs in Germany and received professorial offers from Heidelberg, Greifswald, Frankfurt, and eventually Strasburg. In parallel, he became a member of the ss in April 1933 and rose through the ranks of the ss medical service to the position of colonel (*Sturmbannfuehrer*) in the Nazi executive organization.[52] During his time at the Reichsuniversitaet, between 1941 and 1944, Hirt became interested in osteological research based on racial-anthropological assumptions about evolutionary skeleton developments (see also figure 6.1).

Hirt's "research program" sought to arrange a collection of skeletons with racial variances in different stages of development. It became infamously known, since he had selected more than fifty corpses from among the inmates of the concentration camp Struthof close to the Vosges Mountains.[53] As director of the department of anatomy, he encouraged neuroanatomical research in his associates such as the institute assistant Dr Anton Kiesselbach (1907–1984) in their work on the sympathetic innervation system as well as the spinal ganglia with their histological organization.[54]

Most of the brain science innovations at the Reichsuniversitaet had nevertheless been instigated through the laboratory in the department of physiology between 1935 and 1941, under the headship of Hans Lullies (1898–1982), yet another member of the NSDAP, NDLB, and SA, who subsequently became the dean of the medical faculty at the University of Cologne. Lullies investigated the periodic bursts of action potentials alongside the nervous membranes. This interdisciplinary program was also supported by specialized assistants from the department of anatomy who worked on the histological structure of the myelin sheets of the nerves, which became a milestone for his physiological career.[55] Lullies's colleagues in the institute of physiological chemistry further analyzed the chemical changes in electrically stimulated peripheral nerves, eliciting, for example, the interdependence of spreading potentials and the tonus upkeep in muscle reflexes in frogs and crabs.[56] Lullies's membership in three major Nazi organizations, however, had nearly no effect on the continuation of his career in leadership positions in West Germany following World War II, where he became an early dean of medicine at the University of the Saarland in Homburg.[57] Further research in neuromorphology was carried out by the head of the pathology department, Helmut Kaiserling (1906–1989), who likewise was a keen member of the NSDAP and

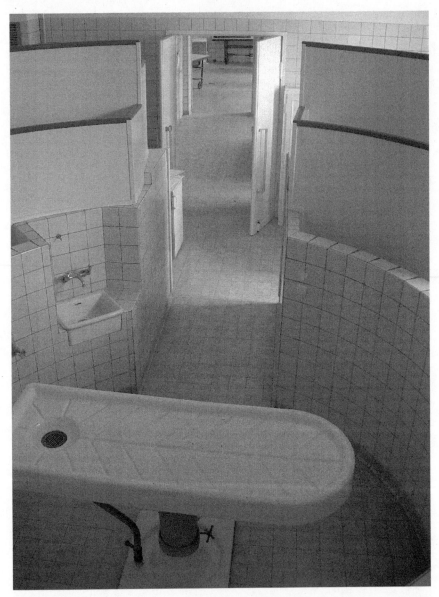

6.1 The previous anatomical dissection room of the Reichsuniversitaet Strassburg (in the double-department building for anatomy and physiology of the Medical Faculty), in which August Hirt's osteological preparations were pursued (shortly before its complete reconstruction in 2005). Coll. Frank W. Stahnisch. © 2008 Frank W. Stahnisch, Calgary, Alberta.

influenced various search committees toward the acceptance of Nazi professors for academic positions. Kaiserling pursued research on inflammatory diseases of the nervous system together with his team of neuropathologists.[58] This group of researchers included Theo Soostmeyer (b. 1898), Erich Fischer (b. 1916), and Willy Ochse (b. 1920).[59]

The largest investments of funding in the brain research field through the Nazi government in Alsace-Lorraine, however, were in two autonomous research institutions of medical science. Both had been planned to emphasize the research orientation of the University of Strasburg once again, while explicitly relating it back to the tradition of the Kaiser Wilhelms University before World War I, as a politically motivated endeavour to showcase the achievements of German science. The first of these advanced scientific institutions was the Central Research Institute of the Medical Faculty, which was conceived on the model of the KWI for Medical Research in Heidelberg.[60] Here, in particular, researchers were brought together to initiate collaborative large-scale projects and to promote networking between the natural sciences and biomedical investigations regarding radioactivity, radiation, and oncology. Likewise, strong support came from the military research side, since this central Faculty Research institute was associated with the Institute for Applied Research in Military Science (Institut fuer wehrwissenschaftliche Zweckforschung) and Heinrich Himmler's (1900–1945) foundational *Ahnenerbe*, the think tank with its office in Berlin-Dahlem.[61] Also a participant in this research institute was the Munich physiologist Sigmund Rascher (1909–1945), an adjunct researcher in the "Division R[ascher]," who had murdered inmates from the concentration camp Dachau during his *Luftwaffe* seawater freezing and high altitude experiments.[62] The data that he gathered provided the research material for Rascher to write his *Habilitation* thesis, which was submitted to the medical faculty of the University of Strasburg in 1944. Anatomist August Hirt was likewise involved in the "Division H[irt]," where his group's research activities spanned oncological questions and applied problems of Wehrmacht medicine.[63] These included research on the functional properties of the sympathetic nervous system. Other notable members of the central research institute were the internist and NSDAP and member, pharmacologist Otto Bickenbach (1901–1971); the dermatologist and NSDAP, SA, and SS member Ernst-Heinrich Brill (1892–1945), who returned to Rostock University but kept collaborating with the Strasburg group; the anthropologist Gustav Weigand (b. 1908?), and the physicist and NSDAP and SA member Rudolf Fleischmann (1903–2002) (see figure 6.2.).[64]

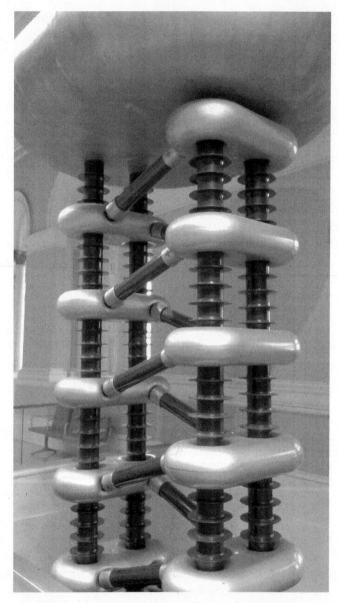

6.2 Model reconstruction developed after Professor Rudolf
Fleischmann's 1944 high voltage generator (1.5 million Volts),
which produced ionized radiation for radiological applications in
oncology and was also used for producing ionized heavy water for
the German nuclear physics reactor (part of the central research
institute of the faculty of medicine of the Reichsuniversitaet
Strassburg), 1944. The model is part of the collection of the
National Museum of Scotland, Edinburgh. Coll. Frank W.
Stahnisch. © 2018 Frank W. Stahnisch, Calgary, Alberta.

Even though it is difficult to identify a specific focus on neuroscientific themes in the biomedical programs of the central research institute in the Strasburg medical faculty, a number of research problems crossed boundaries with racial anthropology, military research, and applications in oncology and war medicine. Most of the basic psychiatric research continued to be supervised by brain psychiatrist Bostroem, even after he had been dismissed as curator of the Reichsuniversitaet. The large numbers of approved dissertations with neurological and psychiatric research themes – sixteen out of 125 dissertations in total (13 percent) between 1941 and the closure of the medical faculty – are indicative of the continued high level of neuroscientific activities in Strasburg at that time. Most of these projects, however, were pursued in conjunction with other interdisciplinary research fields, and racial and eugenic discriminations as well as the murderous impetus of human experimentation and euthanasia are also visible here (see chapter 4).[65]

With the approach of the Western allied armies in October 1944, the Reichsminister for science, education, and culture, Bernhard Rust (1883–1945), ordered that Strasburg University be evacuated and its faculty relocated in the heart of Germany at the University of Tuebingen. In a first phase of this move, the military-related plants and equipment were deconstructed or even destroyed, so that they could not be captured by the American troops and US Alsos Mission of Field Intelligence Agency, Technical.[66] While the clinical physiologist and gynaecologist Otto Busse (1896–1960), physicist Fleischmann, psychiatrist Jensch, and anatomist Kaiserling were immediately interned through French military officials, who knew exactly whom to look for, anatomist Hirt and paediatrician Kurt Hofmeister (1896–1989) were the only representatives of the Strasburg faculty who managed to reach Tuebingen by the end of 1944. Ten days before allied troops marched into the Swabian university town, on 9 April 1945, the medical faculty of the Reichsuniversitaet Strassburg was officially closed.[67]

The situation at the University of Leipzig is similarly illustrative of the development of the brain sciences during the Third Reich. The social deterioration of the early Leipzig brain sciences landscape with the advent of the National Socialist period is instructively reflected in a report that the neuropathologist Richard Arwed Pfeifer was ordered to draft for the Soviet Military Administration on 7 May 1946, one year after the war had ended. Suffice it to say that the Nazis' ever-tightening grip on all institutional and social aspects of the Third Reich had led to an oblique system of nepotism, obscurity, and arbitrariness, through which personal intrigues, blackmailing, and political traps brought university professors in contact with the GeStapo. When the new Soviet administration came in, the Red Army officials wanted to investigate Pfeifer's role in the psychiatric patient euthanasia programs between 1933 and 1945. Specifically, they had been made aware of the fact that prior to the armistice, Pfeifer had assumed the position of acting director in the Flechsig Institute and the clinical department of psychiatry and neurology, after Paul Schroeder had passed away on 7 June 1941. This report reveals some of the questionable views that researchers at the University of Leipzig had held of themselves. Pfeifer began by mentioning that historically the Brain Research Institute had developed from a small laboratory within the clinical department of psychiatry and neurology, where it was established when the hospital opened (see also chapter 1). Following the celebrations surrounding the eightieth birthday of Paul Flechsig in 1927, the institute became autonomous, with Flechsig continuing the somatic tradition of brain research and psychiatry based on the "assumption that all mental diseases are in fact diseases of the brain."[68]

Written in the vein of a *kowtow* to the Soviet administrators, Pfeifer's report hastened to emphasize that the neuroscientific positions of the Russian physiologist Ivan Petrovitch Pavlov (1849–1936) would "have always been maintained" and that Pavlov had personally benefited from his continued exchanges with Flechsig since an earlier visit to Leipzig in 1877.[69] Pfeifer also mentioned that the Russian neurologist Vladimir Michailovitch Bechterev (1857–1927) had received postdoctoral training in Flechsig's clinical department from 1885 to 1886. Yet it was not only by means of alluding to "the great Russians" that Pfeifer tried to equilibrate the perception of the early neurosciences at Leipzig. He made a point of mentioning that "the great Jewish scholar" Paul Ferdinand Schilder (1886–1940) had likewise trained under Flechsig between 1920 and 1925. What Pfeifer certainly did not mention was that Leipzig neurologists and psychiatrists were quite reluctant to keep their Jewish colleague among their ranks – even before the Nazis had come to power – so much so that Schilder had to submit his resignation and seek a new scientific career outside Germany at New York University's School of Medicine in 1929.[70]

With regard to Pfeifer's personal antagonisms with Schroeder, the director of psychiatry, however, and the latter's attempts to blackmail him *vis-à-vis* the Nazi government, Pfeifer remained very quiet in his report. He simply described the technicalities of how Schroeder had reintroduced earlier histopathological research on the central nervous system since

1926. Pfeifer attributed this orientation to Schroeder's prior training with the neurohistologist Nissl at the clinical department of psychiatry and neurology at the University of Heidelberg. The report only alluded to the circumstance that Schroeder had created an autonomous histopathological laboratory for the study of nervous diseases in children and adults. While pointing to Bostroem's brief headship of the Leipzig clinical department, Pfeifer made absolutely no mention of their membership in the NSDAP or any other Nazi organization.[71] Likewise, he spared any comments to the Soviet officials about the personal involvement of these psychiatrists and neurologists in the Nazi euthanasia program, which had ordered the murder of patients with mental and neurological diseases. Particularly, he omitted to mention that Schroeder and his assistant physicians Hans Buerger-Prinz (1897–1967), as well as Jensch, had been commended in 1940 to the "hereditary health court" (*Erbgesundheitsgericht*), where they had become directly involved in the decision-making processes for the forced sterilizations of numerous psychiatric patients and asylum inmates.[72] Of course, a transparent report on the involvement of Leipzig psychiatrists in the Nazi medical atrocities would have cast a negative light on Pfeifer himself.[73]

What is more, the noted neurologist Oswald Bumke, who had been a Leipzig professor in the Paul Flechsig Institute from 1921 to 1924, was subjected to disciplinary action following the war. Bumke had succeeded Kraepelin in the chair at Ludwig Maximilians University. And due to the fact that Munich clinical neuroscience institutions had been involved in the National Socialist euthanasia program, he was subjected to a thorough "de-Nazification" program.[74] However, Bumke was able to return to his chair in 1946 after "personal clearance" from the US Military Court, soon after which he retired from his clinical duties.[75] Already since the early 1920s, he had introduced significant changes to the organization of psychiatric care in the University of Leipzig's clinical department. He had still based his own psychiatric theorizing on materialist interpretations of brain function and concentrated further neuromorphological research on nervous regeneration phenomena and histopathological changes in dementias. In addition to these areas of laboratory research, however, his clinical department also offered psychological and genetic research activities. Pfeifer later wrote:

[With Bumke], a strictly psychologically oriented psychiatrist, a versatile administrator and writer had arrived, whose textbooks are a good read even today. The changes in the clinical department, however, were drastic and complete, while Bumke would really have liked to ban the neuromorphological laboratory from the institute of anatomy.[76]

Such a "ban of brain anatomy" from the activities of the Leipzig clinical department of neurology and psychiatry only happened at the end of the war, and with the restructuring of the local scientific landscape in the founding years of the German Democratic Republic after 1949.[77]

Given the scientific renown of Pfeifer and his increasing alignment with Soviet administration officials, clinical neuroscience at Leipzig was completely regrouped in the immediate postwar period. The acting head of the clinical department of neurology and psychiatry moved Flechsig's Brain Research Institute out of the hospital grounds and reintegrated it as an autonomous neuroscience research institute of the university in 1946.[78] A year later, the outpatient department was likewise reorganized as a separate unit closer to the vicinity of the city.[79] When the German Democratic Republic was founded on 7 October 1949, the neurosurgical service was likewise formed as an autonomous division, which included twenty hospital beds, first as a unit of neurosurgery and as a proper department in the faculty – the first of its kind in Eastern Germany.[80]

ON THE SOCIO-POLITICAL CONTEXT DEVELOPMENTS WITHIN THE NAZI MEDICAL CORPS

Discussion of the general issues of health care in this chapter takes an epistemological and contextual perspective rather than a perspective of social history. Yet, not to give a false impression: my aim is to outline some of the relevant socio-political contexts of the Third Reich that influenced the process of marginalizing specific areas in medicine that the Nazis saw as alien to their health care philosophy, while promoting those seen to be in line with the new political goals.[81] The area of early neuroscience did not represent a stable subject; the contours of what counted as brain research, neurology, and psychiatry had, as I have shown in the preceding chapters, shifted greatly since the end of the Wilhelminian Empire. A closer historiographical observation reveals the dimension and scope of these changing forms of political decision-making on the growth of this field, first under explicit Nazi political auspices, and later during the financial, material, and human resource constraints imposed on neuroscience and brain psychiatry in the war effort of World War II.

Given the importance of basic biological views in medicine and health care during the first decades of the twentieth century, it is not surprising that physicians had been strongly attracted to the Nazi movement since the 1920s. This attraction is reflected, for instance, in the nearly three thousand doctors (representing 6 percent of the profession), who joined the National Socialist Physicians League (Nationalsozialistischer Deutscher Aerztebund / NSDAeB) in the first month after the Nazis seized power.[82] In their social alliances with various branches of the party system, German doctors and medical researchers chose to belong to a number of organizational groups, the most important being the NSDAeB, the National Socialist German Workers Party (NSDAP) itself, and the National Socialist German Teachers League (NSDLB) for university faculty members and teachers, the SS, and medical columns of the SS (including the medical corps, cavalry, air force, and so forth). This is not the place to discuss the involvement of all of these organizations in the medical sector; that has been done by other scholars.[83] Rather, what I intend to examine, in describing the changing boundaries of the field of neuromorphology, is the fact that a large proportion of German physicians and health care workers felt attracted to the NSDAeB, indicating their outright endorsement of the political ideals of the new Nazi government.

The NSDAeB was formed as a professional union during the later Weimar years – in 1929 – to serve as a lobby group for medical doctors in support of their professional and monetary interests (largely represented in the conservative physicians' *Hartmannbund*).[84] It later emerged as an influential social platform that introduced eugenic, national public health, and militaristic concepts into the framework of new Nazi reform initiatives. Internally, the NSDAeB was seen as a defence mechanism against socialist plans to change the status of physicians to become public employees and thus reduce their freedom of choice in opening general practices (see also chapter 4). Outright anti-Semitism was exhibited widely in the German medical corps, as it was perceived that Jewish physicians themselves were overrepresented by a factor of ten to one, at a time when 10 percent of all non-Jewish doctors were unemployed. However, by 1939 the NSDAeB was eclipsed by the party itself, with nearly 45 percent of all physicians in Germany and Austria rushing to join the NSDAP. In the eyes of younger doctors, as a lobbying instrument for their professional purposes, the NSDAeB had already done its job, since the Nazis had risen to power on 30 January 1933.[85]

This perception of success was mainly due to the "Law of the Restoration of a Professional Civil Service," passed only three months later on 7 April 1933. The law directed that all state officials who criticized the new regime, along with those considered "of non-Aryan descent," had to be dismissed from office. Nazi ideology regarded it as unacceptable and even dangerous for Aryans to be taught by Jews, and as a result many university professors, teachers, and doctors in the public health service lost their positions in the civil service. Even honorary officials of science boards were released from their duties. Hence this law cut deeply into the developed culture of science and medicine in Weimar Germany, now in a political climate where Nazi legal programs and actions were manifested through the dominance of racial hygiene, eugenics, and later even patient euthanasia.[86] What is crucial with regard to the emergence of the new research field of the neurosciences was the active expulsion of what the Nazis saw as a "Jewish form of medicine and health care," particularly exemplified by the psychoanalytic tradition in psychiatry, socialist health programs, and the emergence of medical sexology.[87] The normative context of medicine and psychiatry in the Third Reich was such that physicians stepped out of their traditional doctor-patient relationships and abandoned deeply ingrained professional behaviour of mutual respect, showing open antagonism toward their Jewish colleagues and toward physicians who opposed the increasing radicalism and inhuman shape of the medical system.

"DE-JUDIFICATION" OF THE GERMAN BRAIN SCIENCES AND THE EXODUS OF GERMAN-SPEAKING MEDICAL DOCTORS

The changes in the political and organizational structure of the German-speaking medical system during the Third Reich can be linked to the specific elements of Nazi politics and the philosophy of the increasingly co-ordinated and lockstepped (*gleichgeschaltet*) medical corps. The primary focus of public health was the provision of health care for Aryan Germans. Resources were cut for non-Aryans, and handicapped patients, as "unworthy eaters," became less and less supported through the health care system.[88] These attitudes were also reflected in the medical corps itself, which during the purges of 1933 and 1935 was cleansed of non-Aryan doctors and researchers. Oppositional health care professionals were either put under arrest or became increasingly supervised by colleagues who had been rigorous members of the NSDAP party. It was only a "logical" next step in this system for the process of the expulsion and later the murder of Jewish and non-conformist doctors in concentration camps to begin.[89]

However, the historical literature has been concerned primarily with the biographical developments and criminal activities of Nazi doctors, while the particular cultural context of this period has been only marginally discussed with respect to the "de-judification" process in the German-speaking brain sciences.[90] These developments in the Nazi period are important for my narrative, however, since they allow us to follow, for example, the loss of licences to practise medicine for individual doctors and medical researchers, and to understand the restraints upon Jewish neurologists and psychiatrists in the exercise of their professional rights. The closure of mental asylums, social care facilities, and health education institutions in the same period was an important prelude to what extended into the greatest exodus of scientists and doctors in European history (see figure 6.3).[91]

It needs to be re-emphasized, nevertheless, that not all clinical neurologists, psychiatrists, and laboratory neuroscientists who left Germany and Austria after 1933 were of Jewish origin. Although the numerical data vacillate on this point, between 10 and 20 percent of science émigrés decided to leave Europe also for other reasons. Among these reasons was the fear that their relatives could be imprisoned on account of their former political opposition as socialists, communists, or pacifists; or merely the fact that they had been abroad on research fellowships and decided that things could only get worse if they returned to their homelands.[92] This was the case for Berlin biophysicist Max Delbrueck (1906–1981), for example. He later conducted important neuro-membrane research in the United States and became a prominent professor at the California Institute of Technology in Pasadena. Likewise, Hungarian-born and Viennese-trained Stephen Kuffler (1913–1980), who worked on single nerve-muscle preparation, joined Johns Hopkins University in Baltimore. Previously, in his first country of exile, Kuffler had passed an extensive period in the laboratory of John Eccles (1903–1997) at the University of Otago in New Zealand, where he investigated the neurophysiology of nerve dendrites.[93] Also in this category is the clinical psychiatrist and geriatric physician Erich Lindemann (1900–1974), who arrived in America in 1927, and through other appointments later became the chairman of psychiatry at the Massachusetts General Hospital.

A brief look at the numbers of the émigré neuroscientists reveals that approximately two thousand scientists and professors were expelled from Germany before 1938.[94] Among them, according to a 1988 survey from the Leo Baeck Institute, were at least six hundred medical researchers and physicians, with half of these researchers being fully trained neurologists and psychiatrists.[95] This sample represents a significant group both with respect to Germany and in comparison to the émigrés' new host countries.

Reichsgesetzblatt

Teil I

| 1933 | Ausgegeben zu Berlin, den 7. April 1933 | Nr. 34 |

**Gesetz zur Wiederherstellung des Berufsbeamtentums.
Vom 7. April 1933.**

Die Reichsregierung hat das folgende Gesetz beschlossen, das hiermit verkündet wird:

§ 1

(1) Zur Wiederherstellung eines nationalen Berufsbeamtentums und zur Vereinfachung der Verwaltung können Beamte nach Maßgabe der folgenden Bestimmungen aus dem Amt entlassen werden, auch wenn die nach dem geltenden Recht hierfür erforderlichen Voraussetzungen nicht vorliegen.

(2) Als Beamte im Sinne dieses Gesetzes gelten unmittelbare und mittelbare Beamte des Reichs, unmittelbare und mittelbare Beamte der Länder und Beamte der Gemeinden und Gemeindeverbände, Beamte von Körperschaften des öffentlichen Rechts sowie diesen gleichgestellten Einrichtungen und Unternehmungen (Dritte Verordnung des Reichspräsidenten zur Sicherung der Wirtschaft und Finanzen vom 6. Oktober 1931 — Reichsgesetzbl. I S. 537 —, Dritter Teil Kapitel V Abschnitt I § 15 Abf. 1). Die Vorschriften finden auch Anwendung auf Bedienstete der Träger der Sozialversicherung, welche die Rechte und Pflichten der Beamten haben.

(3) Beamte im Sinne dieses Gesetzes sind auch Beamte im einstweiligen Ruhestand.

(4) Die Reichsbank und die Deutsche Reichsbahn-Gesellschaft werden ermächtigt, entsprechende Anordnungen zu treffen.

§ 2

(1) Beamte, die seit dem 9. November 1918 in das Beamtenverhältnis eingetreten sind, ohne die für ihre Laufbahn vorgeschriebene oder übliche Vorbildung oder sonstige Eignung zu besitzen, sind aus dem Dienste zu entlassen. Auf die Dauer von drei Monaten nach der Entlassung werden ihnen ihre bisherigen Bezüge belassen.

(2) Ein Anspruch auf Wartegeld, Ruhegeld oder Hinterbliebenenversorgung und auf Weiterführung der Amtsbezeichnung, des Titels, der Dienstkleidung und der Dienstabzeichen steht ihnen nicht zu.

(3) Im Falle der Bedürftigkeit kann ihnen, besonders wenn sie mittellose Angehörige zu versorgen, eine jederzeit widerrufliche Rente bis zu einem Drittel

des jeweiligen Grundgehalts der von ihnen zuletzt bekleideten Stelle bewilligt werden; eine Nachversicherung nach Maßgabe der reichsgesetzlichen Sozialversicherung findet nicht statt.

(4) Die Vorschriften der Abs. 2 und 3 finden auf Personen der im Abs. 1 bezeichneten Art, die bereits vor dem Inkrafttreten dieses Gesetzes in den Ruhestand getreten sind, entsprechende Anwendung.

§ 3

(1) Beamte, die nicht arischer Abstammung sind, sind in den Ruhestand (§§ 8 ff.) zu versetzen; soweit es sich um Ehrenbeamte handelt, sind sie aus dem Amtsverhältnis zu entlassen.

(2) Abs. 1 gilt nicht für Beamte, die bereits seit dem 1. August 1914 Beamte gewesen sind oder die im Weltkrieg an der Front für das Deutsche Reich oder für seine Verbündeten gekämpft haben oder deren Väter oder Söhne im Weltkrieg gefallen sind. Weitere Ausnahmen können der Reichsminister des Innern im Einvernehmen mit dem zuständigen Fachminister oder die obersten Landesbehörden für Beamte im Ausland zulassen.

§ 4

Beamte, die nach ihrer bisherigen politischen Betätigung nicht die Gewähr dafür bieten, daß sie jederzeit rückhaltlos für den nationalen Staat eintreten, können aus dem Dienst entlassen werden. Auf die Dauer von drei Monaten nach der Entlassung werden ihnen ihre bisherigen Bezüge belassen. Von dieser Zeit an erhalten sie drei Viertel des Ruhegeldes (§ 8) und entsprechende Hinterbliebenenversorgung.

§ 5

(1) Jeder Beamte muß sich die Versetzung in ein anderes Amt derselben oder einer gleichwertigen Laufbahn, auch in ein solches von geringerem Rang und planmäßigem Diensteinkommen — unter Vergütung der vorschriftsmäßigen Umzugskosten — gefallen lassen, wenn es das dienstliche Bedürfnis erfordert. Bei Versetzung in ein Amt von geringerem Rang und planmäßigem Diensteinkommen behält der Beamte seine bisherige Amtsbezeichnung und das Diensteinkommen der bisherigen Stelle.

(Vierzehnter Tag nach Ablauf des Ausgabetags: 21. April 1933)
Reichsgesetzbl. 1933 I

51

The registers of the Royal College of Physicians, for instance, show the presence of around two hundred psychiatrists and several dozen neurologists in the United Kingdom in 1940, and the files of the American Academy of Neurology list approximately five hundred specialists in 1948.[96] The historical problem of emigration-induced change has been researched from many perspectives, including the humanities and social sciences. Not only did these studies draw on individual and collective biographies but they also measured the "hard impact parameters" such as bibliometric methods, association memberships, and statistics on the leading positions in scholarly societies.[97]

This sample therefore represents a significant group of refugee academics. That the massive loss of researchers had a disastrous effect on basic and clinical neuroscience in Germany and Austria is self-explanatory. Some authors have even interpreted these occurrences simply as a matter of "brain loss" for German-speaking science and formulated a *brain gain thesis for the rest of the world*.[98] Although this view might not be entirely off the mark, it fails to account for the complexity of the processes involved; and individual gains too often came at a big loss – for clinical medicine, biomedical research, and psychiatric practice as a whole. Since not much ink has been spilled on the actual problems and obstacles that émigré scientists encountered when arriving in their new host countries, I now shift my focus from a regional to a greater international level and to the long-term effects since the 1930s and 1940s. Although such patterns sometimes point to pre-selective effects, not only of influential individuals like the Frankfurt neurologist Kurt Goldstein and the Breslau psychiatrist Franz Kallmann, or of local scientific milieux at Harvard or Columbia University, these all had a decisive impact on the future development of the neurosciences.[99] With regard to the interdisciplinary field of neuromorphology in the German-speaking countries, my interest is rather on particular areas of biological psychiatry, such as the "emigration" of insulin-shock therapy, electroshock therapy (ECT),[100] psychiatric genetics, and neurological synapse research.[101] The relationship with basic neuroscience now brings the forced migration process closer in touch with the historiographical narrative of the preceding chapters. Some contradictory developments also become apparent, since psychoanalysis, for example, became one of the major adversaries of shock therapies in the wider context of American psychiatry and public health. The double *volte face* from the preference for psychoanalysis over brain psychiatry, to its antagonism with biological psychiatry, and its later rejection due to advances in molecular medicine was a groundbreaking process in the development of modern neuroscience itself.[102]

According to Jack Pressman's book *Last Resort: Psychosurgery and the Limits of Medicine* (1998), the re-evaluation of contemporary psychiatry and neurology toward the development of aggressive surgical and interventional therapies was nevertheless underway during the first half of the 1930s.[103] Somatic forms of therapy had been particularly associated with the psychosurgery of Egaz Moniz (1874–1955) in Lisbon, and with Ugo Cerletti (1877–1963), a former Leipzig psychiatry trainee, at La Sapienza, University of Rome, where he developed electroconvulsive therapy, which later became further adapted as insulin- and cardiazol-shock therapy. The latter two options became concomitantly available when the Nazis took power in 1933, marking likewise a belated introduction of insulin, even though the "calming effect" of this hormone had already been observed in cases of morphine detoxification since the late 1920s. When the Vienna-trained neurophysiologist Manfred Sakel (1900–1957) noticed this effect during hypoglycemic states of drug addicts, where insulin had a positive effect on detoxification, he thought to have discovered a new principle of therapy for patients with schizophrenia and severe depression.[104] In autumn of 1933 Sakel experimented with insulin therapy in his patients at the University of Vienna's clinical department of psychiatry. It was a highly research-driven approach, even though during the coming thirty years it developed into an internationally respected form of psychiatric therapy.[105] It is by way of this mediation through the Swiss psychiatric community that shock therapies became widely applied in psychiatric centres in France and Spain, and in Nazi Germany. At a time when the anti-Semitic sentiments of the Third Reich had been an obstacle to the introduction of Sakel's procedure, a report of the Freiburg psychiatrist Egon Kueppers (1887–1935) to the research ministry of the Reich had nevertheless been received. Kueppers pointed out that the introduction of insulin shock treatment could suspend the need to create new psychiatric hospitals for the next twenty to thirty years. This sat well with Nazi medical philosophy, which viewed psychiatric patients and the mentally ill merely as "useless eaters." It captured the new determination prevailing in the German medical, neurological, and psychiatric communities to disband most long-term care facilities for mentally ill and neurological patients. The shock treatments thus offered a resourceful alternative to hospital-based therapy, supplementing public health measures as applied to the organism of "the people."[106]

Despite the welcome reception of his scientific contribution in biological psychiatry, Sakel was forced into exile in North America after Austria had been annexed to the German Reich on 16 March 1938. Once Sakel reached the United States, he became a staff attending physician at the Harlem Valley State Hospital in New York, where his forced migration from Austria led to the unintended introduction of shock therapies into American and Canadian medical communities. The problem of large hospitalization numbers had been recognized as a major strain on North American public health care systems and its demanding treatment situations, which, particularly in state mental asylums, were based on dysfunctional physician- and staff-patient ratios.[107] In this situation, psychiatrists in American psychiatric clinics and asylums perceived shock therapies as a major technological relief, since the economic context did not promise to change for the next decades.[108] While eugenics and psychiatric genetics had paved the way for a widespread application of shock therapies in German-speaking countries, the belief in technological progress stemming from them developed into an enabling ideology in America, which further led to a triumphal procession of shock therapies on the western side of the Atlantic.[109]

THE CULTURAL CONTEXT OF THE FORCED MIGRATION WAVE IN THE BRAIN SCIENCES

Although the main historiographical assumptions and core facts about the exodus of scientists and physicians in the period of German Nazism and Italian Fascism are well known in history of medicine,[110] major incentives to study the case of émigré neuroscientists as part of the narrative of this book have arisen from advances in scholarship of *cultural contexts* and knowledge transfers in the biomedical sciences.[111] Rather than seeing the development of the forced migration wave merely in terms of the process of an escape of large numbers of persecuted neurologists and psychiatrists to North America, the unfolding of an important *bilateral knowledge transfer* needs to be taken into account.[112] This is even more substantial, as one of the consequences of the integration of the differing communities of neurologists and psychiatrists into American scientific cultures was the gradual though very effective transformation of this field into one of the most prolific areas of post–World War II knowledge production.[113] In considering the networks and communication structures of Central European émigré neuroscientists, several historical cases shed light on the cultural contexts of these events.[114] In the same way that American historian John Russell Taylor has described for Hollywood refugee artists in California, émigré neuroscientists found themselves living as "strangers in paradise":[115]

> After all, they had to live somewhere, and on something. They had to deal with local shopkeepers, converse with neighbors, have some sort of social life. And they had to earn a living. Lucky those who, like [Lion] Feuchtwanger [1884–1958], were bestsellers in many languages of the free world and did not have to worry too much about their specific situation. But even great writers like Thomas Mann [1875–1955] were not always so economically fortunate ... at least once they were there it must have been tempting to try to find a place in the industry.[116]

Refugee neuroscientists, like all their compatriots in exile, found themselves in a foreign environment where they had to continue their daily life and learn the communication codes. Changing national immigration regulations (in Canada: 1909; in the United States: 1921), anti-Semitic ideologies (e.g. *numerus clausus* at North American universities), or non-interventionist foreign policies (for instance, American neutrality in World War I until 1917; or in World War II until 1941) had also reverberations for arriving émigré neurologists and psychiatrists in their new host countries.[117] Several trends in the under-investigated collateral histories of the forced migration wave can here be brought into scholarly perspective, one example being local strategies of refusing foreign physicians work permits (through the Royal Colleges of Physicians in the United Kingdom and Canada, as well as the medical boards and the health departments of the United States).[118] Newcomers were often seen as competitors on the medical market.[119] Similarly awkward was the installation of "internment camps" in Britain and later in the self-governing Dominion of Canada, in which refugees from Central Europe were detained along with prisoners of war and Nazi perpetrators.[120] Émigré neuroscientists also found themselves exposed to new environments in North America, where they had to sustain a living and work toward receiving medical relicensing and professional acceptance. In a way, German-speaking émigré neurologists and psychiatrists were as much socialized in their post-Weimar lifeworlds, as had been the German experimental physiologists – such as Emil du Bois-Reymond, Ernst Hallier (1831–1904), and Robert Koch – in the time of the German Empire.[121] Similarly, we see many of the émigré neuroscientists such as Karl Stern and his former colleagues among the Goldstein school in Frankfurt and Berlin – notably Gelb, Franz, and Riese – as having been strongly influenced by their upbringing in the German bourgeoisie with elements of the all-embracing Weimar Culture.[122] For them, the popular quest for "healthy nerves" was no longer an issue of the social and technological burden imposed by industrialization; it became a question of the appropriation of the biological constitution of their patients (see chapter 3).[123]

Many of the proponents of these newly established neuroscientific and psychiatric cultures in the early 1930s, such as the Goldstein group, the Munich school of neurohistology, and the private clinicians in the Berlin urban science spaces, were faced with a ban from their occupations as medical doctors following the loss of their academic working circles in their home countries.[124] Those who were economically in a position to respond decided it was better to leave Germany immediately, often with nothing more in their hands than a suitcase with their clothes and the addresses of relatives and colleagues in their pockets. A 1939 letter from Ernst Silberberg to the émigré German-American experimental patholo- gist Leo Loeb at the University of St. Louis, seeking academic assistance for his brother Martin, tells the tale of many who were displaced:

> Saint Louis Mo., May 15th 1939
> 4535 Lindell Blvd.
>
> My dear Professor [Leo] Loeb [1869–1959],
> My brother [Martin Silberberg] informed me of your kind efforts on my behalf. May I take the liberty to express to you my sincere gratitude for your kind interest and help.
> I shall not fail to call on Dr. Jerome Cook [1884–1964] next Monday [at the Jewish Hospital of St. Louis] as suggested.
>
> Very sincerely yours,
> Ernst Silberberg [1902–1976][125]

In their efforts to survive and rebuild their lost research programs, the immigrating neuroscientists must have seemed like somewhat coherent groups who competed for resources with the members of the medical and scientific establishment in their host countries.[126] When exploring such influences, which émigré researchers and physicians exerted on their receiving cultures in the United States and Canada, the long-term effects on the *neuroscientific community* come into view as well.[127] But rather than look once again the "disastrous effects exerted by vast numbers of exiled neuroscientists," my narrative also looks at some of the bilateral implications of the exiled neuroscientists in America and Germany, trying to meet German philosopher of science Klaus Fischer's earlier challenge[128] that "any consolidated evaluation of its global effects on the growth, content, and international standing of the sciences in the countries of emigration and immigration will have to await further research."[129] With a close study of scientific changes on the cultural, social, and institutional levels, several methodological angles of "emigration-induced scientific change" can be evaluated.[130] These include such questions as: What types of scientific changes can causally be accounted for by characterizing the emigration processes from the perspectives of the home countries as well as the receiving ones? For what types of scientific change will this process have been a modifying rather than a groundbreaking type?[131] And in what ways were central principles of German academic work modified in the readaptation of pre-existing research programs?[132]

Given the fact that many émigrés had virtually nothing with them – having been driven out of their flats in the middle of the night, lost their luggage in European ports, or had to give all their property away to Nazi officials (famously, Frankfurt-born neuropharmacologist Otto Loewi had to hand over his Nobel prize money) – how could they have carried pre-existing concepts, methods, and technologies with them?[133] In 1940 Loewi and his wife Guida (1889–1959) reached New York City without the address of a contact person at New York University, where Loewi was to be hired.[134] On his departure from London in England, he was seen by a consular official, but he was unable to show his dismissal letter from Graz University that would have proven he had held a prior teaching position in Austria. After the Atlantic passage, Loewi handed his sealed papers to the immigration officer and could not believe what he experienced on landing in the United States:

> Upon my arrival in New York harbor, a clerk prepared my papers for the immigration officer. While he was busy doing this, I glanced over the doctor's certificate – and almost fainted. I read: "Senility, not able to earn a living." I saw myself sent to Ellis Island and shipped back to Mr. Hitler. The immigration officer fortunately disregarded the certificate and welcomed me to this country.[135]

Emigré neuroscientists did have positive experiences, but the failures, backlashes, and hostilities that many of them experienced in their private and working lives tell much about the situatedness of incoming researchers and physicians in their new living and working contexts. This was particularly true for those who were greeted by an anti-German and often outright anti-Semitic climate. Many met with exclusion from the professional job market and cultural misunderstandings as to their positions, and suffered from a low language proficiency that created many disturbances among their peers.[136] In addition, there was also a widespread mood of resignation among many German-speaking émigrés, particularly in the first three years of the war when the *Blitzkrieg* seemed to take over the whole European continent.[137] Driven by their need to find support and allies – as with many other contemporary immigrant groups – German-speaking émigrés would seek out their compatriots in neighbourhoods such as New York's Lower East Side, the Clayton neighbourhood of St. Louis, or the Pacific Palisades near Los Angeles. Their complaints about American culture and ongoing exchanges about experiences from previous lives in Europe were legendary. In their social gatherings there was no separation between scientists, artists, and writers, all of whom served the basic functions of moral and practical support in interdisciplinary exchanges (among the Goldsteins in New York, with members of the New School of Social Research, or the Deutsches and members of the Harvard and Tufts medical faculties).[138]

The personal decisions of the émigrés to stay in America and find positions had often been influenced by their level of education, relationships with colleagues, and family support networks.[139] An interesting case in this respect is the professional couple of Martin (1895–1969) and Ruth Silberberg (1906–1997) from Breslau, where pathologist Ruth Silberberg had to work for four years without receiving any salary. At the same time her neurohistologist husband had to move from one low-paid position to the next – working first in Halifax in Canada for three years until 1936, then in New York and finally at Washington University Medical School in St Louis in the United States (see figure 6.4).

The Silberbergs eventually became naturalized Americans, and both of them received professorships, developing quite successful academic careers in American pathology communities. In an exchange of letters with his mentor, the biologist Leo Loeb on 4 August 1938, Martin Silberberg was frank about his disappointment with their working situation:

Dear Dr. Loeb,
   I am sick and tired of moving around, unless it means a definitive step forward ... Herefore [!] I cannot risk any more adventures.[140]

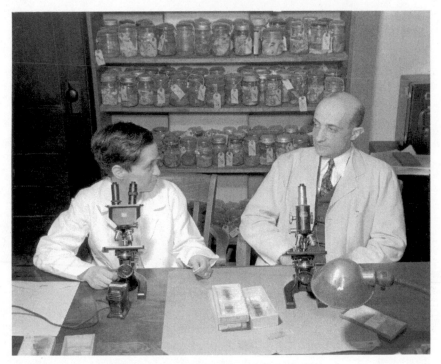

6.4 The professional émigré couple Ruth and Martin Silberberg in their lab, 1949.
(VC412 SilberbergR-SilberbergM-01). © Courtesy of the Visual Collections, Rare Books
Collection and Archives of the Becker Medical Library, Washington University School of
Medicine, St Louis, USA.

And even the Silberbergs' move to the Rockefeller Institute for Medical
Research (founded in 1901) in New York City had offered little relaxation
of their demanding life circumstances:

> Dear Doctor Loeb,
>   Nothing has been heard of promotion or raises of salaries, since
> Dr. [Irving P.] Graef's [1902–1979] departure. I am pretty sure that
> no changes will take place. It is the policy of the school to exploit
> everybody and to make use of everybody's plight. The school has the
> highest percentage of Jewish [!] students, who are glad to pay fees
> that are about 30% higher than Yale's or Harvard's ... But, what can
> we do, if the difficulties to obtain a fairly decent position are unsur-
> mountable [!]? The only good aspect is that Dr. [William C.] Von
> Glahn [1900–1961] lets us have our own ways in research.[141]

The case of the Silberberg couple can be seen as one of many examples of the pragmatic difficulties that arriving neuroscience refugees had to surmount before they could eventually resume their clinical and research work. This group of émigrés in North America was rather more hetero-geneous than has been thought in the past:

The distinction between those "migrating" and those "emigrating" from Germany between the two world wars is, to this extent, con-ceptually muddled, as it may obviously lead to unintended disqualifi-cations. It makes a cleavage where none really exists, or conversely builds a single category where cases are in fact incommensurable.[142]

As Fischer has suggested, it is not useful to limit too closely the definitions of "theory change" in the reintegration of émigré neuroscientists in North America. Truly, the very hiring of a refugee scientist or physician was *per se* an example of scientific change, in so far as newcoming colleagues spoke a foreign language, had different research experiences, and used methods foreign to their American peers.[143] This also pertains to émigrés' frequent observations about what appeared to them as underdeveloped medical care systems, particularly in smaller cities of Canada and the United States, as they compared these work situations with the intensive communities in such leading places as Breslau, Frankfurt, or Berlin.[144] It is important to note the paradoxical cases of émigrés' readaptation, since their prior train-ing was often of no direct help to them in obtaining a position and re-establishing a major research program comparable to their home countries. This is striking in the case of the unsuccessful application of Jaroslav Otakar Pollak (1906–1974), a versatile neuropathologist from Czechoslovakia, who sought a faculty position at Washington University School of Medicine in St Louis. Pollak had received his MD from the University of Bruenn in 1930 and managed to immigrate to the United States as a university teacher, starting out as an associate in legal medicine at the Massachusetts General Hospital between 1938 and 1941.[145] Although his department head at the Harvard University School of Medicine contacted colleagues in St Louis and wrote letters of support to the committee, Pollak's application was still turned down because he was perceived as "so alien:"

10 December 1938

Dr. David McK[enzie]. Rioch [1900–1985]
Department of Anatomy

Harvard Medical School
Boston, Massachusetts

Dear Rioch:
I intended to present to the Executive Faculty at the meeting on December 7 the matter of appointing Pollak to the post in neuropathology[, since ...] the Faculty had expressed doubt as to the advisability of taking action mainly because of the vacancy on the Chair of Pathology ... Also *doubt has been expressed about the advisability of appointing a German émigré* whose personal characteristics are unknown first hand to any member of the Faculty.[146]

Such adverse reactions from search committees were by no means uncommon incidents, since many observations of the sort could be found in administration records in the hiring American university hospitals and departments.[147] The same holds true for autobiographical accounts from émigré neuroscientists who returned to Europe termporarily or for good.[148] This can be gleaned from the story of another refugee from Czechoslovakia – the psychiatrist and neuropathologist Robert Weil (1909–2002), who immigrated to Canada before the outbreak of World War II in 1939. While giving his later address as the president of the Canadian Psychiatric Association, Weil emphasized his comfort with his integration into the Canadian academic landscape. At the same time, he mentioned that he could barely have given a presentation in English five years before:[149]

Before I finish my *personal introduction* I wish to express my gratitude to the Canadian people, which gave not only me alone a new faith in mankind. From the first day I ... we – and I speak here for me and my wife – felt quite at home in this sociable and friendly country ... I spoke a little while ago about *my insufficiencies in the English language* and therefore I hope you will excuse my maltreatment of your mother tongue. 5 years ago I would have called everybody, who would have told me, that I am going to speak at this time before a english speaking [!] Masonic gathering as fantastic at least [!][150]

The lessons that we can draw from such problematic occurrences, such as language problems, lack of social integration, and methodological alienation or theoretical incommensurabilities, as well as from the many productive instances of the integration of émigré neuroscientists into pre-existing working groups, are largely related to the specific actors involved. One example is the community roles played by kinship relationships and professional contacts, which emerged as decisive factors in the integration of neuroscientific émigrés into research communities in the host countries. A particular social support role was assumed by individuals who had visited the United States or Canada prior to 1933. Psychosomatic physician Franz Gabriel Alexander at the University of Chicago, neurologist Leo Alexander at Tufts Medical School in Boston, or psychoanalyst Sándor Radó at Columbia University in New York, for instance, all played important roles in mentoring forced migrants from the large German, Austrian, Hungarian, and Czech medical centres to follow their personal examples.[151] Among those later émigrés who were helped by the first group of transatlantic travelers were representatives of non-analytical brain psychiatry, such as geneticist Kallmann from Berlin and the above-mentioned pioneers of somatic treatment approaches, Sakel from Vienna as well as Budapest's Ladislaus von Meduna (1896–1964).[152] Their examples stress the importance of the role played by intermediaries and matching institutions. This early process was further amplified through the institutional involvement of the Rockefeller Foundation after 1934–35 and its close ties to the research institutions since the Weimar Republic as well as the American Emergency Committee in Aid of Displaced Foreign Physicians.[153]

Published disciplinary histories and available oral history accounts by scientific refugees have pointed to major achievements and landmark methodological events. Their contributions can be analyzed here by looking at the alignment of émigré neuroscientists with research groups involved in developments such as laboratory progress in neural regeneration research, new classifying approaches of tumour pathology, or the introduction of electron microscopy in histological nerve cell research, to name only a few.[154] When we align this historiographical analysis carefully with the early interdisciplinary approaches in German-speaking neuroscience, a number of similar observations emerge, as Ute Deichmann has pointed out in her work on emigration-induced changes in experimental biology: "The emigration of scientists after 1933 caused, with a higher probability, significant scientific change within novel fields of research rather than within the established ones."[155] For neuromorphology and its neighbouring disciplines, this was also the case; examples are the development of biological and genetic approaches, along with progress in regeneration research or advances in neurochemistry.[156] Among the elements that fostered such theory-changes in the neurosciences, official and unofficial networks within the Deutsche Forschungsgemeinschaft, the KWG, and the early Deutsche Forschungsanstalt for Psychiatry were crucial. They played major roles in the support, placement, and sustaining of continued relationships between the émigré neuroscientists in the United States and Canada, and fostered multifaceted patterns of clinical and basic research linkages.[157]

7

On Cultural and Professional Contexts of Theory-Change in the Neurosciences Due to the Forced Migration Wave since 1933

Germany/Austria – United States/Canada

SOME CONSEQUENCES OF THE EXODUS OF CENTRAL EUROPEAN NEUROSCIENTISTS

Hitler is my best friend ... He shakes the tree and I gather the apples.
Walter Cook[1]

The expulsion of Jewish and non-conformist researchers and physicians from the health care system in the German-speaking countries had similar major consequences for the scientific and professional practices in the emerging field of neuroscience on both sides of the Atlantic.[2] From this perspective, two things stand out about the 1930s and 1940s, and the immediate postwar period. First, research into mental illness and clinical neurology in both America and Europe changed dramatically during and after their expulsion in such great numbers, significantly altering the foundations of modern biomedicine as well as the politics of research in the twentieth century. A look at the example of brain research activities in Germany, Austria, and their neighbouring countries shows us how precisely the Nazi *Machtergreifung* destroyed many of the career plans of the proponents of neurology, psychiatry, and neuropathology.

Second, after their forced migration to North America this group of émigrés came into pre-existing clinical and research settings that, of course, had their own backgrounds of conceptual, personal, and organizational interactions related to different research cultures.[3] The effects of forced migration on modern brain research and the transplantation of European concepts into the scientific community on the western side of the Atlantic are quite apparent in cases described elsewhere.[4] I shall therefore concentrate here on some less well known émigré neuroscientists, their emigration process, and their support networks, along with the cultural difficulties they encountered when establishing new lives in the United States and Canada.[5]

Yet, rather than evaluate these occurrences merely in terms of an escape of large numbers of émigrés, we can see them as the development of an important *bilateral knowledge transfer*. In fact, it is viable to examine the readaptation of German-style research programs in certain postwar neuroscience contexts. This does not pertain solely to exchanges between major research traditions, in which distinct German-speaking protagonists became key players in American and Canadian medical communities too.[6] In particular, émigré neuroscientists introduced useful research approaches (such as innovative methodologies in neurogenetics, biological therapies in psychiatry, and forms of early neurorehabilitation, for instance) that could be added to the pre-existing and established methodologies in their new host countries.[7] They also brought about creative and encompassing educational programs, which materialized in a push of innovation in the emerging field of neuroscience. Many of the émigrés, however, had to await prolonged relicensing periods and were often excluded from regular positions during the war. Quite typical in this respect is the case of psychiatrist Grete L. Bibring (1899–1977), who became chief of psychiatry at the Boston Beth Israel Hospital only in 1946, a year after the war. Yet after that, she contributed considerably to the field of clinical psychiatry.[8]

When seen in the context of forced migration, however, the case of the Harvard psychiatrist Bibring is remarkable. She was able to benefit from the broad clinical training in neurology, psychiatry, and psychoanalysis that she had received in Austria. She managed to translate her expulsion from her former position as a staff-attending physician in Vienna into a major success once she rekindled her career in the American research community during the postwar period. Not only was she successful in continuing her clinical work and her research in her former field of psychoanalytic psychiatry but she rose through the ranks to become a full professor, later department head at Harvard, and even president of the American Psychoanalytic Association.[9] This career path was extraordinary not only in relation to Bibring's peer female psychiatrists and neurologists in the United States but also *vis-à-vis* her compatriot émigré colleagues. Most women émigré neurologists and psychiatrists had to give up their scientific work and medical practices (see figure 6.3) – many needed to change into nursing, as did the Berlin psychiatrist Hertha Nathorff, *née* Einstein (1895–1993), since they were not relicensed in medicine.[10] By withdrawing from their own career aims and taking on nursing, laboratory assistance, and care-provider positions, they often enabled their partners to prepare for their respective examinations. Others experienced obvious career changes, as in the examples of Breslau neuropathologist Ruth Silberberg in St Louis (see figure 6.4), the Berlin neurologist Herta Seidemann (1900–1984) in New York City, or the psychiatrist Hertha Riese, *née* Pataky (1892–1981) in Richmond, Virginia.

The study of such collective biographies of émigré neuroscientists, institutional histories, and related networks thus serves as a distinctive mirror of global history in specific local milieux. As in the case of Seidemann, entire research schools were often expelled from the German-speaking countries. An intriguing example is the group of the academic co-workers of Karl Bonhoeffer, the director of the department of clinical psychiatry at the Berlin Charité (between 1912 and 1938). Nearly a third of his longtime research associates fled to the United States.[11] This illustrious group of psychiatrists and neurologists included Paul B. Jossmann (1891–1978), who went to the Veterans Administration Outpatient Clinic in Boston; Lothar Bruno Kalinowsky (1899–1992), who continued his clinical work at the Mount Sinai Hospital in New York; Kallmann, who led the Genetics Laboratory of the New York State Psychiatry Institute between 1938 and 1961; and Fred Quadfasel (1902–1981), who worked also at the Hospital of the Veterans Administration in Boston, where he served as a chief aphasiologist from 1958 to 1961. Seidemann likewise went to New York, where she took up the post of a staff attending physician in the experimental psychology division headed by Goldstein at Montefiore Hospital in the Bronx.[12] Erwin W.M. Strauss (1891–1971), the only physician from the former Berlin group to settle in the state of Kentucky, was made a director of the Veterans Administration Hospital and professor at the University of Kentucky College of Medicine (1949–63).[13]

Understandably, the personal education and training in medicine that these émigrés had received before they actually left Germany, Austria, Czechoslovakia, Poland, or other countries, is quite important to understanding the developments in neurology and psychiatry prior to the phase from 1933 to 1945. The exodus of the vast number of physicians and scientists from Nazi Germany has been the subject of considerable research, which has investigated the impact of politics on academic societies and medical practice.[14] This can serve as a good point of departure for a further step in the analysis – an exploration of the overlapping spheres

of psychiatry and neurology in the guise of *Nervenheilkunde* that had
been typical for many of the European émigrés arriving in North America
after 1933. Many of these émigrés had been trained in the basic sciences,
such as neuropathology, neuroanatomy, or neurophysiology, while gaining
substantial proficiency in psychiatry in pre-eminent venues such as Berlin,
Leipzig, Breslau, or Strasburg, among many others (see chapters 2 and
3). The lines of this development must be further mapped. By focusing
on a multitude of biographies and clinical histories, we can gain a valuable perspective on the involvement of German-speaking émigrés in various sectors of the US and Canadian health care systems. To be more
specific, I use the subdevelopment of émigré neurologists and psychiatrists
as an instructive example to gain in-depth knowledge of the impact of
such differences on cultural codes and professional and research practices.
This process shaped the development of an advanced scientific and clinical
field that encompassed neurology, psychiatry, neurosurgery, and psychoanalysis also in North America. Analyzing the development of a preliminary typology of refugees from German-speaking neuromorphology
touches also on important recent discussions regarding the international
brain drain in the biomedical sciences.[15]

THE "LAW FOR THE RESTORATION OF A PROFESSIONAL CIVIL SERVICE" (1933) AND THE FORCED MIGRATION OF PSYCHIATRISTS, NEUROLOGISTS, AND BASIC NEUROSCIENTISTS[16]

What ultimately defined the role of the neurosciences in the overall development of Nazi medicine was the involvement of the mentally ill and
neurologically handicapped as prime targets of racial hygienists and
eugenics activists, begun in 1933 but markedly aggravated during the war
years (1939–45).[17] In addition, various areas of psychiatry and neurology
became rejected, because they were seen as particular forms of "Jewish
science" that fell short of racial, eugenic, and medical National Socialist
ideals.[18] On the one hand, a large number of doctors had what the Nazis
considered "Jewish family backgrounds." On the other hand, many physicians who had materialistic views were suspicious of the unclear boundaries between neurology, psychiatry, and even psychoanalysis that were
typical in the *Nervenheilkunde* field of the German-speaking countries.[19]
The attacks of Nazi party officials and doctors on many progressive brain
scientists led in several steps from 1933 to 1935 and 1938 to the expulsion of up to a third of the field's leading physicians from Central Europe.[20]

The initial impulses for these anti-Semitic and likewise also "anti-psychiatric" tendencies in Nazi medicine came with the inauguration of special laws, legal instruments that were released soon after the NSDAP took power. These groundbreaking political changes during the National Socialist period had a major influence on brain research in the 1930s. In April 1933, the so-called Law for the Restoration of a Professional Civil Service (see figure 6.3) came into effect, mandating the expulsion of all non-Aryan and politically oppositional faculty and staff from state-supported academic and research positions.[21]

Shortly thereafter, the establishment of the Nuremberg Race Laws on 15 September 1935 further contributed to the expulsion of thousands of medical doctors and scientists from their offices. It widened the circle of individuals who were considered non-Aryan and in consequence also decreed that Jewish physicians would no longer be allowed to care for their Gentile patients.[22] Following this law, the government of the Reich added more articles aimed at expelling Jewish scientists and doctors from universities and other state-funded institutions:[23]

For the re-establishment of a national professional civil service and for the simplification of administration, officials may be discharged from office according to the following regulations (the detailed criteria of exclusion), even when the necessary conditions according to the appropriate law do not exist.[24]

The Law for the Restoration of a Professional Civil Service effectively maimed the highly developed research culture in Weimar Germany and shook the international standing of German medicine.[25] In a government administrative list published regularly from 1934 onward, it was recorded that 614 university teachers in medical science were dismissed.[26] It is interesting to note that three German universities – Berlin, Frankfurt am Main, and Breslau – conspicuously accounted for 40 percent of the total number of academic staff released.[27] Of the approximately fifty-two thousand doctors in Germany when Hitler came into power in 1933, about 16 percent had Jewish ancestry, a total of about eight to nine thousand physicians.[28] About 30 percent of physicians and faculty members belonged to the group of consultants in neurology and psychiatry or had at least some considerable training in *Nervenheilkunde*, before working in internal medicine, neuroanatomy, neurosurgery, pathology, and other neighbouring disciplines.[29] Further insight is gained by looking at the keynote addresses to the German Association of Neurologists and

Psychiatrists (Gesellschaft Deutscher Nervenaerzte) since 1907, which reads somewhat like the "Who's Who" of contemporary European neurology; the list includes many names of Jewish-German neuroscientists such as Ludwig Edinger, Hermann Oppenheim, Adolf Wallenberg, Otto Marburg (1874–1948), Kurt Goldstein, and Friedrich Heinrich Lewy.[30] The scientific changes that followed the forced migration after 1933 were processes with marked results that few could have predicted at the outset and which would transform North American medicine and neuroscience in lasting ways.

THE EMIGRATION OF KURT GOLDSTEIN'S GROUP TO THE UNITED STATES: "PHYSICIANS, PSYCHOLOGISTS, OR PHILOSOPHERS?"

A particularly good example of the impact of the changes on contemporary neurologists and psychiatrists in the early National Socialist period is the development of Kurt Goldstein's holistic approach – with its integration of philosophical theories and aspects from social psychiatry, as well as its introduction of neuroscientific innovations. After his expulsion from his professorship and his onward migration through Switzerland and the Netherlands, Goldstein eventually reached the United States, where he exerted considerable influence on the communities of psychiatry and neurology during the period of his exile. Following his earlier move from the Frankfurt Institute for Research into the Effects of Brain Injuries to the Charité teaching hospital in Berlin Moabit during the latter Weimar years (see also chapter 3), Goldstein was engaged in restructuring the department of neurology in Berlin into an interdisciplinary research centre under his chairmanship. His research program and clinical service attracted an illustrious group of accomplished experts, who joined this centre from all parts of Germany. Among them, from 1931 to 1932, was the Bavarian-Jewish neurohistologist Karl Stern, who had worked as a young house officer in the Frankfurt Edinger Institute. Its research facilities soon made Moabit Hospital one of the most renowned hospitals in the country with the neurosurgeon Moritz Borchardt, Adhémar Gelb as head of the experimental psychology laboratory, and Ludwig Pick as the head of neuropathology. In this way, Goldstein's holistic approach went far beyond a mere philosophical orientation; it had become a formal program. It was thus not a huge surprise that the members of the Goldstein group became a prime target for the Nazis and the research centre at the Berlin Moabit Hospital was later dissolved.[31] Yet it was on the basis of the research findings of his group in Berlin, and particularly in Frankfurt before, that Goldstein was able to finish *The Organism*, his seminal book on the philosophy of holistic neurology, during his exile in Amsterdam (figure 3.6).[32]

Eventually in 1935 Goldstein reached New York, where he could continue his clinical work as a neurologist in private practice. However, as a result of losing the organizational basis for his research program and the collaboration of the Berlin group of intellectually oriented neuroscientists, the continuation of Goldstein's program was nearly suspended. It proved a major disadvantage that Goldstein was already fifty-seven when he arrived in the United States, an age that seriously impeded his integration into the faculty ranks at Columbia and inhibited the re-establishment of a department of neurology. This is not to say, however, that Goldstein did not have had some academic success – quite the opposite is true, showing the remarkable aptitude of this highly exceptional clinical neuroscientist.[33] Yet, this adjustment took place in the face of external constraints with which Goldstein had to cope. Being forced to practise for his living and the survival of his family, Goldstein also started to lecture in New York, Boston, Cambridge (Massachusetts), and at diverse venues on the East Coast, activities that proved very time-consuming. Furthermore, with his arrival in America, he further extended his research interests into the areas of psychology and empirical sociology, thus straining the time and resources he could devote to neurology.

With regard to the intricate process of reviewing Goldstein's scientific aspirations in the United States, his biographer Harvard psychologist Margarete L. Simmel (1923–2010) has stated that Goldstein did not find the right scientific culture he was looking for.[34] In her view, he never felt really at home, mainly because of his broader interests in the arts, his distinctly European worldview, and his harmonious personality. Goldstein was deeply rooted within the German academic culture, which had laid the foundation for his neuroscientific identity during the previous three decades. His move brought about a cultural disruption, which younger émigrés likewise often mentioned but more easily mastered by assimilating to the more empirical and applied research styles in North America.[35] This is not to say that Goldstein was unaware of the difficulties this assimilation entailed – quite the opposite was true for this highly self-reflective intellectual. In his letters to his secretary Bella Sack (1921–1977), for instance, and to his research assistant Martin Scheerer, he was explicit in thanking them for making his English "more readable" or expressing his gratitude for their "untiring assistance in the elaboration of lectures and courses."[36] Other instances include his reflections about the overly pragmatic context of American psychology and clinical psychiatry, and his frequent references in conversations with friends to the family's financial hardship.

With our cultural perspective on the scientific and clinical practices addressed here, it is certainly possible to see Goldstein's example as typifying the cases of other émigré neuroscientists who landed in America during the last decade of their active career. It further poses a test case for clashing assumptions about neurological theories and effective forms of research organization. In Goldstein's case, this plays out in contrast between the interdisciplinary collaboration under the holistic paradigm and the disciplinary formation of many traditional neurology departments at both Columbia University and the Montefiore Hospital in Brooklyn, where Goldstein established his "laboratory for experimental psychology" for investigating aphasic stroke patients.[37] In hindsight, Goldstein's case shows that the biographies of individual émigré neuroscientists can tell us a great deal about the actual makings of brain research even from a methodological point of view.[38] This observation ties in well with recent discussions in the field of history of science, characterized by an influential article penned by University of California historian Mary Terrall, entitled "Biography as Cultural History of Science."[39] In this work, Terrall has drawn the attention of historians of medicine back to using collective biographies as a historiographical tool for explaining the interests, turns, and directions that medicine often takes in response to unanticipated influences.[40] Attaining the high goal of uncovering "all the multifarious strands of scientific work [that] were used by this individual to make his way in science and in the world" is a laborious and very sophisticated undertaking. Yet further exploration of *some* of the contingencies in individual émigré biographies can nevertheless be an inspirational exercise. Or perhaps, to be more explicit, the subsequent explorations of two groups of émigrés in the United States and Canada, namely the collaborators *in the holistic neurology research program* and émigré neuroscientists who had engaged *in neurodegeneration and nerve trauma studies*, can shed important light on the continuities and breaks in the emerging field of neuroscience. In a nutshell, Goldstein exemplifies the individual experiences of many medical and non-medical scientists who had previously opposed Nazism and the destructive programs enacted to marginalize the mentally ill and neurologically handicapped – or, to use Edwin Black's title, Germany's *War Against the Weak*.[41] Nazi doctors had generally criticized the contemporary fields of psychiatry and neurology for their "negative features" – "liberalism, individualism, mechanistic-materialist thinking, Jewish-communist human ideology, lack of respect for the blood and soil, neglect of race and heredity, emphasis on individual organs, and the undervaluing of soul and constitution."[42]

The more than seventy thousand patients murdered in mental asylums and psychiatric clinics (related to *Aktion T4*), as well as the parallel with the chronology of the war events, bear witness to this condemnation.[43] Through the expulsion of innovative and leading neuroscientists such as Goldstein and the members of his group, the important tradition of holistic neurology, which had contributed many impulses to neurology, aphasiology,[44] experimental psychology, psychoanalysis, and psychophysiology, was prevented from continuing as a major tradition in Germany. It would have acquired that scientific status, had the Nazis not driven its proponents out of the country or killed them in concentration camps, as in the tragic cases of pathologist Ludwig Pick and psychoanalyst Karl Landauer, among other prominent researchers.[45] Subsequently, holistic neurology almost ceased to exist in German-speaking countries. Since such vast numbers of highly skilled émigré neuroscientists fled to North America, nearly all institutions of higher learning took in some of them, wherever positions were vacant. It is one of the tragic facts of the emigration process, however, that, while individual researchers did find new homes and work places, many coherent and functioning interdisciplinarity research groups were scattered all over the continent.[46] In the case of the emigration of the Goldstein group, comprising Karl Stern, Walther Riese, Adhémar Gelb, and others, they were dispersed from the University of Idaho to the Virginia Medical School, or – as in the case of Gelb – they had died or were interned before they could leave Germany, Austria, or their neighbouring countries.[47]

In the "New World," émigré neurologists and psychiatrists maintained connections with the preceding networks in the German-speaking countries to the extent possible, but they also made many new acquaintances with leaders of the emerging field of American neuroscience with whom they engaged in significant collaborations. Among Goldstein's friends in the United States we could include, for example, the Harvard social psychologist Gordon W. Allport (1897–1967), the psychologist Gardner Murphy (1895–1979) at City College New York, the humanist Abraham Maslow (1908–1970) at Brandeis University, and the psychologist Carl Rogers (1902–1987). Rogers was at the University of Rochester in upstate New York, when they first met. These acquaintances contributed to the process of reinstituting Goldstein's former scientific program. And they

were likewise instrumental in fostering the reception of his holistic neurological work, at least in the expanding world of clinical psychology.[48]

Goldstein's alliances with many leading American psychologists rather
than neurologists came at considerable expense both for the support of
his contemporary research program in New York and for the later US
reception of his holistic neurology. The uneven uptake of Goldstein's ideas
was paralleled by the disintegration of the holistic and interdisciplinary
program of neurology. During his exile Goldstein had to divide his interests
into various disciplinarily organized areas, such as social psychology,
laboratory experimentation, clinical neurology, and even empirical sociology. Nevertheless, his book The Organism (see figure 3.6.) and his ties to
the Gestalt movement became well known, especially to psychologists
and neurological aphasiologists. Although he and his collaborators persisted in their work on aspects of several of these areas, these programs
had to be pursued at very different institutions – with varying groups and
often without financial support. What the German-born socialist professor of comparative education Robert Ulrich (1890–1977) said retrospec-
tively about him, when reviewing the "William James Lectures" in
Cambridge, Massachusetts, is fitting for many other émigrés as well:[49]

[Americans] wondered suspiciously about his many-sided interests,
which extended from medical research to psychology and philosophy. What was he really, they asked: a physician, a psychologist or
a philosopher?[50]

There were both revolutionary and modifying change-processes at work.
The modifying type can be regarded as the usual situation, when the group
of émigré researchers and physicians mobilized its existing practical,
methodological, and human resources in adjusting to the new working
contexts (including for example émigrés' research skills, therapeutic experiences, personal acquaintances, or foreign language proficiencies). In the
case of Goldstein, his medical research background translated into a basic
research program in holistic neurology and the introduction of a great
background of clinical experience, along with interdisciplinary exchanges
with psychologists, psychiatrists, and neurologists.[51] These not only
included the New York medical community, but extended to the New
School for Social Research, the New York Psychoanalytic Institute, the
support programs of the National Institutes of Health, and the American
Academy of Neurology. The contributions that the individual members
of the group themselves made neurology, experimental psychology,

linguistics, and aphasiology were received in *prima facie* unrelated fields such as philosophy, *Gestalt* theory, and psychosomatics circles. From there, they rarely fed back into the primary neurological literature. As for the east side of the Atlantic, some erratic psychologists and psychiatrists had continued to apply elements of holism and biological Gestaltism, but in a more nationalistic and modified guise, as exemplified by the case of Matthias H. Goering at the Institute of German Research in Psychology and Psychotherapy in Berlin.[52] However, the rise of Nazi medicine had virtually destroyed the research basis for neurological holism and Gestalt theory in German-speaking countries. And neither the United States nor Canada had developed an interdisciplinary terrain of neuroscience (see chapter 1),[53] despite the permeability of American neuroscience to foreign investigators who went on to reverse their previous academic travel direction from North America to Europe.[54]

Although it has been expressed in disciplinary histories of neurology, psychiatry, and neuroanatomy that one of American neuroscience's defining features was that it was so receptive to external impulses, émigré neuroscientists were also fully aware of the cultural differences that existed in research expectations, concepts of open exchange, and problem-solving attitudes, as neurophysiologist Eric Kandel (b. 1929) astutely captured:

> [What] makes science so distinctive, particularly in an American laboratory, is not just the experiments themselves, but also *the social context, the sense of equality between student and teacher, and the open, ongoing, and brutally frank exchange of ideas and criticism.*[55]

On the contrary, the work of the holistic neurologists in exile certainly valued broad social and paedagogical endeavours of education and healing over the applied accounts of neurological diseases and treatment, which they faced in American and Canadian scientific communities.[56] During their years in Europe, the members of the Goldstein group had been actively involved in workers' unions and provided free care to the poor proletariat and their families. Examples were the Gallus community in Frankfurt am Main as well as in Moabit and the "Red Wedding" in Berlin. Above all, many were educated in *Gymnasium* high schools and valued arts, music, and literature while they were politically liberal and had incorporated the social democratic ideals of the young Weimar Republic. Many of these values resurfaced later in the process of scientific forced migration in general and, for the Goldstein group in particular, translated into émigré neuroscientists' research programs, clinical approaches, and attitudes toward medical education and health care practices.[57]

I now want to trace some landmarks of the communicative topography of these individual neurologists, neuroanatomists, psychiatrists, and psychologists in their American diasporas from the 1930s to the 1950s.[58] I map these out as a way of better understanding how international acquaintances, personal relationships, and institutional networks helped facilitate the difficult transatlantic emigration process. As Goldstein's biographer Simmel has pointed out:[59]

He was grateful to the country where he and so many others had found asylum first, and a new home – but it was still a home in exile. When he appreciated things American, or criticized them, it was always as an outsider, a spectator ... he would often comment on the lack of tradition on this side of the Atlantic. I remember once replying that all the tradition in the world would not help anyone to even the tiniest hamburger, be it here or in Europe. His immediate reply was "Ach was," followed by "The younger generation thinks only of its stomach," and, finally by "You are probably right, and that is just what is so awful." I never could argue him out of that final adjective.[60]

What appears here as the central problem for émigré neuroscientists was the cultural difference in scientific aims and their search for a new work place with their readjustment to the pre-existing research cultures, working groups, and academic milieux they encountered, perceiving them literally as a *New World*. Continuous comparisons with their former European experiences were always present, and the exaggerations of modern life in their host countries were constant subjects of conversation and complaint.[61]

The members of the Goldstein group certainly proved to be no exception, no matter what their influential contributions to neurology, psychiatry, psychology, or matters of the philosophy of science had been. In talking about this still informally associated group of researchers, I include the earlier collaborators from Frankfurt and Berlin, who had all fled to different destinations in North America. Walther Riese emigrated to Richmond, Virginia; Frieda Fromm-Reichmann (1889–1957) became a psychiatrist at the Chestnut Lodge mental asylum in Maryland; and Karl Stern joined the Allan Memorial Institute in Montreal, Quebec.[62] Goldstein's closest friend, Adhémar Gelb, had been expelled from his chair at Halle University and was just about to leave Germany, in 1936, for a position at Kansas State University when he succumbed to a tuberculosis infection. Gelb was only forty-nine when he died in a sanatorium clinic in the Black Forest.[63] Another deplorable fate of one of the collaborators of Goldstein was that of the psychoanalyst Karl Landauer from Frankfurt's Psychoanalytic Institute. While Goldstein left the country immediately after the secret police had incarcerated him in 1933, Landauer himself remained in Germany for another decade. He simply did not anticipate that the Nazis would do a university professor any harm. In 1943, however, he was arrested and deported to Bergen-Belsen in Lower Saxony, where he perished in 1945 at the age of fifty-eight, just months before the camp was liberated by the British 11th Armoured Division on 15 April 1945.[64]

Despite the dispersion of the remaining researchers over the university landscape in the United States and Canada, the new East Coast network of the Goldstein group reinstituted effective intellectual exchanges in their new exile. Goldstein himself continued an intellectual relationship with his cousin, the émigré philosopher Ernst Cassirer, at Columbia University for another decade. This influence of Cassirer's "functional philosophy" is prominently documented in Goldstein's "William James Lectures," entitled "Human Nature in the Light of Psychopathology," at Harvard in the academic year 1937–38.[65] These lectures summed up Goldstein's earlier Frankfurt observations together with results from patient observations and histories in his monograph *Effects of Brain Injuries in War.* This work, published following a five-year grant from the Rockefeller Foundation, gave Goldstein the opportunity to resume the position of a respected professor for theoretical neurology at Tufts Medical School in Boston until his retirement in 1945.

After his retirement from his teaching position at Columbia, Goldstein, together with German-born psychologist Martin Scheerer, his former PhD student at Columbia, inaugurated an experimental psychology laboratory at Montefiore Hospital in the Bronx, NY. In this lab, where Scheerer had a postdoctoral research role, they continued experiments with neurological patients suffering from brain lesions and aphasic symptomatologies. Interestingly, they followed many of the protocols and experimental arrangements that Goldstein had developed in collaboration with Gelb. Likewise, Goldstein maintained letter exchanges with his other brother-in-law, Hans Rothmann (1899–1970), who after his own emigration to the United States held an adjunct position in neuroanatomy at the University of California in San Francisco. Rothmann worked particularly on the organization of the cortex in dogs and the influence of the pineal gland on corticogenesis. Two other influential names that deserve mention in this context are the Harvard scholar of education Robert Ulrich on matters of the rehabilitation of patients with brain injuries, and the phenomenologist philosopher Aron Gurwitsch (1901–1973) at Brandeis University.[66] Although the group of collaborators was evidently heterogeneous and the interactions among them varied markedly, their work relationships, the conceptual enrichment the contributed, and the reception of their writings show that they re-established some degree of complementarity in their scientific activities on the western side of the Atlantic:

> It was primarily through the close conjunction of Goldstein the neurologist with Gelb the psychologist that neuropsychology flourished in the Frankfurt Institute ... Goldstein had a much firmer grasp of general neurology together with clinical intuition and a sense for broad questions. He also found it easy to write and had an encompassing writing style, which set him apart from many clinical neurologists and laboratory medical scientists. On the contrary, Gelb was more of the experimenter ... A portrait of Gelb hung above Goldstein's desk, together with his favorite [Johann Wolfgang von] Goethe portrait.[67]

A number of institutional cross currents will help further elucidate our understanding of the ways in which the subjective experiences of "America" impinged on the German-speaking émigrés and their continued research efforts. Here, a number of aspects from counterfactual historiography come into play, since disciplinary histories of neurology have often alluded to the fact that Goldstein's life could not be understood without taking adequate account of the transition of "1933." The question has repeatedly been raised as to what would have happened to Goldstein's approach if he had had the chance to continue to work in Germany, acknowledging his and his collaborators' ties and intellectual backgrounds in the European academic landscape.[68] More helpful than to reinstate this particular question will be to re-examine the potential of the interactions present in the leading German-speaking centres in the brain sciences and analyze the often underscored factors in the functional milieux of holistic neurology. Nearly all the group members continued in varying degrees to search for comparable work conditions, once they had been forced out of their prior institutions in Frankfurt, Berlin, Munich, and elsewhere. At the same time, their future destiny was obscure to these refugees, since few of their former experiences in the German-speaking contexts applied to academia in the

United States and Canada.[69] Yet of course, Goldstein's own biography is in various respects quite similar to those of others who are less well known, including his former pupil Karl Stern from Frankfurt, who eventually fled to Montreal in Canada.[70] Their biographies both reveal an unfortunate double obstacle to the careers of these accomplished holistic neurologists, first through the effect of Nazi politics and second through the impediments of the pre-existing programs that they encountered in the North American research landscapes.

It is fair to ask why members of the Goldstein group were accepted in some institutions of higher learning but not in others. When letter exchanges, phone conversations, and telegrams are analyzed, it appears that this is more than a simply a rhetorical question. These communications circulated, for example, between the headquarters of the Rockefeller Foundation in New York, the Emergency Committee in Aid of Displaced Foreign Physicians, university deans' offices, and many job-search committees throughout the country. In consequence, quite an intriguing view of American academia emerges for this period compared to what is preserved in the standard biographies, curricula vitae, and academic dictionary entries.[71] If we take a more in-depth look at Goldstein's story, we can with all validity ask what American neuroscience would have looked like in the 1950s and 1960s if, with the help of the American Committee on the Placement of Exiled Scientists and Scholars and the Rockefeller Foundation, the Institute for Advanced Study at Princeton had accepted him as a faculty member. In fact, Princeton was very close to hiring Goldstein in late 1939, when even the illustrious Abraham Flexner became involved in the effort to convince the institute director, Franklin Ridgeway Aydelotte (1880–1956) to create a new academic position:

At the suggestion of Dr. [E. Michael] Bluestone [1891–1971] I call AF [Abraham Flexner] to know if there would be any possibility of G's [Goldstein] being given facilities for work at the Institute of Advanced Studies along with the necessary support ... [Flexner] says while the question should properly go to his successor Aydelotte, he knows that the answer is "No." The Institute is not in a position to add a new department. AF advises me to speak frankly with G. on the question of his family obligations.[72]

Similar developments related to Goldstein and his collaborators indeed lead to legitimate speculation about the influence of specific groups and academic networks when assessing the general impact of émigré neurologists and psychiatrists on the field of American neuroscience.

The story of Stern is much similar. Although he, like Goldstein in the United States, appreciated his reception in Canada, he could not really continue the mutual research program with his mentor in an uninterrupted form.[73] Despite being a much younger researcher, arriving in Canada only at the age of thirty, Stern encountered seemingly incompatible programs at McGill University, where he worked for the first fifteen years. At the Montreal Neurological Institute, the eminent Canadian neurosurgeon Wilder Penfield, who had been four times nominated for the Nobel Prize, organized all the clinical and laboratory divisions around one central research program on the cortical architecture of the human brain.[74] Likewise, at the Allan Memorial Institute, the psychiatrist D. Ewan Cameron (1901–1967), who had previously refused to join Penfield in the latter's institute, pursued his own research program on schizophrenias.[75] This psychobiological research left only limited space for a broad German-style *Hirnforschung*, as appreciated by Stern, Goldstein, and others. On the clinical side too, the ongoing medical programs at McGill's research centres did not connect very well with an interdisciplinary form of neurology, which Goldstein and his pupils conceived as an encompassing integration of neurology, psychology, behavioural therapy, and even philosophy.[76]

As an early collaborator of Goldstein in Frankfurt in the years 1930–31, and then a pupil of the tumour specialist Walther Spielmeyer at the Deutsche Forschungsanstalt for Psychiatry in Munich in 1931–32 and a staff attending physician with Goldstein in Moabit, Stern supplemented the neurohistological expertise at the Montreal "Neuro." Soon after the Allan Memorial Institute (AMI) opened in 1943, he was given a position there as a geriatric psychiatrist in Cameron's service. He began to work explicitly at the Geriatric Unit (the first one in Canada) and taught courses as a research assistant and later as an assistant professor of psychiatry. Stern always referred back to his classic humanist education in German high school and to the widespread culture of learning during his medical studies and his immersion in Goldstein's holistic neurology as a direct extension to his philosophical and anthropological leanings. Subsequently, however, he decided to leave to become the head of psychiatry at Ottawa University in 1957.[77] Stern could certainly be viewed as an important case example of an émigré neuropathologist who, after being a basic laboratory researcher had become a fervent clinician and, above all, an influential university teacher. He touched the lives of approximately ten dozen administrators, academics, and leading physicians in the Anglo- and French-Canadian psychiatric, psychoanalytic, and medical communities.[78]

As for Goldstein, he continued his clinical work as a neurologist in his private practice in Manhattan, commuting between New York and Boston, where he resumed lecturing at Tufts Medical School. Having lost his organizational basis and the group of intellectually minded co-workers from Frankfurt and Berlin through the rise of Nazism, Goldstein did not succeed in fully re-establishing the diversified German working group again as a full interdisciplinary centre. Being forced to practice medicine all along in order to provide for his family (since his wife had fallen chronically ill), lecturing at diverse places and broadening his interests into psychology and sociology led to a shift away from the neurological research that he had pursued in his home country.

This shift is reflected in the telling description by Simmel, who met Goldstein in Boston in 1942. Quite forthrightly she stated in his biography that the forced migration process had ruined Goldstein's scientific career as a clinical neurologist[79] because Goldstein could no longer find the academic culture that he sought from his earlier career. To her mind, he had never felt at home, chiefly because his relationship with the German-speaking culture of philosophy, literature, and the arts that had contributed so substantially to his whole identity for almost four decades of his professional career had been disrupted. This culture had marked the most productive time of his life and contributed to his *raison d'être* as an intellectual neurologist. The gist of his generally encompassing approach to holistic neurology is still reflected in Goldstein's "William James Lectures," which he delivered two years after his emigration to North America:

> Ultimately all failures in social organization are caused by an under-estimation of the significance of the abstract attitude and by the misjudgment of the detrimental influence which can emanate from human traits if one changes them through artificial isolation. With the help of the abstract attitude the fallacy that is basic to all false social organization can be disclosed.[80]

In these lectures, Goldstein deliberately compared the functioning of types of "social organization" with the physiological action of the human body.[81] Quite frankly, this was not really a new thought, nor was it even revolutionary with respect to Goldstein's subject of "Human Nature in the Light of Psychopathology," as it addressed social organization in a psychopathology context.[82] At Harvard the proponent of holistic neurology spoke mainly to an audience interested in general psychological questions, with few attendees from medicine and a heterogeneous group of participants originally from Germany.[83] They came to hear an illustrious émigré professor speak on his research on the eve of one of human history's most severe catastrophes: World War II. Although Goldstein was advocating for the right "abstract attitude," which he presented to his Harvard audience, he was in fact campaigning for patient-centred clinical medicine. He was quite aware of the difficulties this approach implied, in speaking about the overly pragmatic and applied context of American psychology and psychiatry, which he saw as "organ-centred," "repair-oriented," and unmistakably "mechanistic."[84]

By 1940, even before America's declaration of war on Japan and Germany, Goldstein had decided to become a naturalized US citizen. In his continued communications with former co-workers in his American exile, he also expressed an immensely personal interest in the course of the war. He had written reference letters, for example, to the Rockefeller Foundation to support Walther Riese his application for a fellowship in Lyon, France, where Riese assumed an instructor's position at the University of Lyon's medical school until the German army invaded France.[85] Goldstein remained in contact with Riese after the latter had immigrated to the United States in 1940 via Casablanca, which was the last open harbour in unoccupied North Africa.[86] Yet like Goldstein himself, who shifted away from holistic neurology to find appropriate niches for his work in applied experimental psychology, Riese was no longer working as the neuromorphologist he had been trained to be in Koenigsberg by Ernst Meyer, Jr (1871–1931). Needing to find himself a research area alongside the disciplinary neurology and neuropathology fields, Riese gave neuroanatomy courses and ventured into theoretical neuropsychology, and later even into medical history.[87] The tragic decline of Goldstein's holistic neurology was visible as well in the decreasing productivity that is evident in the output of his former colleagues' medical writings during and after the war.

The Goldstein school took on a quite different aspect during the exile of its members in the United States and Canada, compared to what it was before 1933. Its members continued to stay in contact as best they could over often long distances and met from time to time during lecture series and workshops at various institutions, particularly on the American East Coast. After Goldstein's arrival in New York in 1935, however, he was mainly occupied with his private practice in neurology and psychiatry in downtown Manhattan, from which his manifold engagements and affiliations in New York, Boston, and elsewhere unfolded. In the period immediately after becoming a landed immigrant, he tried to keep up his contacts and relationships with many former colleagues and friends in their North American exile, among them, for example, the neuropatholo-gist Riese, with whom he continued exchanges at the Medical College in Richmond, Virginia, about neuroanatomical matters of language process-ing, as well as theoretical discussions about clinical neurology. Yet like Goldstein, Riese also had to move a large part of his activities away from holistic neurology, since the he could only find a teaching position in neuroanatomy, and he increasingly ventured into theoretical neuropsy-chology to collaborate with the Virginia aphasiologist Ebbe C. Hoff (1929–1968). Later, Riese even delved into medical history, in which context he came into close contact with the Swiss émigré and doyen of modern social history of medicine, Henry E. Sigerist (1891–1957) at the Institute of the History of Medicine at Johns Hopkins University.[88]

Thus, looking at the *cultural perspective* of scientific and clinical prac-tice, it is certainly possible to see the stories of Goldstein, Stern, and Riese representing those of many others of this group, and not simply as addi-tional, singular biographies related to the forced migration wave from Germany. In hindsight, it becomes evident that their lives and the local *acculturation* narratives tell us much more about the actual makings of clinical practice and research at the time.[89] On the one hand, Goldstein's group was just about to make the Moabit Hospital in Berlin into one of the country's major centres for neuroscientific research, with interdisci-plinary contributions from neurosurgery, neuroanatomy, and neuropa-thology in the various divisions of this teaching hospital of the Charité. With the Nazi *Machtergreifung*, however, their plans were decimated, leading physicians and researchers ousted, research units closed, and many members expelled.[90] On the other hand, in their countries of refuge – Switzerland, The Netherlands, France, the United Kingdom, the United States, and even Canada – they all came into pre-existing settings with their respective interplays of conceptual, personal, and academic relations, in which, as Stern wrote, "*methods became mentalities.*"[91] The stories of many younger neurologists and psychiatrists – among them Riese, Stern, Franz, and Fromm-Reichmann – as well as psychologists, especially Gelb, Landauer, and Scheerer, who had been strongly influenced by the approaches of holistic neurology, played out in similar ways.

When reflecting on the medical situation in the aftermath of World War I and the sociopolitical dimensions of the Weimar Republic (see chapters 2–4), it becomes clear that the aura around holistic concepts had already begun to dim. In fact, discourse on neurodegeneration was about to shift from the traditional clinical problems relating to the rehabilitation of brain-injured veterans to the investigation of underlying nutritional processes. At the same time, the bourgeoning tradition of eugenics became critical of the holistic concentration on the mentally ill and neurological cases as uneconomic, while racial hygiene and Nazi medicine after 1933 sought to annihilate the work of Goldstein and his co-workers, which appeared marginal to the party's aims. It becomes evident that it was, rather, the special cultural context of the early Weimar period that had given rise to Goldstein's interdisciplinary collaboration among the holistic neurologists.[92] The neuropsychologist Hans-Lukas Teuber, the elder (see figure 8.4), from the Massachusetts Institute of Technology perceptively identified these historical distortions, which accompanied the refuge of the Goldstein group in America and affected the postwar reception of this work:

> The incredibly rapid development of our field in the 50's and 60's of this century was bound to make Goldstein into an historical figure, seemingly before his time, but history has a curious way of reaching into the present and of replaying half-forgotten themes in the future.[93]

In hindsight, then, it can be said that holistic neurology ceased to exist as a consequence of the death of members of the group and the emigration of many of its protagonists, who were geographically scattered all over North America. They continued their research and educational work in often very dissimilar contexts of psychology, neuropathology, or psychoanalytical psychiatry. One respective interpretation, which has become the most dominant one in the literature, is that holistic neurology represented a case of failure to adapt culturally to the pre-existing research communities in North America.[94] It is imperative, however, if we wish to achieve a more balanced picture of the influences on the emerging field of neuroscience, to also take the international transfer relations themselves closely into account. Such patterns seem to point to sometimes pre-selective effects – not only with regard to influential émigrés like Goldstein, or local cultural milieux such as Columbia University or Tufts University's School of Medicine. Yet they all had a relevant effect on the neuroscience refugees' future.[95] Even under the challenging circumstances, the informally related Goldstein group in exile still gave rise to far-flung ramifications in the American context.[96] Such indirect consequences were also remarked upon by Teuber immediately after Goldstein's death:

Such subterranean influence [Teuber alludes to the Wisconsin sorting test by émigré psychologist Egon Weigl (1902–1979) and the clinical description of frontal lobe signs in patients with brain injuries], an indirect success of Goldstein's teaching, is often overlooked by those who say, with some justification, that Goldstein remained a guest in his new country, that he never took roots again or played as large a role as he had at the height of his career in Germany.[97]

Teuber's emphasis on the "subterranean influence" of Goldstein and his collaborators is even more pertinent when reports by his contemporary peer researchers are taken into consideration. Eyewitness accounts remark, for instance, on Goldstein's formidable talent for relating to many interdisciplinary researchers during lecture tours and workshops, and in his extended letter exchanges.[98] With regard to the younger psychiatrists and neurologists who had been involved in the group, such as Fromm-Reichmann and Stern, their accomplishments as academic teachers and supervisors have been re-emphasized in historical vignettes.[99]

According to such accounts, Goldstein, Riese, Fromm-Reichmann, and Stern had interested a whole new generation of medical and psychology students in a broad array of perspectives on the brain and nervous system. These perspectives included neurohistological studies, clinical psychopathology, and psychoanalytic therapy, as well as psychophysiology. They also extended their reach into their teaching toward a humanist attitude on the part of the medical doctor, a concept of which they themselves were the best conceivable role models. Even though many contemporary colleagues might not have agreed with this humanistic and even psychoanalytical orientation, neuropathologist and psychiatrist Stern in Montreal made a point of signalling the attraction of the holistic perspective in teaching and methodical education:

When I look back today at my years as a student of Medicine in Munich, Berlin, and Frankfurt, I see that the true influence did not come from the curriculum of learning but from something outside. [The Heidelberg psychiatrist] Karl Jaspers [1883–1969] has pointed out that all academic learning presents one of three elements. First, the pure transmission of knowledge and of factual material. Secondly, the teaching of the Master ... When Freud traveled to Charcot, he got more out of it than neurology ... Thirdly, there is the Socratic Method.[100]

As the examples from the Goldstein group illustrate, émigré neuroscientists did not simply succumb to new cultural codes when they had to radically alter the direction of their research. Their acculturation took place in an environment that many exiled medical researchers and physicians understood in the same way as Swiss-American medical historian Sigerist saw it. He had noted in his widely read book *American Medicine* in 1934 that: "There are still large sections of the population that do not receive the medical attention they need. Splendidly equipped technically, American medicine is still backward socially."[101] Viewing the forced migration process in its wider cultural dimension thus leads to a more comprehensive account of the role of émigré neuroscientists in the research cultures in the United States and Canada. Together with the émigré doctors also travelled the scientific methods and attitudes from their earlier work in Central Europe. The international network of the Goldstein group is a good example for such culturally laden research styles, which became highly visible in the adaptation and acculturation process of the émigré neuroscientists. In this sense, "America" had an effect on their neuroscience at the same time as they were in the process of leaving their imprint on neuroscience on the western side of the Atlantic.[102] The émigrés mobilized their methodological, conceptual, and biographical resources and reconstructed them when they set out to find new jobs, continue their interests, and settle into somewhat alien research surroundings.[103] As could easily be anticipated, this process was not only a quasi-linear history of scientific adaptation or success. The exodus of scientists from German-speaking Europe resulted in considerable professional changes, even the sudden ending of medical careers, tragic personal circumstances, and sometimes deep experiences of "culture shock."[104]

ARRIVING IN THE UNITED STATES YOUNG: FRANZ JOSEPH KALLMANN AND ERIC E. KANDEL – "DISTINCTIVE SCIENCE IN AN AMERICAN LABORATORY"

I have shown above just how intertwined the political and organizational experiences of the German-speaking neurologists and psychiatrists had been with the health care systems from the Weimar Republic to the National Socialist period. There are two other individuals whose stories serve to illustrate even more vividly just how the émigrés' backgrounds affected their acculturation process in America. Psychiatrist Franz Joseph Kallmann from Berlin and neuroscientist Eric Kandel, originally from Vienna, belonged to a different generation, arriving in their new host country considerably younger than Goldstein and many of his Frankfurt associates. Kallmann presents an example from biological psychiatry in which an individual researcher transitioned rather seamlessly between the political and cultural systems of the Weimar Republic and the National Socialist period. His example testifies to the fact that research in the wider biomedical area had by the 1930s assumed a very important international character.

Franz Kallmann was born in the Prussian province of Lower Silesia as the son of the Jewish surgeon Bruno Kallmann (1861–1941), who in the latter half of the nineteenth century converted to the Christian faith. Soon after Kallmann's high school graduation, he was conscripted into the German Army and took part in the counter-defence against the Russian troops on the eastern front in Prussia in February of 1915. Wounded on the battlefield, he returned to Breslau, and in the final year of the war took up medical studies at some of the German research hotspots interested in the experimental investigations of human genetics – the University of Bonn and the University of Breslau. Kallmann received his MD degree from the latter university in 1919 and continued his postgraduate training with eminent psychiatrist Karl Bonhoeffer in Berlin and neuropathologist Hans Gerhard Creutzfeld in Munich.

From 1928 onward, Kallmann worked as a neuropathologist in the asylum of Berlin-Herzberge and thereby collaborated with Ernst Ruedin, the director of the Munich Deutsche Forschungsanstalt for Psychiatry, on questions relating to the inheritance of schizophrenia, becoming one of the most well known protagonists of genetic psychiatry on an international scale.[105] Ruedin, however, who turned out to be an active protagonist of Nazi eugenics, acted as quite an ambivalent mentor to Kallmann. This became more pronounced when it emerged that Kallmann was "half-Jewish" with respect to the Nazi Nuremberg Race Laws of 1935. One year later, Ruedin was so worried that he might lose Kallmann – or worse, his exceptional genetic "know-how" – that he suggested that Kallmann flee. Ruedin advised Kallmann strongly to seek exile and a new position in North America, from which they could still continue their collaboration without Kallmann's life being endangered.[106]

This was not at all an easy decision for Kallmann, however, since he wholeheartedly approved of eugenics and most of the restrictive programs of the Nazi public health service. In fact, as a geneticist he considered these concepts and programs to be very rational and medically advanced, associating with them the benefits of social psychiatry and neurological genetics. But his own risk, and even more so his parents' uncertain future in Germany, finally led him to seek refuge in the United States in 1936. All along, Kallmann maintained close ties to his former colleagues and researchers throughout Nazi Germany – colleagues such as Ruedin himself, Bonhoeffer in Berlin and Theobald Lang (1898–1957), who had formerly been a scientific member of the Deutsche Forschungsanstalt for Psychiatry in Munich. It was at the New York State Psychiatry Institute that Kallmann took up his new position and published his hallmark study, *The Genetics of Schizophrenia*, in 1938. This work became the reference publication for psychiatric and neurological twin studies and was a seminal textbook for the foundation of modern psychiatric epidemiology.[107] The material basis of *The Genetics of Schizophrenia* was constituted from the earlier data from Berlin-Herzberge that Kallmann had brought with him in his luggage on the ship to Ellis Island.[108] The research data showed that siblings of schizophrenics have a ten times increased risk for being diagnosed with the disease as well, while the likelihood for other relatives of schizophrenics was only slightly higher than in the normal population.

During the same time period, when Ruedin was at the Deutsche Forschungsanstalt in Munich, and Otmar Freiherr von Verschuer (1896–1969) at the Berlin KWI for Anthropology, Human Heredity and Eugenics was collaborating with the SS physician Josef Mengele (1911–1979) at the Institute for Hereditary Biology and Racial Hygiene in Frankfurt on twin studies in psychiatric asylums,[109] Kallmann also embarked on his own twin studies of schizophrenia and manic-depressive illness. This work was based on a new dataset of seven hundred siblings in various New York State hospitals and was financially supported by the state's Department of Mental Hygiene. For many years, these findings, in conjunction with the former Berlin research, provided the major evidence for the influence of genetic factors on schizophrenic and manic-depressive illnesses.[110] Kallmann thus very quickly resumed his central role as a major international player in human psychiatric genetics. This was further emphasized when he became a co-founding member and later even president (1950–51) of the American Society of Human Genetics, and in 1955 assumed the directorship of the New York State Psychiatry Institute. The annual reports of the National Institute of Mental Health offer insights into the support given to Kallmann's research program based on collaborative investigations with the Laboratory of Psychology in the intramural program (from 1952 to 1965).[111]

Kallmann's work was well received among American geneticists, but the idea of inherited differences in human behaviour at first garnered little support from the psychiatric community. Despite its initial successes, an interesting twist appears in Kallmann's emigration story, when compared with another development influenced by Nazi politics.[112] Clearly, the political intentions of Nazi medicine were vastly different from those of the US mental health care system in the postwar period, but the similarities in the scientific approaches in the research landscapes on both sides of the Atlantic need also to be considered. Medical scientists were among the very practitioners who pursued eugenic research on pedigree charts, conducted statistical assessments of disability and disease prevalence in social subgroups, invented racial hygiene and anthropological body measurements, and broadened the study of genetics theoretically. Yet the idea of genetically caused differences in human behaviour found only little support among psychiatrists during the 1940s and 1950s.[113] It is exactly at this point that the contribution of the National Institutes of Health becomes so important for the advancement of interdisciplinary thought in the growing field of neuroscience and its overlap with biological psychiatry in the United States. These dynamics are reflected in the introductory editorial to the annual report of 1954 of the National Institute of Mental Health, written by its director, Seymour S. Kety (1915–2000). Kety's editorial clearly expresses his discontent with the institute's and its advisory committee's reluctance to support and foster genetic research in the psychiatric and psychological communities of the time:

As a result of the concern expressed by the National Advisory Mental Health Study Section over the failure of past research efforts to produce more definite results in relating the biological sciences to the field of mental health, a committee was established ... A continuing concern of the Committee has been *the biophobic and psychophobic attitudes* of representatives of the behavioral and biological disciplines, respectively, and the problem of communication that exists between one field and another.[114]

As eminent American historian of psychiatry Gerald Grob (1931–2015) has shown, such biophobic attitudes were largely a result of the influence of another group of medical refugees: psychoanalysts. Psychoanalysts probably shaped the field of psychiatry, mental health, and psychology more than any other aspect of forced migration in America from the 1940s to the 1960s. They also established an important new cultural trend, in which genetics played no significant role and which, after Nazi atrocities had become widely known, was often regarded as a dangerous form of knowledge.[115] As clinical psychoanalysis and mental health research were strongly supported through the extramural program of the National Institutes of Health and sustained important ties with the clinical research branch, frictions between the various disciplines surfaced within the orientation of the institutes.[116] The historical case of Kallmann thus reflects the intricate relation between psychiatric genetics and contemporary forms of eugenics in the public health field in the Third Reich before he was forced to leave Germany and his working context in Central Europe. At the same time, Kallmann's career is indicative of strategic research decisions taken by the directors of the individual National Institutes of Health on the west of the Atlantic. What his example further shows can be interpreted as a double fracture of historical events: medical scientists in America were among the social protagonists who pursued their research aims also under the spread of Nazi philosophies on an interconnected international level.[117] They became major inventors of racial hygiene, which largely subsumed medical genetics as a scientific foundation for eugenic and mental health applications. Neurologists and psychiatrists likewise took part in the precarious movement that drove a considerable part of their Hippocratic brethren out of office and into exile, where diverging scientific traditions came to meet again under grossly changed hierarchical contexts.[118]

With respect to the cultural backgrounds and biographical resources mobilized by individual émigré neuroscientists in North America, the story of the millennium Nobel Prize winner in Physiology or Medicine Eric Kandel – himself a refugee who left Austria as an adolescent – is another one that stands out. It reveals some important factors that helped émigré neuroscientists fall on their academic feet, after entering research and clinical work in the emerging field of the neurosciences in the United States and Canada. Kandel, son of a shopkeeper in Vienna, was born in November 1929, during the Great Depression. His childhood during the interwar period was still touched by the intellectual culture the Habsburg Empire left behind in its former capital.[119] Preventing his entry into medical training at the University of Vienna, however, which would naturally have followed after his Gymnasium graduation, Hitler's march into Vienna on 12 March 1938 brought with it the same race laws already in existence in the German Reich.[120] Kandel's parents, for whom it was a difficult decision to leave their home country, their close family, and thriving business, eventually made up their minds. They agreed that the situation in occupied Austria had become too dangerous and that further suppression of Jews would arise the longer they stayed. So, in 1939, they left for New York on the basis of a legal document signed by an American guarantor (an affidavit), just months before the outbreak of World War II.[121]

In his autobiography, Kandel repeatedly emphasized how much he felt that the experiences of the vibrant cultural city of Vienna helped him determine his later research interests in the human mind and memory investigations.[122] Quite intriguing in this respect is that Kandel, a basic laboratory neuroscientist, traced his own interest in the biochemical and physiological aspects of memory functions back to his additional exposure to Vienna psychoanalysis. This is not a link usually made by today's neuroscientists, but it is remarkable in that it points to similar perspectives of intellectual interest, as well as to the parallel origins of late nineteenth-century neuropathology as those mapped above (see chapter 1). As was the case with Ludwig Edinger in Frankfurt and Oskar Vogt in Berlin, Freud too aligned his neuroscientific considerations with the techniques of hypnosis, after staying in Paris with Charcot in 1885:

> Freud did not define the ego, the id, and the superego as either conscious or unconscious, but as differing in cognitive style ... Although Freud did not intend his diagram to be a neuroanatomical map of the mind, it stimulated me to wonder where in the elaborated folds of the human brain these psychological agencies might live ... I found it ironic and remarkable that I was now being encouraged to take that journey in reverse, to move from an interest in the top-down structural theory of mind to the bottom-up study of the signaling elements.[123]

In ways similar to Kandel's description of it in *The Search of Memory* (2006), many émigré neuroscientists related their own research orientation in neurology, psychiatry, and public health to their former experiences in their home countries, having worked in some of the leading European brain science centres before their persecution and expulsion.[124]

After his graduation from Erasmus Hall high school in Brooklyn, Kandel entered Harvard College in 1944, initially wanting to take a degree in history and literature. Eventually, however, he befriended a fellow student, Anna Kris (b. 1931) from a fellow émigré circle; and perhaps because her parents, Ernst Kris (1900–1957) and Marianne Kris-Rie (1900–1980), had been prominent psychoanalysts and were well acquainted with Freud's work, Kandel changed his mind. He began to study medicine at New York University's Medical School, aiming to become a clinical psychiatrist himself.[125] In the summer of 1955, he started an elective period at Columbia University in New York with a German-speaking émigré from Minsk in Belarus, Harry Grundfest (1904–1983), who was then a neurology professor at Columbia University's College of Physicians and Surgeons.

Kandel initially approached the somatically oriented Grundfest with the idea of learning more about the "biological underpinnings of psychoana-lytical memory theory," which for the Columbia-trained neurologist seemed an awkward endeavour to pursue. It is very likely that their dif-ferent upbringings – in Vienna in the middle of the hotspots of psycho-analysis and interdisciplinary neuroscience, in the case of Kandel, and in a peripheral commercial town in Galicia, in the example of Grundfest – also shaped their different approaches to neuroscience, its scope, and its limits.[126] The subsequent argumentation between the Columbia mentor and his young mentee indicative of the many irritations among émigré neuroscientists once they had landed in North America and had begun to contribute to the communities of their new host country.

Accordingly, the elective period with Grundfest turned out to be decisive for Kandel in two ways. On the one hand, it was a cathartic experience for him during which he learned that it was rather hopeless to reduce psychoanalytic theory to neuronal cell physiology. On the other hand, new political circumstances changed his career path considerably. While one major political event (the Nazis' seizure of power in Austria) had forced him out of his home country, another political event – the outbreak of the Korean War (1950–53) – brought him to work in the new National Institutes of Health (see figure 7.1). Since Kandel had interned in Grundfest's laboratory for two extended training periods, the latter nominated him for a continuing position in Bethesda, Maryland. Work at the National Institute of Mental Health counted as an alternative service to the general conscription of physicians for the medical corps deployed in Korea.[127] The founding of the National Institutes of Health shortly before, in 1948, and particularly the research conducted on mental health since the 1950s were further landmark events that shaped this phase of transformation toward the formation of early neuroscience research activities. Conversely, there were now additional job opportunities for many émigré doctors, once they had been relicensed and intended to resume professional work in American postwar neuroscience institutions.[128] The inauguration of the National Institutes of Health was significant for the postwar careers of many émigrés in that it provided additional funding support when the reorientation of the Rockefeller Foundation's support initiatives away from biomedicine toward global health led traditional funding streams to dry out.[129] The Rockefeller Foundation had been instrumental in sus-taining a great number of leading researchers throughout the years 1933 to 1945, but following the war it elected to put its funds into programs with greater relevance to population and global health.[130]

On the basis of Grundfest's recommendation, Kandel was eventually accepted by the neurophysiologist Wade Marshall (1907–1972) to work in his experimental laboratory from 1957 to 1960. Marshall was the chief of neurophysiology and was interested primarily in a mapping program of the functional organization of the human cortex. As principal investigator, he had previously received numerous grants from the National Institutes of Health to investigate dendrite morphology and the neurochemical effects of curare-like substances, research into which he integrated Kandel as a new laboratory worker. Since the advent of the 1950s, the National Institutes of Health had been on a steep rise to become one of the liveliest places for biomedical research in the country, and in fact the world. This attracted many aspiring visitors to work and reside in Bethesda for a term – and often many years.[131] That particular research milieu brought Kandel into contact with leading neuroscientists of the time. Among them were: the émigré neurophysiologist Karl Frank (1916–1993), pioneering the examination of intracellular neuronal recordings; W. Alden Spencer (1931–1977), who began to work on hippocampus physiology and neurogenetics; and the prolific Japanese-American biophysicist Ichiji Tasaki (1910–2009). Tasaki had joined the National Institutes of Health from Keio University, following his postgraduate training at the University of Uppsala in Sweden, to experiment on the electrophysiology of the sense organs. As in Kallmann's case, the prevailing spirit of biological reductionism at the National Institute of Mental Health also proved to be highly influential to young Kandel when he began his research for a tractable system for studying learning.[132] This research materialized later, when he came across an appropriate model in the sea slug Aplysia while visiting biological marine laboratories in Southern France. He had joined the group around the Czech-born neurophysiologist Ladislav Tauc (1926–1999) for a year-long visiting period, which laid out for him a path for new findings in neurophysiology.[133]

What becomes clear from his case is the effect that major contextual political developments had had on Kandel's career in the neurosciences (see figure 7.1). This was evident in his entry into the field through the "back door" of psychoanalytic psychiatry, the contingent identification of Aplysia as his main biological model, and subsequent visiting periods in French research institutes. Furthermore, what could have been perceived as a logical succession of ensuing research steps from Aplysia to the study of the role of memory in mice would not have turned out as positive if the National Institute of Mental Health had not become such an integral catalyzer of biomedical research at the middle of the century. These rather undirected developments need to be seen as enhanced forms of science communication and the transfer of ideas from senior to junior scientists since the late 1940s. Culturally socialized in the late Habsburg capital of Vienna, Kandel had experiences in his home country that gave rise to "a fascination with memory, a fascination that focused first on history and psychoanalysis, then on the biology of the brain, and finally on the cellular and molecular processes of memory."[134] After Kandel had immigrated to the United States with his parents and brother, he developed a remarkably prolific career, which was to a large extent a reflection of the new prominence of North American research institutions. Certainly, the intensity of research exchanges and collaborations, the culture of scientific and political liberalism on US campuses, and above all the breathtaking technological advances of postwar academic institutions ultimately made Stockholm possible for Kandel in the year 2000.[135]

As with other émigré neuroscientists, it was most obvious to Kandel that the cognitive understanding of scientific subjects and professional practices had varied markedly with the influence of time and culture. Émigré researchers were themselves strongly aware of such a *cultural dimension of science*, due to their experiences of leaving their home countries and starting fresh in new academic contexts. This is manifest, for example, in Kandel's recollections, as he ponders on the background of Vienna in his autobiography:

Vienna's culture was one of extraordinary power, and it had been created and nourished in good part by Jews. My life has been profoundly shaped by the collapse of Viennese culture in 1938 – both by the events I experienced that year and by what I have learned since about the city and its history. This understanding has deepened my appreciation of Vienna's greatness and sharpened my sense of loss at its demise. The sense of loss is heightened by the fact that Vienna was my birthplace, my home.[136]

Most émigré scientists in North America probably agreed with Kandel's emphasis on the considerable effect that the culture of their home countries exerted on their personal and scientific lives, regardless of whether they were forced to emigrate from Berlin, Frankfurt, Leipzig, Breslau, Munich, or Vienna. Émigrés soon began to realize that forms of research organization, scientific conduct, and the use of new investigative methods overseas were different from what they had been accustomed to.[137] Nevertheless, these reflections needed time to emerge and ripen. Many landed

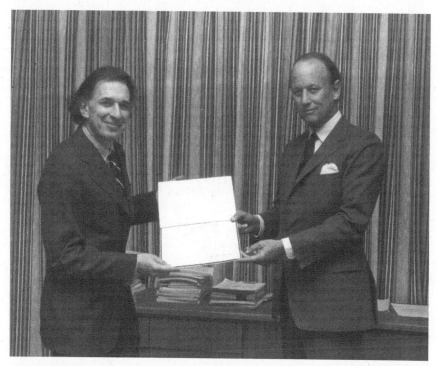

7.1 Eric R. Kandel (left), director of the Center for Neurobiology and Behavior at Columbia University, is standing with Donald S. Fredrickson (1924–2002), director of the National Institutes of Health (right). They are holding an award at a medical event in Bethesda, MD, 1978. © Courtesy of the US National Library of Medicine, Bethesda, Maryland, USA.

professional immigrants of the mid-1930s had to strive to sustain their families, and it was necessary for them to accept all sorts of practical, health care, and clinical forms of work in order to guarantee their survival in their host countries. They arrived in North America in a period following the economic downturns of the Great Depression, during which continuous employment in the postsecondary sector was very scarce.[138] Yet, even when they were successful in entering North American universities to continue their professional careers, they had to face the difference in the lifeworlds they encountered, as the German-Canadian neuropathologist Stern eloquently put it in 1965 when reflecting on his exile in the cultural climate of Montreal:

If you asked me to state quickly what is wrong with "modern thinkers," I would say that methods became mentalities. This happened,

for example, in the case of Darwin or of Freud. The method, with its
pristine clarity and compactness, is processed and diluted into something penetrating and pervasive, which makes up a climate.[139]

In keeping with such lines, the respective narratives from the massive
exodus of Jewish and oppositional neuroscientists from German-speaking
Europe consist of much more than just an alignment of events that
occurred in the academic sphere of contemporary research in neurology
and psychiatry. Influential individuals like Kandel or Kallmann, as well
as local scientific and cultural milieux – Columbia University and New
York University, or the National Institutes of Health in Bethesda, for
instance – proved to have considerable influence on the future development of the neurosciences in the twentieth century. Of course, there were
several long-term consequences from the massive exodus of Central
European émigré researchers and physicians since the 1930s. Some were
of a more groundbreaking sort (such as the first use of synthetic psycho-
active drugs in clinical settings, the introduction of somatic therapies, or
the spread of psychoanalysis in psychiatry). Others were of a rather
"ameliorating" type (the introduction of the idea of a brain research
centre, the promotion of general educational programs, or the contingent
interchanges between individual neurologists and psychiatrists) (see also
the Introduction). These brain researchers would probably never have
met and collaborated if the forced migration process had not taken place.
The late neurophysiologists Horace Magoun (1907–1991) and Louise
Marshall (1910–2004) have drawn attention to these changes in the field
of neuroscience in their book *American Neuroscience in the 20th Century*,
pointing out:

> This counter-current effectively enlightened and instructed both
> young and old scientists and accelerated the diffusion of functional
> concepts of the nervous system into the traditional morphological
> studies. With new research ideas and teaching programs, the transfer
> of apparatus and methodologies became a major element in the
> growth of neuroscience in the United States.[140]

The forced migration process of Central European neuroscientists quite
often resulted in profound changes of orientation along with innovative
forms of rearrangement of preceding traditions in the German-speaking
countries, as Kandel's example has shown: crossover programs between
psychoanalysis and neurophysiology; clinical brain psychiatry and public

mental health initiatives; and holistic neurology and experimental psychology, to name only a few. These new research directions were instigated by so many creative academics, such as the neuropathologist Riese in Richmond, Virginia, the neurologist Goldstein in New York, or the psychiatrist Stern in Montreal. In their efforts to adapt to pre-existing North American scientific research styles, the arriving émigré neuroscientists began to substantially enrich them.

A GATEWAY TO THE NEW WORLD: TRAUMA RESEARCH IN THE TRANSATLANTIC EXILE – "AMERICA WAS A RELIEF AS WELL AS A SHOCK"

Unlike the Berlin neurotraumatologist Max Bielschowsky, who had been a senior scientist during the 1930s and was spared immediate extradition from his position as he had been an army captain in the Great War (exception for *Frontkaempfer* in the Law for the Restoration of a Professional Civil Service), most of the psychoanalytical trauma researchers were persecuted by the Nazi regime early in its rule. Prominent researchers were forced out of Germany and Austria, seeking refuge mainly in the United Kingdom. This move across the English Channel is prominently exemplified by the Vienna neurologist and "father of psychoanalysis" Sigmund Freud and by the psychosomatic physician and founder of "focal psychotherapy" Michael Balint (1896–1970), the Hungarian pupil of Sándor Ferenczi.[141] Others had either tried to immigrate directly to the United States or had travelled to America shortly before the outbreak of World War II via earlier exiles in Germany's neighbouring countries. This wave of émigrés included the neurologist Ernst Simmel and the psychiatrist Helene Deutsch (1884–1982) from Berlin, the Cologne psychiatrist Gustav Aschaffenburg of the university mental asylum Lindenburg, and the German-American neurologist and psychiatrist from Wuerzburg William G. Niederland (1904–1993). By 1937, twenty-seven psychoanalysts had fled to the United States, a trend that increased significantly by the time the Americans actively entered the war in 1942.[142] As was the case with many doctors in the German-speaking field of *Nervenheilkunde* – with its shifting boundaries between neurology, psychiatry, psychoanalysis, and allied disciplines – psychoanalysts found themselves to be prime targets of Nazi defamation either as "Jewish" or as "socialist physicians." What is more, they were seen as doctors who had shown an interest in helping and caring for individuals whose "lives were not worth living" (Binding and Hoche: see also figure 5.2).[143] From the new public health perspective of the so-called *Volksmedizin*, the work of traumatologists and psychoanalysts was denigrated as being completely useless; it could only result in prolonging the lives of patients with mental illnesses and inherited neurodegenerative diseases. Following the institution of the general alignment policy (*Gleichschaltungspolitik*) of the Nazi regime and the ever more violent attacks from street mobs in the build-up to the *Reichskristallnacht* pogroms on 9–10 November 1938, about two-thirds of the psychiatrists and psychoanalysts in Germany and Austria had found themselves forced to leave and seek refuge in a US or Canadian exile.[144]

As I have shown, neurological, psychiatric, and psychoanalytical approaches to trauma research had been part of earlier and quite different sociopolitical contexts in the German-speaking countries. These contexts had further implications for the scientific conception of "nervous traumas," for what these meant, and for the choice of the most appropriate methodologies to tackle problems associated with such conditions. Vienna-born clinical psychiatrist Heinz Hartmann (1894–1970), for instance, insisted that many of the current societal problems should be treated with psychoanalytical methodologies.[145] This recommendation pertained especially to trauma as a cultural pattern with widespread interpretations in Central Europe during the interwar period. It had received extensive currency from the time of Oppenheim's and Freud's ideas onward. With the uprooting of refugees from their European home cultures, each with its particular subdevelopments on the social, political, and intellectual level, a major transformation emerged in the practices of trauma research among émigré neuroscientists. My plan now is to further trace the reverberations of this transformation in the American context *vis-à-vis* "nervous trauma" and "psychoanalytical trauma," as two of the notions upon which theoretical discourses in neurology, psychiatry, and psychoanalysis hinged in the United States and Canada.[146] These notions were also related to the individual experiences of the émigrés, when most of them could not immediately find new professional and academic homes once they had landed on North American soil.[147]

Through the forced migration of German-speaking psychiatrists and neurologists, psychoanalytical approaches in trauma research were leaving their European cradle. Influential theoreticians such as Hartmann and Simmel had already laid the groundwork for a sustainable reception, so that trauma research could somewhat reconfigure itself on the North American continent under altered existential circumstances.[148] These altered circumstances can be seen both with respect to the newly encountered "American ways of life," as well as in émigrés' own traumatic experiences of persecution and flight, which intensified feelings of cultural uprootedness in many German-speaking psychoanalysts, physicians, and neuroscientists upon first experiencing the North American research context.[149] Many instances of emigration-dependent traumatic experiences figure in the research literature of the time, as Niederland singled out in his book *A Refugee's Life* (1968), from his experiences with traumatized European refugees: (1) the personal shock of having been attacked in their own authority as psychoanalysts; (2) being victimized by Nazi henchmen and secret police agents; (3) being supported by colleagues and friends during the process of flight and new beginning in their exile; (4) reaching North America without no private property and in complete poverty; (5) being forced to sustain themselves and develop new careers in foreign working environments without sufficient proficiency in English; (6) experiencing the indifference or rejection of the pre-existing medical and scientific community, particularly as the arriving émigré physicians and scientists were often perceived as competitors in a tight health care job market; and finally (7) having to cope with the loss of family, friends, and colleagues, who still resided in Europe and had been unable to escape persecution, which raised the question why they had escaped and survived while their loved ones had not:[150] "I shouldn't be here ... Where [should I be]? Where my parents are? Or where my brothers and sisters are? Where my wife is?"[151] According to Niederland, the main questions for the refugees were the circumstances under which they had survived and how they could become valuable members of society again: "Do Americans, the American-born, know what it means to be stateless? A stateless person is not a person – not in the eyes of bureaucrats."[152]

As Gerald Grob has further described, the process of incorporating psychoanalytic approaches into US psychiatric practice had already been underway in the medical community and in an institutionalized form in clinical departments of psychiatry, mental asylums, and state hospitals.[153] With the arrival of more and more German-trained émigré psychiatrists and neurologists, these approaches also became introduced into the pragmatic environments of the North American lifeworlds. Yet despite this quick reception, psychoanalytic trauma researchers found themselves working particularly in clinical contexts as well as integrated into scientific medical discourses. These circumstances did not always lead to acceptance of their therapeutic methods. On the one hand, émigré neurologists and psychiatrists found themselves confronted by a skeptical scientific culture in their host countries, while other forms of psycho- and neurotraumatological research were confined to academic niches. This was prominent in the case of psychophysiological stress research, which Hungarian émigré neurophysiologist Hans Selye (1907–1982) pursued in Montreal, in the department of biochemistry of McGill University.[154] Unable to find a satisfying affiliation with local neurological and psychiatric working groups, he eventually had to leave McGill and its anglophone community after the war had ended, to start a new laboratory at the Université de Montréal, which eventually figured in a much more pronounced medical research context and became the world's leading centre for stress research in a largely French-speaking university.[155]

Another type of situation arose as well, which caused difficulty to the emigrated psychiatrists and psychoanalysts in their American exile. It was well known to non-professional refugees that physicians had received fast-track visas and were admitted to the United States and Canada not solely on the basis of restrictive immigration quota regulations. The Emergency Committee in Aid of Displaced Foreign Physicians or the Psychoanalysts' Emergency Committee had quite often prepared affidavits, as well as economic and social support, to alleviate their emigration process.[156] As self-reflective therapists, they knew that this privileged situation was present among émigré psychiatrists and psychoanalysts, and they coped with this privileged dimension of their own survival while the distressing occurrences in Europe dragged on. Many émigré psychiatrists and neurologists also developed a psychological "survivors' syndrome" themselves, as these cases were clinically analyzed by Niederland himself.[157]

Niederland had previously studied the effects of survival and new beginnings in a foreign country, as well as the separation of émigrés from their families and friends. He published several articles on this subject,[158] which became amalgamated with his own experiences from a year-long flight from his previous exile in Italy, on a British ship to China, and finally to San Francisco in the United States. According to him, the "survivor syndrome" was characterized as a form of traumatic experience that was represented by a "chronic engram highly associated with death and dying."[159] As previously seen in the cases of shell-shocked soldiers, the "nervous traumas" of veterans and their "pension neuroses" during the Weimar Republic, a number of cardinal symptoms were associated with the illness (see chapters 3 and 4). The survivor syndrome was characterized by fear, agitation, distrust, tensions in conduct with other people, and chronically contradicting interests. Niederland called this the "dehumanization"[160] process:

As a clinical physician in the discipline of psychiatry and psychoanalysis, I will focus in the following primarily on medical research results in the field of persecution psychiatry and persecution psychology ... I define the process of dehumanization and the intentional actions leading to it as the systematic attempt to strip a human being of all his psychophysiological functions and abilities in such a way that as the final result of this process – if it can be survived at all – "something" remains that lives, or better vegetates in a human form, Gestalt and species, yet in its psychological dispositions it has become very strongly, if not completely "other."[161]

The phenomenology of alienation that is described here in affected people found its way both into psychotraumatological theory and into the conduct of personal life, not only in the case of Niederland himself. It became highly visible, for instance, in the tragic situation of the Vienna psychiatrist and psychoanalyst Paul Federn (1871–1950). He had received privileged landing papers for the United States, hoping that his loved ones could join him, but his family was not able to obtain visas to follow him to New York. It is likely that Federn's suicide was attributable to this tragic experience.[162] Yet, while the existential situation had major influences on each individual person, external threats could more often be ameliorated, with pre-existing networks, support groups, and families helping the experiences of flight and persecution to be worked through. As a consequence, one's response to such experiences could be interpreted as an "adaption to the new social structures" in which "cooperation as an essential moment of humanity" likewise changed the trauma research approaches.[163]

From this basic notion of the adaptation to new social structures also stemmed the import of certain humanitarian and cultural influences of European psychoanalysis on the American continent, a process through which many émigré psychiatrists could enrich the wider field of the humanities in sociology, art history, and philosophical theory.[164] This trend was so successful culturally that it led to puzzling developments in the postwar neurosciences in the United States and Canada. For example, other "research import products" from émigré neurologists and psychiatrists – such as the psychiatric genetics and epidemiology approach of the Berlin psychiatrist Kallmann, the neurorehabilitative approach of the holistic neurologist Goldstein, or the introduction of psychopharmacological Chlorpromazine therapy, which the Berlin biochemist Heinz Lehmann (1911–1999) after his forced migration to McGill University had promoted to the English-speaking American research community – languished for a long time in the cultural shadow of dominant psychoanalytical theories. In American psychiatry this was the case from the 1940s to the 1960s, before such major advances could develop into important traditions in the neuroscience field.[165]

By looking at the cooperative and network aspects within the context of the forced migration of German-speaking trauma researchers in their exile, it is intriguing to see to what extent many of the developments in neurology, psychiatry, and psychoanalysis had been influenced by the Swiss-American psychiatrist Adolf Meyer.[166] The latter had settled permanently in the States in 1892 after his training at the University of Zurich. Soon he became the head of the clinical Henry Phipps Psychiatric Service of Johns Hopkins University's School of Medicine in Baltimore, Maryland (1913–41). He is often referred to as the doyen of modern US psychiatry and psychopathology.[167] Meyer's status is notable for the fact that he served as an external member in more than a hundred search committees for psychiatric, neurological, and neuropathological positions throughout the States and at major Canadian schools such as Toronto and McGill. Meyer was the president of the American Psychiatric Association and became a member of the boards of many leading American associations in medicine and in the neurosciences. Moreover, he possessed personal contacts with American and Canadian politicians as well as senior members of national funding institutions.[168]

Meyer thus acquired the function of a major node in the North American network of psychiatric and neurological research, including the psycho-analytical and psychopharmacological approaches, as well as neurohistological analyses. He appeared to have been acculturated in these interdisciplinary intentions as a former supervisee of the neuromorphologist Constantin von Monakow, who had been the director of Zurich University's Institute for Brain Research in Switzerland. In influential circles in the United States, Meyer himself now acted as an advisor, moderator, and reviewer. For decades, he was referred to as an elder statesman of American biomedical research and psychiatry in the United States. He had already developed well-established contacts with American colleagues from an earlier research visit in 1891. Once Meyer became the chair of psychiatry at Johns Hopkins, the leading biomedical research university, he was instrumental in fostering the early American network in the clinical neurosciences, developing it from what were rather informal connections among psychiatrists, neurologists, and neuropathologists. Some pivotal institutions, such as the Rockefeller Institute for Medical Research, the Montreal Neurological Institute, and major research universities, acted as the pillars of the emerging field in the US.[169] With respect to the forced migration wave of the 1930s, and as a Swiss expatriate himself, Meyer actively worked to support newly arriving émigré neuroscientists. To further this end, he and others tried to influence and align the Rockefeller

Foundation's fellowships and grants through continuous letter exchanges with Alan Gregg and Rockefeller Foundation senior officials. This ultimately led to considerable support for different kinds of interdisciplinary approaches in psychiatry and brain research in the United States and Canada.[170] Major recipients of the support through the Rockefeller Foundation's established grants-in-aid program were, for example, Kurt Goldstein at Columbia University for his neuropsychiatric work;[171] Halle neurologist Alfred Hauptmann, who assumed a position at the Joseph H. Pratt Diagnostic Hospital in Boston; Robert Wartenberg (1886–1956) from Danzig, who became a professor of neurology at the University of California's School of Medicine in San Francisco; or Berlin's Erwin W.M. Strauss, who directly joined Meyer at Johns Hopkins University.[172]

This type of personal engagement, seconded by several of the above-named groups and institutions, led to the strengthening of pre-existing networks, since many of the more prominent medical scientists and physicians had already been on-site during the interwar period. These transatlantic exchanges were to emerge as the dominant model of internationalization in research areas such as biomedicine and physics between the 1910s and 1930s. Such exchanges were fostered through the vital research support – in both transatlantic directions – of the Rockefeller Foundation, along with participating universities in Germany, Austria, Switzerland, the United States, and Canada (see chapter 3).[173] Some individual researchers and scholars like Franz Alexander from Budapest or Felix Deutsch (1884–1964) and Helene Deutsch from Vienna belonged to the group of "early arrivals" in America during the late 1920s or early 1930s. Their stays were often planned as periods of extended research or lecture tours to North American universities. But many of them decided to hang around, anticipating that the situation in their home countries would deteriorate and only lead to their disadvantage – despite the ambivalence that they felt toward the States: "From a European perspective, America was a relief as well as a shock; Continental culture could be too mannered."[174]

Through the influence of such key players as Meyer and others, the network of relationships among scientists, clinicians, and practising physicians became ever more tightly knit on the American continent.[175] The exchanges nurtured by these networks furthered an intellectual strengthening, and increased the social influence of psychoanalytic and neurological trauma research, which was supported, for example, by the Institute for Psychoanalysis in Topeka, Kansas. This institute, established by the Indiana psychiatrist Karl A. Menninger (1893–1990) in 1919, was augmented by the opening of the Winter Army General Hospital in Topeka after World War II as one of the largest psychiatric training institutions worldwide. Although its primary interest lay in psychoanalytical education, as per its service obligations, it assumed a major role as a foundational research institution in clinical psychiatry at large. All these initiatives and developments led to the connections between traumatology and other neuroscience-related programs becoming ever more pronounced. This was particularly so after the 1940s, when many of the physicians and researchers who had fled from the devastations of the Nazi regime in Germany and its neighbouring countries became further integrated in the ensuing programs. At the preliminary end of this process there also appeared a very modern conception of psychological trauma:

The experience of a vital discrepancy between threatening situational factors and the individual coping abilities of each individual. These are often paralleled by feelings of helplessness and accompanied through defenseless divulgation, finally leading to a continuing unsettledness of the personal self- and world-understanding.[176]

Conversely, the altered conception of "nervous trauma" and "psychological trauma" was accompanied by the individual experiences of many of the émigré psychiatrists, psychoanalysts, and neurologists since the times of their persecution in Europe. In this sense, it is fascinating to consider the surging discourses on modern trauma as an important cultural trope. It connected many of the discourses in medicine, psychoanalysis, art, literature, and even social history in an important network of meanings.[177] It included not only the histories of each traumatized individual subject (i.e., the war-disabled, mental patients, émigré psychiatrists, and neuroscientists) but also the collective memory of a given time, which intricately bonds the contemporary scientific programs to their wider cultural context.[178]

This relationship between individual defences and resilience to various forms of trauma associated with the academic forced migration wave can be seen in many of the émigré psychiatrists, psychoanalysts, and early neuroscientists in their American exile. It can also be seen as a manifestation of an important function of self-protection during intense times of complete reorientation of their cultural self-understanding. On the east side of the Atlantic, the notions of "nervous trauma" and "psychological trauma" had become symbolic of the contradictions and cultural aporias of modernity, as Freud had conceptualized as a psychoanalytical thought figure around the *fin de siècle*.[179] With the introduction of the concept of trauma, Freud had emphasized the wider contours of "modernity" or, as he stated, "the other side of modernity" in the meaning of psychopathology and neuropathology.[180]

It is absolutely striking to see the remarkable ways in which Freud's cultural analysis – still written in the peaceful, civilized, and culturally rich environment of the late Habsburg capital – anticipated the groundbreaking disruptions of the world wars by two and four decades. It drew attention directly to the origin of the horrors and millions of deaths under the Nazi and Fascist regimes in Europe, circumstances under which the researchers themselves should not all be on the side of the victims but shockingly on the side of the perpetrators as well (see chapter 6). In this sense, Freud had importantly mapped the aporias of modernity in their cultural contexts, out of which neither psychiatrists nor neurologists in the 1930s and 1940s could step forth.

"THE END OF A CULTURAL EPOCH":
WORKING IN NEUROPSYCHIATRIC TRAUMA RESEARCH
IN CANADA AND THE UNITED STATES –
ROBERT WEIL, KARL STERN, AND
FREDERIC HENRY LEWY

One neuropathologist whose scientific profile benefited greatly from the new interest in "nervous trauma" was Robert Weil. Weil belonged to a group of German-educated neuroscientists from the fringe provinces of the former Habsburg Empire. He was born into a Jewish family in Bohemia, yet, in his adolescence converted to Lutheranism. He was one of the many clinical psychiatrists of the 1930s who, in his research, displayed a profound interest in a great variety of psychiatric and related areas ranging from the nosology of brain injuries and psychoanalysis, to neuropathology and the histology of brain lesions. Weil graduated with a *Dr. med.* from the German Charles University of Prague in 1933 under the supervision of Ladislav Haškovec (1866–1944). After graduate studies at the Vienna Medical School, he began work as a psychiatrist for the army from 1935 to 1938, first in Prague and then in a small town in Bohemia. This experience of the military psychiatry setting stirred his interest in neurological traumatology early on. However, following the German annexation of parts of Czechoslovakia in 1938, he and his family fled to London, and after his passage to Canada in 1939, Weil shared the fate of many émigré medical scientists.[181] He was transported to a remote area of Saskatchewan, where he was fortunate to be allowed to practise medicine as a family physician between 1939 and 1942, at a time when many of his fellow émigré neuroscientists were often barred from

practising medicine in Canada altogether.[182] To explore this, let us turn
to a letter written by Weil in which he underlined how exceptional it was
for him to intern in neurosurgery at the Saskatoon City Hospital, until
1944, under the supervision of the respected Canadian chief of the surgery
department Arthur LeMesurier (1889–1982).[183] In the last two years of
the war he even managed to work in private practice:

> In 1942 I joined the Mental Health Services of Saskatchewan, my
> first position [in Canada] being a junior psychiatrist in the
> Sask[atchewan] Mental Hospital in Battleford. The medical superin-
> tendent at that time was Dr. J[ack] J. McNeil [b. 1918] – a native
> of Summerside, P.E.I. Dr. McNeil was a great friend of Dr. Clarence
> [M.] Hincks [1885–1965] who visited our hospital almost yearly.
> On one of these visits he was accompanied by Dr. J[ohn D.]. Griffin
> [1906–2001].[184]

Not only did Weil play a major role in Czech psychiatry as a young
researcher and clinician, but he became a leading psychiatrist in the
Canadian community as well.[185] He proved to be a gifted science manager
who introduced new mental health systems approaches to the province
of Saskatchewan, and to Nova Scotia in Atlantic Canada.[186] In a remarkable way, Weil managed to integrate into a regional network of public
health workers in the western prairie provinces too. This integration was
certainly due to the extraordinarily detrimental situation of Saskatchewan
at that time, before it was reshaped under the leadership of its Premier
T.C. (Tommy) Douglas (1904–1986). The health care system had suffered
heavily from the economic downturns in the years after the Great
Depression, and during this time émigré psychiatrists and neurologists
were often readily accepted as replacements for physicians who had
left.[187] Weil's interest in brain research was later curtailed in Canadian
institutional settings, despite his earlier efforts to publish on tumour
neuropathology and other brain research subjects while working at the
German Charles University in Prague. However, he now continued with
some low-level work on nervous traumatology and on immunological
questions related to central nervous system infections. What was much
more important in his work biography was that he created a stimulating
context for laboratory investigations back in Nova Scotia at Dalhousie
University. In Halifax, Weil ardently supported the creation of new posts
for assistant professors and contributed to the promotion and tenure of
a number of associate professors in psychiatry and neurology.[188] These

efforts markedly increased research capacity not only on the Atlantic coast but in the rest of Canada as well. Adding to the traditional power-houses of Montreal and Toronto, Dalhousie emerged as a major neuroscience player during the 1960s. For Weil, who had experienced great diversity in his previous training in brain psychiatry, neuropathology, neurochemistry, and epidemiology, it was crucial that similar multidisciplinary educational structures be introduced at Canadian institutions. At Dalhousie, he suitably advocated for lean hierarchical structures, which put even lower-ranked neuroscientists into autonomous and fairly productive research positions.[189]

Of course, the influence of time and culture played an important role in the acculturation process of émigrés such as Weil in pre-existing North American structures. Émigré researchers and medical doctors were quite aware of the cultural dimension of working life in their new institutions. Their own experiences of oppression and flight from their former home countries put into question many aspects of their scientific and personal life. This is particularly evident in Weil's 1969 presidential address to the Canadian Psychiatric Association:

> Psychiatry – a solution!
> Before I left Europe for England and finally for this country in 1939, I saw the world of my childhood rapidly disintegrate & ideals that have become my second nature destroyed. Like most European observers, I witnessed a process in those eventful years during which a whole *cultural* epoch underwent a complete dissolution. What would follow was not clear. My most pessimistic anticipations ... were many times multiplied by the terrible reality which was to follow after our departure from Europe.[190]

Refugee policy and practice were, in general, often hostile, and the reception accorded émigré physicians by various Canadian provinces and communities often proved to be distancing, if not explicitly anti-Semitic.[191] There were a number of reasons for these types of reactions. First, the early twentieth century witnessed an increasing influence of the state in many areas of public health and the prevention of contagious diseases. In both Canada and the United States, government programs were biased against new immigrants as "potential sources" of infectious diseases, which led to quarantine measures to prevent disease spreading to the local communities. Moreover, mental impairment was conceived as a justification to constrain the immigration of certain foreign groups, including

Jewish refugees.[192] Particularly after the Immigration Act of 1906, Canadian admission policies became selective, including medical and psychological markers as criteria for barring immigrants. These changes had immediate consequences for refugees as well. As ordinary immigrants, they were subject to the same restrictive measures that had recently been introduced. Later on, they became a target for professional regulation policies, mainly through provincial colleges of physicians and surgeons. These immigration policies developed into obvious discrimination actions throughout the 1930s and 1940s.[193]

Thus, Jewish and oppositional neuroscientists who fled Nazi Germany and sought to continue their careers encountered major obstacles. It is quite remarkable that although German medicine enjoyed a high international reputation and its universities and the KWG institutes had frequently been primary venues for North American visiting researchers, émigré physicians often found themselves discriminated against by unyielding relicensing procedures.[194] Although we currently do not have a full quantitative sense of the problem in Canada, preliminary findings from case studies suggest that the procedures were at least as restrictive as in the United States. Between 1933 and 1938, for example, the overall number of foreign-trained physicians allowed to practise in Canada remained almost unchanged from the number before Hitler had come into power.[195] This is remarkable since many North American jurisdictions were still among the most poorly served in the Western world. In the whole province of Nova Scotia, roughly the same size as Ireland, with about half a million inhabitants at the time, there were only six trained psychiatrists including Weil.[196] It was highly disturbing for many of the refugees, having managed to flee the oppressive laws of the Nazi regime, to now find themselves again victimized by discrimination, this time by the selection policies of their North American physician-brethren.

A second reason for the hostile reception of émigrés was the attitude among the members of academia. There are only a few preliminary insights into doctors' immigration to Canada prior to 1935, but one document describes the possible placement of German émigrés in the then Territory of Newfoundland.[197] In the fall of 1933, the British Academic Assistance Council, which the London physiologist Archibald Vivian Hill (1886–1977) had co-founded, was contacted to help with the selection of "a pathologist and a surgeon for a Canadian hospital."[198] Although it is unclear how this transfer unfolded, the Academic Assistance Council was informed that a number of Canadian academics completely rejected the idea of helping their German colleagues by offering them any positions.

In a letter from 1935, the physiologist Frederick Miller (1881–1967) from the University of Western Ontario replied to another of Hill's requests and, although Miller was sympathetic to the idea, he reported that he would not have adequate space in his department. In addition, he reported another difficulty: since the University of Western Ontario Medical School was "a very Scotch, conservative community ... there might be a good deal of criticism of German Jews."[199] What was meant by the notion of "a good deal of criticism" can be inferred from the letters between the Academic Assistance Council and Ardrey W. Downs (1913–1966), head of the Edmonton department of physiology and pharmacology. Although the University of Alberta had only been founded in 1909, showing a great demand for experienced educators, Downs told the Academic Assistance Council executive that he did not want to receive a refugee. After all, there was "the question of character" of such strangers in the academy and there may have been "certain reasons" why the émigré individuals lost their positions in the first place. In his ensuing letter to British historian Walter Adams (1906–1975), Hill expressed that "this is exactly the kind of thing I fear might be common."[200] At best, Canadian researchers and university administrators were indifferent to the experiences of their European colleagues.[201]

A major positive influence, however, was exerted by the Carnegie Foundation. Founded in 1906, it was one of the leading American organizations to immediately respond to the refugee crisis after 1933, in both the United States and Canada.[202] In fact, a number of Canadian universities were invited to apply for financial assistance through fellowship grants as well, which offered help in placing refugee scholars. Dalhousie was one of the first universities to take up this opportunity and in 1934 appointed two "research assistants." The political scientist Lothar Richter (1894–1948) arrived from Berlin; and the neurohistologist Martin Silberberg was hired from Breslau and asked to begin offering student courses in pathology with the beginning of the fall term.[203] In the spring of 1935, the Carnegie Foundation unfortunately had to tell the university administrators that they were forced to cut the funding to two years because of the great demand of fellowships for refugee academics. Although this decreased the attractiveness of external funding for Canadian institutions, overall, none of the philanthropically supported refugee scholars were ever barred from entering the country and starting new careers. Later on, many decided that the lack of funding sources in the Canadian system and the attraction of working in places with larger Jewish communities was worth the move south of the border. Silberberg was part of this particular group and left Halifax together with his wife for a pathology fellowship at Washington University in St Louis.[204]

Finally, while the reception in Canadian institutions of higher learning was already problematic for many German-speaking refugees, settling as an independent specialist or family doctor was nearly impossible until after the war had ended.[205] A search through the archives of the College of Physicians and Surgeons of Nova Scotia – in the Canadian province with the most important seaport of entry to the country at the time – reveals that between 1910 and 1952 neither foreign doctors with non-Canadian passports nor any Jewish physicians had become active officers in the Medical Society of Nova Scotia.[206] It appears that world politics had completely "bypassed" the Atlantic province. Even more astonishing is the fact that about a million people passed through the province's major port of entry – Halifax Harbour – during the whole Hitler period.[207] Looking at all these impediments, it is all the more remarkable that many émigré individuals did manage to adapt to the Canadian health care system over the years.[208] To quote from a retrospective letter from Weil to psychiatrist Charles Roberts (1918–1996), Weil was convinced that his own success had only been possible thanks to his friendship with leading physicians in the field:

> Many of [my] professional activities brought me in close contact with Jack [Griffin], the executive function, the [James S.] Tyhurst [b. 1922] committee ["More for the Mind"], the American Council, or common travel from N.S. to Lima, Peru … all highlights in my psychiatric career.[209]

The particular experience of the differences in mental health care on both sides of the Atlantic can further be deduced from the Hincks Report that brought the Canadian National Committee for Mental Hygiene into being in 1918.[210] Ten years later, this body was granted a Federal Charter with Clarence Hincks (1885–1965) as its first general director, and in 1950 the body was named the Canadian Mental Health Association with the goal of promoting provincial chapters that would address and improve local needs.[211] Weil had entered the Mental Health Service at a time when psychiatric care was "predominantly practiced under poor conditions in mental Hospitals" and the teaching of psychiatry was "uncommon as a subject of study in Canadian universities."[212] By comparison, the disciplines of psychiatry and neurology at the Charles University in Prague had already risen to international recognition under neuropathologist

Arnold Pick (1851–1924) and psychiatrist Ladislav Haškovec, who had made training in neuropsychiatry and psychopathology, as well as social psychiatry and traumatology, compulsory for all medical students.

Weil's broad-based European training in the neurosciences and his experience as a psychiatrist in the Czech army both fostered his adaptation to the Canadian mental health system. His colleagues in Battleford, Saskatchewan, realized that he was capable of making a substantial contribution to psychiatric research in the Saskatchewan Mental Hospital. At this critical juncture in his career, Weil's broad knowledge in psychiatry and basic neuropathology, his involvement in setting up a provincial mental health system, and his social contacts with leading members of the Saskatchewan Health Service and Canadian psychiatric community earned him considerable recognition.[213] His contributions translated, for instance, into the widespread use of statistical methods in mental health research, methods of distributing psychiatric care, the broad clinical training of medical students, and the diagnostic testing of psychopathological conditions as a preventive measure in Saskatchewan and Nova Scotia.[214] With these measures he helped to consolidate the Canadian mental health care system and its basic educational needs.[215] Eventually, Weil was offered a position as the university's first tenure-track professor of psychiatry and stayed at Dalhousie from 1950 until his retirement in 1975 at the age of sixty-six.

Because he was now part of the core faculty of the medical school, Weil could influence its hiring policies and the restructuring of its services in psychiatry, neurology, and neuropathology. By these means he promoted a German-inspired approach to education, requiring residents to develop a broad base of knowledge in psychiatry and all of its related fields – including neurology, internal medicine, and neuropathology.[216] The same attitude materialized in Weil's activities as a founding member and president of the Canadian Psychiatric Association, in his promotion of social psychiatry, and in his interdisciplinary teaching and research approach.[217] Weil's involvement in mental health issues is an excellent example of individual adaptation. Back in Europe his main interests had at first been somatic neurology and then neuropathology. Neither in the Czech army nor in Canadian psychiatry, however, could Weil's post-university interest in morphological research of the brain be fully met again.[218] This particular example demonstrates that he was able to attend to changing demands, and it is quite likely that through his pro-active participation as a scientific referee he began to move at a different pace in both Saskatoon and Halifax.[219] Not only had this highly intellectual psychiatrist reflected on the cultural background of the neurosciences in numerous sociological and philosophical articles, but he reshaped his university's environment in clinical psychiatry and laboratory neuroscience.[220] Although it is hard to find specific experiences of "culture shock" in his case, given that in his letters he reflected mostly on the ease of his adapting to Canada or on his good relationships with patients and his comfortable family life in the Maritimes,[221] we nevertheless find him even after his retirement expressing concern about what he perceived to be the underdeveloped status of psychiatry in Canada:

> From discussions with a number of colleagues I gained the impression that psychotherapy [does not occupy] the same role in the education nor in the practice of psychiatrists as it did in the past [in Europe]. As important [as] psychopharmacology and many of the new discoveries in the neurosciences are, they should not displace totally or particularly the main function-psychotherapy ... [In fact,] a plea for greater emphasis on psychotherapy should be conveyed to the CPA [Canadian Psychiatric Association] and through the CPA to the psychiatric departments of all medical faculties.[222]

It is interesting to look at Weil's relationship with Central Europe during the postwar period. Despite frequent personal letters to earlier colleagues in Prague and Munich, there are no documented lecture tours to German-speaking psychiatric departments. All of Weil's extensive correspondence touches on the surviving members of his family, especially his niece in the Ruhr region. I could only verify one substantial visit to the Old World by Robert and Stella Weil (1914–2012) in the archival material, and it seems to have been of a private nature:

> Last Fall we undertook an extensive tour through the North- and Baltic Sea, visiting Rotterdam, Oslo, Copenhagen, Helsinki, and disembarked from the russian boat ... Over Moscow, Zurich ... eventually reached Munic, in the vicinity of which we visited with old friends.[223]

A lack of formal contact with the scientific community of his former home country such as we find from Weil's correspondence was not uncommon among the group of émigré psychiatrists and neurologists. For many, it was a deliberate choice, in that they had understandably agonized over their expulsion from their positions and their homeland, not wishing to resume professional contacts with the medical and scientific communities that had rejected them in the 1930s.[224] For others, as in the case of Weil, there was simply no need to go back or redeveloping academic ties. They had invested greatly in their North American careers, become widely accepted in their institutions, and as physicians simply could not leave their patients or research programs alone.[225] And, certainly, by the 1950s and 1960s, the academic and medical communities in the German-speaking countries had lost most of their intellectual attraction – precisely *because of* the number of protagonists in cutting-edge fields who had fled the Nazis.

This sense of not looking back becomes even clearer from the biography of another German Canadian neuropathologist who, like Weil, arrived at the end of the 1930s. Karl Stern arrived in Canada following a period of exile in England after his last position at a Charité teaching hospital in Berlin. At first glance, the conditions for a transfer of concepts and methods such as Weil experienced were ideal in Stern's case.[226] After he completed most of his education at the Charité Medical School, Stern graduated with an MD from the University of Frankfurt am Main in 1930. From 1930 to 1931 he worked with Goldstein as a psychiatry resident at the Edinger Institute, at which time the latter had been given the directorship of the Frankfurt Institute for Research into the Effects of Brain Injuries (see figure 1.2).[227] In 1932–33, Stern used a Rockefeller Foundation Fellowship to fund a research project at the department of neuropathology in the Deutsche Forschungsanstalt for Psychiatry in Munich, where he collaborated with the renowned tumour specialist Walther Spielmeyer.[228] In Munich, Stern obtained a personalized position, in which he acted primarily as Spielmeyer's continuing teaching assistant. In order to live up to the high standards of Spielmeyer's expertise in neurodiagnostics, however, an enormous effort was required of Stern in this position. Visiting research fellows expected the same from him as from Spielmeyer, and they were given thorough introductions to the methods of brain histology.[229] Essentially, in Munich, Stern worked at the highest international level of neuropathological education and training.

In the meantime, things had not developed well for Goldstein, his mentor, who did not receive the financial support promised when he succeeded Edinger in his chair.[230] Not being allowed to open a psychiatric ward as planned, Goldstein decided to leave Frankfurt for Berlin in 1930 and invited Stern to join him as a consultant in one of his psychiatry wards and also perform the brain autopsies for the hospital.[231] The Moabiter Krankenhaus was then one of the few academic hospitals with alternative services in neurology, psychiatry, and pathology, which were related to each other as they had been earlier at the Neurological Institute in Frankfurt. Just when everything was in place for Goldstein's clinic, with the prospect of becoming one of the leading centres of German neurology, political catastrophe ensued.[232] Yet despite the fact that Goldstein had been incarcerated in 1933 and fled to Amsterdam that same year, Stern stayed in Germany until 1936. Only then did he decide to seek refuge in London, and there a network of contemporary international scientists came into play. During a lecture tour of the Americas in 1931, Spielmeyer, Stern's mentor from previous Munich days, had met the Montreal neurosurgeon Wilder Penfield and familiarized him with his work.[233] Now, Stern's new acquaintance with a Canadian neurophysiologist at Queen Square – thought to be Herbert H. Hyland (1900–1977), who had visited London for an extended period – helped him make contact with Penfield and leave for Quebec.[234] Once in Montreal, Stern had a position at the Verdun Hospital first, yet soon afterward began working in the pathology service at the Hôpital Nôtre Dame.

Penfield later recommended Stern to D. Ewan Cameron's psychiatry department (see chapter 6), and this recommendation became an important turning point in Stern's continuing career as a mental health expert.[235] Soon after Montreal's Allan Memorial Institute opened in 1943, Stern began to work explicitly in the Geriatric Unit and taught courses as a research assistant and later assistant professor of psychiatry.[236] However, Stern's educational background had centred on a more encompassing approach to psychiatry and neurology. It proved to be quite different to Cameron's views and research interests, which were staunchly empirical and had a solely biological orientation. Stern always referred back to his classic humanist education from the German *Gymnasium* high school and the widespread culture of learning during his medical studies.[237] Stern's holistic view transcended work in the hospital and encompassed social life in general: quite frequently he and his wife organized *soirées* at their home in Outremont, inviting groups of colleagues, students, and interns to listen to Karl's recitals of composer Robert Schumann (1810–1856) or to read psychoanalytic works together by the fireside. The neurochemist Marion K. Birmingham (b. 1921), who later became his assistant, describes her admiration for Stern's accomplishments in the following way:

> Eminent neurologist, psychoanalyst, author, and, oh, what an "amateur" musician! The year is 1948, the place is Karl [Stern's] living

room. His musical evenings are forever engraved in my mind, as are the violent altercations I had with him concerning his views on the Jungian female "anima."[238]

As Stern admits in his autobiographical novel, *The Pillar of Fire* (1951), his interests in neuro-logy and cognitive defects in clinical psychiatry went far beyond the constricted program and routine work of the Montreal Neurological Institute.[239] With the establishment of two separate centres, the close academic links between the clinical fields of neuroscience had now been disrupted, institutionally, at McGill for a long time. The departments of epileptology, neurosurgery, neurology, and neuropathology acted as service units for Penfield's research program on the mapping of the human cortex, with the Montreal Neuro fulfilling the neurosurgeon's needs.[240] By contrast, the Allan Memorial Institute developed into the leading centre on biological psychiatry.[241] On account of the challenging relationship between the renowned Cameron and the émigré psychiatrist on his staff, Stern left Montreal in the 1950s and became a psychiatry professor in Ottawa.[242]

Stern's move to the University of Ottawa's Medical Faculty, which had sprung from the Roman Catholic College of Bytown, must be attributed to a number of factors. Most certainly, the restrictive concept of psychiatry in Cameron's service varied so markedly from Stern's prior experiences, which the latter sorely missed during his working years in Montreal. Stern's conversion from Judaism to Catholicism played another role in his rejection of the biological psychiatry practised at the Allan Memorial Institute, since Cameron did not withhold his personal anti-religious leanings.[243] This was revealed, for example, in an episode from the Montreal visit of the German Christian philosopher Josef Pieper (1904–1997) from the University of Muenster in 1952. While Pieper was participating in a double conference on *The Mission of the University* in Toronto and Montreal, one of the participants introduced him to Stern, whose autobiographical novel Pieper had read earlier. It is remarkable that Stern had reciprocally read Pieper's book *On Hope and Faith* in 1935, while sitting for lunch on a park bench in London near the National Hospital for the Paralysed and Epileptic Queen Square. In *The Pillar of Fire* he even quoted Pieper's book and emphasized how much comfort it had given him during his first year in exile. At the end of their personal meeting in Montreal, Stern's wife brought out the tattered book and handed it to Pieper for his signature. Afterward, while Stern drove him to the bus stop, they engaged in a conversation about Stern's plans to leave Montreal:

[Stern] told me during the short drive about his decision to leave his current position at the world-renowned McGill University and to move to the relatively unimportant Catholic University of Ottawa. I could not understand this decision and asked about his motives ... He told me that it was no longer possible for him to continue to work in an atmosphere of a completely secularized Psychiatry that would be solely guided by the conviction that all of the sources of mental illnesses had to be found in Religion which needed to be eliminated as a psychiatric "complex."[244]

These origins of an overtly differing approach to psychiatry in North America – the approach of what Stern called the "socio-psychoanalytic-therapeutic creation of absolute happiness" – can be found in his own clinical and research program later in Ottawa. At McGill, he had previously cultivated contacts in the francophone community, and a number of residents and interns joined his early Geriatric Unit for individual study periods.[245] Many of these psychiatrists also practised psychotherapy or were classic psychoanalysts. When Stern assumed his professorship at the University of Ottawa, one of the French-trained psychiatrists, Victorain Voyer (1917–1975), joined him in his new department and helped transform it into an important psychiatric educational centre for psychoanalysis and psychopathology, which would be closely associated with the Ottawa Mental Health Centre after 1961.[246] In the same way that Stern included basic psychoanalytic training into psychosocial projects, he also introduced such modules into the psychoanalytic Pavilion Albert Préhost associated with the Université de Montréal in Quebec, where they often held seminars together.[247]

Although the conditions for the transfer of ideas and methods from Germany to Canada had been ideal in Stern's case, his career cannot really be regarded as a "success story" in terms of major advances in the neurosciences. On the one hand, Goldstein's holist neurology group, to which Stern belonged, effectively ceased to exist after the Nazi *Machtergreifung*. When Stern entered the neurosciences in Montreal, like other émigré physicians, he had to deal with distinct research cultures.[248] For the most part, he did not really manage to introduce his own holistic ideas of neurology into the Montreal context. However, this case would be far from complete, if only personal achievements such as the quantity of publications, number of graduate students, or the creation of specifically formalized teaching programs were considered. We need to include the numerous local accounts highlighting Stern's exceptional ability as an academic teacher. He seemed to have interested a whole new generation of medical students in Montreal and later in Ottawa in the histological study of the brain, paired with psychopathology, and the anthropological perspective of psychiatry.[249] He was also influential in his relationships with the younger faculty members who, as the eminent psychiatrist Edrita Fried (1911–1981) emphasized, appreciated Stern's contributions to psychiatry:

> Dean [David L.] Thomson [1901–1964] had an original cartoon by [James] Thurber [1894–1961] above his desk: The psychiatrist with a large rabbit head and floppy rabbit ears is asking his patient: "You said a moment ago that people look like rabbits to you. Now what do you mean by that, Mrs. Sprague?" It was my unrestrained laughter at this marvelous cartoon that got me my first job at the newly founded Allan Memorial Institute of Psychiatry (associated with McGill). Dr. Karl Stern had come to interview prospective biochemistry graduates. He was a musician, a scholar, a psychiatrist, and a most witty person.[250]

These accounts attest to the value of Stern's broad humanistic education, which is often forgotten in the tunnel vision that lauds scientific excellence in a specific discipline alone, disregarding a broad learning foundation as a rich source of future innovations. In Stern's chosen setting there still survived traces of holism; sufficient to impress many of his students.[251] Comparatively minor instances of change in neuroscience and psychiatric knowledge can be attributed to Stern's case, but the historical reconstruction of different styles of neuroscientific research also had an impact at the educational, organizational, and clinical level. The practice of individuals such as Stern in the teaching networks at McGill and the interaction of the individual milieux between Ottawa and Montreal did emerge as a substrate for considerable changes in the regional psychiatric and neuroscientific cultures.[252]

Of all the qualities that successful émigré neurologists and psychiatrists in North America actually possessed, their ability to assimilate to the new disciplinary matrices on the western shore of the Atlantic was of utmost importance. Their ability to cope with the professional constraints and academic setbacks that they encountered was often directly related to the methodological and network resources that they mobilized to resume their scientific work in their new host countries.

This adaptability is very evident in the example of neurologist Friedrich Heinrich Lewy, who, prior to being ousted from his adjunct professorship at the Charité Medical School in 1933, had already built up contacts with many former acquaintances among American medical researchers he had met through academic networks in the KWG and the Rockefeller Foundation. Lewy, the son of a Jewish physician, was born in the Prussian capital of Berlin. He studied medicine in his hometown and in Zurich, and gained a degree of fame with his description of the Lewy Inclusion Bodies in the brain of patients with paralysis agitans (Parkinson's disease) in 1912.[253] This discovery marked only the beginning of a brilliant career as an innovative clinician and neurohistologist who had trained with many illustrious European neuroscientists at the time.[254] His academic pedigree includes such luminaries as the neuroanatomist Constantin von Monakow in Zurich; the clinical neurologist Hermann Oppenheim in Berlin; the psychiatrist Emil Kraepelin; the neuropathologists Franz Nissl and Alois Alzheimer in Munich. Lewy did a lot of scientific fieldwork, then uncommon in experimental neurology, which brought him to the celebrated Italian Marine Station of Anton Dohrn (1840–1909) in Naples to conduct physiological experiments.[255] He also went on extended journeys to Palestine and India, where he successfully carried out research on primate brains.[256] As with many Jewish-born *Privatdozenten* in Berlin, Lewy and his colleague the adjunct professor of neurology Alfred Goldscheider needed to teach at university departments, develop their own agendas at the cutting edge of research, and run private clinics to sustain themselves economically in the outright anti-Semitic environment of the Charité medical faculty (see also chapter 3).[257]

After Lewy was made director of an interdisciplinary neuropathological laboratory at the Neurological Clinic of Breslau, he became head of the clinical department at the Second Medical University Hospital of the Charité in Berlin (see figure 7.3).[258] However, with the *Machtergreifung* came his dismissal from his official university position. Like many neuroscientists fleeing Germany after the "Law for the Restoration of a Professional Civil Service" had been enacted, he decided to emigrate to England in late 1933. He had been seriously constrained in his work by losing his academic affiliation and being forced to accept only Jewish patients in his private clinic and laboratory in the Charlottenburg District of Berlin.[259] He first went to London, where the aid of Sir William Henry Beveridge's (1879–1963) Academic Assistance Council helped him to sustain himself and his family as a research associate. Beveridge, an economist and social reformer, and then director of the London School of Economics, while on a research leave in Vienna in 1933, received information that the German government wanted to release all Jewish academics from their positions in universities, high schools, and other state-run institutions.[260] Appalled by these political developments, Beveridge returned to England and began to create plans to assist displaced academics. He sought help in supporting the natural scientists from eminent Cambridge physicist Ernest Rutherford (1871–1937). The London physiologist Archibald Vivian Hill further complemented and coordinated the assistance program for displaced physicians and researchers in Britain generally.[261]

Lewy received a grant-in-aid to work at the National Hospital for the Paralysed and Epileptic at Queen Square. This grant from the British Academic Assistance Council was in support of applied research in work-related diseases, for investigating brain alterations due to lead poisoning, through animal experiments. Since his grant involved only the support of his salary, Lewy even dared to return to Germany again "to get my apparatus and teaching material" and to bring it to London.[262] He continued his research for about three months and then visited some of the lead workers in their factories in Manchester. Lewy also took blood samples with him to Queen Square for further laboratory analyses. Yet, as with many other Jewish refugee physicians, such as neuropathologist Karl Stern in Montreal or the recognized neurosurgeon Ludwig Guttmann in London,[263] Lewy was not allowed to practise as a clinical neurologist. Surprisingly, this prohibition held even for him, despite his having been a renowned head of a Berlin neurology teaching clinic. Frustrated that he found himself reduced at the age of forty-eight to the work setting of a postgraduate researcher, he wrote a letter on 5 June 1934 to the secretary of the American Emergency Committee in Aid of Displaced Foreign Physicians:

[Could he] visit some of his friends in the United States, to discuss with them what possibilities there are of his obtaining scientific work because he does not possess a British medical qualification that would allow him to engage in clinical practice.[264]

Letters of reference from a number of leading British neuroscientists – including Charles Sherrington (1857–1952), Samuel Alexander Kinnier Wilson (1878–1937), and Gordon Holmes (1876–1966) – eventually facilitated his onward-migration to Pennsburg, Pennsylvania. In studying Lewy's case, one realizes that he had seriously considered coming to Canada. However, having been explicitly dissuaded from going to America's northern neighbour by Rockefeller Foundation officials, he eventually migrated to the United States, where he stayed for the rest of his life. In fact, Rockefeller Foundation officials even warned him about the Canadian government's restrictive immigration policies toward refugee physicians from Nazi Germany (see figure 7.2) – policies that also accounted for the relatively low numbers of émigré researchers enriching the Canadian academy and health care system.[265]

Some scholars have viewed the historical situation as a complete "failure of Canadian academics to aide their colleagues in Germany during the 1930s,"[266] when their numbers are compared to the strong contrast of the scholarly aid associations in the UK (especially the Academic Assistance Council), the United States (the Emergency Committee in Aid of Displaced Foreign Physicians), Switzerland (the Notgemeinschaft Deutscher Wissenschaftler im Ausland), and elsewhere.[267] Those countries had already responded in the year of the Nazi *Machtergreifung*, while in Canada an organized support body became fully functional only in 1939 with the Canadian Society for the Protection of Science and Learning (CSPSL) inaugurated by Canadian faculty associations. By the time of the outbreak of World War II, this concerted endeavour was too late to make a difference in helping the last scholars to escape Nazi-controlled Europe.[268]

. The Rockefeller Foundation officers with whom Lewy had been corresponding were also right about the problem of anti-Semitism in Canadian Medical Schools and Colleges of Physicians.[269] Even the then government of William Lyon Mackenzie King (1874–1950) had been personally influenced by anti-Semitic tendencies, and strong regional differences existed in the Canadian provinces and territories. The acceptance of large numbers of Jewish immigrants was perceived as a threat to society and the prevalent view that Jews were "inassimilable" to a Gentile way of life translated into immigration policies claiming that the integration of even a few Jewish refugees was still "too many."[270] Regarding actual human resource policies, Jewish physicians were marginalized in a system that barely received any foreign and particularly non-British researchers among faculty ranks.[271] In the United States, by contrast, fifteen states, primarily those on the East Coast, continued to permit foreigners to practise medicine after re-licensure. They also offered university positions, whereas the tight *numerus clausus* for Jewish medical students at McGill and Queen's University, for instance, would have made it quite difficult for Lewy to find a position in Canada equal in academic stature, remuneration, and influence to the one he had earlier held in Germany. After careful

THE ROCKEFELLER FOUNDATION
INTER-OFFICE CORRESPONDENCE

From AG's diary:

Tues. June 19, 1934- Munich

Out to Institute with Spielmeyer - we will do nothing to establish Chemische Abteilung. This a German responsibility. Long distance from Rudin who has seen Glum and asks Spielmeyer to ask about it. Rudin has become the important person here - immense activity on records. But in Freiburg now hospitals are beginning to show rapid decrease in number of cases of epilepsy and other nervous diseases because of fear of sterilization drives such diseases away from physicians. Spielmeyer proud of the protests of the Protestants - ashamed of the academic silence. Criticizes Schmidt Ott for lending himself to meetings such as the one day after tomorrow when the subjects will be "What is German in Law - in Art - in Medicine - in Natural Science." Stark running these. University people much worse off than people in the institutes. ? another food shortage next winter.

Loeb money not yet disentangled - may be but very little. To be used as fluid research fund only.

Spielmeyer commends Bielschowsky in the highest terms - still turning out beautiful and important work. Carp solid but not remarkable. Young Williams whom BMP decided to take on fellowship is doing good work and is independent - could do well with a longer training.

Spielmeyer asks if I think he could get a job outside of Germany. Told him I didn't know and advised him to stay at it. He is heartsick and ashamed of his own people. Says people are already buying against probable absence of goods next winter

Met Williams and his wife and took them to dinner. Good impression. Told W to apply for renewal of his fellowship. Tried to make him see what a chance there is for a man of his training and interests. He has done well thus far.

Rudin away - talk with Jahnel who has been in touch with Brumpt and has animals infected with S. Novy which Coutelan brought back. J. has found that a field animal here in Bavaria and Austria called a Siebenschlafer is susceptible to syphilis and it becomes systemic disease even entering the central nervous system.

Lunch with Plaut. He says it will do Spielmeyer good to change his house to Kunigunde 38 and not be distracted by crossing city twice a day. Offering me coffee Plaut added "Perhaps I cannot offer it by next November." Says Swiss newspapers are doing a large business in Germany and gives me Von Papen's speech at Marburg. Plaut rather more philosophical than Spielmeyer. In view of fact that it wasn't a good plan to take detailed notes on the German visits all the above is somewhat vague. I leave with very grave doubts as to stability of Nazis - think the movement will be to the right when it takes place - almost anything can happen but the main test will be the economic and before this time next year. The harvest is not a good one - and export is too difficult. It might be the economic salvation of Germany to go communistic if that would break down resistance in their natural markets to the east. Germany not much of a milieu for science in the near future. Glad we have fellowships in our own hands again for Germany.

7.2 Demonstration of the continued letter exchanges between the headquarters of the Rockefeller Foundation in New York and the American Assistance Council, in 1935 (collection: RF, record group 1.1, series 717, subseries A, box 9, folder 56, Alan Gregg 6/19/34). © Courtesy of Rockefeller Archive Center, Sleepy Hollow, New York, USA.

consideration of the Canadian situation, Lewy was dissuaded and readily accepted a fellowship offer from Pennsburg in 1934, where he arrived with both his wife and his mother. It is hard to find direct evidence about Lewy's personal situation and feelings about living in the States. However, a letter of response dated 27 February 1935, which Max Bielschowsky's wife, Else (1878–1947), wrote back from their London exile to Lewy's spouse in Philadelphia, gives some insight into their adaptation to the American quality of life:

> What you are writing to me gives me the impression that on the other side of the pond, one is much more supportive and helpful to the refugees than they are here. We personally cannot complain, but we are really in an exceptionally good situation. In general, they are very opposed to the strangers here and because these often do not possess enough money to make a decent living ... It absolutely lacerates one's heart if one thinks about what has happed to our beloved fatherland.[272]

After Lewy and his family had settled in Pennsylvania, his initial position was that of a Rockefeller Foundation fellow in the university's neurosurgery department, and between 1943 and 1946 he acquired consultant status to various institutions.[273] This work included consulting for the Surgeon General of the US Army, in which capacity he reviewed severe cases of neurological injuries in former service men. The Surgeon General's Office was, of course, an open door through which Lewy could receive funding for his own neuromorphological program at the University of Pennsylvania and extramural support from the National Institutes of Health as well. This arrangement was quite typical for many émigré doctors, partly because they had to resume working on their initial fellowships of the Rockefeller Foundation and partly because the foundation had created a special support fund for fleeing individuals. During that time, Lewy corresponded with Esther ("Tess") Simpson (1903–1996), secretary to the Society for the Protection of Science and Learning, who followed up with the refugee scholars in an initiative in 1945–46 to inform the society's board about their fate and whereabouts:[274]

> I am happily settled – as you correctly presume – in an Army Barrack, together with 19 Medical Officers, certainly in a congenial surrounding since most of us are professors from various Medical Schools or from the Rockefeller Institute. I am for quite a while on

leave of absence from my Medical School which is spent, anyway, most of the last three years on research in Aviation Medicine for the National Research Council and the Aircorps, aside from my teaching obligations ... Mrs. Lewy has returned to Math and computes range tables for ordinance.[275]

Upon his arrival in Pennsylvania, Lewy changed his name to Frederic Henry Lewy.[276] Even though he had been integrated into many local research projects and clinical groups, and was thus able to pursue his research in conjunction with the National Research Council in Aviation Medicine, it was another twelve years before Lewy became a full faculty member again.[277] In 1946 the Graduate School of Medicine of the University of Pennsylvania appointed him professor of neuroanatomy, and at the same time he continued his work as a neurology consultant at the Cushing General Hospital in Framingham.[278] Lewy's career thereby benefited from his close friendship with the influential neurosurgeon William P. van Wagenen (1897–1961) from the University of Rochester Medical School – the first president of the American Neurosurgery Association – with whom he actively collaborated on peripheral nerve diseases.[279] This positive development is further reflected in a letter dated 13 September 1947, written back to his friend Martha Ursell (1879–1947) in Cambridge, England, who had joined the SPSL to conduct a follow-up letter-based inquiry to gather information about émigrés that the society had supported and helped earlier on:

To complete your list: I am now Professor of Neuroanatomy in the Graduate School of Medicine and Associate Professor of Neuropathology in the Medical School of the University of Pennsylvania, and Consultant to the Surgeon General of the Army. A group of our friends over here talked over the scholars we know and who have come to this country since 1933. The general impression is that everyone has found his nook. During the wartime, even older people were gainfully employed ... Still, I believe that practically everyone makes a living, as small as it may be.[280]

On a personal level, Lewy's example illustrates his socialization in the free-floating culture of ideas, practical experience, and organizational skills in the early German field of the brain sciences. His career was then quite typical for that of the younger Jewish neuroscientists, associate professors, and Privatdozenten in the penumbra of the German medical faculties.[281] Like many former professors who had reached North America in the 1930s, Lewy was an extremely well trained physician and acquainted with a variety of neuroscientific problems, clinical approaches, and methods from neurotraumatology to brain degenerative diseases (see figure 7.3).

As an example of networking, it is striking to see how Lewy's early participation in international conferences, such as the meetings of the International Brain Research Organization since 1931, brought him into close contact with leading neuroscientists of his time.[282] These early contacts grew into manifest networks of international colleagues with whom Lewy corresponded, networks he could build on after his arrival in his country of exile.[283] At major medical meetings, for example, he frequently met with the émigré neurologist Robert Wartenberg, then in San Francisco, or the psychiatrist Erwin Strauss, who had become director of a Veterans Administration hospital in Kentucky.[284] The above-mentioned elements were all enabling factors in the successful implementation of ideas, practical experiences, and organizational skills that many émigré neuroscientists brought from the German-speaking countries to their destinations in exile. And Lewy's contacts at international conferences of brain research clearly helped him to flee the Nazis and to find new research positions in the United Kingdom and the United States. As a highly active émigré neuroscientist, Lewy was able to find his way back into a research and teaching career in the respective neurological and medical professions in the United States.[285]

Overall, it becomes clear that affected refugee neuroscientists did a great deal more than succumb or adapt to academic norms then prevalent in their host cultures. It appears, rather, as an *esprit d'escalier* of twentieth-century history, that for many neuroscientists and psychiatrists the human catastrophe brought about by National Socialism in Germany also created career opportunities and work prospects in new scientific settings – ironically in areas that Nazi officials had sought to destroy forever.[286] The scientific changes following the forced migration after 1933 led to results that few could have predicted at the outset and which would transform North American neuroscience.[287] Many of the American institutions with which émigré physicians became associated thereby developed into major contemporary centres in the neurosciences – examples being the Allen Memorial and the Montreal Neurological Institute (Stern), the University of Pennsylvania's Comprehensive Neuroscience Center (Lewy), and the Neuroscience Institute at Dalhousie University (Weil), which rose to be a prominent neuroscience centre in Atlantic Canada.[288]

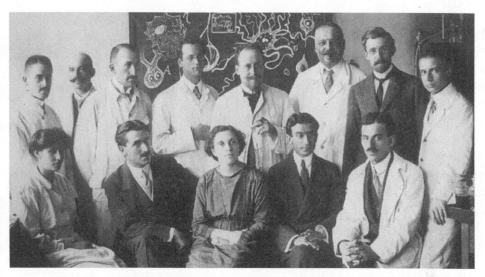

7.3 Friedrich Heinrich Lewy (first bottom right) in Alois Alzheimer's (third top right) laboratory at the Deutsche Forschungsanstalt fuer Psychiatrie in Munich, ca 1911. © Courtesy of the Clinical Department for Psychiatry and Neurology at the Ludwig Maximilians University, Munich, Germany.

The legacies of postwar medical institutions have been extensively addressed in the traditional historiography.[289] At the same time, accounts of the postwar fate of the original institutions with which Weil, Stern, and Lewy were associated in Germany are manifold. Both of the institutions in which Stern worked in the 1920s and 1930s – Edinger's Neurological Institute in Frankfurt and the department of neurology at the general hospital of Berlin-Moabit – continued as research institutions after the war. Most of the divisions of the former Neurological Institute, however, were relocated to a new building at the University of Frankfurt's Centre for Neurology and Neurosurgery. Subsequently the Edinger collection was incorporated on a separate floor into the new Max Planck Institute for Brain Research, when it opened on Theodor-Stern-Kai in 1962. Only the neuropsychological part of the hospital was destroyed after the war in order to make room for an apartment building complex. The neuroanatomist Wilhelm Kruecke (1911–1988) became its first director in the postwar period of 1947. No correspondence with Stern could be found in the historical archives, but Kruecke co-initiated the plan of bestowing a *Doctor honoris causa* in 1959 upon Stern's mentor, Kurt Goldstein – an offer that Goldstein rejected, having been ousted so drastically from his position twenty-six years earlier and told by the SA "to leave Germany forever!"[290] And after Stern's own death in 1975, a street was named in his honour in his Bavarian hometown of Cham.[291] The academic hospital of Moabit continued with a veritable department of neurology, first as a teaching hospital of the Free University of Berlin and, after 1989, as an academic institution of the Charité Medical School before this renowned hospital was closed in 2001.[292]

In the case of Lewy, the major clinical and research institutions he built and headed until the 1930s were almost completely destroyed by air raids on Berlin, as these institutions lay in close proximity to the capital's political centre. Of his three-storey institute, the former workers' clinic of the electromechanical company Allgemeine Electricitaetsgesellschaft at the Hansaplatz in Berlin-Charlottenburg, only the outer walls remained after 1945. Most parts were torn down the very year after Lewy's death.[293] While he had continued his correspondence with fellow émigré neuroscientists in North America, France, and the Netherlands, as well as with British colleagues since the 1940s, postwar letters that show exchanges between him and German colleagues remain to be found. This situation indicates that a reconciliation had not occurred between this great neurologist and the German neurological and psychiatric community, in particular the Deutscher Verein fuer Psychiatrie to which he had belonged in the past.[294] The department of psychiatry and neurology at the German University of Prague, where Weil received his medical training, ceased to exist with the dissolution of the German-speaking university – six hundred years after the latter's inauguration and sixty-three years after the split into a Czech and a German institution of higher learning on 18 October 1945.[295] While researching Weil's papers in the Dalhousie University Archives, I could not find confirmation that he ever returned to Czechoslovakia after the war. He nevertheless maintained contact with a number of colleagues there, as well as with some fellow émigré physicians in Canada and the German-Bohemian Heritage Society in New Ulm, Minnesota.[296]

It seems fitting to end this chapter with a brief look at (some very few) instances of remigration of Jewish physicians and medical researchers to the Federal Republic of Germany (West Germany) or the German Democratic Republic (East Germany). The process of remigration is a highly complex one and it is unknown exactly how many Jewish doctors returned after the war.[297] No statistics are available through Immigration Canada, the German Einwohnermeldebehoerde (Central Immigration Registry), or the Aerztekammern (Colleges of Physicians) as to the exact number of refugees to America who returned to their home country.

Immediately after the war had ended, not more than 5 percent of all émigré physicians are estimated to have considered returning to Europe.[298] Those physicians who did remigrate were a handful of exceptions – mostly psychoanalysts and psychiatrists with decidedly socialist and communist leanings actively trying to rebuild their homecountries from the rubble and ruins that the Nazi regime had left behind.[299] Most émigrés had developed new careers in their host countries. Other than in the case of some well-known philosophers, political scientists, and laboratory researchers, it would have been almost impossible for physicians to re-establish a clinical career back in Germany, Austria, or Czechoslovakia, from which they had been expelled only a few years earlier and where many institutions lay in ruins.[300]

Although hers was a highly unusual situation, it was possible to find one individual among the émigré neuroscientists who reversed her migration direction. An extraordinary pathologist, Ruth Silberberg, a Breslau-trained developmental brain scientist, had fled with her husband, the neurohistologist Martin Silberberg, first to Halifax and eventually to St Louis, where they settled. Ruth accepted invitations from the Deutsche Gesellschaft fuer Pathologie and university institutes to give guest lectures and seminars in Germany during the late 1950s and early 1960s. It was only at Martin's death, however, that she decided to accept an adjunct professorship at the University of Zurich in Switzerland, where she frequently taught during the summer break.[301] Ruth Silberberg represents an émigré researcher who acquired an important voice in both medical communities, yet continued to be torn between the "new" and the "old" world.

Another area in which unintended theory-changes emerged from the wave of forced migrants entering the States, and in which interdisciplinary theories became effectively amalgamated, was the new research field of trauma research. In this field, approaches from various psychoanalytical schools were blended with some of the new neurological advances. In this interdisciplinary working context, new concepts in wound surgery and war-related injuries and diseases became particularly relevant.[302]

The émigré psychiatrists and neurologists who engaged in contemporary trauma research were manifestly situated in their own human subjectivity and were certainly unable to step beyond the continuum established between trauma, psychological health, and well-being as its general reference points. This was certainly the case with respect to their former experiences during what Eric Hobsbawm has called the "Age of the Extremes" in the 1930s.[303] Following the seizing of power by the Nazis,

trauma researchers, like most of the German-speaking psychoanalytic
psychiatrists, psychologists, and holistic neurologists, fled into international exile.[304] Many of the psychoanalysts from German and Austria
been acquainted with the broader social dimension of the trauma concept
for reasons beyond their own experiences of forced migration and exile,
and their developed clinical and psychological work experiences. But, due
to the dramatic development of persecution and flight, the subjective
meaning of trauma moved much closer for many of the psychoanalytically and neurologically oriented trauma researchers themselves.[305] As
individually affected physicians and researchers, many of these émigrés
became the subject of their own scientific pursuit and personal and professional resources, as was prominently the case with the German psychiatrist William G. Niederland in New York.[306] When looking at cultural
modes of the neuroscientific research enterprise, the interplay between
science and everyday life needs to be taken into account *vis-à-vis* the
"trading zones" between groups of émigré researchers and clinicians in
the American research establishment.[307] The unique interplay between
their scientific and ordinary lives becomes very visible in the case of many
of the émigrés who arrived in the new medical and neuroscientific communities in North America.

8

"They Called Me an American Monkey Psychiatrist"

Reanimating German-American Biomedical Research Relations in the Early Postwar Period

A «*STUNDE NULL*» IN GERMAN-SPEAKING MORPHOLOGICAL NEUROSCIENCE?

The human psyche is an inalienable knowledge
(*Ein unverlierbares Wissen aber ist die menschliche Psyche*)

Gerhard Hauptmann[1]

When looking carefully at the developments that led to the emergence of the new research field of the morphological neurosciences between the last decades of the nineteenth-century and the postwar period of the twentieth, we must concede that its legacy in the context of postwar neuroscience in German-speaking countries also comprised various "traumatic normalities."[2] These become particularly visible when we review testimonies from the then-young generation of postwar researchers who witnessed the reanimation of German-American interactions. Their recollections and experiences speak well to the complexity of the history of the emerging field of morphological neuroscience as a merger between the disciplines of psychiatry, neurology, experimental psychology, brain anatomy, and neuropathology – and later behavioural and cognitive sciences – into a single, interdisciplinary field.[3] Applying such a perspective does not, however, relinquish the facticity of historical change.

The devastating effects of the forced migration wave described in the preceding chapters make it evident that this particular history could not be written as a prehistory of the modern neurosciences alone.[4] The areas of research and care for the mentally ill and neurologically disabled were

tightly intertwined with the medical doctrines and ideologies of the changing German political systems.[5] As a consequence of the history of early
neuroscience in the German-speaking countries, a lot more weight had
to be put on the disruption of transatlantic relations and the processes of
reanimating biomedical interchanges. However, a certain caveat needs to
apply here, since the perception of reanimated "biomedical relations"
between West Germany and the United States can only remain a partial
one, in order to allow the narrative to reconnect with the early formation
of the Neuroscience Research Program by Frank Schmitt and his collaborators at the Massachusetts Institute of Technology (MIT) in Cambridge,
Massachusetts. This perspective is crucial, since many neuroscientists
entered the field just after the end of World War II at a time when they
witnessed burgeoning forms of interdisciplinary research collaborations
as part of the war effort.[6]

   Professional medical historiography has only briefly addressed the issue
of the reanimation of German-American biomedical research interaction
during the early postwar period.[7] However, my final considerations can
build on some of the preliminary works. Particularly interesting is the
perspective provided by historian of medicine Carsten Timmermann in
*Americans and Pavlovians: The Central Institute for Cardiovascular
Research at the East German Academy of Sciences*, a case study of biomedical research exchanges between the German Democratic Republic
and the Soviet Union between the 1950s and 1980s. Also noteworthy is
the exploration of historians of science Jean-Paul Gaudillière and Hans-
Joerg Rheinberger into the westward trend between Germany and the
United States in *From Molecular Genetics to Genomics: The Mapping
Cultures of Twentieth-Century Genetics*.[8] What can be gleaned from this
recent scholarship is that the West-German and American relationship in
biomedical science, in particular, was long perceived as following a "normal" course of development on an equal level and above all as a mutually
beneficial process.[9] Yet, apart from the view presented by Quirke's and
Gaudillère's *The Era of Biomedicine* in 2008, that "the growth of biomedical complexes ... characterized by the intensification of research in
the life sciences" was aggravated by regional differences defying "any
description of it as the culmination of a uniform trend,"[10] German-
speaking scholarship in medical historiography has focused mainly on
the internal factors leading to the forced migration of doctors and researchers, or on neurologists' and psychiatrists' collaboration with Nazi politics,
medical institutions, and physician organizations during the Third Reich.[11]
In fact, for the development of the Federal Republic of Germany from

1949 to 1989, Quirke's and Gaudillère's *new ways of knowing* remain largely under-explored territory, and we do not yet have a workable account of the international relations that occurred post–World War II.[12]

OVER THE ATLANTIC – BOTH WAYS?

Israel-based historian Ute Deichmann has provided important perspectives for the postwar reconstruction of the research relationships in the allied field of experimental and molecular biology. In this respect, her historio-graphical analysis can serve as a good heuristic vantage point for my discussion in this final chapter:

> After WWII ... molecular biology as a new interdisciplinary scientific enterprise was scarcely represented in Germany for almost 20 years. There are three major reasons for such a low performance of molec-ular biology: first, the forced emigration of Jewish scientists after 1933 ... Second, German university structures had strongly impeded interdisciplinary research due to an over-focus on medical research disciplines ... Third, the international isolation or self-isolation of German scientists ... was a major obstacle to the implementation of new fields of research developed elsewhere.[13]

Many of Deichmann's findings can likewise be applied to the emerging research field of neuroscience in postwar Germany, from which my final examples are taken. As one can see from the preceding chapters, until the 1930s not only was Germany an international leader in chemistry, bio-chemistry, and other areas of experimental biology, but the development of early neuroscience programs, institutes, and centres in large part took place in the German-speaking world. With respect to the postwar recon-struction of the new research field of neuroscience – quite remarkably – the German-American biophysicist Max Delbrueck was a considerable factor for this community as well. Delbrueck travelled frequently between his home base at the California Institute of Technology and the University of Cologne (see also chapter 6). At the same time, he held a second pro-fessorship in Germany and assumed numerous roles as a science educator and an advisor to research funding institutions, and was also an important mediator between neuroscience communities on both sides of the Atlantic.[14] Moreover, if a similar academic leader among the generation of young progressive brain researchers in Germany were to be found to explain the social efforts for the re-establishment of German-speaking

neuroscience, then this would likely be the 1967 Nobel Prize winner and
longtime director of the Max Planck Institute (MPI) for Biophysical
Chemistry in Goettingen, Manfred Eigen (1927–2019). Through his connections with American neuroscientists, Eigen strongly fostered the merger
between biochemistry, biophysics, and neurology in the Federal Republic
of Germany.[15]

Several factors in the restoration development of transatlantic relations
between Germany and the United States could be related to the US government's overarching Marshall Plan.[16] The economic and social reconstruction plan proposed by US secretary of state George Marshall
(1880–1959), was directed at alleviating financial and cultural strains from
Central European countries after the war.[17] Inaugurated in April 1947, it
further tried to confine the spreading influences of communism after the
war and became instrumental in the reconstruction of academic institutions and the science sphere, as well as laying the groundwork for a normalization process in academic and research exchanges over the next
decades.[18] Despite vital early support through the Marshall Plan for infrastructure programs for higher learning institutions, and despite the return
of formal transatlantic relationships, which were probably most visible in
academia and directly affected the career development and creation of a
"new generation of young (neuro-)scientists,"[19] however, the most profound and direct changes were likely those brought about by specific
contracts under the auspices of the US-German Understandings on Cultural
Exchange, as they were laid out on 9 April 1953, through John Foster
Dulles (1888–1959) – President Dwight D. Eisenhower's (1890–1969)
secretary of state (1953–59) – and West German chancellor Konrad
Adenauer (1876–1967).[20] Adenauer was the foreign minister of the Federal
Republic of Germany from 1951 to 1955 and brought substantial expertise
to his role as the primary representative of West Germany. His engagement
for the reconstruction of international relationships in science and higher
learning can hardly be underestimated, based as it was on the terms of the
1953 US-German Understandings on Cultural Exchange:[21]

1. To encourage the coming together of the peoples of the United
States of America and the Federal Republic of Germany in cultural
cooperation; ...
5. As facilitating the interchange of persons referred to, to look with
favor on establishment of scholarships, travel grants, and other forms
of assistance in the academic and cultural institution within its territory. Each Government will also endeavor to make available to the

other information requested by the other with regard to facilities, courses of instruction or other opportunities which may be of interest to nationals of the other Government.[22]

The ensuing individualized process is intriguing. Highly delicate interactions with research foundations and scientific networks are revealed in the biographical experiences and observations of a number of prominent members of the postwar German-speaking neuroscience field.[23] As one later MPI director of a neuroscience-related institute stated in an interview with the author:

And the Germans had the advantage that Frank Schmitt held Manfred Eigen in high esteem, and the latter was even promoted by him. Eigen received a substantial grant from the *Volkswagen Stiftung*, which the NRP could use whenever it wanted to invite German students and professors ... And because of this, we [German, Austrian, and Swiss neuroscientists] were always incredibly well represented – yes, especially in those founding years of the program ... which was of a great value for us.[24]

In addition to the Volkswagen Foundation, which played such a pivotal role in the resumption of neuroscientific interchanges, the Deutsche Forschungsgemeinschaft, and later eventually the Alexander von Humboldt Foundation, helped with substantial financial support from the late 1940s and early 1950s.[25] The American Rockefeller Foundation also played an active role in the postwar re-establishment of German academic and research institutions by continuing the funding of previous fellows and researchers, giving scholarships to émigré scientists, and also providing infrastructure grants for literature, technical instruments, and the reconstruction of institute buildings destroyed during the war.[26] These institutions enabled – and even fostered – the professional cooperation of German neuroscientists with researchers from Austria, Switzerland, and German-speaking institutions from other Central European countries, along with their American colleagues.[27] Despite the fact that the Rockefeller Foundation had shifted major funding toward the creation of the Rockefeller University in New York City (since 1910), the foundation had maintained contact with several pre-war researchers.[28] Furthermore, émigré neuroscientists in America also played an important role, welcoming and supporting the new generation of young German-speaking neuroscientists who had just arrived to pursue postgraduate training at the National Institutes of Health and major American and Canadian research universities.[29]

In institutional terms, the National Institutes of Health in Bethesda, Maryland, since its inauguration in 1948, gradually took over the Rockefeller Foundation's role in funding American biomedical research and international scientific exchanges after 1948. These funding sources became available on top of the former research fellowships by the Rockefeller Foundation for the ongoing activities in the biomedical landscape, which also brought many leading neuroscientists into close contact and continuous personal and research relationships with this exceptional American institution.[30] As representatives of the US Diplomatic Mission to Germany pointed out, and also as the scientific community perceived it, the National Institutes of Health became the prime mover and shaker of biomedical research in North America during the subsequent decades, from the 1950s to the 1980s:

> Their origin lay in a small, only one room Laboratory of Hygiene from the year 1887. Since then, the National Institutes of Health developed into a global leader in health research and a central institution in medical science on the Federal level of the United States of America ... The National Institutes of Health pursue[d] research not only in their own laboratories, but support[ed] scientific investigations of many non-Federal researchers in universities, medical schools, hospitals, and other research institutions in North America and abroad.[31]

Such self-reflexive rhetorical statements as the one quoted here from a US government agency are also present in many eyewitness accounts by leading German-speaking postwar neuroscientists, when looking back at their own experiences as young postdoctoral researchers in North America. One interviewee, who later became an MPI director in the clinical biomedicine area, travelled to Bethesda in 1956 to work with the neurophysiologist and emotion researcher Paul D. McLean (1913–1977). McLean was one of the most prominent neurophysiologists at the time; as chief of the laboratory of brain evolution and behaviour at the National Institute of Mental Health he was involved in major scientific contributions to the biological understanding of the evolution of the forebrain and related psychophysiological characteristics.[32] For young German neuroscientists during the 1950s and 1960s, the National Institutes of

Health were reputed to be the epitome of leading-edge biomedical institutions:

> There was a high percentage of Jewish researchers in the American neurosciences. It is really astonishing that as a German, especially of that generation, in which I could have done something wrong, that I never experienced any resentments, not even at the National Institutes of Health ... By no means could one say we would have already caught up with their research development. Even ... at the time, when everything was gradually reconstructed, the 68ers marched along and tore it all down again. This was an incredible backlash.[33]

Young German neuroscientists pointed out in particular how, for instance, they later ordered their complete technical equipment for experimental laboratories in Munich and Frankfurt – such as telephone wire, electrical relays, oscillographs, and further measuring instruments – from the United States.[34] In order to better understand both the scholarly and the official political views about the gradual restoration of the research relationships between the Federal Republic of Germany and the United States, I now want to compare researchers' personal experiences with some general developments in the re-established transatlantic support networks, as sketched out above.[35]

PERCEPTIONS AND EXPERIENCES

The narratives of outgoing young neuroscientists among the new postwar generation of German-speaking medical researchers provide striking examples of the inequalities between research and educational centres in the late 1950s and early 1960s.[36] These years marked a time when major German neuroscience institutions in the East and West had just been reopened and literally rebuilt from wartime ruins, or their collections and laboratories reassembled, as in the case of the KWI for Brain Research, which had been scattered over several cities since 1944. These lay hundreds of kilometres apart: the Vogts had founded a new institute in Neustadt (Black Forest) in the 1930s, which then moved to Duesseldorf (Northrhine Westphalia) in 1964;[37] other departments and collections of the Berlin institute moved to Giessen/Dillenburg, Marburg, Goettingen, Munich, Bochum-Langendreer, and Cologne, and later to Frankfurt am Main (Hesse) after 1945.[38]

After they had left their home institutions in Germany, Austria, and Switzerland, the new wave of postwar neuroscientific émigrés felt like "strangers in paradise," as their predecessors had, sometimes for different reasons (new material and technological support), but mostly because they were looking for similar values (freedom of thought and liberal American campus communities):[39]

And the whole summer school took place in an incredible palace of one of the old and wealthy English families, which had to give their properties away ... The house now belonged to the American Academy of Science ... Atmospherically, this was a superb experience and for the German delegates a really great honor ... The booklets, which were printed after the meetings, were very much appreciated by us, as they were inexpensive and the best documents one could get for preparing seminars, talks and similar things.[40]

Furthermore, the challenging research situation in postwar Germany and Austria, along with the urgent need for external help, is bilaterally reflected in researchers' application letters and responses from granting agencies. Executive Rockefeller Foundation administrators such as Alan Gregg (see figure 5.3) or Robert S. Morris (1908–1972?) summed up this "great need of everything" on the west side of the Atlantic:

JHW [Joseph H. Willits, 1889–1979] felt that: (1) other countries in Europe had a prior claim over Germany; (2) working under military government would be difficult; and (3) if we were forced to work only in the American Zone it would inevitably have a political con-notation. On the other hand he did express the opinion that the res-toration of educational and intellectual institutions in Germany was essential to the restoration of the rest of Europe as a whole.[41]

At the receiving end were also two institutions, the clinical department of neurology at the University of Wuerzburg (headed by Georges Schaltenbrand) and the Deutsche Forschungsanstalt for Psychiatry in Munich (Willibald Scholz, a former recipient of Rockefeller Foundation funds, headed the neuropathology department), where researchers had previously been involved in atrocious human experiments or acted as willing recipients of pathological brain specimens from psychiatric patients killed in the *Aktion T4* program from 1939–41 and the "wild euthanasia" actions during the Nazi Period.[42] These circumstances were already known to the investigators of the Alsos Mission of Field Intelligence Agency, Technical, as well as to expert witnesses to the Nuremberg Doctors Trials during the 1940s.[43] The single Austrian institution that received Rockefeller Foundation funding during the immediate postwar period was Graz University's institute for zoology, headed by the ethological researcher Karl von Frisch (1886–1982), who later received the Nobel Prize for Physiology or Medicine in 1973 for his research on synchronized social behaviours of honey bees.[44]

A highly politically driven funding initiative within the Rockefeller Foundation's portfolio was its support for the psychosomatic researcher and psychoanalyst Alexander Mitscherlich (1908–1982), immediately after the political creation of the Federal Republic of Germany in 1949.[45] Émigré psychiatrist Mitscherlich had been an expert witness at the Nuremberg Medical Trials, where he detailed the Nazi atrocities of patient murder, forced sterilization, and coerced human subject experimentation for the first time, which were to appear in the internationally acclaimed book *Doctors of Infamy: The Story of Nazi Medical Crimes* (*Medizin ohne Menschlichkeit*), which was published soon after the Nuremberg Medical Trials had ended in 1947. Through this experience, Mitscherlich became an invested researcher on the authoritarian character and human social group behaviours, research toward explaining the enthusiasm and coercion of social masses for Nazism and Fascism in Europe.[46] American politicians and the Rockefeller Foundation further tried to develop Heidelberg University as a model academy, to serve as a landmark institution for re-educating the new elites of democratic West Germany.[47]

Renewed Rockefeller Foundation research grants during the postwar period were paid out primarily as institutional aids and were tightly concentrated on the support of approximately ten excellent individual researchers working in the area of neurology, psychiatry, and psychology. These included: the pharmacologist Wolfgang Heubner (1877–1957) at the Berlin Charité, the physiologist Karl Thomas (1883–1969) in Erlangen, Georg Schaltenbrand and the neurologist Juerg Zutt (1893–1980) in Wuerzburg, neuropathologist Hugo Spatz at the reinaugurated Max Planck Institute for Brain Research in Dillenburg and Giessen, the psychiatrists Ernst von Weizsaecker, Ernst Kretschmer (1888–1964), and Karl Jaspers in Heidelberg, the pharmacologist Sigurd Janssen (1891–1968) in Freiburg, the internist Franz Volhard (1872–1950), and the neuro- and orthopaedic surgeon Joerg Rehn (1918–2003) in Frankfurt.[48] Many of

these researchers and physicians had already been funded by the
Rockefeller Foundation before the war, while it seemed to have escaped
the American funding institutions that individuals such as Drs Volhard,
Heubner, and Schaltenbrand had been dedicated NSDAP members, had
supported war-related research on nutrition and drug actions, and – as
in the prominent case of Schaltenbrand – had pursued coerced human
subject experimentation in neurology that led to the willing acceptance
of the death of hospitalized patients.[49] Already in November 1947, the
Rockefeller Foundation had sent out a memorandum, drafted by its Paris
officer Robert S. Morrison and related to the US Army Military administration's policies, which strongly emphasized the necessity for continued
financial support for German scientific and academic institutions:

> My [Lucius D. Clay's, 1897–1978] first impulse last year was to
> regard the question of RF aid to Germany as in no way different
> from that of aid to any European country. Such a course would have
> been in line with AG's [Alan Gregg's] proposition that a physician
> does not censure or punish his patients ... For some time to come the
> primary and, to me, the only task which should engage our energies
> in Germany is the nurture of a stable democratic society.[50]

Moving ahead with little resentment – and often with too little security
– the re-establishment of prewar personal relationships by American-
known educators became an important factor in the new academic and
scientific reconstruction process.[51] The internal planning decisions of
the Rockefeller Foundation sought to identify and cultivate a new group
of recipients for science funding, by labelling them as candidates and
"trustworthy good men."[52] Often, however, the Rockefeller Foundation
had to refer back to prewar communications, such as an earlier central
document about the most promising neuroscience institutions and interdisciplinary working groups in the German-speaking landscape, which
prominent Munich neuropathologist Walther Spielmeyer had put
together and sent to the New York office at the beginning of the National
Socialist period in 1935.[53] It emerges that, when the dust had settled
after the end of the war, the Spielmeyer list was simply dug up again
and Rockefeller Foundation officers worked from it to determine the
whereabouts of those scientists and find out whether they were still
active in their brain research endeavours. Although many of these alleg-
edly "trustworthy good men" had been forced out of Germany and

Austria in the 1930s, however, a good number of ethically highly problematic neuroscientists, such as Schaltenbrand, Spatz, and Hallervorden – who had continued their work under the murderous Nazi auspices of the past[54] – remained on the Rockefeller Foundation list for potential future funding of "good men." Not only had they decided to stay in Germany after 1933, but they very successfully aligned with military funding streams, profiting in their procurement of brains and nerve specimens from the euthanasia program under the murderous Nazi auspices of the past.[55] Despite participating in the dreadful human experiments, and receiving dedicated research benefits through the murderous *Aktion T4* and the euthanasia program involving psychiatric patients and disabled children,[56] they were now again perceived as "the best-trained researchers" and "German leaders in neurology," serving as the primary go-to academics for the postwar reconstruction of the neurosciences in the 1950s and 1960s:

This was the situation after the war. Nothing new [in starting our research programs] was created. During the war, most of the Jewish colleagues had been murdered or forced out of the country. More than a third of all our academic personnel – and to my mind those were the best – were lost during the war. And then there were those who could not get along with the Nazis – those who belonged to old bourgeois professorial families – and they also left their academic positions and the country. And the remaining ones, they did not advance much further. Then the borders were closed and nothing could come in from abroad, no visitors, and there was no exchange. And the death knell to our field [of early neuroscience] was that all the young people – in medicine – they had joined the army, served in military hospitals and thousands of young students and physicians [the interviewee spoke of physicians in general] became war casualties and, of course, they were also lost for neuroscience. This was the whole tragedy with the Nazis. And this was still the situation in the 1950s and 1960s, when we began.[57]

The present chapter is not the place to delve further into the actual living and working conditions of the new wave of young neuroscientists who had travelled for research training to the United States and Canada. What is quite illuminating, however, is that most postwar émigré researchers made their experiences in the vibrant American styles of experimental and clinical neuroscience investigations highly thorough and promisingly beneficial.[58]

Historians of science, along with contemporary eyewitnesses of the postwar wave of young migrating neuroscientists and physicians, have repeatedly emphasized the differences in the local and national contexts prevailing on both sides of the Atlantic. After their own scientific collaborations and the ensuing friendships between German and American neuroscientists in this "exciting new world," for many their return to the Federal Republic of Germany appeared as an "absolutely great decline."[59] Returning researchers had not anticipated finding the German research situation and landscape so different from their American – and sometimes British and Israeli – experiences.[60] Their remigration to Germany required a deeply traumatic readaptation in the universities, laboratories, and clinics of the Federal Republic of Germany, which were still in the process of reconstruction:

> And there was this incident, which deeply impressed me, when
> I returned to Marburg after a number of years at the National
> Institutes of Health. It must have been in 1959 or 1960 – I had
> come back from the National Institutes of Health and should give
> a talk in the Medical Society. [Yes ... it was] criticized that I had the
> hand in the pockets of my trousers, and also it was said that I obviously could not speak German any longer ... *They even went so far
> as to call me an American monkey psychiatrist.*[61]

Such misunderstandings, hostility, and open attacks at guest presentations toward both returning exchange researchers and also the small group of émigrés who had fled the German-speaking countries[62] during the Nazi period but wished to return for lecture series or summer academies after 1945 were often nurtured by stern academic hierarchies, continued right-wing nationalism among professors, and even personal envy over the international working opportunities from which these neuroscientists had benefited.[63] Most important for the development of the early field of neuroscience, however, were the prevailing irritations based on the use of different research methods and changes in research themes between the United States and West Germany. These differences had emanated both from the forced migration of leading researchers and from the military investments in adjacent research fields in America throughout the war:

Well, for the time after [19]45, one has to see that it took fifteen – yes at least fifteen years – before our neurosciences [in the German-speaking countries] reached the American standard again. In my field, psychiatry [in Germany] for example, the big names were [Ernst] Kretschmer, who is barely mentioned today, [Hans] Buerger-Prinz [1897–1976], who [is] even less mentioned, and who had introduced the anthropological – hermeneutic-anthropological – method into psychiatry. At no point had laboratory experimentation been involved – this was no longer accepted; well, experimentation even became a dirty word.[64]

For the majority of returning young neuroscientists, neurologists, and psychiatrists, however, the then-existing cultural, political, and technological differences between the research traditions in North America and West Germany proved to be a tremendous obstacle during their remigration to the Federal Republic of Germany, when they sought to acquire continuing university positions in the traditional university-based research system. Their German peers had been trained in completely different milieux, protected and promoted by former faculty mandarins who still dominated the academic system at that time. In the German-speaking neurosciences, these were different "schools"; for example, "die Toennis-Schule" (neurosurgery), "die Vogt-Schule" (neuroanatomy), "die Nonne-Schule" (neurology), "die Schneider-Schule" (brain psychiatry), "die Scholz-Schule" (neuropathology), whereby postgraduate trainees were all decidedly overrepresented in the chairs and professorships of postwar neurosciences in the Federal Republic until the 1970s.[65] At the same time, German universities gave continuing work opportunities to a large number of ex-Nazi professors and doctors.[66] Consequently, in postwar years, there was in German medical faculties almost a taboo on historiographical research on medicine and science related to the 1930s and 1940s.[67]

For the young generation of returning neuroscientists, the re-establishment of the Max Planck Gesellschaft in 1948 eventually offered a safe haven for many,[68] and the building boom of Max Planck Institutes from the 1960s forward (1962: Frankfurt am Main – brain research; 1961–62: Munich – psychiatry clinic and neuropathology;[69] 1982: Cologne – clinical neurology) and the society's international research

institutes, offered a new array of research positions outside the German
university system:

> Especially in this house [the MPI for Psychiatry], where no clinical
> department existed for twenty years ... and the *Nussbaumstrasse* [the
> university clinical department of psychiatry] – and he [Kurt Kolle,
> 1898–1975] had consultants, such as [Karl Friedrich] Scheidt [1906–
> 1945], who were strongly oriented towards experimentation, but
> they proposed biochemical views. He [Scheidt] had tried to identify
> and reclassify the psychoses in biochemical terms ... There was only
> one man in Frankfurt [am Main] ... [Edwin] Rausch [1906–1994],
> who developed experiments in the older tradition of German
> *Gestaltpsychologie*. But in general, Gestalt theory barely had any
> followers in [German] psychiatry.[70]

Drawing primarily on a set of first-rate oral history interviews with
selected German researchers in leadership positions in the interdisciplinary postwar neurosciences, I have ventured to give a few historical perspectives about the "second wave" of young neuroscientists, who travelled
to North America in the 1950s and 1960s. Although heuristic in nature,
this attempt can nevertheless be seen as quite illuminating. These considerations intriguingly show that "normalization" of transatlantic relationships in the research field of neuroscience was far from a smooth process;
it suffered notable breaks, disruptions, and distortions along the way.
Written documents and institution-based archival materials are rather
silent on the specific adjustment difficulties, personal problems, and
instances of "culture shock" in that transition, which rendered it a "traumatic normalcy" that paralleled the reunion and the *Wiederanschluss* of
German and US biomedical research.[71] Higher political developments
stimulated particular initiatives of student and professorial exchanges or
conferences, while administrators and officers of major funding institutions revised their judgments about universities and research institutes in
Germany, Austria, and Switzerland.

Political rhetoric, however, did not always meet the needs of individual
neuroscientists: For German-speaking researchers, travelling to the United
States or Canada was a considerable financial risk, if not an actual impedi-
ment until the 1960s – when additional foundations stepped in and filled
the support gap.[72] While the "American experience" of the younger generation of German neuroscientists proved for many to be highly gratifying
and very stimulating, their re-entry into German academia was not always

an easy enterprise: research traditions that were now important in postwar America had emigrated with the neuroscience refugees of the 1930s and were now disrupted or even completely defunct in their home countries.[73] In neuroscience-related areas, this was the case with experimental psychology, Gestalt psychology, psychoanalytic psychiatry, and holist neurology. Young researchers who travelled to North America were often perceived by the older generation of West German professors as having fraternized with an undesirable "scientific enemy."[74] Disciplinary order, obedience to academic hierarchies, and proper displays of social behaviour were often ranked much higher in postwar German academia than bridge-building between scientific disciplines or even active interdisciplinary cooperation across the Atlantic.

THE SCIENTIFIC RELAY FUNCTION OF THE BURGEONING NEUROSCIENCE RESEARCH PROGRAM

The interdisciplinary enterprise of the Neuroscience Research Program in the United States undoubtedly shaped today's biomedical research landscape much more than any other single scientific development during the twentieth century. As the organizers of the Neuroscience Research Program in Cambridge, Massachusetts, George Adelman (1926–2015) and Barry Smith (b. 1930), have described, it was the vision of the American neurophysiologist Frank Schmitt at the end of the 1950s to overcome pertinent constraints in research and training within the American medical and science faculties. Schmitt's influence – and thereby also his and his co-workers' attraction to young research trainees from the German-speaking countries – extended far beyond the fact that he coined the very term "neuroscience" in a research proposal to the National Institutes of Health in 1962; he also laid a most fruitful societal foundation for the general scientific endeavour when the Neuroscience Research Program was created at the Massachusetts Institute of Technology.[75]

Disciplinary margins were still prevalent at that time, perpetuated from nineteenth-century forms of research organization in physics, physiology, and pathology.[76] In their scholarly work on the postwar development of American neuroscience, William Bechtel, Lily Kay, Judith Swazey, and Fred Warden have drawn attention to the influences of Schmitt's interdisciplinary biophysics approaches.[77] With his integrative stance on the creation of the "Neuroscience Study Program," Schmitt managed to bring together an international group of eminent researchers from various disciplines.[78] This program at first spanned physics, chemistry, information and computer science, and it later expanded to experimental biology and psychology to stimulate their productive interaction in the study of the nervous system:[79]

> Perhaps the most significant overall influence of the [Neuroscience Research Program] organization has been its catalytic role in creating and promoting *the growth of a neuroscience community* ... In much the same way that a physics community developed in the mid-nineteenth century, a neuroscience community has begun to emerge since the early 1960s, formed by the joining together of specialists from a number of previously separate communities in the shared pursuit of penetrating the complexities of the human brain and behavior.[80]

Schmitt, who in 1955 received the honour of being named institute professor at MIT, can be seen as an influential pioneer in the political and scientific organization that laid the groundwork for the modern field of neuroscience in the twentieth century.[81] He had indeed been ingenious in using the technical term of the sciences of the brain and nerves – "neuroscience" *avant la lettre* – in planning the Neuroscience Research Program in 1962.[82] Nevertheless, various precursor versions of the term "neuroscience" had already been used in the 1950s, as in the work of Stanford neurophysiologist Ralph Waldo Gerard (1900–1974), who nevertheless did not have in mind a fully fledged plan for a new research field. In Gerard's use, the word referred primarily to a theoretical category rather than an educational program of an emerging neuroscientific community of scholars.[83]

In the following quotation from his autobiography, *The Never-Ceasing Search* (1990), Schmitt presents a breathtakingly broad perspective on the neurosciences as including complementary input from clinical and theoretical psychology, public mental health, and even relevant aspects from the social sciences. Schmitt was quick to describe a dramatic underlying shift in the field of neuroscience shortly after World War II, and – by promoting his own influence in that development – he even dubbed this process "*a scientific revolution,*" bringing it well in line with Harvard historian of science Thomas S. Kuhn's term that was still much in vogue in both the social and natural sciences throughout the 1990s:[84]

> Clinical payoffs from basic research, and progress in fundamental knowledge of brain mechanisms, suggested that neuroscience was

reaching a watershed [in the late 1950s] and that a revolution was already underway in prevention and treatment of disorders such as schizophrenia, manic-depressive psychosis, multiple sclerosis, stroke, mental retardation, and many other genetic and developmental disorders of the nervous system. Perhaps, even more importantly, neuroscience offered hope that a better understanding of the biological roots of human nature would enhance prospects for well-being, social welfare, and even the survival of human life on this planet.[85]

Schmitt's words are certainly framed in a strong rhetorical way in order to promote his own work as well as the academic standing of the newly emerged research field of the neurosciences in North America.[86] Yet, despite prevailing historical accounts of that time, Schmitt certainly played an important role in these profound changes regarding the sciences of the brain and nervous system, as has been acknowledged even by some of his critics, such as Marcus Raichle or Bill Lampard from Washington University in St Louis.[87] Schmitt's influence also extended to laying a most fruitful societal foundation for the general scientific endeavour, when the Neuroscience Research Program was created at MIT (see figure 8.1).[88]

In a series of articles from 1960 to 1964, *Time Magazine* even went so far as to dub Frank Schmitt as "Mr. Neuroscience."[89] His tremendous impact extended not only to the establishment of interdisciplinary work in the laboratory set-up at MIT; it also hinged largely on his administrative involvement in many scientific and medical fields throughout the United States. Moreover, the Neuroscience Research Program advocated for new research facilities for graduate students, trainees, and visiting neuroscientists in the organization of this new academic research field.[90] It is certainly not an exaggeration to view Schmitt's intention to create the program as an extension of his earlier engagement with multidisciplinary approaches in biophysics.[91] This was more than merely an idiosyncrasy of Schmitt's own work from the fringes, as it were, dating from the period in the 1950s when he intensively pursued electrophysiological recordings in giant squid axons.[92]

His early research career had in fact taken him to frequent visits of European research institutions during the interwar period. After being awarded a fellowship from the National Research Council to pursue his postdoctoral studies, Schmitt first visited the biochemistry department of Jack Drummond (1891–1952) at University College London in England, and then went on to visit major laboratories in Germany between 1927 and 1929.[93] These visits became an important source of inspiration to him. During his sojourn in Berlin, Schmitt worked, for example, in the

Volume 17, Number 4/December 1979
Published by The MIT Press
ISSN 0028-3967

NEUROSCIENCES
Research Program Bulletin®

CELLULAR MECHANISMS IN THE SELECTION AND MODULATION OF BEHAVIOR

Eric R. Kandel   Franklin B. Krasne
Felix Strumwasser   James W. Truman

PARTICIPANTS

Hugo Aréchiga   Eric R. Kandel   Allen I. Selverston
Michael V.L. Bennett   Andrew Kramer   Felix Strumwasser
Theodore H. Bullock   Franklin B. Krasne   Duncan Stuart
William J. Davis   Irving Kupfermann   Paul Taghert
Alan N. Epstein   Earl Mayeri   Richard F. Thompson
Edward V. Evarts   Keir G. Pearson   James W. Truman
Robert Hawkins   Donald W. Pfaff   Frederic G. Worden
Graham Hoyle   Francis O. Schmitt   Robert H. Wurtz

8.1 Front cover of the *Neurosciences Research Program Bulletin*, 1979 (personal copy). Coll. Frank W. Stahnisch. © 2012 Frank W. Stahnisch, Calgary, Alberta.

physiological chemistry laboratories of several German Nobel laureates, notably Otto Warburg (1882–1970) at the KWI for Cell Physiology, and Otto Meyerhoff (1884–1951) at the KWI for Biology in Berlin-Dahlem. In the physical and chemical colloquia in which Schmitt participated, he came into contact with many illustrious scientists of the time, such as the Nobel Prize laureates physicist Max Planck, Walter Nernst (1864–1941), Albert Einstein (1879–1955), and chemist Fritz Haber (1868–1934). Like many other of his countrymen he enjoyed the collegial atmosphere, particularly that of Meyerhoff's laboratory, which focused on the scientific analysis of glycolysis in biological tissues, along with the social events of the Dahlem "beer evenings" at the guest house of the KWG and nearby pubs, at which he made a number of continuing, lifelong relationships. From a research organizational perspective, Schmitt was impressed by the way in which Meyerhof managed "*his* KWI"[94] and how well the latter related to the research associates by giving them a substantial amount of individual freedom to pursue their own work.[95]

The episode of Schmitt's visits to the KWG Berlin is quite telling. Apparently, the international academic relations of the 1920s and 1930s were quite often portrayed as having been significantly disrupted by military aggression and academic hostilities, along with the later process of forced migration during the Fascist and Nazi period in Central Europe.[96] This view in scholarly literature is appropriate to some extent, yet it should not be overlooked that important prewar forms of exchange relations were first and foremost sustained by people: the scientists, physicians, trainees, administrators, and politicians of the time. Schmitt can be seen as a good representative of this group, who continued to maintain their personal contacts on the international level after World War I. Scientists like Schmitt became important players in the reanimation of previous transatlantic exchanges in the early neurosciences, and many were instrumental in knitting together the safeguarding nets for vast numbers of émigré neurologists and psychiatrists who were forced to emigrate to the United States and Canada after 1933.[97] These personal relationships endured even after the second catastrophe of the twentieth century – World War II. And they led to revitalized academic relations in the postwar period in both parts of Germany, the Federal Republic of Germany in the west as well as the German Democratic Republic in the east.

During the reconstruction of research institutions and universities in Germany, Schmitt again set out on month-long journeys to visit Central European science institutions, concomitant with the planning process of the Neuroscience Research Program. These visits had been meticulously planned through letter and telephone exchanges with scientific peers, while a number of Schmitt's contacts came from his personal interest in the field and ongoing work in his laboratory. For example, his visit to the MPI for Medical Research in Heidelberg was motivated by his primary interest in the "molecular biology" of the time. Also, at the MPI for Biophysical Chemistry in Goettingen, he visited the renowned biochemist Manfred Eigen, who was working on the kinetics of nucleic acids in biological cells.[98] The men became good friends, and Schmitt later designated Eigen as an honorary associate of the Neuroscience Research Program. As they had been during the years of the Weimar Republic, researchers' international relationships became very intimate and lively again in the postwar period of the 1950s.[99] As Schmitt reveals in *The Never-Ceasing Search*, meeting young Eigen in Goettingen, and again in Heidelberg later that year during a workshop with the neurophysiologist Hans Hermann Weber (1896–1974), gave rise to continuous exchanges over the planning of the Neuroscience Research Program. Eigen also invited Schmitt to a legendary workshop gathering (with his associates and graduate students) with recreation activities in the hiking and spa town of Hahnenklee in the Harz Mountains. This experience served as an important model for Schmitt's conference activities of the Intensive Study Program in Neuroscience (see figure 8.2) at the University of Colorado at Boulder.[100]

It was certainly beneficial that Schmitt and Eigen shared a love for extended mountain hikes, as well as for private chamber music presentations, activities through which they became personally very close. Yet over and above, they held similar views about the foundations of the emerging field of biophysics;[101] and it is probably much more than mere anecdote that Schmitt became excited by Eigen's research on proton-conduction. This tied in with the work of the Belgian neurophysiologist Leo de Maeyer (1927–2014) at the MPI for Biophysical Chemistry, since Schmitt favoured the idea that nerve axons themselves had to be proton conductors. Thus, the preliminary results of his European colleagues' investigations served as leitmotifs, while anticipating the direction in which he was to move.[102]

THE NEUROSCIENCE RESEARCH PROGRAM

From the perspective of contemporary German-speaking neuroscientists, the United States was a major point of reference, even more so after the devastation or loss of leading research institutes during World War II.[103] Yet America itself had experienced a genuinely boundless development

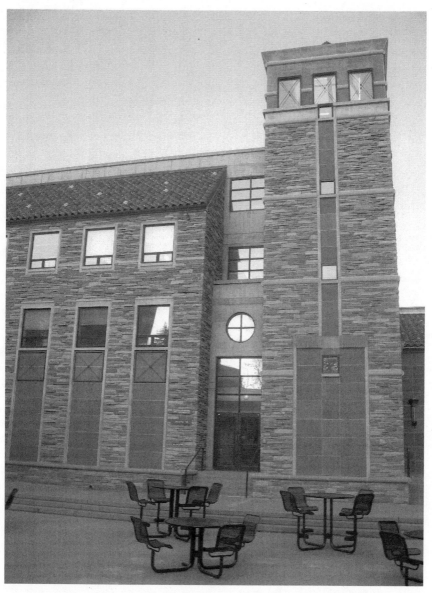

8.2 Lecture halls 140–142, University of Colorado Department of Chemistry & Biochemistry, where the first Interdisciplinary Study Program meetings were convened by Francis O. Schmitt. Coll. Frank W. Stahnisch. © 2012 Frank W. Stahnisch, Calgary, Alberta.

of biomedical science in the early decades of the twentieth century. This
process was based largely on the restructuring of its universities following
the influential report of Johns Hopkins–trained administrator and politician Abraham Flexner since the 1910s. Fostered through increased state
funding, vast amounts of philanthropic money, and the rapid growth of
its institutions since the end of the Great War, American scientific output
had risen to breathtaking dimensions.[104] With the end of World War II,
the international focus of researchers had shifted away from the German-
speaking countries primarily to the United States. Financial opportunities
and technical supplies for the Intensive Study Program in Neuroscience
and later the Neuroscience Research Program, for example, were mind-
boggling to young German neuroscientists who tried to pursue their
postgraduate training in the States during the postwar period.[105] Since
the inception of the Neuroscience Research Program, Schmitt had also
inaugurated a private support organization: The Neuroscience Research
Foundation, the bylaws of which were modelled after those of the
Massachusetts General Hospital. It created sustained funding for the
program and its activities. The senior German Neuroscience Research
Program associates who had been asked to organize themed work sessions
were also overwhelmed by the opportunities given to them. The affluence
of the program was extended not only to the Boulder Intensive Study
Program summer conferences (see figure 8.2) but also to the laboratories
in Cambridge, Massachusetts. Several members who took part in the
Neuroscience Research Program as senior fellows at Brandegee Mansion
in the Boston neighbourhood of South Brookline, described it almost as
a "palace." It appeared to them like "a museum of Roman and Greek
art," and early German participants were "jealous" about the affluence
they encountered. Brandegee Mansion offered many rooms, a dining hall,
and a ballroom for social gatherings. There was even the possibility of
staying to work in the library.[106] In many respects, this Massachusetts
conference venue was similar to the Harnack Guest House of the KWG
in Berlin (see figure 8.3), as it had been planned between 1926 and 1929,
at the time when Schmitt worked in Warburg's and Meyerhof's
laboratories.[107]

   Although Brandegee Mansion had served as a small research institute
in addition to the laboratories at MIT, the number of resident scientists
there was comparatively small. The young generation of postwar German
neuroscientists thus perceived it as a great honour to be invited as visiting
fellows of the Neuroscience Research Program.[108] Other associates or
visiting scientists stayed in the laboratories close to MIT, or in Schmitt's

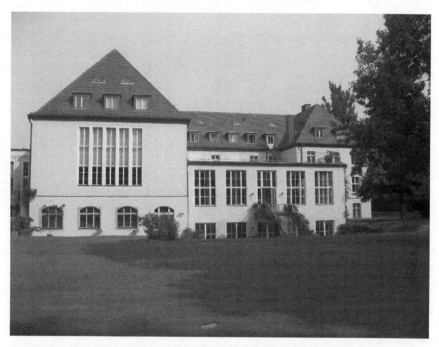

8.3 The Harnack Guest House of the Kaiser Wilhelm Society in Berlin (built in 1929). Coll. Frank W. Stahnisch. © 2008 Frank W. Stahnisch, Calgary, Alberta.

department of biology, thus forming a distributed community in the Boston area. The personal experiences of those who took part in the dedicated Neuroscience Research Program work sessions played a significant role in reconstituting the interdisciplinary neuroscience field in postwar Germany. Schmitt, who himself had German ancestors in Missouri, maintained sympathies for the country of his grandparents and continued to maintain personal relationships with Eigen and a number of his prewar mentors in the KWG.[109] Eigen himself became an enthusiastic supporter of the Neuroscience Research Program and helped advance biomedical brain science during the 1960s from his vantage point of the physical chemistry of membrane proteins.[110]

The financial involvement of the Volkswagen Foundation, facilitated through Eigen's influence, helped tremendously in establishing what could be called a transatlantic research school. It offered travel allowances to many young investigators, enabling them to participate in Neuroscience Research Program meetings as well as the legendary summer schools on the University of Colorado's Boulder campus. The Boulder meetings were composed of both *planned meetings* and *informal work sessions* which brought over two hundred international researchers, graduate students, and postdocs, together with their invited families, to a stunning venue in Colorado's Rocky Mountains. During the evening soirées everyone stayed together at the Hallett Residence Hall, attended chamber music presentations – often with Manfred Eigen at the piano in the lounge hall – and went on extended excursions to Flagstaff Mountain for recreational activities and prolonged discussions.[111] The first Boulder Meeting, convened by the Colorado biophysicist Richard Henry Bolt (1911–2002) and focusing on biophysical science, took place in 1958.[112] These Boulder meetings likewise served as a template for the Intensive Study Program in Neuroscience, which hosted meetings in 1966, 1969, 1973, and 1977. The resulting publication efforts marked a milestone for the *Big Books of Neuroscience*, which were later published by MIT Press and made widely available to international students, who experienced the Boulder summer schools as the "Neuroscience Olympic Games" of their times.[113]

Associates and Neuroscience Research Program scientists were chosen for their genuine research interest as well as the prominence of their publications. The program committee came mainly from the United States, yet individual chairs for the work sessions were often recruited from international working groups. Schmitt himself was looking for prominent scientists or "good men" (in the expression of the time), such as German-born neurobiologist Heinrich Kluever (1897–1979) from the University of Chicago. These academic scouts would then inform him about other "interesting men" in their field. The selection of new Neuroscience Research Program associates usually took place via secret poll, but when chosen most of the young researchers were eager to attend. The networking opportunities proved so promising to them that an invitation to the Neuroscience Research Program meetings was seen as a major opportunity to make acquaintances across international borders, institutions, and scientific disciplines.[114] For young German participants, involvement in the research activities of American neuroscience was invaluable, since they had witnessed that the forced migration of Jewish neurologists and psychiatrists, along with the devastations of World War II had led to a monumental demise of Central European brain research activities. As one contemporary neuropathologist stated in an oral history interview: "Nobody knew anymore how science had to be done; they were all away! – There was no other alternative than going to the US to develop oneself intellectually."[115]

The German participants came because they wanted to learn autoradiography, new techniques in electron microscopy, chemical analyses of the synapse or the axon membranes, for instance, that were much more advanced than those used in their home institutions.[116] Critical voices nevertheless declared that Schmitt had only "used the names" for promotion purposes – "superstars" like the Nobelists Manfred Eigen, the Norwegian-born neurochemist Lars Onsager (1903–1976) at Yale University, and Gerald Edelman (1929–2014) from the Rockefeller University in New York – which he incorporated in his core group of thirty-six persons in the beginning years.[117] Critics were perhaps correct with regard to the inclusion of Onsager, who was completely "alien to the field" at first. Subsequently, however, he came to fruitfully integrate other contributors' perspectives on the nervous system into his own experimental analyses of chemical synapses – advances through which he contributed to Neuroscience Research Program's scientific mandate.[118] Things could change rapidly, since the program was set up such that, every year, the associates themselves organized one session. They could then elect five new members into their circle, a process that guaranteed a frequent turnover of personnel.[119]

The *Neurosciences Research Program Bulletin* (see also figure 8.1) presented the published proceedings of the individual meetings of the Neuroscience Research Program, which included many cutting-edge themes that emerged from the meeting discussions.[120] Each volume was written by the chairperson of the respective workshop, who produced a synthetic overview of their neuroscience topic.[121] The *Neuroscience Research Program Bulletin* came at a reasonable price and was much appreciated by American students, who used the individual volumes as learning materials for exam preparations.[122] Into the 1980s, the field of neuroscience was still consolidating; hence, a relative lack of information contributed to the eagerness of many investigators trying to acquire access to the Neuroscience Research Program Bulletin. During the immediate postwar period in German-speaking countries, neuroscientifically oriented journals, such as *Psychiatria et Neurologia; Nervenheilkunde; Archiv fuer Psychiatrie und Nervenkrankheiten; Anatomischer Anzeiger; Der Nervenarzt; Der Pathologe; Journal fuer Psychiatrie; Neurologie und Neurochirurgie; Glia; Neuropsychologie; Fortschritte der Neurologie – Psychiatrie (und ihrer Grenzgebiete)*; and *Neuroforum*, did not address the topics of the innovative Neuroscience Research Program in any corresponding way. There were impressive quantitative as well as qualitative differences between the postwar American and German brain science traditions.[123] In fact, the Intensive Study Program distinguished itself by including leading-edge subjects such as "components of the nervous system," "brain correlates of functional behavioural states," "development of the nervous system," "complex psychological functions," "electron microscopical analyses of the nervous system," and "molecular genetic neuroscience," to name only a few.[124]

As in the interwar period during the 1920s and 1930s, insufficient provision of research journals, thinned library collections, and a lack of international publications prevented German biomedical research from seamlessly reconnecting with global trends.[125] This lag was assessed as lasting one to two decades until the establishment of the Neuroscience Research Program allowed Germany to reconnect with the international level of neuroscientific research after World War II.[126] Schmitt's program provided an important forum and networking opportunity with the international scientific community: "Nearly everyone who received a professorship in German neuroscience during the 1970s and 1980s had actively taken part in the legendary Boulder meetings."[127] Yet the gap in postwar neurosciences between North America and the German-speaking countries consisted of more than the differences in their infrastructures: the period of reconciliation in research endeavours was also characterized by profound cultural divergences. This was strikingly captured by the case of a returning postgraduate trainee, who later became a star researcher in German-speaking neuroscience: "'neuro-' was even a dirty word; I was called a veterinary psychiatrist on my return back home to Germany ... Not by everyone, and often jokingly, but nevertheless. It was really interesting: experiment, experiment – animals, and animals are not humans."[128] In North America, at the same time, the sources of funding for the Neuroscience Research Program ran dry, and the program came to an end in the 1980s after two decades.[129] To a large extent, it even fell "victim to its own accomplishment."[130] It had been so extraordinarily successful that five presidents of the Society for Neuroscience – after its foundation in 1971 – had been former Neuroscience Research Program associates: Edward R. Perl, 1968–70; Walle J.H. Nauta, 1972–73; Theodore H. Bullock, 1973–74; Eric R. Kandel, 1980–81 (Nobel Prize, 2000); and David H. Hubel 1988–89 (Nobel Prize, 1981).[131] The enormous impact of the Neuroscience Research Program is also highlighted by the fact that out of seventy-five former associates, a total of thirteen went on to win a Nobel Prize.

The international networks that had been established gave rise to two further landmark events in the history of neuroscience: the foundation of the International Brain Research Organization in Paris in 1960 and the 1969 inauguration of the American Society for Neuroscience. At the same time, of course, this had important repercussions on the gradual *re-establishment of interdisciplinary centres* in the German-speaking countries. From methodological and conceptual perspectives alike, the Neuroscience Research Program had created the modern outlook of the emerging field.[132] It also helped in establishing the international Society for Neuroscience, of which more than 2,500 early members had taken part in the Neuroscience Research Program during the twenty years that Schmitt chaired its regular meetings in the United States.[133]

In 1966 the *Journal of the Intensive Study Program* openly addressed the conceptual question, "What is neuroscience?" by highlighting the hybrid nature of this new field. Aiming toward a program similar to American historian of science Thomas S. Kuhn's concept of a *disciplinary matrix*, which involved researchers, scientific objects, institutes, and societies, the hybrid nature of Neuroscience Research Program's knowledge economy made it much easier for new ideas and practices to develop in this interdisciplinary melting pot.[134] These occurrences gave rise to scientific developments in a new research field that otherwise would barely have developed.[135] In this respect, it is also remarkable that many of the early neuroscientists of the 1930s and 1940s, either as visitors or as exiled academics, acted as important facilitators in this new acculturation process for young West German scientists and physicians who found their way to North America. The working groups of the following have often been mentioned, for example, in emphasizing their continuous support for the young postwar investigators: German-born neuropsychologist Werner Schneider (1900–1935?) at Columbia University, the neurophysiologist Alvin M. Liberman (1917–2000) at the National Institutes of Health, who was the descendent of German immigrants, and the psychologist Teuber, the elder, at MIT, who was an émigré from Berlin (see figure 8.4).[136]

RE-ESTABLISHING INTERNATIONAL
RESEARCH RELATIONS

In hindsight, then, a visionary conceived the Neuroscience Research Program itself, and Schmitt's major contribution to the history of

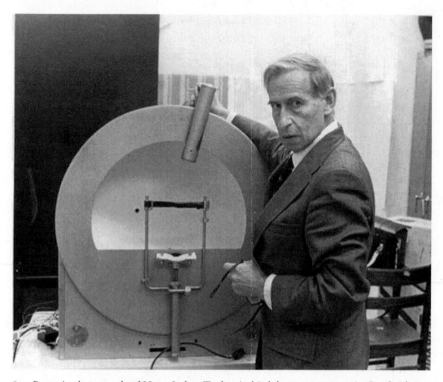

8.4 Portrait photograph of Hans-Lukas Teuber in his laboratory at MIT in Cambridge, MA (ca. 1970), with a periscopic physiological research device. © Courtesy of the MIT Museum, Cambridge, Massachusetts, USA.

neuroscience was primarily of a social and organizational nature. All too often, however, scientists and historians of science erroneously downgrade the importance of accomplishments such forging, transforming, and sustaining research fields by viewing organizational achievements as "merely social."[137] However, natural science and biomedical research constitute a form of knowledge pursuit only insofar as they are social endeavours themselves; there would be no inspiration of ideas, no publications, no prizes, if it were not for the benefit of a particular group of scientists or modern society at large. This is evident when surveying Schmitt's ongoing effect on the emerging field of neuroscience. The strength of both the Neuroscience Research Program and the legendary Boulder meetings at the University of Colorado are now fairly well known to neuroscientists and historians of neuroscience alike.[138]

Today, circumstances have changed rather profoundly. During the founding years of the 1950s and 1960s, there were major obstacles for a "normalization process" in contemporary biomedical research and in the interdisciplinary field of neuroscience. In this respect, it proved to be a major asset that Germany and Austria had not been internationally isolated again.[139] Many of the returning young scientists and scholars later developed very successful careers during the 1960s, often made possible through their membership in Frank Schmitt's Neuroscience Research Program:

> Well, everyone who was later appointed as a chair [in the neurosciences] in Germany, they had all participated at least once at the conferences [of the Intensive Study Program or the Neuroscience Research Program]. Whether it was [the neurophysiologist Otto-Joachim] Gruesser [1932–1995], [the neuropathologist Hans Gerhard] Creutzfeld or the [biologist] Dietrich Schneider [1919–2008], they had all been there. Everyone of distinction, also my student Wolf Singer [b. 1943], who was at that time just a postdoc and a very young man, or the retina group [Heinz Waessle (b. 1943) and Leo Peichl (b. 1950)] from Frankfurt.[140]

Yet, apart from the glowing view about the normalization process of the reanimation of transatlantic biomedical relations that I present here, many open questions remain, which contemporary historians of medicine and science will need to address in the future. Why, for instance, was the number of returning forced migrants, even for summer academies and lecture series, so small during the 1940s and 1950s?[141] Why was this group not more actively approached by senior biomedical researchers and officials recruiting them to act as piloting mentors for the new transatlantic relationships? Why was there no "Max Planck of the Brain Research Field," who would have publicly apologized[142] for the expulsion of Jewish neuroscientists immediately after the war? Why was the potential of returning neuroscientists not better used for the reconstruction of the research landscape in the German-speaking countries?[143] Notwithstanding the questions as to how many researchers and scholars there were, who were those who did not move on to positions at MPIs and remained either in subaltern positions at university institutes and in larger institutions of the Helmholtz Association of German Research Centres or in the pharmaceutical industry, with their potential perhaps never fully utilized in the "normalization processes" after 1949?[144]

Even though today's historians of medicine rarely refer to *The Open Society and Its Enemies* (1945), the positivistically inspired book by the

Austro-British philosopher Karl Popper (1902–1994), in concluding I consider it relevant to direct our attention here to some of the major theses in his book:

> We can interpret the history of power politics from the point of view of our fight for the open society, for a rule of reason, for justice, freedom, equality, and for the control of international crime. Although history has no ends, we can impose these ends of ours upon it ... History itself – I mean the history of power politics, of course, not the non-existent story of the development of mankind – has no end nor meaning, but we can decide to give it both. We can make it our fight for the open society and against its antagonists.[145]

The Open Society and Its Enemies was also written during Popper's own exile in New Zealand as a lecturer at Canterbury University College, Christchurch, from 1937 to 1945. It is valuable to remind ourselves that the lessons profiled in the book were learned gradually, often not explicitly but sub-cutaneously, during individual encounters, experiences, and personal relations.

Similarly, the insights emanating from the previous chapters were gradually learned in the early interdisciplinary neuroscience community, even though often rather subconsciously during individual encounters, experiences, and personal relationships and friendships. This learning process quite often took place the hard way and could be termed a healing process from the "traumatic normalities"[146] that the history of the interdisciplinary field of the neurosciences in the German-speaking countries between the 1880s and early 1960s had left in its wake. Looking at the firsthand experiences of postwar German neuroscientists helps shed light on the gradual reanimation of transatlantic exchanges between the Federal Republic of Germany and the United States after World War II, as these were intended to stabilize the research cultures in the new "Free World."[147] My narrative about the emergence of the interdisciplinary field of neuromorphology in the German-speaking countries can serve as an instructive example to reappraise the status, organization, and – last but not least – the social situatedness of neuroscience as one of the most exciting and complex fields of modern biomedicine today.

9

Conclusion: The Development of Interdisciplinary Work in the Neurosciences

Subject Constraints, Social Necessities, and the Development of Research Networks

In Germany, the view that function is an attribute of form seems to have dominated neuroanatomy since Oscar and Cécile Vogt.

Former MPI director[1]

The makeup of the emerging interdisciplinary field of neuroscience in the German-speaking countries between the 1880s and the 1960s strongly reflected the changing influences and protracted legacies of the historical context of the three political and cultural periods directly preceding the end of World War II: the late Wilhelminian Empire, 1880s–1918 (with its end during World War I), the social experiment of the Weimar Republic, 1919–33, and eventually the National Socialist period, 1933–45 (including the war). As the narrative of the creation of this new research field is embedded in a more comprehensive and cultural context, I have extended the exceptional situation of the years between 1933 and 1945 by including earlier historical scholarship on psychiatry and neurology in Germany and Austria.[2] With the advent of the "age of nervousness" in Germany from the Wilhelminian Empire to the rise and demise of National Socialism, the prevailing practical and social demands made it necessary to deal with what leading neurologists and psychiatrists had perceived as a rise in the number and impact of nervous diseases instigated by urbanization and mechanization in the highly competitive modern German society of the time.[3] These problems brought an increasing number of bourgeois, male, and high-performing individuals into the clinics, hospitals, and asylums of the neurologists and psychiatrists from the first decades of the last century. When parallel discourses about "nervous exhaustion" and "nerve degeneration" rose to the fore in response to the medical situation after World War I and during the Weimar Republic, the allure of holistic concepts in medicine and psychiatry became increasingly attractive, and the preoccupation with neurodegeneration research was transformed. Attention was redirected from clinical problems of the rehabilitation of casualties and war-traumatized veterans toward inquiries into the underlying nutritional processes and constitutional factors of individuals in their specific social milieux.[4]

Basic researchers and physicians became engaged in these social discourses, not only *in the public sphere* but also in their day-to-day clinical and laboratory routines, when political and economic concerns pushed early neuroscientists to find answers for the problems of war injuries, nervous exhaustion, and malnourishment in the early years of Weimar German society. Neurologists, psychiatrists, and brain researchers in their laboratories felt quite motivated by the possibilities made available by recent methodological and technical advances. They were approached by science administrators to analyze particular research questions, while the military, the recently created Deutsche Forschungsgemeinschaft, and international funding agencies such as the American Rockefeller Foundation offered new and sustained support for experimental neuroscientific investigations. Researchers in traditional clinical fields (neurology, psychiatry, internal medicine, and clinical psychology), and also brain anatomists, neuropathologists, neuroserologists, and neuroradiologists, felt that they were noticeably gaining from such a contribution to the postwar values of the Weimar Republic. In this context, neuropsychiatry and laboratory brain science became part of an entire system for the restitution and regeneration of the society after the Great War. This impetus resonated well with researchers' programs to analyze the neuromorphological bases of respective diseases, a project in which many (since the times of von Recklinghausen, Edinger, and Weigert, and their peers) had been engaged under the epistemological aegis of the Wilhelminian Empire, when issues of nerve lesions, oncology, and war injuries loomed large for Imperial Germans as well as Austro-Hungarians.[5] The resulting knowledge assets and medical practices then found a place in the new Weimar preoccupation with nervous regeneration and healing, as neurological and psychiatric findings were integrated into the development of a functional public health and injury pension system – following the paradigm of restoration of German postwar society at large.[6] In all these areas, factors from social and racial hygiene combined with eugenics ideals began to play major roles. These became even more prominent toward the end of the Weimar Republic. Such trends were reflected in the biographies of many of the early neuroscientists in the neuromorphology field when they offered their services to the research programs of the Deutsche Forschungsgemeinschaft in support of activities that were to strengthen the eugenics enterprise and contribute to the marginalization of the nervously "degenerated" within the new Nazi medical philosophy.[7]

Yet, at the beginning of the 1920s, this context also offered an increasing opportunity for medical specializations such as neurology and psychiatry to distinguish themselves as fields separate from their original discipline, internal medicine. Although the driving forces behind these divisions were manifold, they were sometimes balanced by new interdisciplinary endeavours that tackled social problems in more comprehensive, holistic ways. Several important factors played a role here: among them were new ways of knowledge production in specialized neuroscience laboratories, changed clinical and diagnostic practices, and sociopolitical factors in particular.[8] This specialization process was represented in the establishment of dedicated journals (see chapters 1 and 8), the creation of separate academic societies from the 1900s, new university chairs, and by the development of specialized instruments, therapeutic practices, and certainly pivotal textbooks in the field.[9] Despite such observable differences in the diagnostic, treatment, and research practices of the new brain research communities, clinical approaches in general remained a traditional combination of neurological and psychiatric techniques. Apart from these disciplines' continuing separation from internal medicine, however, it took a relatively long time in the German-speaking community of Nervenheilkunde for the two areas of psychiatry and neurology to become completely separated. In fact, the separation was incomplete even after the Gesellschaft Deutscher Nervenaerzte (founded in 1907) was politically dissolved in 1934 and forced to join the Deutscher Verein fuer Psychiatrie,[10] which had been independently founded in 1903, as the Deutsche Gesellschaft der Neurologen und Psychiater (which lasted formally until 1954).[11] Dictated by the new NS government, this merger was designed to bring both communities under better control and hence more in line with Nazi medical philosophies, in which the psychiatrically and neurologically ill were marginalized as "nervous degenerates." The same move further anticipated the drastic eugenics and euthanasia measures that Karl Binding and Alfred Hoche had already outlined and presented in their manifesto, Allowing the Destruction of Life Unworthy of Life:

Its Measure and Form (*Die Freigabe der Vernichtung lebensunwerten Lebens. Ihr Mass und ihre Form*), as early as 1920.[12]

The separation of academic neurology and psychiatry from their original discipline, internal medicine, along with the growth of the encompassing field of *Nervenheilkunde* as an interdisciplinary clinical and research field, offered a considerable niche in the German-speaking health care system. It attracted particularly Jewish and other medical students from non-traditional backgrounds, often with social democratic and socialist political leanings, into these areas. During the 1920s and 1930s, when the scientific hierarchies and administrations of many medical faculties in the German-speaking countries were still dominated by anti-Semitic sentiments, innovations in neurology, psychiatry, and the early interdisciplinary field of neuroscience were due largely to the *reorganization of research at the medical fringes*. However, such fringes proved to be a fertile ground for many scientific advances – in topological diagnostics, clinical elecrophysiology, and neurosurgery, for example[13] – which allowed this *revolutionary* work to be transformed into *normal* applications.[14] As I have shown by concentrating on some very influential researchers–and their respective institutions – Heinrich Obersteiner in Vienna, Paul Edinger in Frankfurt, Oskar and Cécile Vogt in Berlin, Paul Flechsig in Leipzig, and Emil Kraepelin in Munich – the racialized academic situation after the turn of the century proved to be a roadblock to the engagement of Jewish neuroscientists. Bypassing these obstacles, they actively tried to find places in niche research fields such as paediatrics, dermatology, psychiatry, neurology, or neuropathology in German-speaking medical faculties.[15]

The unique situation of working at the fringes of established medical fields can hardly be overemphasized and it did not emanate from the early neuroscientists alone. Rather, it ensued from the sheer necessity of social assimilation and the ascent of Jewish scientific, artistic, and economic groups in the permeable society of the Wilhelminian Empire. The establishment of formal anti-discrimination laws against all religions by individual federated states of the Empire made school and university systems more accessible for Catholics and Protestants alike,[16] since religious discrimination prevailed there as well. Subsequently the children of the ascending mercantile and administrative classes of society entered the universities in German-speaking countries in higher numbers than ever before.[17] Yet Jewish students and lecturers entering the institutions of higher learning in the Wilhelminian period continued to experience strong anti-Semitic and often anti-democratic sentiments among the established professoriate.[18] This made it rather impossible for Jewish academics to assume roles as the "mandarin types" of German professors (see also my Introduction), as most lacked the academic mentorship, particularly in traditional medical and scientific disciplines. Not to mention that long-term positions in the emerging fields of neurology, psychiatry, and experimental biology were rather scarce at the time.[19] For many of this cohort of aspiring students with interests in research approaches of neuromorphology, this meant that they had to give up their aspirations and dreams and become general practitioners (*Haus-* and *Landaerzte*) or work in non-research fields, or medical advertisement, for example. The limitation of academic positions at medical faculties in general, and research-directed fields in particular, made it imperative to excel in order to retain their chances of attracting patients, funding support, and internal political patronage in the academy.[20]

An additional option for some highly committed individuals such as Gregor Mendel, Max Lewandowsky, and Max Borchert was to set up their own private laboratories and clinics *outside the established university system*, often with external funding support from well-to-do philanthropists.[21] This historical background, then, helps us to understand not only why most of the innovative centres in German-speaking interdisciplinary neuroscience were developed in the penumbra of established communities and only later became affiliated with medical and science faculties that sought to incorporate their potential and piggyback on their academic renown. As an aside, it also explains why the knowledge and collective academic memory *vis-à-vis* such comprehensive neurological institutes (of Obersteiner, Edinger, the Vogts, and Brodmann) are scarcely present today (see the presentation in the Introduction).

Rather, clinical departments of neurology and psychiatry, along with research institutes of anatomy and pathology, had been dominated by academic mandarin-type professors until the early 1900s, which often meant that underlying anti-Semitic sentiments had also ruled in the Imperial university research institutions. In the whole state of Bavaria, for instance, only one Jewish anatomist, Jakob Herz (1816–1871), and one Jewish physiologist, Isidor Rosenthal (1836–1915), received full professorships in research institutes within the three existing medical faculties during the nineteenth century.[22] The tide began gradually to turn, however, as shown in above discussion regarding developments in the medical faculties of Frankfurt am Main (see the Introduction), Strasburg, Leipzig (chapter 2), and Berlin (chapter 3). Becoming more prominent by the 1890s, the emerging interdisciplinary community in early neuromorphology began to accommodate young researchers from outside, although granting them merely a "temporary right of academic residence" for two or three pre- or postdoc years, before they had to leave the institutes for anatomy and pathology again and continue faculty assistantships in the clinical departments of psychiatry and neurology, and *vice versa*. Even when academics were endowed with large publication lists, multiple academic accolades, and top marks, many of the early neuroscientists still had to leave their contract positions again and were henceforth lost to the whole scientific endeavour, despite the material and personal resources that had been invested in their participation in the field.

THE SOCIOPOLITICAL DIMENSION OF "BIG SCIENCE" AND A NEW SELF-DESCRIPTION OF BRAIN RESEARCHERS, 1920S TO 1930S

The medical field hospitals, pathology units, and specialized mental and neurological rehabilitation units for war veterans instigated after the Great War gave rise to an increasing incorporation of young neurologists and brain psychiatrists in the research-minded culture of neuromorphology in the German-speaking countries. Through historical contingencies, these early neuroscientists worked primarily in institutions of modern formats and largely outside the widely acclaimed research universities. Considering the discussion above, it is then not surprising that the two largest German research centres in Berlin and Munich were each located miles away from their respective medical schools (e.g. figure 4.3). They had received their start-up funding exclusively from outside ministerial sources, which was notoriously symbolized by the last-minute withdrawal of funding from the Prussian Ministry of Science, Arts, and Culture for the brain research institute in Berlin-Buch. The ensuing integration of the extra-university laboratories into the institute system of the KWG, after its creation in 1911, often took place against a background of outright animosity on the part of the research groups in the Deutsche Forschungsanstalt for Psychiatry – fearing research competition and loss of its status as the most prominent and singular research institute in the early brain sciences field in Germany – and the KWI for Brain Research, toward the established clinical departments in the university system. Only with the end of World War I did Jewish and other fringe neuroscientists (such as Goldscheider, Goldstein, Von Weizsaecker, and others) acquire chairs in the university system in any numbers and gradually begin to transform the established research institutes from within and often from the bottom up.

In addition to the stimulation of their academic positions, most German-speaking neuroscientists received their intellectual inspiration from a variety of other sources. Researchers working in the tradition of Carl Weigert often developed their staining techniques in collaboration with industry chemists from Hoechst and Chemische Fabrik Griesheim and other companies[23] – and thus not primarily with their scientific peers in the university (see the case of Bielschowsky and the paths to developing his own silver stain in chapter 3).[24] Psychiatrically oriented neuroscientists often set up their own experimental units, which served general hospitals and other institutions (as in the case of the established experimental psychology programs of Adhémar Gelb in Frankfurt and Berlin; see chapter 6). Furthermore, many of the non-mandarin type of younger brain scientists displayed a high degree of sophistication in the arts and humanities, which served them well for their theoretical projects in neurology and psychiatry (as for example in Kurt Goldstein's holistic program or Viktor von Weizsaecker's medical anthropology; chapter 4).[25]

For these scholars, in particular, interdisciplinarity in early neuroscience involved not only the use of extra-mural medical or biological approaches, but also the inclusion of new philosophical concepts: for instance, Kantian functionalism, further developed and expounded by philosopher Ernst Cassirer in his *Philosophie der Symbolischen Formen* (*The Philosophy of Symbolic Forms*) in 1923 and received in the medical writings of his cousin, the neurologist Kurt Goldstein; social theory (the form of social neurology practised by Walther Riese in Frankfurt or Karl Stern in Berlin); and even linguistic approaches, as Von Weizsaecker integrated them into the psychiatric treatment of patients with speech disorders:

> Thus, degeneration and regeneration are both a building principle and a destructive drive. The striving for health and for disease resembles a will for life and death already in the first processes of a biological cell, of the organ systems, and the physiological functions. The statement, that the aim of a medical *action* would be to restore the ability to work and to enjoy life in each patient, cannot be seen as a definition of the therapeutic process, but it is essentially a description of a *social state* and its ideal interpretation.[26]

These assumptions further came to bear on a new self-definition on the part of many of the early neuroscientists in their urge to contribute to Weimar society. It was often exemplified by an all-embracing approach of the "intellectual researcher" (in the *Bildungsbuerger* tradition) as a member of the new democratic Weimar society. Neurologists and psychiatrists such as Goldstein, Stern, or Karl Landauer openly and expressively emphasized the social role of medicine, much to the chagrin of their adversaries in the nationalist political camp and the rising eugenics-minded Nazi physicians.[27] It should not go unnoticed here that for similar reasons, yet from a completely antagonistic political standpoint, progressivist Nazi psychiatrists and neurologists such as Max De Crinis and Ernst Ruedin also argued for a stronger involvement of neuroscience in the "new medical ethics" and the social programs of public health – *Volksmedizin*.[28] They prepared the way for the subsequent Nazi programs of forced sterilization, child euthanasia, and *Aktion T4*, which killed tens of thousands of asylum inmates and hospital patients, whose bodies were intentionally used in the "interdisciplinary" research programs of the Nazi times.[29] The major figures of these murderous Nazi programs were also brain researchers who had been trained during the preceding liberal periods of the Wilhelminian Empire and the Weimar Republic. They now came to personally identify with the materialistic, *voelkisch*, and exclusivist (albeit murderous) ideals of Nazi medicine and health care, which they also integrated into their neuroscientific research programs.[30]

INTERDISCIPLINARY VISIONS OF NAZI BRAIN
RESEARCHERS, 1930S TO 1940S

Nazi medical philosophy during the 1930s and 1940s concentrated exclusively on improving the health of what was seen as the "Aryan German people," and excluded Jews along with Sinti and Roma from the aegis of the public health system.[31] Early progressivist neuroscientists and psychiatrists, such as Ruedin at the Deutsche Forschungsanstalt for Psychiatry and De Crinis in the Berlin clinical department of psychiatry at the Charité, came to outright identify with the Nazi reconstruction of the biomedical research enterprise toward the end of the Weimar Republic. For them, there was no conceptual break with former "progressivist" social ideals and scientific aims at the beginning of the National Socialist period, but rather a continuum under changed political contexts emerging after 1933; that is, the continuing provision of medical care exclusively for Aryan Germans, which marginalized the disabled and mentally ill and gradually shifted its research focus toward military medicine, oncology, and nutrition.[32] As German social historian Hans-Walter Schmuhl has shown, particularly during World War II, when public attention was diverted to the occurrences in the war theatres, Nazi physicians and researchers "used the patient material," from hundreds of murdered hospital inmates from the euthanasia programs targeting the mentally and neurologically ill for neuropathological and neurophysiological purposes. This practice included such prominent science institutes as the KWI for Brain Research and the Deutsche Forschungsanstalt for Psychiatry, as well as renowned university anatomy, pathology, and clinical neurology departments in Berlin, Wuerzburg, Leipzig, and others.[33]

Such activities likewise became a "new form of interdisciplinarity" in neuroscientific research and were created through tight personal and institutional networks, which had already been formed in the brain research, neurology, and psychiatry communities of the Weimar Republic (see chapters 3 to 5). Researchers in the KWG and university departments (many of whom had close links to the KWIs through research cooperation or prolonged visits as guest scientists) actively sought to link their scientific work to the Nazi euthanasia program in various ways. This structure made it possible for the system to function without the necessary involvement of centralized leadership bodies (though the Reichsforschungsrat, Deutsche Forschungsgemeinschaft committees, and the KWG board of regents exerted considerable organizational influence within the German scientific and medical communities too).[34] These mutually beneficial relationships supported the functioning of the "supply system," so that the provision of brains, spinal cords, nerve tissue preparations, and patients for coercive experimental purposes did not stop. Instead, it continued in most efficient ways so that the respective neuroscientists did not even need to ask twice to be provided with "study material," which they desired for the continuation of their programs at the brain science centres.[35]

The promptness with which the medical system in the early neuroscience field opened itself up to the new racist and eugenic philosophies, and the reception of stern Nazi physicians and researchers in influential leadership roles, was fostered by an incipient generational change. A number of the old-school Wilhelminian professors such as Walther Spielmeyer in Munich and Paul Flechsig in Leipzig had died, and anti-Nazi academic leaders (such as Oskar Vogt and Max Bielschowsky) were ousted from their headships of institutes and departments toward the end of the 1930s. This change in managerial structures of relevant KWG institutes and university research departments also led to a conceptual transformation of the ongoing programs and their institutional reorganization.[36] In Berlin, Munich, Strasburg, Vienna, and other places, very tight networks of brain anatomists and pathologists developed in conjunction with local clinical units, as well as military research structures. Two such important cases, which illustrate the readaptation of the new form of interdisciplinarity under Nazi pretexts, are the cities of Strasburg and Munich – with their inclusion of the nearby concentration camps – Natzweiler-Struthof in Alsace and Dachau near Munich – as "feeder institutions" for human experimentation activities at departments of physiology, anatomy, and pathology.[37] This was by no means always a directed, top-down process prompted by the Nazi government and military command structures themselves.[38] Rather, such cases proved to be interdisciplinary endeavours to which neuroscientists and psychiatrists themselves actively contributed, emphasizing the "unimaginable research opportunities, the necessity to use the patient material for research purposes since the victims were to die anyway,"[39] and the particular "contribution to racial anthropology and evolutionary biology which could be gained from researching under-developed populations of non-Aryan hereditary stock."[40]

Besides the benefits for individual research programs that many anatomists and pathologists, such as August Hirt in Strasburg, Ludwig Aschoff in Freiburg, or Julius Hallervorden in Berlin, saw in getting access to Nazi oppression systems (such as torture prisons of the secret police, orphan homes, closed mental asylums, and more),[41] for leading psychiatrists (such as Hoche, Ruedin, De Crinis, and Schneider) and neurologists (such as Schaltenbrand and Spatz), a much larger medico-philosophical project was underway.[42] It actively placed post-1933 basic and clinical brain research at the very centre of the emerging field of eugenics and racial discrimination.[43] This transformation of the system included drastic negative eugenics measures (compulsory genetic counselling, marital segregation laws, and surgical and radiological forced sterilizations), which eventually led to outright murder of neurological and psychiatric patients (many of whom, such as the "socially deprived," "alcoholics," and post-traumatic "epileptics," were not even diagnosed with hereditary disease at all).[44]

In the various chapters of this book, I have looked at additional influences of cultural aspects on scientific practice as they gave rise to new interdisciplinary advances in brain research after the early 1880s. When this early history of the emerging neuroscience field is further placed in the context of Nazi medicine, it becomes clearer why the mentally ill and neurologically handicapped in particular were excluded from the health care system in Nazi Germany and why, subsequently, neurologists and psychiatrists were antagonized by their peers also because of the high percentage of Jewish doctors in this area.

In fact, the emerging interdisciplinary field of neuroscience, with its contributions from clinical neurology, brain psychiatry, neuropathology, neuroanatomy, experimental psychology, and allied disciplines, must be regarded as an important aspect of the history of medicine and health care in the National Socialist period. It gives us insights into the shaping of the modern biomedical enterprise along with the political coordinates of the public health service. In chapter 6, I have drawn attention to certain problems inherent in the historiography and scholarship of this period. When Nazi medicine is not viewed in terms of its broad effects and implications for modern biomedical research, but is simply denigrated as "ideological," "perverted," or "murderous," then an important perspective on the intrinsic mechanisms of modern medical science endeavors is missed.[45] By applying the distorting mirror of Nazi medical science to the historical developments in the early neuroscience field in the 1930s and 1940s, I have attempted to develop a much broader picture of the scientific foundations, cultural encodings, and social and economic contexts of modern biomedicine. Even the atrocious war crimes (such as military-related research in synapse- and autoregulation-pharmacology, pressure- and temperature-related experiments in aviation physiology, and nerve gas development for chemical warfare) or human experimentation in mental asylums, penitentiaries, and concentration camps (such as malnutrition, stress, and sibling research) need to be contextualized within the deadly framework of Nazi medical philosophy, which built largely on internationally developed and applied eugenic beliefs.[46] Far from being passive pawns in the new political system of the National Socialist period, physicians, psychologists, and neuroscientists became actively involved in bringing the racial hygiene program to its full life. They assumed roles as intellectual and administrative planners, while becoming scientific beneficiaries of research grants, program support, and social awards in the transformed German and Austrian societies after 1933 and 1938 respectively.

Conversely, some historiographical groundwork during the past two decades has grown increasingly critical in regard to postwar legends about Nazi medicine between 1933 and 1945. This literature has highlighted the involvement of small elite groups as protagonists – in the public health system, oncological and nutritional research, military medicine, and human experimentation in psychiatric asylums and concentration camps, among others. It has further mapped the interplay of racial hygiene, *voelkisch* ideology, and social economic considerations within the Nazi eugenics movement. The social and biological field of eugenics, which had risen to central awareness of physicians, biologists, and sociologists

since the 1900s, played an important contextual role for the development
of early interdisciplinary endeavours in the neurosciences because many
diseases of the brain were inherited or suspected to result from hereditary
dispositions.[47] In this context, it is also interesting to notice from the
perspective of collective biography that a number of physicians in the
eugenics movement during the Weimar Republic had strong previous
inclinations toward social medicine and psychiatry. For them, neurology
and psychiatry developed to become "in the true sense of the word a
healing medical discipline," for which the actual therapeutic repertoire
proved to be fairly limited at the time.[48] In the case of the National
Socialist period, emerging interdisciplinary trends in the neuroscience
field did not simply cease to exist with the year of 1933. On the contrary,
since right-wing physician groups, racial hygiene researchers, the military,
and the pharmaceutical industry acted as important stakeholders in further
developing this multidisciplinary but increasingly murderous field, by
making chemicals available for testing or profiting from basic research
carried out in coercive laboratory and clinical contexts.[49] The healing of
the sick and the extinction of the weak now coincided with barbarous
approaches pursued by medical doctors and other health care professionals, who helped transform neurological and psychiatric areas in order to
contribute to the Nazis' "War against the Weak."[50] The role of early
neuroscientists among the medical corps and the public health service
during the Third Reich makes it very clear that developments between
1933 and 1945 cannot be regarded merely as historical contingencies,
but were a direct expression of a modern knowledge pursuit that – according to Alexander Mitscherlich and Fred Mielke (1921–2015), witnesses
of the Nuremberg Doctor's Trials – had lost its human face: "*Medizin
ohne Menschlichkeit*" ("Medicine without Humanity")![51]

CONTINUITIES AND BREAKS IN THE EMERGING FIELD
OF GERMAN-SPEAKING NEUROMORPHOLOGY

Despite the different cultural contexts of the three succeeding sociopolitical
systems in the period from the late nineteenth century to the first half of
the twentieth century, similar forms of interdisciplinarity remained intact
across these political changes. For example, alliances between the scientific,
the economic, and the military spheres affected the growth of the early
neuroscientific community from the late Wilhelminian era onward. The
strength of these relationships certainly varied during this period, as exemplified by the fluctuation in the influence of the military system, which was

reduced after the end of World War I yet regained its impact again toward the end of the Weimar Republic and during World War II. Major exchanges, personal acquaintances, and collaborations on scientific programs tended to continue further, leading to a highly functional early neuroscientific work in the research communities in the German-speaking countries at the time. I have suggested in the Introduction and chapter 1 that, from evidence in the institutional files of prominent research universities, the origins and the success of the early interdisciplinary field of neuroscience were based on a *free-floating culture of ideas, practical experiences, and organizational skills*.[52] Intellectual migration rates were high from the beginning of the century, when a significant percentage of the novices and young researchers had studied at many universities, and more than half of the middle-rank assistants had held several positions before entering other university services in psychiatry, anatomy, and pathology to contribute to the interdisciplinary neuroscientific research field. Apart from the organizational structure of contemporary research institutes and neurological and psychiatric clinical departments, even general career developments in neuromorphology were not specifically mapped out. The future scientific elite was severely exposed to job restrictions and often sought to leave the hierarchical institutional structures at their earliest opportunity. The resulting precarious social organization of the brain research community in the German-speaking countries not only became the context for but also developed into an important precondition of the growth of interdisciplinary work projects, programs, and units contributing to the emergence of the new research field.

In the course of this historiographical account of the development of interdisciplinary structures in research, teaching, and exchange relationships as these were influenced by different spheres of social life from the Wilhelminian Empire to the National Socialist period and beyond, I have given considerable attention to the early development of brain research centres after the creation of Obersteiner's first institute for neuroanatomical and neurophysiological investigations in Vienna in 1882.[53] In seeking to ascertain what prompted the emergence of interdisciplinary neuroscience programs and centres, I found that, in German-speaking neuromorphology in the first half of the twentieth century, changing research practices often arose from changes in the structures of pre-existing traditions of academic research. While breaking with organizational forms of the nineteenth century, prominent scientists and physicians such as Obersteiner in Vienna, Edinger in Frankfurt, Flechsig in Leipzig, Kraepelin in Munich, or the Vogts in Berlin helped to foster new trends by developing group-oriented activities outside pre-existing medical and science faculties. Eventually such activities also arose within the university system itself, while the groups and institutes involved subsequently changed the overall landscape in this biomedical field in an irreversible way. The new organizational forms of the neurosciences now became represented in formerly unseen units such as "neurobiological laboratories," "brain research divisions," and "neurological institutes," as well as through the physical juxtaposition of specific groups on similar levels and floors at more established university research departments (see figure 2.2).[54] Particularly in chapters 2 and 3 I have demonstrated how innovative impulses for this new research field came from professional and economic sources, as well as from network structures and international funding support outside the university system. Later research centres developed primarily from preceding private laboratories that were often augmented by a potpourri of added buildings and structures such as technical workshops, chemical laboratories, and animal facilities.[55]

Early brain researchers' work places were frequently the living rooms of their private homes (as in the case of Edinger and the Vogts) (see figure 3.4), or were developed from the clubs and collections of learned bourgeois societies (such as the Senckenberg Society in Frankfurt) with no direct academic affiliations (see figure 3.1). Even in the few cases where the established university system did play a role in these developments, as in the examples of Obersteiner at the University of Vienna (see figure 1.1), Flechsig at the University of Leipzig (see figure 2.3), or Foerster at the University of Breslau (see figure 1.3), the first working places and laboratories had also been established outside preconceived departmental structures. The need for these arrangements is strikingly represented by the grudging provisions for the innovative beginnings of contemporary neuroscientific research: the marginal space that was "graciously" offered under the anatomical dissection tables of the Vienna pathology department; the chair of brain pathology that became established "within" the clinical psychiatry department in Leipzig, and the neurological laboratory "stowed" into the basement of Breslau University's Faculty of Dentistry. In focusing on the demanding social problems reflected in the interdisciplinary attempts of the neuromorphological sciences between 1910 and 1945, my analysis shows how important a new form of interdisciplinary and collaborative work became, in order to make these research endeavours in the neurosciences possible against great odds. It has thus made possible a better understanding of the scientific, organizational, and cultural innovations as these came to influence the burgeoning brain research field at large.[56]

MIGRATING MINDS AND METHODS AFFECTING
THE INTERNATIONAL (RE-)FORMATION
OF MODERN NEUROSCIENCE

The argument I have put forward in regard to the developments and changes in the landscape of the early field of neuromorphology in the German-speaking countries could not have been adequately understood without taking the embedded networks among brain researchers, physicians in their private practices, and wealthy philanthropists into account. From these networks developed important extra-university research settings that transformed into fruitful and supportive relationships with philanthropists and funding bodies, as well as international research and training relationships, thereby preparing the ground for a truly transatlantic research environment.[57] This perspective necessitated a new look at the situation of émigré neuroscientists before they were forced out of the German-speaking countries during the National Socialist period. Yet beyond the level of the individual and collective biographies of individual émigré neuroscientists and their arrival and acculturation process in the American neuroscientific communities, it appeared necessary here to place these developments in a larger context of interdisciplinary exchanges through which new forms of scientific practice have emerged. The resulting perspective has helped to better understand the underlying issues of knowledge-transfer in brain research, along with the complex process of receiving émigré neuroscientists and psychiatrists in their new home countries.

In the case examples presented (particularly in chapters 7 and 8), I have concentrated especially on postwar neuroanatomy, neurology, and public mental health, to illustrate the specific tensions among three different kinds of medicine: laboratory research, clinical medicine, and social health care. These relationships varied from arm's-length distance to mutual interdependence, and – more rarely – to solid collaboration with one another (quite visibly in the cases of Weil in rural prairie Canada and Kallmann in the metropolitan setting of New York City). Then, of course, there were variations due to different local, regional, and national contexts. Whether these affected the status of medical services, the relationship between health professionals and the state, or the evolution of medical specialties, these differing contexts nevertheless influenced the evolution of the emerging biomedical complexes to which the émigré neuroscientists actively contributed.[58]

It should by now have become clear that the invention of the mere word "neuroscience" and its subsequent uses must be viewed as a testimony to above-mentioned differences (see also the Introduction). The prominence acquired by the term since the 1960s coincided with the appearance of a new system of medical innovation in relation to biology and health policy.[59] Cultural differences, divergences in the use of research methods, and their theoretical reframing, along with the political constraints of international collaboration, have been described in the latter chapters. They were important in fostering – but also hindering – the process of "normalization of international relations" (*Normalisierung der internationalen Beziehungen*)[60] during the later political reconstruction of the Federal Republic of Germany and the formation of new global political systems between 1945 and 1965.[61] The moral and political economy of the postwar period stimulated the rapid internationalization of biological research. Acknowledging this complex history may be helpful for understanding the current wave of "biomedicalization"[62] as less radical and unexpected than social analysts have assumed. And it can also help us appreciate West- and East German relations with respect to biomedical interchanges and the development of new academic resource systems in different political landscapes.[63]

As I described in the Introduction, the shared views and thoughts of currently active neuroscientists were of considerable interest to me in my research: When speaking, on the one hand, to my colleagues in Germany, the idea of "neuroscience centres" was often associated with recent creations of larger scale institutes in the 1990s, while giving the impression that the creation of such centres must have been an invention by American neuroscientists, later introduced back to the German biomedical system (see also the Introduction of this book). On the other hand, when I asked North American neuroscientists about the substantial differences between their institutions and the older German counterparts – such as the Edinger Institute in Frankfurt am Main, the Deutsche Forschungsanstalt for Psychiatry in Munich, or the KWI Brain Research Institute in Berlin – they often seemed uninformed about the local contexts of the universities, urban spaces, or research institutions in which the neuroscientific contributions of such luminaries as Edinger, Flechsig, or the Vogts had taken place, even though they were of course quite familiar with their published works. Nevertheless, such earlier perspectives remain rather neglected in the scholarship of today.

I have described here how surgeons, pathologists, internists, serologists, psychologists, and philosophers worked collaboratively on early topics of the brain sciences from the mid-nineteenth century to the mid-twentieth. It should by now be clearer why indeed contemporary philosophers discussed with experimental neuroanatomists, why neurologists collaborated with Gestalt psychologists, or how neuropathologists supported neurosurgeons in their endeavours. These considerations established the common ground for my narrative, which has spanned from the first brain research institute in Vienna 137 years ago to the modern neuroscience centres in North America, as started by Cushing in Boston, Schmitt in St Louis and Cambridge, Massachusetts, or Penfield in Montreal.[64] All these American and Canadian founders had visited and trained in the early neuroscience research centres of the German-speaking countries between the 1910s and 1930s. At the same time, their approaches and models served in many ways as important templates for later influential American brain researchers, whose programs strongly reshaped the manner in which research investigations in the biomedical sciences took place in the twentieth century. It is in this sense that the bold claims – such as the curability of many psychiatric and neurological conditions, a fuller understanding of the complexity of brain processes, and complete elucidation of human cognitive functioning – made in Schmitt's autobiographical account, *The Never-Ceasing Search*, had their repercussions in the interdisciplinary field of the brain sciences – not only in the later coining of the term "neuroscience" but also in the creation of the societal basis for this endeavour through the Neuroscience Research Program, which so considerably shaped today's landscape.

As for individual programs in the brain sciences, however, scientific practices and theories had already arisen through new forms of interdisciplinary settings in the German-speaking countries between 1882 and 1962. Breaking with the discipline-bound and discipline-dominated set-up of brain research in the nineteenth century, which had been largely confined to research in specialized institutes for physiology, anatomy, neurological clinics or psychiatric clinics, new centres for interdisciplinary brain research developed in the penumbra of universities and medical schools.

I have tried here to give some explanations for the fundamental social, philosophical, and technological changes that helped foster new trends toward group-oriented neuroscience activities *avant la lettre*, which later gave rise to the innovative changes that the biomedical field underwent from the nineteenth to the twentieth century.[65] Although postwar American research centres such as Frank Schmitt's Neuroscience Research Program at MIT brought the modern field to prominence in the specific contexts of Central Europe. In so doing, I have proposed some historical answers as to the place, time, and culture in which these trend-setting changes in early neuroscience had emerged. The evolving relationships between medical

and research disciplines – such as anatomy, neurology, psychiatry, physiology, serology, and neurosurgery – helped shape new epistemological and
social contexts for brain research under the specific influences of changing
political conditions in Germany, Austria, Switzerland and their neighbouring countries that affected the development of the neurosciences.

My subsequent analysis has pertained to a most relevant sub-develop-
ment of these processes by drawing attention to the marginalization and
later expulsion of a large number of Jewish and oppositional German-
speaking émigré neuroscientists, and their move to North America. The
forced migration wave of neurologists, psychiatrists, neuropathologists,
and many other medical researchers in this field indeed provides us with
ample perspective on the effect of culturally laden research styles, the
enhancement of knowledge, and the advancement of particular areas of
the neurosciences. But rather than see this development merely as a result
of the flight and or expulsion of large numbers of émigrés, it has become
manifest that major reassessments were well underway from the 1910s
to the 1930s in Central Europe. Their pace was accelerated, however, and
they were thoroughly transformed through their integration into the
pre-existing medical and scientific cultures of émigré neuroscientists' new
host countries, the United States and Canada. Yet, of course, historians
of forced migration have long since investigated the extraordinary event
of "intellectual migration" during the Nazi era and pointed to the effect
of the massive exodus of German-speaking doctors.[66] In this endeavour,
the complementary input of clinical and theoretical psychology, public
mental health, or relevant aspects from the social sciences has also been
pointed out for the early research field of neuromorphology. While some
scholars have interpreted the forced migration process merely as an issue
of "brain loss" for German-speaking science and "brain gain" for the rest
of the world, they have thus far neglected to acknowledge the complexity
of the processes involved.[67] Large parts of the history of transatlantic
transfers in medicine and bioscience during the early postwar period still
remain to be written; yet I have ventured to give some tentative answers as
to the historical place, time, and culture in which these cutting-edge visions
and transitions took place within the early field of neuroscience.[68]

Graphic Representations

This numbered list of graphic representations is provided to aid readers in their appreciation of the numerous individuals, research units, centres, and institutes in Central Europe and North America, which are described as the main focus of this book. First, a graphic overview representation of genealogical relationships between mentors and students with the lineage of influences (considered were supervisory, traineeship-, and close working relationships; places are provided for training institutions) is provided. Second, a graphic representation of individuals who were in the same place during the period under investigation (geographic distribution refers to cities with emergent brain science centres) is added for readers' convenience, to help them follow the lineage of influences over time between individuals, and network reception *vis-à-vis* the same places and contemporary time periods of the geographical analysis. These tables are certainly not exhaustive in nature. They are meant primarily as graphic overview representations to enhance the individual and collective biographies as well as clarify the institutional relationships described in the book.

Table 1 (Parts a, b, c, and d): Graphic overview representation of genealogical relationships between mentors and students with lineage of influences (considered were supervisory, traineeship-, and close working relationships; places are provided for training institutions)

(a) Later 1880s to WWI / Coll. Frank W. Stahnisch. © 2019 Frank W. Stahnisch, Calgary, Alberta.

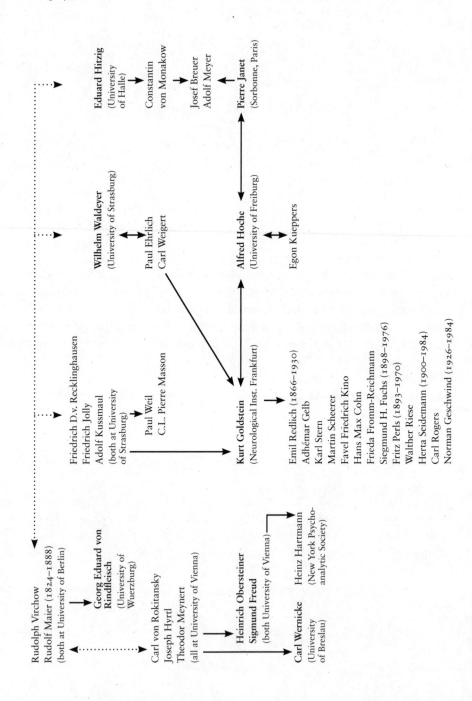

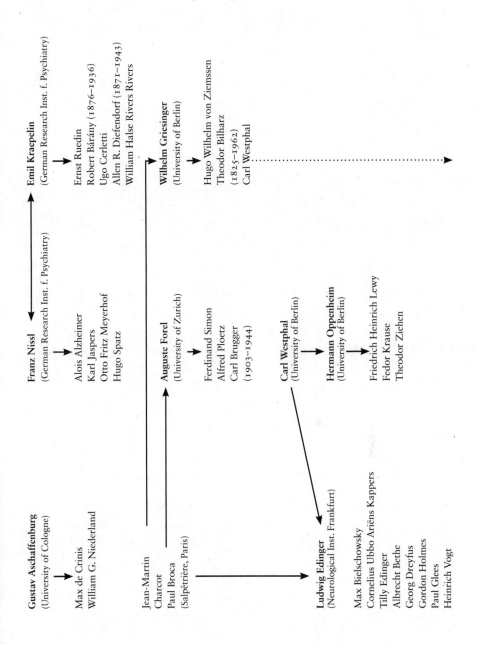

Emil Kraepelin
(German Research Inst. f. Psychiatry)

Ernst Ruedin
Robert Bárány (1876–1936)
Ugo Cerletti
Allen R. Diefendorf (1871–1943)
William Halse Rivers Rivers

Wilhelm Griesinger
(University of Berlin)

Hugo Wilhelm von Ziemssen
Theodor Bilharz
(1825–1962)
Carl Westphal

Franz Nissl
(German Research Inst. f. Psychiatry)

Alois Alzheimer
Karl Jaspers
Otto Fritz Meyerhof
Hugo Spatz

Auguste Forel
(University of Zurich)

Ferdinand Simon
Alfred Ploetz
Carl Brugger
(1903–1944)

Carl Westphal
(University of Berlin)

Hermann Oppenheim
(University of Berlin)

Friedrich Heinrich Lewy
Fedor Krause
Theodor Ziehen

Gustav Aschaffenburg
(University of Cologne)

Max de Crinis
William G. Niederland

Jean-Martin
Charcot
Paul Broca
(Salpêtrière, Paris)

Ludwig Edinger
(Neurological Inst. Frankfurt)

Max Bielschowsky
Cornelius Ubbo Ariëns Kappers
Tilly Edinger
Albrecht Bethe
Georg Dreyfus
Gordon Holmes
Paul Glees
Heinrich Vogt

(b) 1910s to 1930s / Coll. Frank W. Stahnisch. © 2019 Frank W. Stahnisch, Calgary, Alberta.

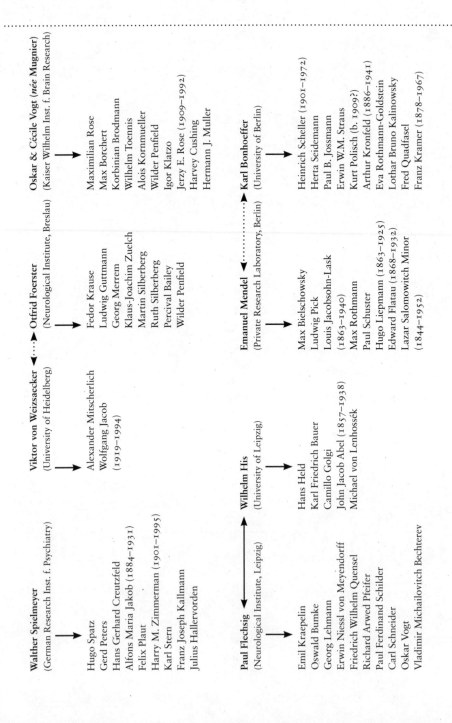

(c) 1930s to 1940s / (d) WWII to early 1960s / Coll. Frank W. Stahnich. © 2019 Frank W. Stahnisch, Calgary, Alberta.

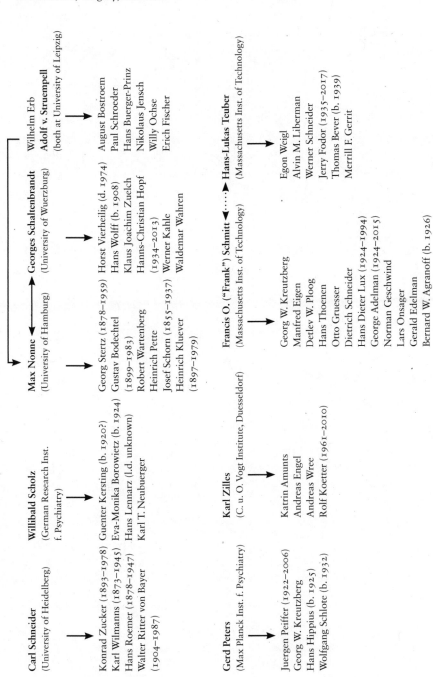

Note

Table 1 shows the connections between leading researchers and their students in the key brain research units, centres, and institutes in Central Europe and North America from the 1880s to the 1940s. Direct relationships are indicated by arrows and include supervisory, apprenticeship, and close working relationships. Indirect collaborations and strong reception of works and concepts are given as dotted-line arrows. Life dates are included for individuals who are mentioned only in the table but not in the book. Part (a) covers the period from the late 1880s to World War I, showing relevant and leading researchers and institutions during these years. Part (b) covers the 1910s to 1930s. Part (c) covers the 1930s to 1940s. Part (d) covers the period from World War II to the early 1960s. University/ research locations are provided here only for the group of supervisors and mentors, not for the group of trainees and pupils.

Table 2 (Parts a, b, c, and d): Graphic representation of individuals who were in the same place during period of investigation (geographic distribution refers to cities with emergent brain science centre)

(a) Later 1880s to WWI / Coll. Frank W. Stahnisch. © 2019 Frank W. Stahnisch, Calgary, Alberta.

University of Vienna, Austria

Maximilian Leidesdorf (1816–1889)	Doeblinger Mental Asylum, Vienna
Joseph Hyrtl	Anatomy Dept.
Carl von Rokitansky	Pathology Dept.
Ernst von Bruecke	Physiology Dept.
Richard Heschl	Dean's Office, Faculty of Medicine
Theodor Meynert	Psychiatry and Neurology Clinic
Sigmund Freud	Private Practice, Vienna
Heinrich Obersteiner	Institute for Anatomical and Physiological Studies of the CNS
Graf Leo von Thurn und Hohenstein	K&K Ministry of Education & Cultural Affairs, Austrian Government

KWU Strassburg, Germany

Richard Freiherr von Krafft-Ebing Friedrich Jolly	Clinical Dept. of Psychiatry
Gustav Schwalbe / Christian F.W. Roller / Wilhelm Waldeyer / Franz Keibel / Paul Weil / Andreas Forster	Anatomy Dept.
Adolf Kussmaul / Ludwig Edinger	Buergerhospital Strassburg Dept. of Internal Medicine
Friedrich D. v. Recklinghausen Arnold Chiari	Dean's Office, Faculty of Medicine Pathology Dept.
Friedrich Goltz	Physiology Dept.
Robert Wollenberg Claude L.P. Masson	Pathology Dept., (Émigré to Canada)
Jacques Felix Pfersdorff	Neurology Professorship

University of Leipzig, Germany

Carl Ludwig	Physiology Dept.
Wilhelm Wundt	Philosophy Dept. (later: in a separate Psychology Inst.)
Theodor Fechner	Philosophy Dept.
Wilhelm His / Hans Held / Camillo Golgi / Karl F. Bauer / Bernard Katz	Anat. Dept. (Golgi: Italian Visitor) (Katz, 1911–2003: Émigré to UK)
Paul Flechsig / Emil Kraepelin Oswald Bumke / Georg Lehmann Erwin Niessl von Meyendorff Friedrich Wilhelm Quensel	Neurological Institute, Leipzig
August Bostroem / Paul Schroeder / Heinrich Klien/ Carl Schneider / Wilhelm Erb	Clinical Dept. of Psychiatry & Neurology / Polyclinic

(b) 1910s to 1930s / Coll. Frank W. Stahnisch. © 2019 Frank W. Stahnisch, Calgary, Alberta.

University of Frankfurt, Germany

Ludwig Edinger	Senckenberg Pathology Institute
Carl Weigert	Senckenberg Anatomy Institute
Paul Glees	Long-term Visiting Res. Associate in the Anatomy Dept. (from NL)
Heinrich Vogt	Neuropathology Div. Edinger Institute
Richard Wachsmuth (1868–1941)	Inaugural University President
Albrecht Bethe	Physiology Dept.
Tilly Edinger	Neuropalaeontology Division, Senckenberg Museum
Kurt Goldstein	Institute for Research into the Effects of Brain Injuries
Georg Dreyfus	Outpatient Dept., City Hospital Sachsenhausen, Frankfurt
Heinrich Hoffmann	Child Psychiatry Div., Frankfurt

Neurol. Centr. Station (NCS), Berlin

Oskar Vogt (also Director of the KWI for Brain Research (until 1936) / Cécile Vogt (*née* Mugnier)	Neurological Central Station / KWI for Brain Research (since 1914)
Max Borchert / Max Lewandowsky	Clinical Practice, Berlin
Maximilian Rose	Tissue Prep. & Culturing, NCS
Max Bielschowsky (Émigré to UK)	Neuropathology Division
Korbinian Brodmann	Neurophysiological Brain Mapping, NCS
Wilder Penfield	Visiting Researcher in Neurophysiology, NCS (from Canada)
Marguerite Vogt	Trainee, Anatomy Division
Marthe Vogt (1903–2003)	Neurochemistry Division
Jan F. Toennies	Engineer, Neurophysiology Div.
Hermann J. Muller	Visiting Researcher in Inheritance Research, NCS (from USA)
Wilhelm Toennis	Cooperation in Neurooncology
Wilhelm von Drigalski	Accredited City Physician, Berlin

KWI for Brain Research, Berlin-Buch (after 1937)

Hugo Spatz	Director, who succeeded Oskar Vogt in 1937
Wilhelm Kruecke (1911–1988)	Neuropathology trainee (Arrived with Spatz in 1937)
Julius Hallervorden	Neuropathology Dept. / Branden-burg-Goerden state asylum
Nicolai Timoféeff-Ressovsky / Helena Alexandrovna Timoféeff-Ressovsky	Neurogenetics Dept.
Max Heinrich Fischer	Neurophysiology Dept.
Thea Luers	Technical assistant, Neuropathology Dept.
Alfred Krupp von Bohlen und Halbach	Industry philanthropist (Essen)
Gertrud Soeken (1897–1978) / Eberhard Zwirner (1899–1984)	Research Clinic, Buch Campus
Alois E. Kornmueller (1905–1968)	Neurophysiology Dept. / Third City Lunatic Asylum (Hufeland Hospital)
Heinrich Scheller (1901–1972) / Paul Vogel (1900–1979)	Third City Lunatic Asylum (Hufeland Hospital)

Neurological Institute, Breslau

Otfrid Foerster	Neurological Laboratory
Ludwig Guttmann	Neurosurgical Ward, Wenzel-Hanke-Hospital (Émigré to UK)
Fedor Krause / Georg Merrem	Neurosurgical Ward, Wenzel-Hanke-Hospital
Klaus-Joachim Zuelch	Neurophysiology Division, BNI
Martin Silberberg / Ruth Silberberg	Neuropathology Division, BNI
Wilder Penfield	Visiting Researcher, Neurology Institute (from Canada)
Oswald Bumke	Cooperation (Textbook Project)

(c) 1930s to 1940s / Coll. Frank W. Stahnisch. © 2019 Frank W. Stahnisch, Calgary, Alberta.

University of Wuerzburg, Germany

Georges Schaltenbrand	Clinical Department of Medicine & Neurology
Werner Heyde (1902–1980)	Mental Asylum of Werneck, Franconia
Wilhelm Toennis	Physiological Laboratory / Continued Cooperation in Aeronautic Neurology
Juerg Zutt (1893–1980)	Clinical Dept. of Psychiatry (Arrived from Berlin in 1946)
Waldemar Wahren (b. 1896)	Monkey Laboratory Wuerzburg Clinical Campus
Hans Georg Bammer (b. 1921)	Chief of Service, Clinical Department of Medicine & Neurology
Horst Vierheilig (d. 1974)	Physiology Laboratory / Clinical Department of Medicine & Neurology
Hans Wolff (b. 1908)	Monkey Laboratory Wuerzburg Clinical Campus

Reichsuniversitaet Strassburg (RUS), Germany

August Bostroem Nikolaus Jensch	Curator's Office, RUS / Dept. of Neurology
Hans Kurt Eisele (1913–1967) Niels Eugen Haagen (1898–1972)	Concentration Camp Natzweiler-Struthof, Alsace
August Hirt / Anton Kiesselbach	Anatomy Dept.
Hans Lullies	Physiology Dept.
Helmut Kaiserling / Willy Ochse Theo Soostmeyer / Erich Fischer	Pathology Dept.
Otto Bickenbach	Pharmacology Dept.
Ernst-Heinrich Brill	Clinical Dept. of Dermatology
Kurt Hofmeister	Clinical Dept. of Paediatrics
Gustav Weigand	Anthropology & Palaeontology Dept., RUS
Rudolf Fleischmann	Physics Division, Clinical Campus

University of Leipzig, Germany

Paul Schroeder	Clinical Dept. of Psychiatry & Neurology
August Bostroem (Departure to the RSU in 1942)	Clinical Dept. of Psychiatry & Neurology
Hans Buerger-Prinz	Consultant, Psychiatry Clinic / Hereditary Health Court, Saxony
Heinrich Klien / Carl Schneider	Staff Attending Physicians, Psychiatry Clinic
Richard Arwed Pfeifer	Neuropathology Dept. / Clinical Dept. of Psychiatry & Neurology
Paul Ferdinand Schilder	Flechsig Institute (Émigré to USA)
Max Clara (1899–1966)	Anatomy Dept.
Werner Catel (1894–1981)	Clinical Dept. of Paediatrics
Georg Renno (1907–1997) Paul Nitsche (1876–1948)	Mental Asylum, Leipzig Doesen, Saxony

(d) WWII to early 1960s / Coll. Frank W. Stahnisch. © 2019 Frank W. Stahnisch, Calgary, Alberta.

KWI/MPI for Psychiatry, Germany

Ernst Ruedin (until 1945)	Director, KWI for Psychiatry / Demographic Study Unit
Friedrich Schmidt-Ott	President of the DFG
Franz J. Kallmann (Émigré to USA)	Demographic Study Unit
Felix Plaut (Émigré to UK)	Neuroserological Dept.
Johannes Lange (1891–1938) / Werner Scheid (1909–1987)	Staff Attending Physicians, Psychiatry Clinic
Karl T. Neubuerger (1890-1972) (Émigré to USA)	Neuropathology Dept.
Willibald Scholz (leading the institute back into the MPG, 1954)	Director, MPI for Psychiatry
Guenter Kersting (b. 1920?) / Eva-Monika Borowietz (b. 1924) / Hans Lennarz	Neuropathology Dept.
Juergen Peiffer (1922–2006) Wolfgang Schlote (b. 1932)	Former Trainees in Neuropathology
Gerd Peters (successor to Prof. Scholz)	Director, MPI for Psychiatry, 1961–74
Edith Zerbin-Ruedin (1921–2015)	Genetics Division
Georg W. Kreutzberg	Neuropathology Dept.
Werner Wagner (1904–1956) Detlef Ploog / Dietrich Schneider Hans Hippius (b. 1925) Paul Mattusek (1919–2003)	Clinical Psychiatry Dept. Biology & Psychotherapeutic Research Programs
Feodor Lynen (1911–1979)	Cellular Chemistry Dept.
Otto Creutzfeldt (1927–1992)	Neurophysiology Dept.

C. & O. Vogt Inst. f. Brain Research, Duesseldorf

Oskar Vogt	Insect Collection, Neustadt i.S. (until 1959)
Cécile Vogt (*née* Mugnier)	Pathology Division, Neustadt i.S. (until 1962)
Igor Klatzo (1916–2007)	Anatomy Division, Neustadt i.S. (until 1947)
Heinz A.F. Schulze (1922–2015)	Visitor, Charité Berlin (from GDR)
Adolf Hopf (1923–2011)	Neuropathology Division U of Duesseldorf, since 1964
Anton Kiesselbach (1907–1984)	Anatomy Dept., University of Duesseldorf, Curator of Vogt Collection since 1964
Karl Zilles (b. 1944)	Neuroscience Chair, C. & O. Vogt Inst. f. Brain Research
Rolf Koetter (1961–2010)	Computational Neuroscience Div., C. & O. Vogt Inst. f. Brain Research
Katrin Amunts (Successor to Prof. Zilles in 2013)	Neuroscience Chair, C. & O. Vogt Inst. f. Brain Research

MIT, Cambridge, MA, USA

Francis O. ("Frank") Schmitt / George Adelman (1926–2015)	Dept. of Biophysics
Hans-Lukas Teuber	Dept. of Psychology (Émigré from Germany, 1941)
Georg W. Kreutzberg	Visitor, MPI f. Psychiatry (Germ.)
Manfred Eigen	Visitor, MPI f. Biophysical Chemistry (from Germany)
Detlev W. Ploog	Visitor, University of Marburg (from Germany)
Hans Thoenen	Visitor, University of Bern (from Switzerland)
Otto Gruesser	Visitor, Free University of Berlin (from Germany)
Dietrich Schneider	Visitor, MPI f. Psychiatry (Germ.)
Hans-Dieter Lux (1924–1994)	Visitor, University of Goettingen (from Germany)
Lars Onsager (1903–1976)	Visitor, Yale University (USA)
Gerald M. Edelman (1929–2014)	Visitor, Rockefeller Inst. f. Medical Research (from USA)

Note

These tables list noteworthy (active/leading) researchers in the brain sciences, from the 1880s to the 1960s, and their institutional affiliations in Central Europe and later in North America. The tables are arranged chronologically to show which individuals were working together or in close proximity during the same period. The first column identifies the relevant researchers based in each university or research institute. The second column indicates the researchers' departmental and/or professional affiliations. Life dates are included for individuals who are mentioned only in the table but not in the book. Part (a) covers the period from the late 1880s to World War I. Part (b) covers the 1910s to 1930s. Part (c) covers the 1930s to 1940s. Part (d) covers the period from World War II to the early 1960s. University/research locations are provided here only for the group of supervisors and mentors, not for the group of trainees and pupils.

Notes

PREFACE

1 Cf. Machamer, McLaughlin, and Grush, *Theory and Method in the Neurosciences*, 200–30.
2 Choudhury and Slaby, *Critical Neuroscience*, 27–52.
3 See, for example, Stahnisch and Russell, *Forced Migration in the History of 20th-Century Neuroscience and Psychiatry*, xi–xiv.
4 The first meeting of the Neuroscience Research Program took place in February 1962, introducing the notion to a wider scientific community in the second half of the twentieth century. Schmitt, *The Never-Ceasing Search*, 222.
5 An instructive theoretical discussion is provided in: Fitzgerald, Littlefield, Knudsen, Tonks, and Dietz, "Ambivalence, Equivocation and the Politics of Experimental Knowledge," 701–21.

CHAPTER ONE

1 Penfield, *No Man Alone*, 265.
2 Holmes, Ghaderi, Harmer, Ramchandani, et al. "The Lancet Psychiatry Commission on Psychological Treatments Research in Tomorrow's Science," 237–86.
3 Yeung, Goto, and Leung, "The Changing Landscape of Neuroscience Research, 2006–2015," 1–10.
4 Habermas, *Erkenntnis und Interesse*, 27.
5 Breidbach, *Die Materialisierung des Ichs*, 15–22.
6 Jacobson, *Foundations of Neuroscience*, 16–53.

7 On the historiographical frame, see for example in: Ash, "Wandlungen der Wissenschaftslandschaften im fruehen Kalten Krieg," 29–65.

8 Kreft, Kovacs, Vogtlaender, Haberler, Hainfellner, Bernheimer, and Budka, "125th Anniversary of the Institute of Neurology," 439–43.

9 Berghahn, "The Debate on 'Americanization' among Economic and Cultural Historians," 107–30.

10 The contemporary notion of "brain research" (*Hirnforschung*) was widely used. It comprised both basic and clinical disciplines, from the anatomy and physiology of the nervous system to clinical neurology, psychiatry, and neuropathology, etc. See also Breidbach, *Die Materialisierung des Ichs*, 11–14. The terms "brain research" and "neuroscience" during the first half of the twentieth century will be used here interchangeably. It is my intention to explore some of the important developments that since the late nineteenth century have helped nurture the emergence of neuroscience as an encompassing interdisciplinary field of research.

11 Most scholarly investigations of interdisciplinarity have thus far been confined to discussions in the philosophy of science and the sociology of knowledge rather than the historiography of medicine and science. In these areas of scholarship, there already exists an extensive body of literature that focuses on the meanings of interdisciplinary knowledge structures and the social constraints of interdisciplinarity in both science and biomedicine. At the same time, preceding studies have singled out several areas that deserve careful scrutiny before advanced analytical approaches can be further developed: to what extent does the concept of interdisciplinarity depend on the concept of scientific disciplines? What are the exact boundaries of pro-, trans-, inter-, and multidisciplinarity? And in what ways is interdisciplinarity a theoretical notion rather than a heuristical tool? See, for example, Lepenies, "Toward an Interdisciplinary History of Science," 45–69; Thompson Klein, *Interdisciplinarity*, 17–76; and Koetter and Balsiger, "Interdisciplinarity and Transdisciplinarity," 87–120.

12 On the notion of a "scientific problem field," see Laudan, *Progress and Its Problems*, 28–39.

13 Included among the most influential studies are: Weinberg, *Reflexions on Big Science*, 159–71; Hughes, *The Manhattan Project*, 105–21.

14 For a recent study of the emergence of neurophysiological trends out of the military traditions during wwii, see the instructive thesis by Stadler, "Assembling Life," 137–248; a similar argument is also expanded in Rose and Abi-Rached, *Neuro: The New Brain Sciences and the Management of the Mind*, 180–9; as well as in Gavrus and Casper, *The History of the Brain and Mind Sciences*, 1–24.

15 Harwood, *Styles of Scientific Thought*, 1–45.

16 Here I will make use of the interpretation given by historians Gerald L. Geison and Timothy Lenoir in their foregoing works. See, for example: Geison, *Scientific Change*, 20–40; Lenoir, *Instituting Science*, 1–21.

17 Methodological specification and discipline formation around identifiable educational and research processes can be seen as a defining feature of the German-speaking natural science system from the eighteenth to the nineteenth century. See also the seminal historical and sociological study by Stichweh, *Zur Entstehung des modernen Systems wissenschaftlicher Disziplinen*, 356–439.

18 For the increasingly challenging functional tradition in nineteenth-century neurophysiology, see Clarke and Jacyna, *Nineteenth-Century Origins of Neuroscience Concepts*, 157–211.

19 Schmuhl, *Die Gesellschaft Deutscher Neurologen und Psychiater im Nationalsozialismus*, 293–8.

20 In fact, this research question necessitates historiographical *analysis on a meso-level* (i.e. political influences on research administration and funding institutions; demands from military officials, patient groups, and war-injured veterans, etc.). Cf. Stahnisch, "Psychiatrie und Hirnforschung," 76–93. For a sociological model, see Latour, "One More Turn," 276–90.

21 The German notion of *Nervenheilkunde* is a term non-translatable into the English language. The historical concept, which approximates it in a strong way is the nineteenth-century usage of "nervous *and* mental diseases," as in the oldest specialized American *Journal of Mental and Nervous Disease* (founded in 1874). As shown here in my book, the technical term of "neuroscience" only came into existence in the early 1960s. For the scope of the German notion of *Nervenheilkunde*, see Breidbach, *Die Materialisierung des Ichs*, 15–22.

22 Cf. John Fulton, *Selected Readings in the History of Physiology*, 56–8.

23 Also in Stahnisch, "Psychiatrie und Hirnforschung," 76–93.

24 Ibid.

25 Ringer, "Toward a Social History of Knowledge," 45–212.

26 Ibid.

27 For example, in Stadler, *Assembling Life*, 197–248.

28 Hagner, *Homo cerebralis. Der Wandel vom Seelenorgan zum Gehirn*, 252–7.

29 Stadler, *Assembling Life*, chapters 1 and 2.

30 Schmitt, *The Never-Ceasing Search*, 214–17.

31 See further, in Vidal and Ortega, *Being Brains*, 71–105.

32 Nagel, *The View from Nowhere*, 13–27.

33 Lovejoy, "The Meaning of Vitalism," 610–14.

34 In a published form, see also Kreutzberg, "Interview," 244–7.

35 Rolando del Maestro, *Interview* (5 May 2007) with author. For all interviews referenced in this book, written consent has been requested and received in light of international practices and regulations. For some tape-recorded oral interviews, which were pursued as pilot interviews, consent was only received orally before recording. These are also referenced here, but in an anonymized form, providing just the role, institution, and location of the neuroscientists and assistants.

36 At least six of the German neuroscientists I spoke with were aware of the institutional histories of their own research centres. The individual answers are not identified here; yet much background information was gained through interviews (formal and informal exchanges) with the following individuals: Ingo Bechmann (19 February 2007); Volker Bigl, (15 September 2004); Karl Max Einhaeupl, (27 August 2001); Hermann Handwerker (13 June 2003); Bernd Holdorff, (2 October 2007); a former MPI director, (14 November 2003); Georg W. Kreutzberg (†) (18 May 2017); Winfried Neuhuber (28 October 2004); Robert Nitsch (28 November 2010); Leo Peichl (26 April 2004); Ruediger Lorenz (†) (15 May 1999); Olaf Ninnemann (14 June 2001); a senior scientific member of the Max Planck Gesellschaft, (26 April 2004); a former MPI director (†) (21 November 2003); the director of a university anatomical institute (10 July 2002); Gebhard Reiss (10 July 2002); Wolfram Richter (†) (27 July 2001); Bert Sakmann (20 May 2017); Hartmut Wekerle (25 May 2017); another senior scientific member of the Max Planck Gesellschaft (†) (14 November 2003); an academic archivist of the Max Planck Gesellschaft (20 November 2003); and a former director of a brain research institute of the Helmholtz Society (6 March 2005).

37 Cf. Siefert, "Den Kranken dem Leben zurueckgeben," 20–35; Holdorff and Winau, *Geschichte der Neurologie in Berlin*, 157–74; or Kaestner, "wurde Leipzig zu einer der Hauptstaetten neurologischer Forschung," 81–100.

38 Singer, "Auf dem Weg nach Innen," 20–34.

39 Gaudillière, "Making Heredity in Mice and Men," 181–202; see also Krige and Pestre, *Science in the Twentieth Century*, xxi–xxxv.

40 Quirke and Gaudillière, "The Era of Biomedicine," 442 (author's emphases).

41 Da Solla Price, *Little Science, Big Science*, 92–115; and Harwood, *Styles of Scientific Thought*, 1–45.

42 Two detailed and differentiated tables with relevant genealogical influences of nineteenth- and twentieth-century mentors and supervisors as well as the local distributions and networking connections between contemporary

neuroscientists are provided in the appendix of this book. They may help and guide the reader in appreciating the connections and relationships between the many early brain scientists in the German-speaking countries together with their international associates and visitors (see appendix).

43 The underlying conceptual innovations were already in existence on the European continent; in the footnotes of his autobiography, Schmitt himself acknowledged the contributions from the German centres in the former Kaiser Wilhelm Society in Berlin and Munich. Schmitt, *The Never-Ceasing Search*, 80–4. See also Freemon, "American Neurology," 605–12.

44 Harrington, *Reenchanted Science*, 103–39; Hagner, "Gehirnfuehrung," 144–76; Borck, *Hirnstroeme*, 85–140.

45 Knorr-Cetina, "Das naturwissenschaftliche Labor," 85–101.

46 Also in Schmidgen, Geimer, and Dierig, *Kultur im Experiment*, 7–14.

47 See, for example: Stahnisch, "Zur Bedeutung der Konzepte der 'neuronalen De- und Regeneration,'" 243–69; Weber, *Ernst Ruedin*, 223–51; or Kreft, *Deutsch-juedische Geschichte der Hirnforschung*, 167–222.

48 The American Neuroscience Research Program also included a number of émigré neuroscientists such as the neurohistologist Alvin M. Silverstein (b. 1935) from Silesia, the biochemist Felix Haurowitz (1896–1987) from Czechoslovakia, and the neurophysiologist Eric Kandel, who had emigrated from Vienna to New York as a teenager with his parents.

49 Knorr-Cetina, *Epistemic Cultures*, 2–11.

50 Cf. Kreft, Kovacs, Voigtlaender, Haberler, Hainfellner, Bernheimer, and Budka, "125th Anniversary of the Institute of Neurology," 439–43.

51 This had not been emphasized in Obersteiner's title of the professorship. However, it is most prominently reflected in sixty-six publications from his institute altogether. Physiology had thereby not taken the central place that he had wished it to assume (because an animal stable and an operation room, to be built according to the original plan for his institute, were still missing). Heinrich Obersteiner, *Letter* (27 March 1883) to the Habsburg minister of education and cultural affairs, Graf Leo von Thurn und Hohenstein, AMUW, Obersteiner Collection; author's translation.

52 Bechmann, *Heinrich Obersteiner (1847–1922)*, 8–31.

53 Obersteiner, *Beitraege zur Kenntnis vom feineren Bau der Kleinhirnrinde*, 101–14.

54 Freud, *Ueber das Rueckenmark niederer Fischarten* (1881).

55 The Dean of the Vienna Medical Faculty, *Letter* (no day given, November 1882) to Heinrich Obersteiner, AMUW, Obersteiner Collection, n.p.

56 Bechmann, *Heinrich Obersteiner (1847–1922)*, 30–1.

57 Zierold, *Forschungsfoerderung in drei Epochen*, 42–361.

58 Stahnisch, *"Flexible Antworten – offene Fragen,"* 56–62.

59 Cf. the collection fonds of the German National Archives in Koblenz
    (BA KO R. 73) on questions of the financial support of research organiza-
    tions through the Deutsche Forschungsgemeinschaft.

60 Lenoir, *Instituting Science*, 19–20.

61 Ibid., 17.

62 See also Anctil, *Dawn of the Neuron*, 208–17.

63 Vom Brocke, *Schmidt-Ott, Friedrich Gustav Adolf Eduard Ludwig*, 165–7.

64 Additional research grants by the Rockefeller Foundation helped to stabi-
    lize the early neuroscientific research programs after WWI. Europe officer
    Edwin R. Embrée, *Diary Entry* (10 November 1922), Rockefeller Archive
    Center (RAC) in Sleepy Hollow, NY, Rockefeller Foundation (RF) Archives,
    RG 1.1, series 717, box 7, folder 36; all the citations used follow the signa-
    ture system of the RAC.

65 Schneider, *Rockefeller Philanthropy and Modern Biomedicine*, 208–22.

66 Alan Gregg, *Letter* (no day or month given, 1935) to the RF New York
    Office, RF Collection MS Germ. Disp. Schol. 1935–36, RAC, RF Archives,
    KG 6.1, series 1.1, box 4, folder 46, 8f. (emphasis in original). American
    funding altogether continued to orient and shape German-speaking brain
    science until the 1930s and early 1940s. Since 1925, the Notgemeinschaft
    der Deutschen Wissenschaft had addressed the pressing issue of funding
    large-scale endeavours with greater societal relevance, which – right from
    the start – required expensive technical equipment such as in nuclear phys-
    ics, aviation engineering, or modern experimental medicine.

67 "The NG [Notgemeinschaft] has the task of serving the interest of German
    science through the following means: (a) to (d) mention the support of
    individual researchers and institutions (e) ... through vital increase and
    support of Group Research Activities (*Gemeinschaftsarbeiten*), which
    are of particular interest to the national economy, public health
    (*Volksgesundheit*), and public well-being (*Volkswohl*)." Notgemeinschaft/
    DFG [German Research Council], *Praesidium Minutes* (no day or month
    given, 1920), BA KO, Collections on the Deutsche Forschungsgemeinschaft
    R 73/69, 63.

68 As described in the preface, the technical term "neuroscience" did not his-
    torically exist before the 1960s. While a theoretical meaning of "neurol-
    ogy" and the contemporary notion of brain research had been in scientific
    use, these were marginal disciplines in the perception of most funding
    agencies. Research in these areas was nevertheless funded among the more
    traditional disciplinary groups of surgery, internal medicine, the fields of

oncology, or experimental biology, etc. See also Proctor, *Racial Hygiene*, 79–82.

69 See, for example, Cottebrune, "Die Deutsche Forschungsgemeinschaft," 354–78.

70 Vom Brocke, "Die Kaiser-Wilhelm-/Max-Planck-Gesellschaft," 1–32.

71 Kroener, *Von der Rassenhygiene zur Humangenetik*, 16–39.

72 Ibid., 28f.

73 Weber, *Ernst Ruedin*, 114–56; Roelcke, "Programm und Praxis der psychiatrischen Genetik," 21–55.

74 Ernst Ruedin, *Letter* (16 January 1930) to Se. Exc. Herrn Staatsminister Schmidt-Ott, Historisches Archiv des Max-Planck-Instituts fuer Psychiatrie, RAC, International Finance Corporation [in alliance with the Rockefeller Foundation], KWIBR [Kaiser Wilhelm Institute for Brain Research], America's Great Depression Portfolio, 45–6 (author's emphasis).

75 Oskar Vogt, *Letter* (2 December 1930) to the President of the DFG Friedrich Schmidt-Ott, HAMPIP [Historical Archive of the Max Planck Institute for Psychiatry, Munich], RAC, IFC, KWIBR, AGD Portfolio, 64–5; author's translation (author's emphasis).

76 Historical Précis of the institute assistant Thea Luers, *Geheimnisse des Gehirns* (ca. 1950), 31–4, HAMPG [Historical Archive of the Max Planck Society, Berlin], KWIBR fonds.

77 Stahnisch, "Psychiatrie und Hirnforschung," 76–81.

78 Alan Gregg, *Letter* (6 November 1928) to the RF New York Office, HAMPG, RAC, RF Collection International Finance Corporation, KWIBR, America's Great Depression, 27.

79 Luers, *Geheimnisse des Gehirns*, 34.

80 Doehl, *Ludwig Hoffmann. Bauten fuer Berlin*, 76–83.

81 Satzinger, *Die Geschichte der genetisch orientierten Hirnforschung*, 87–95.

82 Suffice it to say that for rhetorical and political reasons he did not publicly mention Obersteiner's earlier institute in the Austrian capital. Some insights into the earlier planning of the Viennese laboratory can also be gleaned from Hughlings-Jackson, "Gulstonian Lectures on Certain Points in the Study and Classification of the Diseases," 210.

83 Zilles, "Brodmann: A Pioneer of Human Brain Mapping," 3262–78.

84 Satzinger, *Die Geschichte der genetisch orientierten Hirnforschung*, 191–8.

85 Ibid.

86 Ibid., 93–5; Stahnisch, "Timoféeff-Ressovsky," 323–4.

87 Luers, *Geheimnisse des Gehirns*, 37.

88 See also in Radkau, *Das Zeitalter der Nervositaet*, 9–18.

89 Bethe, "Neue Versuche ueber die Regeneration," 385–478; Edinger, "S. Ramón y Cajal (Madrid), Studien ueber Nervenregeneration," 128; Bielschowsky, "Ueber Regenerationserscheinungen an zentralen Nervenfasern," 131–49.

90 Vom Bruch, "Kontinuitaeten und Diskontinuitaeten in der Wissenschaftsgeschichte," 1–15; Kevles, "Into Hostile Political Camps," 49; Harwood, *Styles of Scientific Thought*, 138–80.

91 Finkelstein, *Emil du Bois-Reymond*, 272–73.

92 See, for example, Stahnisch, "Der 'Rosenthal'sche Versuch,'" 1–30.

93 Stahnisch, *Transforming the Lab*, 44–5.

94 Friedrich Jolly, *Letter* (no day or month given, 1895) to Carl Fuerstner, ADAS [Archives départementales [du Bas-Rhin] à Strasbourg], AL 103 / No. 1158 / Pa. 239, Collection on the Medical Faculty, Clinic of Psychiatry, vol. V (January 1894–August 1901), n.p.

95 Harwood, *Styles of Scientific Thought*, 147–8 (round brackets and emphasis in original).

96 Ibid.

97 Leipzig 1934, Film 443, UAL, Collection on the Medical Faculty, B III 1a/ vol. 1 – Anatomy Chair (1849–1917), n.p.; Strasburg 1898–1918, ADAS, AL 103 / No. 1200 / Pa. 254, Collection on the Medical Faculty, Department of Anatomy (January 1898–October 1918), n.p.

98 Radkau, *Das Zeitalter der Nervositaet*, 9–15.

99 Radkau, "The Neurasthenic Experience in Imperial Germany," 205.

100 Ibid.

101 For example, Cajal, *Studien ueber Nervenregeneration*, 99; and Bielschowsky, "Ueber Regenerationserscheinungen an zentralen Nervenfasern," 131–49.

102 Hagner, *Homo cerebralis*, 105–10.

103 Cajal, *Degeneration and Regeneration of the Nervous System*, 56–7.

104 Shepard, *Foundations of the Neuron Doctrine*, 127–38.

105 Cf. Thompson Klein, *Interdisciplinarity*, 109.

106 Auerbach, "Die Aufbrauchtheorie und das Gesetz der Laehmungstypen," 449; author's translation.

107 He specifically called it phenomena of active *Nervenzerfall* (active nerve deterioration). Edinger, "Aufbau und Funktion," 26; author's translation.

108 Bielschowsky, "Die Silberimpraegnation der Neurofibrillen," 186.

109 Ibid., 187.

110 Ibid. 186–7.

111 Zuerner, *Von der Hirnanatomie zur Eugenik*, 211–14.

112 Stahnisch, "Ludwig Edinger," 147–8.

113 Stadler, *Assembling Life*, 310–23; and Vidal, *"Brains, Bodies, Selves, and Science,"* 930–74.

114 Latour, Mauguin, and Teil, "A Note on Socio-Technical Graphs," 33–6.

115 Holmes, *Hans Krebs*, 234–423; and *Hans Krebs*, 277–440; Todes, *Pavlov's Physiology Factory*, 119–254; *Ivan Pavlov*, 140–95; Rheinberger, *Toward a History of Epistemic Things*, 28–31.

116 Jacyna, *Medicine and Modernism*, 99–142.

117 "I [Penfield] wrote to Foerster, asking permission to visit his clinic as a graduate student, and [Edward] Archibald [1872–1945] to postpone arrival in Montreal until September. But we did not wait for answers. I managed to get a Rockefeller Fellowship from [Richard Mills] Pearce, [Jr, 1874–1930] who was in charge of the foundations' medical philanthropy for Europe and Canada. It amounted to only one hundred eighty-two dollars a month but it added a grant for travel expenses for me. That would enable me to take trips to all the medical centres of Europe. When I wrote to Dean [Charles F.] Martin [1868–1953] at McGill to tell him the change of plan, he sent an immediate check of a thousand dollars towards our expenses. He thought highly of medical science in Germany, remembering his own graduate years there." Penfield, *No Man Alone*, 160.

118 As an indication of the magnitude of these exchanges, there were two hundred North Americans alone at the Deutsche Forschungsanstalt. Kraepelin himself spoke of the educational value and role of building national identity through "his institute" only in the highest forms of praise: "I am pleased that I could help to bring this work [the creation of the DFA for Psychiatry] into existence, as the necessity for such research [an interdisciplinary exploration of the various perspectives in brain psychiatry] has probably not been more obvious than at any other time in our history. We hope that the intended further development of this haven of German science will help to reconstruct our national integrity effectively." Kraepelin, *Memoirs*, 190.

119 Allan, *The Ideology of Elimination*, 13–39; Dyck, *Facing Eugenics*, 55–83.

120 Eight interviews of senior neuroscientists (between 27 July 2001 and 28 November 2010) with author – from the list of interviewees provided in the appendix.

121 As in many instances of the time, and particularly in the emerging field of the neuromorphology during the 1920s and 1930s, such professional relationships were paralleled by deep personal friendships and continuous collaborations. Penfield remarked in his autobiographical notes that he was impressed with Foerster as a charming and warm colleague and friend: "Today we went to Prof. Foerster's home for dinner. They live in

a very nice apartment near the medical school, and not far from the Zoo.
He [Otfrid Foerster] is a rather tall, stooped man who has kindly manners
and a rare but beaming smile. His mother was there, quite proud of her
deceased husband [Richard Foerster, 1843–1922]. He also was a professor but of philology in Kiel. Frau Professor Doktor, for such is her title, is
very charming. She has blond hair just turning gray … They were cul-
tured and pleasing. The professor's room was an astonishing picture –
journals and books piled all over the floor and chairs, but in perfect order
and no dust anywhere. He knew just where to put his hand on anything
in any part of this room. He was writing in a book on the experiences
learned from the war by surgeons on both sides – in neurology … He
loves coffee and we had it several times a day, lingering long over it. I am
learning how to sit and talk or not talk. He has the best mind with which
I have come in contact, with the exception of [Charles Scott] Sherrington
[1857–1952], and their mental type, simplicity, accuracy, and logic, are
very much alike. Neither has any pretense." Wilder Penfield (4 April
1928), *Neurosurgeons I Have Known*, Osler Library of the History of
Medicine at McGill University, Wilder Penfield Fond/W/U 117, 8.
122 Wilder Penfield (no day or month given, 1928), "Report to McGill
University," Osler Library of the History of Medicine, Wilder Penfield
Fonds/P 142, 6 (author's emphasis).
123 Penfield, *The Significance of the Montreal Neurological Institute*, 3.
124 Stahnisch, "The Essential Tension," 162–3.
125 Feindel, "The Montreal Neurological Institute," 8212; Rolando del
Maestro, *Interview* (5 May 2007) with author.
126 Director David Colman of the Montreal Neurological Institute, *Interview*
(26 May 2007) with the author.
127 Penfield, *The Significance of the Montreal Neurological Institute*, 3.
128 See also the excellent article by Annmarie Adams, "Designing Penfield,"
207–40.
129 Feindel and Leblanc. *The Wounded Brain Healed, 1934–1984*, 79–128.
130 Penfield, *The Significance of the Montreal Neurological Institute*, 5. A first
semi-public sketch of the institute originated around 1930 in interchanges
of Penfield with the architectural office. It was largely based on Penfield's
previous observations in the Breslau Neurological Institute headed by
Foerster. See in Osler Library of the History of Medicine, General
Collection/E/VN 1, 2, n.p.) (see figure 1.4).
131 Stahnisch, *German-Speaking Émigré-Neuroscientists*, 36–68.
132 See, for example: Nicosia and Huener, *Medicine and Medical Ethics*,
1–15; Proctor, *The Nazi War on Cancer*, 45–51 and 74–83; Cornwell,
Hitler's Scientists, 71–90.

133 Proctor, *Racial Hygiene*, 3.

134 Ibid., 5.

135 Holloway, "Totalitarianism and Science," 231–50.

136 Cf. Kuehl, *The Nazi Connection*, 27–36.

137 Fischer, *From Kaiserreich to Third Reich*, 38–9.

138 Cf. Weindling, *Health, Race and German Politics*, 61–154; Kuehl, *The Nazi Connection*, 18–39; Proctor, *The Nazi War on Cancer*, 248–78.

139 See, for example, Shevell, "Neurosciences in the Third Reich," 132–8.

140 Hayward, "Germany and the Making of 'English' Psychiatry," 67–90.

141 Klee, *Auschwitz, die NS Medizin und ihre Opfer*, 434–6.

142 This has been shown by recent scholarship both for the United States since 1900 and Germany after 1905. Kuehl, *The Nazi Connection*, 27–63.

143 Weindling, *Health, Race and German Politics*, 305–98, and more recently in Hildebrandt, *The Anatomy of Murder*, 258–9.

144 Proctor, *Racial Hygiene*, 5; Dickinson, "Biopolitics, Fascism, Democracy," 1–48; Esposito, *Terms of the Political*, 100–11.

145 Proctor, *Racial Hygiene*, 6.

146 Ibid., 1.

147 Cf. Bliss, *The Making of Modern Medicine*, 5–94.

148 Proctor, *Racial Hygiene*, 1.

149 Barnes and Edge, *Science in Context*, 65–6.

150 Mendelsohn, *Human Aspects*; Barnes and Edge, *Science in Context*; Ash, "Von Vielschichtigkeiten und Verschraenkungen," 91–105; and Fee and Brown, *Making Medical History*, 288–311.

151 When work for this book began, little scholarly literature was available that focused on the specific theory structure and changing uses in the neurosciences. One valuable book, however, was Marcus Jacobson's *Foundations of Neuroscience* (1993), as it sought to address the interdisciplinary nature of neuroscience by placing great emphasis on the singular use of the word in designating one unified body of knowledge about the brain and the mind, along with bringing certain theories about function, morphology, and genetics more closely together. Jacobson, *Foundations of Neuroscience*, 16–53.

152 Benjamin, "On the Concept of History," 392.

153 This holds, despite the fact that the "axis powers" and the United States had rebuilt their international partnerships after the end of World War I. Kevles, "Into Hostile Political Camps," 47–60.

154 A fruitful historiographical approach for this endeavour is the comparative perspective offered by German-American historian of higher education, Fritz K. Ringer (1934–2006). Particularly his book, *Fields of*

Knowledge, 1–32, offers an appropriate cultural framework on changing mentalities and knowledge economies of academic disciplines.

155 Kater, *Doctors Under Hitler*, 12–34.

156 On the issue of *voelkisch*-oriented public health, eugenics, and immigration policies in Nazi Germany, see the excellent study by Strippel, *NS-Volkstumspolitik*, 105–93; for the implications for the disciplines of psychiatry and neurology, refer for instance to Weindling, *John W. Thompson*, 3–10.

157 The somewhat euphemistic notions of "émigré scientists," "Central European émigrés," or the "wave of forced migrants" are seen here as to transport neutral meanings. These may not be at all adequate for the description of the processes of persecution and struggle for survival of many of the individuals expelled from the German-speaking countries. However, the aforementioned notions are fairly established in the research literature, so I continue to use the terms as neutral and descriptive terminology.

158 Strauss and Roeder, *International Biographical Dictionary of Central European Émigrés*, vol. 2; Ash and Soellner, *Forced Migration and Scientific Change*, 1–19.

159 Jelliffe, Link, and Mendelsohn, *Fifty Years of American Neurology*, 3–103; Magoun, *American Neuroscience*, 405–10.

160 Cf. Stroesser, *Deutsche Gesellschaft fuer Neuropathologie und Neuroanatomie*, 12–13.

161 Strasser, "Institutionalizing Molecular Biology in Post-War Europe," 533–64.

162 Lehrer, "How the Brain Reacts to Financial Bubbles," MM 24.

163 Magoun, *American Neuroscience*, 405–10; Rasmussen, *Picture Control*, 102–96.

164 Cf. Bliss, *The Making of Modern Medicine*, 5–94.

165 See Adelman, "The Neurosciences Research Program," 15–23.

166 Magoun, *American Neuroscience*, 151–3.

167 Engstrom, *Clinical Psychiatry in Imperial Germany*, 194–8; Roelcke and Engstrom, *Die "alte Psychiatrie?"* 9–25; Vom Bruch, *Kontinuitaeten und Diskontinuitaeten in der Wissenschaftsgeschichte*, 9–18; Hofer, *Nervenschwaeche und Krieg*, 209–52; Kloocke, Schmiedebach, and Priebe, "Psychological Injury in the Two World Wars," 43–60; or: Richter, *Das Kaiser-Wilhelm-Institut fuer Hirnforschung*, 349–408; Harrington, *Reenchanted Science*, 102–39; and Borck, *Hirnstroeme*, 85–139.

168 Recent historiographical studies have pondered on the cultural contexts of biomedical laboratory research and shown that these experimental

investigations depend on local traditions, influencing scientific and experimental approaches alike. See: Knorr-Cetina, "Das naturwissenschaftliche Labor," 85–101; Knorr-Cetina, *Epistemic Cultures*, 26–45.

169 Peiffer, "Die Vertreibung deutscher Neuropathologen," 99–110; Peiffer, "Zur Neurologie im 'Dritten Reich,'" 728–33; Burgmair and Weber, "Das Geld ist gut angelegt, und Du brauchst keine Reue haben," 343–78; Roelcke, "Wissenschaften zwischen Innovation und Entgrenzung," 92–109; and Roelcke, "Programm und Praxis der psychiatrischen Genetik," 21–55.

170 For a recent methodological approach to biographies as a valuable perspective for the cultural historiography of science, see Terrall, "Biography as Cultural History of Science," 306–13.

CHAPTER TWO

1 Flechsig, *Die Localisation der geistigen Vorgaenge*, 7; author's translation.
2 Mommsen, *Imperial Germany*, 1–100.
3 Cf. Crawford, Olff-Nathan, Walker, Strauss, Weiss, Burkhard, Olivier-Utard, and Bonah, *Sciences et Cultures nationales*, 29–35 and 121–34.
4 Fischer, *From Kaiserreich to Third Reich*, 3–38.
5 Ibid., 37–8; author's translation.
6 Ringer, *The Decline of the German Mandarins*, 14–80.
7 Ibid., 1 (author's emphasis).
8 These are of specific interest today in the application of what has come to be termed the "knowledge translation field," also in the modern neurosciences. See in Brosnan and Michael, *Enacting the 'Neuro' in Practice*, 680–700.
9 Braitenberg, "Hirnforschung," 43–8; Parnes, "Trouble from Within'," 425–54.
10 Troehler, "Theodor Kocher and Neurotopographic Diagnosis," 203–14; Finger, *Origins of Neuroscience*, 438–40; Stahnisch, "Making the Brain Plastic," 413–35.
11 Millett, "Hans Berger," 522–42.
12 See, for example: Kroener, *Von der Rassenhygiene zur Humangenetik*, 16–39; Kater, *Hitler's Early Doctors*, 25–53; and Proctor, *Racial Hygiene*, 1–45.
13 Daston, "The Moral Economy of Science," 4 (emphasis in original).
14 Roelcke, "Programm und Praxis der psychiatrischen Genetik," 21–55.
15 See, for example: Bonah, *Les sciences physiologiques en Europe*, 86–132; Angermeyer and Steinberg, *200 Jahre Psychiatrie an der Universitaet Leipzig*, 81–154.

16 Departments of neurology and psychiatry did simply not want to remain the only institutions that did not have "*a scientific laboratory*" (*wissenschaftliches Laboratorium*). Koenig, "A Detour or a Shortcut?" 47–65. Such a narrative can be elicited in the researched archival collections of the Archives départementales du Bas-Rhin and the Archives of the Medical Faculty of the Université Louis Pasteur in Strasburg. See, for example, Friedrich Jolly, *Letter* (no day or month given, 1895) to his colleague Carl Fuerstner, ADAS, AL 103 / No. 1158 / Pa. 239, Collection on the Medical Faculty, Clinic of Psychiatry, vol. V (January 1894–August 1901), n.p.

17 Weisz, *The Medical Mandarins*, 3–32.

18 Craig, *Scholarship and Nation Building*, 100–35 and 195–225.

19 Cf. Stahnisch, "Die Neurowissenschaften in Strassburg zwischen 1872 und 1945: Forschungsaktivitaeten zwischen politischen und kulturellen Zaesuren," 227–62. *Nota bene*: The German name of "Strassburg" (in American English typewriter spelling for Straßburg) is used in connection with the official German names of the Kaiser Wilhem Universitaet and the Reichsuniversitaet Strassburg, whereas Strasbourg in French spelling is here used for the Université de Strasbourg and other official institutions during the interwar period, while Strasburg in neutral English spelling is applied throughout the main text.

20 Roscher, *Die Kaiser-Wilhelms-Universitaet Strassburg*, 1–103.

21 The contemporary rhetoric was to develop the new Kaiser Wilhelm University of Strasburg as a "first-rate German university." Ibid., 133–41.

22 Pearson, "U.N. Cries 'Uncle,'" 37.

23 Roscher, *Die Kaiser-Wilhelms-Universitaet Strassburg*, 29–32.

24 Winkelmann, "Wilhelm von Waldeyer-Hartz," 231–4.

25 Ibid.

26 Loetsch, *Christian Roller und Ernst Fink*, 31–47.

27 Strasburg 1898–1918, ADAS, AL 733 / 734. Collection on the Medical Faculty, Schwalbe, Gustav, 1886–1916. Personal file: Gustav Schwalbe, (1844–1916), n.p.

28 Edinger, *Mein Lebensgang*, 60.

29 López-Muñoz, Boya, and Alamo, "Neuron Theory," 391–405.

30 Ammerer, *Seelenheilkunde und Wissenschaft*, 48–54.

31 Strasburg. 1877–1882, ADAS, AL 103 / No. 1154 / Pa. 238, Collection on the Medical Faculty, Department of Psychiatry (January 1877–March 1882), vol. II, n.p.; Department of Anatomy (January 1898–October 1918), n.p., AL 103/No. 1154/Pa. 254.

32 Baeumer, *Von der Physiologischen Chemie*, 183–287.

33 Weisz, *The Development of Medical Specialization*, 165.

34 Cf. Bonah, *Les sciences physiologiques en Europe*, 84 and 117.

35 The Chancellor of the Reich in Berlin, Theodor von Bethmann Hollweg (1856–1921), *Letter* (5 May 1911) to the Governor of Alsace-Lorraine, Karl Leo Julius Fuerst von Wedel (1842–1919), ADAS, AL 103 / No. 1423 / Pa. 335, Collection on the Curator of the Kaiser Wilhelms University in Strasburg, Professorial Exchange Program with America (May 1911, Sect. II, No. 25), n.p.

36 Weisz, *The Medical Mandarins*, 1.

37 University Curator Christian Riele, *Public Lecture* (28 August 1905). Strasburg 1898–1918, ADAS, AL 103 / No. 1200 / Pa. 254, Collection on the Curator of the Kaiser Wilhelms University (January 1898–October 1918), n.p. (author's emphasis); author's translation.

38 Baeumer, *Von der Physiologischen Chemie*, 183. The fonds of the collections of the BA KO R. 73 relate to questions on the financial support for research and institutional organizations by the Deutsche Forschungsgemeinschaft. In particular, see BA KO R73/II *Einzelfall- und Foerderakten* 10 002-16 017, with forty-six medically oriented research programs in neuromorphological subject areas being supported in Germany, Austria, and with collaborations from Switzerland and even the Netherlands.

39 Cf. University Curator Christian Riele, *Public Lecture* (28 August 1905). Strasburg 1898–1918, ADAS, AL 103 / No. 1200 / Pa. 254, Collection on the Curator of the Kaiser Wilhelms University (January 1898–October 1918), n.p.

40 Stahnisch, "Ludwig Edinger," 147–8.

41 Strasburg. 1877–1882, ADAS, AL 103 / No. 1154 / Pa. 238, Collection on the Medical Faculty, Department of Psychiatry (January 1877–March 1882), vol. II, n.p.

42 Crawford, Olff-Nathan, Walker, Strauss, Weiss, Burkhard, Olivier-Utard, and Bonah, *Sciences et cultures nationales*, 33–4.

43 Compare also in: Harwood, *Styles of Scientific Thought*, 170–1.

44 Stahnisch, "Transforming the Lab," 46–8.

45 Department of Anatomy (January 1898–October 1918), n.p., AL 103/ No. 1154/Pa. 254.

46 Franz Keibel (1861–1929), *Letter* (3 December 1915) to the Dean of the Medical Faculty Strasburg 1898–1918, ADAS, AL 103 / No. 1200 / Pa. 254, Collection on the Medical Faculty, Department of Anatomy (January 1898–October 1918); author's translation (author's emphasis).

47 Nipperdey, *Deutsche Geschichte*, 696–7; author's translation.

48 Eckart and Gradmann, *Die Medizin und der Erste Weltkrieg*, 1–7.

49 Collection on the Medical Faculty, Dissertations fonds. ADAS, AL 103 / No. 1200 / Pa. 254.

50 Keibel likewise became the acting head of the institute for pathology after the *Ordinarius* of pathology had been ordered to the Western Front. Keibel, *Letter* (26 July 1915) to the University Curator Georg Karl Emil Petri (1852–1918) at the Kaiser Wilhelms University. ADAS, AL 103 / No. 1200 / Pa. 254, Collection on the Medical Faculty, Department of Anatomy (January 1898–October 1918); author's translation.

51 Gleichen, *Die Theorie der modernen optischen Instrumente* (1911).

52 Wollenberg, *Ich gedenke mit Wehmut und Ruehrung*, 100–10.

53 He then moved to the University of Munich. Universitaet Muenchen, Personen- und Vorlesungsverzeichnis, 107.

54 Cf. Craig, *Scholarship and Nation Building*, 195–225.

55 Wechsler, *La Faculté de Médecine*, 21–31.

56 During his research visit to the New York Presbytarian Hospital, where Penfield had worked earlier, Masson was offered a professorship of neurology in Montreal. He first got to know Penfield from the latter's neurological research laboratories. Penfield was later quite helpful in the bringing Masson to the Université de Montréal in Quebec. Genty, "Masson, Claude Laurent Pierre," 272–3; also, see Pierre Masson, "Le Dr Penfield vu par un ami, le Dr P. Masson. L'éminent professeur français fait l'éloge de son esprit encyclopédique," *Le Canada* (6 October 1933): 10. Osler Library of the History of Medicine, General Collection/E/K 33-10-6, 1.

57 Crawford, Olff-Nathan, Walker, Strauss, Weiss, Burkhard, Olivier-Utard, and Bonah, *Sciences et cultures nationales*, 10–13.

58 Moulin, Clarac, Petit, and Broussolle, "Neurology Outside Paris Following Charcot," 170–86.

59 Flexner, *Medical Education in Europe*, 12.

60 A clear stance on the cultural development of scientific disciplines has been advanced by Lenoir, who emphasized the nature of science as a cultural practice. Likewise he treated the formation of disciplines and scientific institutions as particular sites for constructing forms of social and cultural identity in relation to other cultural frames, focusing especially on the creation of new disciplines and the problematic relation between science, industry, and the state. This development was already tangible in the wake of World War II and in the immediate postwar period in the biomedical sciences as well; see Lenoir, *Instituting Science*, 239–94.

61 Cf. Weindling, *Health, Race and German Politics*, 441–564.

62 Cranefield, "The Organic Physics of 1847 and the Biophysics of Today," 407–23.

63 See, for example, the very insightful methodological atlas published by the St Petersburg and Koenigsberg physiologist Elie de Cyon (1843–1912), *Methodik der physiologischen Experimente*, 316–555.

64 Helga Sprung and Lothar Sprung, "Wilhelm Maximilian Wundt," 343–50.

65 Lothar Pickenhain, *Letter* (13 September 2004) to the author. Wundt, *Grundzuege der physiologischen Psychologie* (1859–1862).

66 Nicolas and Ferrand, "Wundt's Laboratory at Leipzig," 194–203. Wundt's general influence was certainly not confined to Leipzig alone. Very prominent, for example, is his attempt to convince Kraepelin that he should write a concise textbook of psychiatry, which later lay the groundwork for an eminent career in brain psychiatry. Compare: Kraepelin, *Memoirs*, 20.

67 Also, the Leipzig institute was funded through French war reparation payments, similar to the building situation at the Kaiser Wilhelms University in Strasburg. Hagner, "Cultivating the Cortex in German Neuroanatomy," 542.

68 Stahnisch, "Griesinger, Wilhelm," 582–3.

69 For a contextual background of the psychiatric health care system discussions of the time, see particularly Sammet, *Ueber Irrenanstalten und deren Weiterentwicklung*, 87–153.

70 Stahnisch, *Medicine, Life and Function*, 131–74.

71 Flechsig, *Irrenklinik der Universitaet Leipzig*, III; author's translation. He particularly described the organizational models in terms of annexes to larger academic hospitals (such as those in Berlin, Wuerzburg, and Strasburg) or to bigger general hospitals (e.g., Munich, Erlangen, Marburg, Goettingen, and Halle), which were often far from the institute buildings of the local universities.

72 Wagner and Steinberg, *Neurologie an der Universitaet Leipzig. Beitraege zur Entwicklung des klinischen Fachgebietes von 1880 bis 1985*, 4.

73 Also, Edinger's parallel emphasis that he had modelled his own institute at the University of Frankfurt am Main on the organizational sketch of the Obersteiner Institute in Vienna gave rise to continuous and well-developed debates among the later members of the Edinger Commission, who sought to find an adequate successor after his death in 1918, so that the interdisciplinary legacy of the Frankfurt institute could be further developed after WWI; Werner Friedrich Kuemmel, *Interview* (17 October 2005) with author. See the collection on the "Edinger Commission" in the UAF [University Archive Frankfurt], as a partial collection in the Frankfurt Institute for the History and Ethics of Medicine: "The Neurological Institute of the University of Frankfurt am Main had been founded by Ludwig Edinger. Beginning with a very small workshop of Edinger in the

Senckenberg Institute for Pathology, it had been developed to a world
famous research unit and was received as a central reference institute
among the circle of international brain research institutes." (p. 1) (Edinger
Commission. *Petition to the Medical Faculty in Frankfurt am Main*, 1919,
8 pp. with lit.); author's translation.

74 The end of wwii brought the destruction of the clinical departments of
psychiatry and neurology through the bombing raids of the Royal Air
Force between 1943 and 1945. Lothar Pickenhain, *Letter* (13 September
2004) to author.

75 Angermeyer and Steinberg, *200 Jahre Psychiatrie an der Universitaet
Leipzig*, 272.

76 Mentally ill King Ludwig II had invited his personal physician von
Gudden for a promenade near the Wuermsee (Lake Starnberg), where both
drowned under still unknown circumstances. Burgmair and Weber, "Dass
er selbst mit aller Energie gegen diese Hallucinationen ankaempfen muss,"
27–53.

77 Thereafter, Lehmann continued to work on questions of general psycho-
patholgy, probably under the influence of Bumke himself. See, for example,
Lehmann, "Zur Casuistik des Inducirten Irreseins," 145–54.

78 See, for example, Niessl von Meyendorff, *Die aphasischen Symptome und
ihre corticale Lokalisation* (1911); Niessl von Meyendorff, *Ueber die
Prinzipien der Gehirnmechanik* (1926).

79 It concerned the *Heilanstalt fuer Nerven- und Berufskranheiten der
Knappschafftsberufsgenossenschaft Bergmannswohl-Schkeuditz* in the
nearby mining area of Altscherbitz in northern Saxony.

80 Angermeyer and Steinberg, *200 Jahre Psychiatrie an der Universitaet
Leipzig*, 274. See also the following certificate, which Flechsig signed for
one of the trainees, which proved very helpful for continuing research
work and finding positions in regional clinical hospitals:

Flechsig, Paul, Psychiatrist (b. 28 June 1847, in Zwickau):
Certificate for the Candidate in Medicine, Johannes Kuehn (Dresden):
   It is certified in this letter that he had conducted research as an elective
   student in the Department of Psychiatry during the semester between
   1 Jan and 31 Jan 1919 and that he had been fully employed during this
   time.
Leipzig, 31 January 1919
The Director of the University Clinical Department of Psychiatry and
Neurology.
Flechsig

Flechsig certificate, Leipzig 1919, UAL, Exceptional Collections 38 (Taut: Scholars); author's translation.

81 The Flechsig Institute became independent during the interwar period, in 1926, and continued as an internationally recognized institution of the German Democratic Republic after WWII; it still bears the same name today. See, for example, in Becker, Feja, Schmidt, and Spanel-Borowski, *Das Institut fuer Anatomie in Leipzig*, 8–9.

82 His, "Beschreibung eines Mikrotoms," 229–32.

83 Stahnisch, "His, Wilhelm, the Elder," 653–4; Stahnisch and Bulloch, "Mihály (Michael von) Lenhossék," 1901–03.

84 Cf. Stahnisch, "Mind the Gap," 101–24.

85 Ibid., 107.

86 At the time, there was rarely any evidence for chemical transmission mechanisms for nerve conduction. Bennett, *The Early History of the Synapse*, 107–16.

87 Ley, "Bauer, Karl-Friedrich 1947–1974," 8–9; A former anatomy department head, *Letter* (13 March 2003) to author.

88 Berlin histologist Stieve became highly criticized for his subsequent human experiments with murdered inmates of the political concentration camp Ploetzensee. The former president of the German Association of Anatomists, Wolfgang Kuehnel, *Letter* (15 February, 2002), to author; while it took the professional anatomical society almost another decade to support ongoing history of medicine research into the matter. Please see Winkelmann and Schagen, "Hermann Stieve's Clinical-Anatomical Research," 163–71; Hildebrandt, "The Women on Stieve's List," 3–21.

89 See, for example, the article that Bauer co-authored with the Erlangen pathologist Erich Mueller (1903–1984), "Die Zellenlehre," 171–2.

90 Spanish neuroanatomist Javier de Felipe, *Letter* (18 November 2001) to author. On the Leipzig morphological school and Hans Held, see particularly Becker, Feja, Schmidt, and Spanel-Borowski, *Das Institut fuer Anatomie in Leipzig*, 10–60.

91 Ley, "Bauer, Karl-Friedrich 1947–1974," 8–9.

92 Bauer, "Das Reliefbild des Nervengewebes," 351; author's translation.

93 The Erlangen department of anatomy experienced a period of extensive research output between 1947 and 1974 under Bauer's leadership, when he also worked with neuro-ophthalmologist Johannes Wolfgang Rohen (b. 1921). Particularly the multi-volume series of *Basic Medical Science* (*Medizinische Grundlagenforschung*) offered a forum in which publications from major American, Swedish, and Swiss researchers appeared. Bauer had kept in contact with them after his research period at the

Rockefeller Institute for Medical Research from 1937 to 1938 in New York. Nevertheless, the neuroscientific tides had turned, and, because of his insistence on the "neurencytium theory," Bauer increasingly lost his international acceptance. This is in itself an interesting fact, since the Erlangen department had not been destroyed during World War II bombings, as one of the few remaining and intact postwar German departments of anatomy, and it already possessed a sophisticated electron microscope and latest up-to-date technological equipment. See also the account given in Stroesser, *Deutsche Gesellschaft fuer Neuropathologie und Neuroanatomie*, 12–13; Stahnisch, "Mind the Gap," 101–24.

94 Wilhelm Heinrich Erb in Heidelberg, *Letter* (2 February 1919) to Adolf von Struempell in Leipzig; qtd. after Peiffer, *Hirnforschung in Deutschland*, 400. Unfortunately, the building has since disappeared, having been completely destroyed in World War II.

95 Cf. Steinberg, "Oswald Bumke in Leipzig," 348–56.

96 Dohm, *Geschichte der Histopathologie*, 288–9.

97 Ibid., 285–6.

98 Karenberg, "Klinische Neurologie in Deutschland," 20–9.

99 For more on the influences from Obersteiner's Institute in Vienna and the Leipzig neuroscience centre, see Edinger, *Mein Lebensgang*, 90–101.

100 Hagner, "Cultivating the Cortex in German Neuroanatomy," 541–63.

101 The funding strategy was similar to the cases of Munich, Breslau, and Berlin. Earlier publications had emphasized the purely philanthropic intention of the Rockefeller Foundation's engagement in biomedical research, a perspective from which my discussion diverges, when looking at the Rockefeller Foundation's investment for early neuroscience education. Cf. Fosdick, *The Story of the Rockefeller Foundation*, 123–55.

102 This lively tradition of exchanges with American students, visiting scholars, and faculty continued from the Wilhelminian period until the beginning of World War II. Burgmair and Weber, "Das Geld ist gut angelegt, und Du brauchst keine Reue haben," 368–73.

103 Von Lenhossék, "Die Nervenendigungen," 92–100; von Lenhossék, "*Der feinere Bau*," 121–7.

104 Stahnisch and Bulloch, "Mihály (Michael von) Lenhossék," 1901–03.

105 Angermeyer and Steinberg, *200 Jahre Psychiatrie*, 279.

106 The so-called *Aktion T4* program killed more than 70,000 psychiatric patients and asylum inmates in the German Reich. See, for example, the article by Rotzoll, Roelcke, and Hohendorf, "Carl Schneiders 'Forschungsabteilung,'" 113–22.

107 Leipzig 1926, Film 1339, UAL, Collection on the Human Resources Department PA 48 (Richard Arwed Pfeifer), 12–13.

108 Ibid., 14.

109 Paul Schroeder, *Letter* (2 July 1926) to the Medical Faculty. Leipzig 1926, Film 1339, UAL, Collection on the Human Resources Department PA 48 (Richard Arwed Pfeifer), 36; author's translation.

110 Paul Schroeder, *Letter* (13 June 1934) to the principal of the University of Leipzig. Leipzig 1934, Film 1339, UAL, Collection on the Human Resources Department PA 48 (Richard Arwed Pfeifer), 58. Long after Pfeifer had received the chair and set up his own research program, Schroeder seized the opportunity that presented itself when the Nazi government came into power. In an attempt to blackmail him, Schroeder wrote to the principal of the university on 23 June 1934, mentioning: "I may assume that the superior ministry has assembled enough material in its files to reach a final judgment about Herrn Professor Pfeifer" and signed with "*H[eil]. H[itler]*.! Yours very sincerely [*Euer Spectabilitaet ganz ergebener*] P. Schroeder." Ibid., 59.

111 Thompson Klein, *Interdisciplinarity*, 107.

112 As a hallmark multi-volume textbook, it fostered the disciplinary separation of neurology from psychiatry; a continuation of the first series of handbooks (1910–14) and supplements (1922–29) was later published by the German-Jewish neurologist Max Lewandowsky in Berlin. Holdorff and Winau, *Geschichte der Neurologie in Berlin*, 193–205. Lewandowsky's immense publication and editing efforts in clinical neuroscience materialized further when he became the chief editor of *Zeitschrift fuer die gesamte Neurologie und Psychiatrie* in 1910, after Alois Alzheimer had stepped down from the editorship in chief.

113 Vein and Maat-Schieman, "Famous Russian Brains," 583–90.

114 Stahnisch and Koehler, "Three Twentieth-Century Multi-Authored Handbooks," 1067–75.

CHAPTER THREE

1 Edinger, "The Relations of Comparative Anatomy to Comparative Psychology," 437.

2 For a discussion of the concept of a "neuroculture" in comparing differing research programs on similar scientific problems, see Frazzetto and Anker, "Neuroculture," 815–21.

3 See also the discussion of the long-lasting impact of World War I on the belligerent societies during the 1920s and 1930s, with their many attempts to care for, reintegrate, and reanimate their injured, frail, and war-tired populations, in Geroulanos and Meyers, *The Human Body in the Age of Catastrophe*, 34–137.

4 This specific relationship of external and internal factors of science as an interpretation of the research pursuit in its larger context has been pointed out by Barnes and Edge, *Science in Context*, 8–9: "It is often thought that there is a unique and specific kind of barrier which protects science, and particularly scientific judgment, against the intrusion of so-called 'external influences' … Certainly, the evidence presently available suggests that 'external' influences upon scientific judgment are neither unusual nor necessarily pathological, and that the barrier which such influences have to penetrate is not fundamentally different from the boundaries surrounding other sub-cultures."

5 Latour, Mauguin, and Teil, "A Note on Socio-Technical Graphs," 33–6.

6 Cf. Sulloway, *Freud, Biologist of the Mind*, 3–21; Borck, "Visualizing Nerve Cells and Psychic Mechanisms," 75–86.

7 Reisner, "Trauma: The Seductive Hypothesis," 381–414.

8 Stahnisch, "Zur Bedeutung der Konzepte der 'neuronalen De- und Regeneration,'" 243–69.

9 See also Werner, Zittel, and Stahnisch, *Ludwik Fleck. Denkstile und Tatsachen*, 41–259; Knorr-Cetina, "Das naturwissenschaftliche Labor," 85–101.

10 Morel, *Traité des dégénérescences physiques, et intellectuelles et morales*, 23–46; Geroulanos and Meyers, *The Human Body in the Age of Catastrophe*, 111–37.

11 Radkau, "The Neurasthenic Experience in Imperial Germany," 205. See more recently Clark, *The Sleepwalkers*, 359–60.

12 See also Canning, Barndt, and McGuire, *Weimar Publics/Weimar Subjects: Rethinking the Political Culture of Germany in the 1920s*, 153–74.

13 This was more a self-organizing process than a planned development. Brunner, "Psychiatry, Psychoanalysis and Politics," 352–65.

14 Blackshaw and Wieber, *Journeys into Madness*, 1–42.

15 Wells, *The War That Will End War* (1914).

16 Perry, *Recycling the Disabled*, 4–5.

17 Stahnisch, "Ludwig Edinger," 148; Crouthamel, *Invisible Traumas*, 166–70.

18 Stahnisch, "Making the Brain Plastic," 413–35.

19 Bohleber, "Die Entwicklung der Traumatheorie," 797–839; Tutté, "The Concept of Psychoanalytical Trauma," 897–921.

20 For an insightful case study on the British psychiatrist William Halse Rivers (1864–1922), see for example Young, "W.H.R. Rivers and the War Neuroses," 359–78.

21 Sulloway, *Freud, Biologist of the Mind*, 31–49; Borck, "Visualizing Nerve Cells and Psychic Mechanisms," 75–86.

22 Penfield, *No Man Alone*, 174.

23 Cf. Bethe, "Neue Versuche ueber die Regeneration," 385–478; and Bielschowsky, "Ueber Regenerationserscheinungen an zentralen Nervenfasern," 131–49.

24 Habermas, *The Structural Transformation of the Public Sphere*, 9.

25 Roelcke, "Electrified Nerves," 177–97.

26 Holdorff, "Die nervenaerztlichen Polikliniken in Berlin vor und nach 1900," 127–40.

27 Lenoir, *Instituting Science*, 6–7.

28 Holdorff and Wolter, "Ueber die Kontroversen Oskar Vogts," 413–27. See also Sven Dierig's work for a case study from electrophysiology or Christoph Gradmann's discussion of microbiology: Dierig, "Urbanization, Place of Experiment and How the Electric Fish Was Caught," 5–13, and Gradmann, *Laboratory Disease*, 171–233.

29 Nyhart, *Biology Takes Form*, 80–90, on similar occurrences in experimental biology.

30 Roelcke, "Electrified Nerves," 185–91.

31 Griesinger, *Mental Pathology and Therapeutics*, 94–113, here 113.

32 Eulenburg, "Catalepsy," 370.

33 Morel, *Traité des dégénérescence physiques, et intellectuelles et morales de l'espèce humaine*, 1–7.

34 Engstrom, *Clinical Psychiatry in Imperial Germany*, 194–8.

35 Ackerknecht, *A Short History of Psychiatry*; Roelcke, "Wir ruecken Schritt vor Schritt dem Tolhause naeher," 56–67; for an instructive comparative example regarding this intricate relationship between eugenics and psychiatry in Western Canada, see Stahnisch and Kurbegović, *Psychiatry and the Legacies of Eugenics: Historical Perspectives on Alberta and Beyond*.

36 From an earlier manuscript draft of von Monakow and Mourge, *Introduction Bioloqique à l'Étude de la Neurologie et de la Psychopathologie* for the *Zeitschrift fuer Psychologie* (1921), 403–10, esp. 403–4. Archive of the Institute for Medical History and Museum of the University of Zurich; Monakow, Constantin von, Correspondenz, Box 2.

37 Ganesh and Stahnisch, "The Gray Degeneration of the Brain and Spinal Cord," 506–8.

38 Roelcke, "Electrified Nerves," 190–2.

39 Kraepelin, "Psychiatric Observations on Contemporary Issues," 256–69.

40 Kraepelin, *Psychiatry*, 394; author's emphasis.

41 Kraepelin, "Zur Entartungsfrage," 745–51. See a general account in Killen, *Berlin Electropolis*, 81–126.

42 Schmiedebach, "Post-traumatic Neurosis," 27–57.

43 Kraepelin, *Psychiatry*, 53.
44 Lerner, *Hysterical Men*, 223–48.
45 For example, see Kraepelin, *Psychiatry*, 208.
46 Kraepelin, *Psychiatrie*, 1973–74; vol. 1, 53–4; author's translation.
47 Helmchen, *Psychiater und Zeitgeist*, 13–9.
48 Vogelsaenger, "Auf den Spuren der psychosomatischen Medizin," 259–64.
49 Schmiedebach, "The Public's View of Neurasthenia," 219–22.
50 Radkau, "The Neurasthenic Experience in Imperial Germany," 199–217.
51 It is important that intellectual concepts of modern life, as having a nega-
    tive impact on health – particularly brain health – were not restricted to
    the German-speaking countries, but became widely available in the
    Western World. They were also shared by many British, American,
    Canadian, and French authors on the effects of wartime stresses on the
    brains of civilians. Foley, *Encephalitis Lethargica*, 435–40.
52 Cajal, *Studien ueber Nervenregeneration*, 1–86; and Bielschowsky, "Ueber
    Regenerationserscheinungen an zentralen Nervenfasern," 131–49.
53 Stahnisch, "Making the Brain Plastic," 422–6.
54 Borck, "Fuehlfaeden und Fangarme,"144–8.
55 Ramón y Cajal and Camillo Golgi were awarded the Nobel Prize in
    Physiology or Medicine in 1906 for this approach. Bracegirdle, *A History
    of Microtechnique*, 57–110; Stahnisch and Nitsch, "Santiago Ramón y
    Cajal's Concept," 589.
56 For such innovative technology-based visualization processes, see
    Cambrosio, Jacobi, and Keating, "Phages, Antibodies and
    'De-Monstration,'" 131–58.
57 Luers, *Geheimnisse des Gehirns*, 31–2.
58 Hagner, "Cultivating the Cortex in German Neuroanatomy," 541–63.
59 Cajal, *Degeneration and Regeneration of the Nervous System*, 56–7. Cajal
    himself did report regeneration phenomena in several CNS areas, such as
    the lower spinal cord or the visual cortex, while making his observation in
    experimentally lesioned rabbits and puppies. In terms of his discussion of
    nervous regeneration, it was primarily the fact of a re-establishment of fibre
    connections at the lesioned junction, rather than the quantity and quality
    of restored nerve cell endings in these wounds, which interested him.
60 Javier de Felipe, *Letter* (18 November 2001) to author.
61 Harrison, "Experiments in Transplanting Limbs," 239–81; Brazier,
    A History of Neurophysiology in the 19th Century, 144.
62 Keshishian, "Ross Harrison's 'The Outgrowth of the Nerve Fiber,'" 201–03.
63 For the technical term, see in: Galison, *Image & Logic*, 783.
64 Auerbach, "Die Aufbrauchtheorie und das Gesetz der Laehmungstypen,"
    449; author's translation.

65 Dierig, Lahmuncd, and Mendelsohn, "Toward an Urban History of Science," 1.

66 Kreft, *Deutsch-Juedische Geschichte und Hirnforschung. Ludwig Edingers Neurologisches Institut in Frankfurt am Main*, 48–56.

67 Hoeres, "Vor 'Mainhattan,'" 71–97.

68 Stahnisch, "Ludwig Edinger (1855–1918)," 147–8.

69 Mann, "Senckenbergs Stiftung," 244.

70 Efron, *Medicine and the German Jews*, 234–64.

71 A former MPI director, *Interview* (21 November 2003) with author.

72 Edinger, "Ueber die Schleimhaut des Fischdarmes," 651–92.

73 Edinger, *Mein Lebensgang*, 59–67.

74 Stahnisch, "Ludwig Edinger," 147–8.

75 Edinger, "Ueber die Schleimhaut des Fischdarmes," 685; author's translation. This is remarkable, given the focus on the cortex in neuroanatomy throughout the nineteenth century.

76 Edinger, *Untersuchungen zur Physiologie und Pathologie des Magens* (1881).

77 Emisch, *Ludwig Edinger*, 62–5.

78 See, for example, Stahnisch, "Der 'Rosenthal'sche Versuch,'" 1–30.

79 Efron, *Medicine and the German Jews*, 50–1.

80 Klausewitz, *175 Jahre Senckenbergische Naturforschende Gesellschaft*, 311–18.

81 The Senckenberg Society of Natural Scientists is still an active research institution today. It comprises a large botanical garden, a museum with zoological collections, the Edinger Institute, the institute of anatomy and pathology, and the institute for the history and ethics of medicine of the Johann Wolfgang.Goethe University. Ibid.

82 Edinger, *Mein Lebensgang*, 101; author's translation.

83 Cf. Goldstein, *Selected Papers*, 4–5.

84 Emisch, *Ludwig Edinger*, 56–78.

85 Edinger, *Mein Lebensgang*, 102; author's translation. Further, on the procurement of embryological material see Weigert, "Zwei Faelle von Missbildungen eines Ureters," 531–2.

86 Edinger, *The Anatomy of the Central Nervous System of Man and of Vertebrates in General* (1885–99). It went through eight editions and two translations before 1908.

87 Mann, "Senckenbergs Stiftung," 244–63.

88 Ibid.

89 "All scientists who worked at the 'Senckenberg' contributed to what could be called a small community. They felt at home in the collections, laboratories, and the library, the latter being easily accessible. Shortages were quickly handled and requests were put through directly to a person who

could respond to them." Edinger, *Vorlesungen ueber den Bau der nervo-esen Zentralorgane*, 3; author's translation.

90 Stahnisch and Hoffmann, "Kurt Goldstein and the Neurology of Movement," 283–6.

91 Goldstein, *Selected Papers*, 1.

92 Glees, "Ludwig Edinger (1855–1918)," 254.

93 Edinger even went so far as to call Wallenberg his "anatomical conscience." Edinger, *Mein Lebensgang*, 190.

94 Glees, "Ludwig Edinger (1855–1918)," 251–5.

95 Bertelmez, "Charles Judson Herrick," 77–108.

96 Haines, "Santiago Ramón y Cajal at Clark Unviversity," 463–80.

97 Herrick, "Editorial Announcement," 1.

98 Stahnisch, "Ludwig Edinger," 147–8.

99 Hammerstein, *Die Johann Wolfgang Goethe-Universitaet*, 14–24.

100 Peiffer, "Die Vertreibung deutscher Neuropathologen," 102.

101 Goldstein, *Die Behandlung, Fuersorge und Begutachtung*.

102 Ibid.

103 "In the brain-injured patient, we encounter changes of structure. Resulting from this, a whole series of earlier and normal action-realizations can no longer be sustained and previous viable tasks no longer resolved. When the patient is confronted with them, however, various abnormal action-realizations occur, which I call the 'catastrophic reactions' [*Katastrophen-reaktionen*], i.e., an irritation of the body and mind that can lead to the disruption of other well-organized reactions and the characteristic phenomenon of angst." Goldstein, "Zum Problem der Angst," 238; author's translation.

104 Danzer, *Vom Konkreten zum Abstrakten*, 11–70.

105 Harrington, *Re-Enchanted Science*, 103–8.

106 Teuber, "Kurt Goldstein's Role," 301–2.

107 The situation in the United States and the United Kingdom was quite different in this respect, since the societal separation between neurology, psychiatry, and neurosurgery had already taken place before World War I. Cf. Gavrus, *Men of Dreams and Men of Action*, 57–92; Casper, "Atlantic Conjectures," 650.

108 Up to 30 percent of all neurologists and psychiatrists had been of Jewish descent in prominent university cities. Peters, "Emigration deutscher Psychiater nach England," 161–7.

109 Sieg, "Strukturwandel der Wissenschaft im Nationalsozialismus," 255–70; van Rahden, *Jews and Other Germans*, 21–63; Gruettner and Kinas, "Die Vertreibung von Wissenschaftlern," 123–86.

110 See also Stahnisch, "Psychiatrie und Hirnforschung," 76–81.

111 Karenberg, "Klinische Neurologie in Deutschland," 20–9.

112 Reichswehrministerium, *Heeres-Sanitaetsinspektion*, vol. 3, 46–53.

113 Goldstein, *Selected Papers*, 3.

114 Benzenhoefer and Kreft, "Bemerkungen zur Frankfurter Zeit," 31–40.

115 Edinger Commission (UAF collection). *Petition to the Medical Faculty in Frankfurt am Main*, 1919, 1–3.

116 Ibid.

117 Hammerstein, *Die Johann Wolfgang Goethe-Universitaet Frankfurt am Main*, 45.

118 Bay HstA [Bavarian Main State Archive], MK 8/I Ministry of Science, Education and Art, 20980, Medical Research, n.p.

119 See the collection on the "Edinger Commission" in the UAF, as a partial collection in the Frankfurt Institute for the History and Ethics of Medicine (Edinger Commission, *Petition to the Medical Faculty in Frankfurt am Main*, 1919, 8 pp. with lit.).

120 Plaenkers, Laier, and Otto, *Psychoanalyse in Frankfurt am Main*, 180–94.

121 Benzenhoefer and Kreft, "Bemerkungen zur Frankfurter Zeit," 31–40.

122 Magoun, *American Neuroscience*, 31–2.

123 Neumaerker and Bartsch, "Karl Kleist," 411–58.

124 Kleist, "Ueber die gegenwaertigen Stroemungen in der klinischen Psychiatrie," 389–93; author's translation.

125 Hossfeld and Olsson, "The Road from Haeckel," 293–6.

126 Ibid.

127 Neumaerker, "Karl Kleist," 411–58.

128 Kohring and Kreft, *Tilly Edinger. Leben und Werk einer juedischen Wissenschaftlerin*, 21–298.

129 Letter exchanges between Tilly Edinger and the director of the Frankfurt Institute of Neurology Wilhelm Kruecke (7 June 1960 to 26 February 1961). In Peiffer, *Hirnforschung in Deutschland*, 1041.

130 Bechmann, Nitsch, Pera, Winkelmann, and Stahnisch, "Zentrales Nervensystem," 355–550.

131 Ashwal, *The Founders of Child Neurology*, 616–18.

132 Emisch, *Ludwig Edinger*, 120–30.

133 Guttmann and Scholz-Strasser, *Freud and the Neurosciences*, 37–46.

134 Goldstein, *Selected Papers*, 5.

135 Stahnisch and Hoffmann, *Kurt Goldstein and the Neurology of Movement*, 283–86.

136 Goldstein, *Selected Papers*, 5.

137 Emisch, *Ludwig Edinger*, 87–119.

138 Edinger often called this the "correlative identity of form and function." See also the description of new organizational patterns of biomedical research institutions in Lenoir, *Instituting Science*, 179–293.

139 Glees, "Ludwig Edinger (1855–1918)," 254.

140 *Homo cerebralis*, 232–40.

141 Stahnisch, *Medicine, Life and Function*, 153–200; Finger, *Origins of Neuroscience*, 32–50. For the technical notion, see Lakatos, *Criticism and the Growth of Knowledge*, 116.

142 Stahnisch, "The Emergence of Nervennahrung," 405–8.

143 Edinger, "Aufbau und Funktion," 26; author's translation.

144 Radkau, *Das Zeitalter der Nervositaet*, 9–15.

145 Edinger and Fischer, *Ein Mensch ohne Grosshirn*, 337; author's translation.

146 Craver, *Explaining the Brain: Mechanisms and the Mosaic Unity of Neurosciences*, 232–7.

147 Edinger, "Ueber die Regeneration des entarteten Nerven," 769.

148 Ibid.; emphasis in original; author's translation.

149 Emisch, *Ludwig Edinger*, 79–103.

150 Goldstein, *Selected Papers*, 4.

151 Edinger, "Ueber die Bedeutung der Hirnrinde," 350–2; Edinger, *Mein Lebensgang*, 150–5.

152 Wallenberg, "Ludwig Edinger," 997–1008; Glees, "Ludwig Edinger," 254; Kruecke and Spatz, "Aus den Erinnerungen von Ludwig Edinger," 35–41.

153 Hammerstein, *Die Johann Wolfgang Goethe-Universitaet*, 14–24.

154 See, for example, Douglas, *How Institutions Think*, 9–68.

155 Thompson Klein, *Interdisciplinarity*, 107.

156 Cf. Stahnisch, "Ludwig Edinger," 147–8.

157 See also, recently, Heynen, *Degeneration and Revolution*, 251–85.

158 Weitz, *Weimar Germany*, 7–40; and Crouthamel, *War Neurosis Versus Savings Psychosis*, 163–82.

159 A famous definition of mental and racial hygiene by the Zurich neuropsychiatrist Auguste Forel in 1905. Kuechenhoff, "Der Psychiater Auguste Forel und seine Stellung zur Eugenik," 19–36.

160 See the works of Alfred Hoche from Freiburg in the 1920s or Oswald Bumke from Leipzig in the early 1930s. Hoche, *Handbuch der gerichtlichen Psychiatrie*, 211–21; Bumke, "Klinische Psychiatrie und Eugenik," 394–5; Hofer, "War Neurosis," 250–5.

161 Stahnisch, "The Emergence of Nervennahrung," 405–8.

162 In response, Edinger conceived there to be some rehabilitative potential in changes to the environment, such as physical moves from unhealthy living conditions, the practice of gymnastics or temperance in alcohol

consumption, which he even separately recommended to his patients. Edinger, *Der Anteil der Funktion an der Entstehung von Nervenkrankheiten*, 45–57.

163 Stahnisch, "Zur Bedeutung der Konzepte der 'neuronalen De- und Regeneration,'" 243–69.

164 Both Edinger and Kraepelin had pursued postgraduate studies with Flechsig at the Leipzig institute, where they refined the methodological knowledge that they applied to their subsequent research programs in Frankfurt and Munich. Kaestner and Schroeder, *Sigmund Freud*, 166.

165 Bielschowsky, "Die Silberimpraegnation der Neurofibrillen," 186–7.

166 Ibid.; author's translation.

167 Stahnisch, "Zur Bedeutung der Konzepte der 'neuronalen De- und Regeneration,'" 255; author's translation.

168 Zuerner, *Von der Hirnanatomie zur Eugenik*, 21–3 and 39–43.

169 Cf. Stahnisch, "Making the Brain Plastic," 414–16.

170 Canguilhem, *The Normal and the Pathological*, 144.

171 See Kaufmann, "Science as Cultural Practice," 125–44; and recently, for the Weimar context, Geroulanos and Meyers, *The Human Body in the Age of Catastrophe*, 3–77.

172 In order to realize this intricate psychiatric knowledge transition "from bed to beside," a well-planned interdisciplinary structure of the units of the new Munich research centre was anticipated: "The research institute should be opened at the beginning of April, 1918. Unfortunately, we were not able to install all the departments intended. Our former psychological laboratories were still partly used for other purposes, or had to serve anatomical purposes and a replacement could not be found for the time being. Moreover, I was preoccupied with my clinical activities and lacked an assistant, who could have supported my methodological instructions for psychological studies. The installation of a chemical laboratory also caused great difficulties. In order to gain room for the serological depart-ment, we had been forced to move the chemical laboratory to the top floor of the clinic, but now, under the pressure of war conditions, the nec-essary building alterations could not be made and the needed equipment could not be supplied ... We therefore decided to satisfy ourselves for the time being with the installation of two histopathological departments under Nissl and Spielmeyer, a topographic-histotological one under Brodmann, a serological one under Plaut, and a genealogical one under Ruedin and to leave further development to the future." Kraepelin, *Memoirs*, 182.

173 Stahnisch, "Transforming the Lab," 46–8.

174 Bielschowsky, "Ueber Regenerationserscheinungen an zentralen Nervenfasern," 131–49.

175 American historian of science Anne Harrington has drawn considerable attention to this work. Harrington, *Reenchanted Science*, 103–39.

176 Goldstein, *Ueber Rassenhygiene*, 461; author's translation.

177 For the analytical historiographical notion see in Loewy, "The Strength of Loose Concepts," 371–439.

178 Churchill, "Regeneration," 126–9, for an account of the basic neuroexperimental approaches.

179 Bumke, *Lehrbuch der Geisteskrankheiten*, 609; author's translation.

180 Doeblin, *Berlin Alexanderplatz*, 7; author's emphasis and translation.

181 Casselman, Dingwall, and Casselman, *Dictionary of Medical Derivations*, 197.

182 Klahre, *Die Psychiatrie profitiert von der Hirnforschung*, 12.

183 For general medical developments in Berlin, see Winau, *Medizin in Berlin*, 196–269; and for the particular history of the contemporary neurosciences, consult Holdorff and Winau, *Geschichte der Neurologie in Berlin*, 193–216.

184 Cf. Goschler, *Wissenschaft und Oeffentlichkeit in Berlin*, 7–28.

185 See, for example, in Richter, *Das Kaiser-Wilhelm-Institut fuer Hirnforschung*, 352–72.

186 French biologist and Nobel Prize winner François Jacob (1920–2013) wittily coined the word "like in a real laboratory" for this phenomenon. Cf. Jacob, *The Statue Within*, 9–11.

187 Bernard, *Einfuehrung in das Studium der experimentellen Medizin*, 201; author's translation.

188 Schulze, "Hirnlokalisationsforschung in Berlin," 59–62.

189 Richter, *Das Kaiser-Wilhelm-Institut fuer Hirnforschung*, 384–87.

190 Danek and Rettig, "Korbinian Brodmann," 555–62; Kreft, *Deutsch-Juedische Geschichte und Hirnforschung*, 223–83.

191 Harrington, *Reenchanted Science*, 259–371; Eisenberg, Collmann, and Dubinski, *Verraten – Vertrieben – Vergessen*, 7–17.

192 Klatzo, *Cécile and Oskar Vogt*, 18–27.

193 See also: Luers, *Geheimnisse des Gehirns*, 31–4 (author's emphasis); author's translation.

194 Ramón y Cajal, *Recollections of My Life*, 602 (author's emphasis).

195 Dejong, "The Century of the National Hospital," 676–9.

196 Luers, *Geheimnisse des Gehirns*, 31–2.

197 Satzinger, *Die Geschichte der genetisch orientierten Hirnforschung*, 66–78.

198 Luers, *Geheimnisse des Gehirns*, 31–2 (author's emphasis); author's translation.
199 Stahnisch, "Zur Bedeutung der Konzepte der 'neuronalen De- und Regeneration,'" 243–8.
200 Richter, *Das Kaiser-Wilhelm-Institut fuer Hirnforschung*, 367–73.
201 Burgmair and Weber, "Das Geld ist gut angelegt, und Du brauchst keine Reue haben," 368–73.
202 The visit took place on 6 November 1928. Historisches Archiv des Max-Planck-Instituts fuer Psychiatrie, RAC, International Finance Corporation, KWIBR, America's Great Depression, 27.
203 Stahnisch, "Psychiatrie und Hirnforschung," 76–81.
204 Luers, *Geheimnisse des Gehirns*, 37.
205 Cf. Doehl, *Ludwig Hoffmann. Bauten fuer Berlin*, 28–48.
206 Alan Gregg, *Letter* (5 May 1926) from Germany to the RF headquarters in New York. RAC, RF Archives, RG 1.1, series 717A, box 10, folder 64, 1.
207 Anon., *Manuscript* "Germany" (May 1926). RAC, RF Archives, RG 1.1, series 717A, box KWIBR, 8. [It is an anonymous document, and the original quotation is in American English. From the writing style, though, it is possible to assume that it was Gregg who was the author of this brief report.]
208 Satzinger, *Die Geschichte der genetisch orientierten Hirnforschung*, 191–2; author's translation.
209 Luers, *Geheimnisse des Gehirns*, 83–4.
210 Stahnisch, "Timoféeff-Ressovsky," 323–4.
211 Hagner, *Geniale Gehirne*, 249–66.
212 Klatzo, *Cécile and Oskar Vogt*, 42–52.
213 Alan Gregg, *Cable* to New York RF headquarters; Historisches Archiv des Max-Planck-Instituts fuer Psychiatrie, RAC, 717A KWIBR, IOC–AG (July 31, 1933), 71.
214 Schuering, *Minervas verstossene Kinder*, 101–9.
215 Bielka, *Die Medizinisch-Biologischen Institute Berlin-Buch*, 157.
216 Schulze, *Persoenliche Erinnerungen*, 399–403. The brain research institute and the bumblebee project ceased to exist after Cécile Vogt's death in 1962. The collections and archival materials were however later given to the University of Duesseldorf, where the C[écile]. & O[skar Vogt]. Institute for Brain Research was inaugurated in 1991. It still aims to continue neuroscientific investigations in the tradition of the Vogts. Karl Zilles, *Interview* (6 March 2005) with author.
217 Holdorff, "Founding Years of Clinical Neurology in Berlin," 223–38.
218 Zilles, "Brodmann: A Pioneer of Human Brain Mapping," 3262–78.

219 Danek and Rettig, "Korbinian Brodmann," 557–8.

220 Fix, *Leben und Werk des Gehirnanatomen Korbinian Brodmann*, 95–108.

221 Wahren, "Oskar Vogt. 6.4.1870-31.7.1959," 363–4.

222 Stahnisch, "Zur Bedeutung der Konzepte der 'Neuronalen De- und Regeneration,'" 244–8.

223 Luers, *Geheimnisse des Gehirns*, 30–1; author's translation.

224 Garey, *Brodmann's Localisation*, 2–9.

225 Nitsch and Stahnisch, "Neuronal Mechanisms Recording the Stream of Consciousness," 1–9; Rolando del Maestro at the Montreal Neurological Institute, *Interview* (5 May 2005) with author.

226 Penfield, *No Man Alone*, 168.

227 Richter, *Das Kaiser-Wilhelm-Institut fuer Hirnforschung*, 382–3.

228 Penfield, *The Difficult Art of Giving*, 249. For the neurosurgical work, which they both did together, see Foerster and Penfield, "The Structural Basis of Traumatic Epilepsy," 5399–419.

229 B.B. "Duesseldorf erhaelt Hirnforschungsinstitut. Akademie gewann Wettlauf der Hochschulen – Neuer Lehrstuhl geplant," 9; Karl Zilles, *Interview* (6 March 2005) with author.

230 In: Haymaker and Schiller, *The Founders of Neurology*, 14; author's emphasis.

231 Cf. Brodmann, "Beitraege zur histologischen Lokalisation der Grosshirnrinde," 79–107 and 287–334.

232 Wahren, "Oskar Vogt. 6.4.1870-31.7.1959, 370–1"; see also the archival materials in the UAHUB [University Archives of the Humboldt University of Berlin], Collection on the Human Resources Department, BAB 1503, pertaining to Brodmann's personal file.

233 Karenberg, "Klinische Neurologie in Deutschland," 20–9.

234 Fix, *Leben und Werk des Gehirnanatomen Korbinian Brodmann*, 87–93.

235 Garey, *Brodmann's Localisation in the Cerebral Cortex*, xv.

236 Fix, *Leben und Werk des Gehirnanatomen Korbinian Brodmann*, 87–93.

237 Belz, "Kurt Goldstein (1878–1965)," 11–70.

238 Harrington, *Reenchanted Science*, 259–371.

239 Stahnisch, "Ludwig Edinger," 148.

240 Jung, "Ueber eine Nachuntersuchung des Falles Schn.," 353–8.

241 Gelb and Goldstein, *Psychologische Analysen hirnpathologischer Faelle*, 324; author's translation.

242 Meyer and Geroulanos, *Experimente im Individuum*, 94–7.

243 Villa Sommerhoff (figure 1.2) was built in 1804 by a Frankfurt patrician family on the grounds of a medieval cemetery – which lay outside the former city walls – for witches, illegitimate children, and people who had committed suicide. With the beginning of World War I, it was

reappropriated to serve as a hospital for the German Army. Goldstein's sanatorium continued as an autonomous rehabilitation centre until its complete destruction during the US Air Force bombings of Frankfurt am Main in 1944. Today, only a few stepping stones to the villa entrance and approximately fifteen metres of the eastern park's surrounding wall remain. The area is now home to an old people's residence and a professional training school, while one third of the previous estate serves as a nice municipal park (*Sommerhoff Park*).

244 Kreft, "Zwischen Goldstein und Kleist," 131–44.

245 "My idea was to build an institution which offered the opportunity *to observe the patients' everyday behaviour and to study them in all respects*. Accordingly I organized in Frankfurt am Main, under the administration of the government, a hospital which consisted of a ward for medical and physiotherapeutic treatment, a psychophysiological laboratory for special examination of the patients and theoretical interpretation of the observed phenomena, a school for retraining on the basis of the results of this research, and finally workshops in which the patient's aptitude for special occupations was tested and he was taught an occupation suited to his ability. I was assisted in this work by younger neurologists, teachers, and psychologists. Here the cooperation of my late friend, the psychologist A. Gelb, for over ten years proved to be of the greatest significance ... *This intensive cooperative work yielded many results of practical and theoretical value for medicine and psychology*." Taken from Goldstein, *Notes on the Development of My Concepts*, 3 (author's emphases).

246 Pick was a proud German patriot, who had served in the military during World War I. His personality and strong sense of identity made it impossible for him to leave his beloved home country, and he was later deported to the concentration camp of Theresienstadt, where he was killed in 1944. Simmer, *Der Berliner Pathologe Ludwig Pick*, 217–30.

247 Stahnisch, "Zur Zwangsemigration deutschsprachiger Neurowissenschaftler," 441–72.

248 Goldstein, *Selected Papers*, 11–12.

249 Stern, *Pillar of Fire*, 79–80; Crome, "The Medical History of V.I. Lenin," 3–9.

250 Cf. Harrington, *Reenchanted Science*, 291. On the dreadful attitude of the Nazi medical philosophy particularly toward the mentally ill and neurologically handicapped, see also Weindling, *John W. Thompson*, 3–10.

251 Heinrich Pette, quoted from Klee, *Das Personenlexikon zum Dritten Reich*, 457.

252 Goldstein, *Selected Papers*, 10.

253 Harrington, *Reenchanted Science*, 291–97.
254 However, Goldstein had been forced by Nazi officials to sign a document that he would never return to Germany. Belz, "Kurt Goldstein (1878–1965)," 28–33.
255 Anon., "Displaced Scholars" (1935). RAC, RF Archives, RG 1.1, series 717A, box 2, Spec. RAF. The Emergency Committee conceded to a payment of a sum of US$1,500 for his purpose.
256 Another such example of the problematic situation of finding positions in the North American medical system is represented in the search for an associate professorship in psychiatry at Washington University School of Medicine, a position that came to be filled by a German-trained émigré from Czechoslovakia. In the communications legitimizing the search, institutional and experiential factors played a great role together: "For the position of Associate in Neuro-Psychiatry it is proposed that a well-trained man be secured. It is believed that such a man is available. He is Dr. Michael Kasak [1888–1967?]. Dr. Kasak is a graduate of Washington School of Medicine and was a former assistant in the Department of Neurology. Since 1919 he has been Docent in Psychiatry at the University of Riga, Latvia. He has had a thorough continental training and had studied in Berlin, Paris, and Munich. He is well qualified by taste, experience, and study for the position. As part of his preliminary training he worked with Dr. Southard [it is probable that Elmer Ernest Southard, 1876–1920, is alluded to here; yet Kasak's direct training with Southard appears to be an error on the part of the Washington University School of Medicine committee chair, since Southard had already died in 1920, even though Kasak had stayed at the Boston Psychopathic Institute] at the Boston Psychopathic Institute … Dr. Kasak has also worked with Dr. [Egon] Lorenz [1891–1854] at the University of Wisconsin, and has published work while there." This unsigned letter was supposedly written by the chemist Philip A. Shaffer (1881–1960), who was the dean of Washington University's School of Medicine between 1937 and 1946. Archives and Rare Books Division of the Becker Library, WUSM [Washington University School of Medicine] (RG 01c, central administration records, subgroup 1: Office of the Dean, ser. 2, box 15, Medicine, School of, Department of Neurology and Psychiatry, Subdepartment of Neurology under Direction of Sidney I. Schwab [1871–1947]), 3–4.
257 Simmel, "Kurt Goldstein 1878–1965," 9.
258 Cf. Stahnisch, "Zur Zwangsemigration deutschsprachiger Neurowissenschaftler," 449–53.
259 Ulrich, "Kurt Goldstein," 15.
260 Lethen, *Lob der Kaelte*, 289.

CHAPTER FOUR

1 Wilhelm Erb, *Ueber die wachsende Nervositaet unserer Zeit*, 1; author's translation.

2 Hofer, *Nervenschwaeche und Krieg*, 45–88; Roelcke, "Electrified Nerves," 177–97; Kloocke, Schmiedebach, and Priebe, "Psychological Injury in the Two World Wars," 43–60.

3 Cf. Casper, "One Hundred Members of the Association of British Neurologists," 338–56.

4 Karenberg, "Klinische Neurologie in Deutschland," 20–9.

5 Tubbs, Loukas, Salter, and Oakes, "Wilhelm Erb and Erb's Point," 486–7.

6 Ibid., 487–8.

7 Schmiedebach, "The Public's View of Neurasthenia in Germany," 219–38; Eckart, "Die wachsende Nervositaet unserer Zeit," 9–38; Hofer, "War Neurosis and Viennese Psychiatry," 243–60.

8 Cf. MacMillan, *The War that Ended Peace*, 358–60.

9 The Freiburg neurologist Alfred Hauptmann (1881–1948), *Letter* (30 December 1917), to Max Nonne in Hamburg, qtd from Peiffer, *Hirnforschung in Deutschland*, 394; author's translation.

10 For the Austro-Hungarian context, see Blackshaw and Wieber, *Journeys into Madness*, 1–42.

11 The Berlin psychiatrist Fritz Mohr (1874–1957), *Letter* (26 August 1915) to Max Nonne, qtd from Peiffer, *Hirnforschung in Deutschland*, 861; author's translation.

12 As theatre director Max Reinhardt (1873–1943) so strikingly captured in his work at the time (1932), qtd from Weitz, *Weimar Germany*, 27.

13 Fritz Mohr, *Letter* (26 August 1915) to Max Nonne, qtd from Peiffer, *Hirnforschung in Deutschland*, 861; author's translation.

14 Mommsen, *Imperial Germany*, 1–100.

15 Taylor, *Grandeur et misère de la modernité*, 11 and 20 (author's emphasis).

16 Eckart, *Man, Medicine and the State*, 73–87.

17 Saretzki, *Reichsgesundheitsrat und Preussischer Landesgesundheitsrat*, 50–3.

18 Roelcke, "Electrified Nerves," 190–2.

19 Bumke, *Ueber Nervoese Entartung*, 104–5; author's translation (emphasis in original).

20 Radkau, *Das Zeitalter der Nervositaet*, 416–27; Zweig, *Erziehung vor Verdun*, 569.

21 Beard, *American Nervousness*, 23–6.

22 Ibid., 26.

23 Ibid., 76.

24 Heinrich Erb, *Letter* (2 February 1919) to Adolf von Struempell, qtd from Peiffer, *Hirnforschung in Deutschland*, 400; author's translation (emphasis in original).

25 Cf. Killen, *Berlin Electropolis*, 6–7 and 34–42.

26 Heinrich Erb, *Letter* (2 February 1919) to Adolf von Struempell, qtd from Peiffer, *Hirnforschung in Deutschland*, 400.

27 Weingart, Kroll, and Bayertz, *Rasse, Blut und Gene*, 251.

28 Kraepelin already used the term *Volkskoerper*, which later received high currency among Nazi physicians and public health workers. Bleker and Eckelmann, "'Der Erfolg der Gleichschaltungsaktion kann als durchschlagend bezeichnet werden," 87–96.

29 Kraepelin, *Memoirs*, 178–84.

30 Kraepelin, *Zur Entartungsfrage*, 745–51.

31 See, for example, Ruedin, *Studien ueber Vererbung*, 254–6; Hoche, *Handbuch der erichtlichen Psychiatrie*, 114–18.

32 Kraepelin, *Memoirs*, 118–29.

33 Hofer, "War Neurosis and Viennese Psychiatry," 258–9.

34 Cf. Ruedin, "Ueber den Zusammenhang zwischen Geisteskrankheit und Kultur," 741.

35 Finkelstein, *Emil du Bois-Reymond – Neuroscience, Self, and Society in Nineteenth-Century Germany*, 272–3.

36 Also, see Kraepelin, *Psychiatry*, 20–2 and 53.

37 Reichswehrministerium, Heeres-Sanitaetsinspektion. *Sanitaetsbericht ueber das deutsche Heer*, vol. 3, 46–53.

38 Weitz, *Weimar Germany*, 167–8.

39 See also Crouthamel, *Invisible Traumas*, 103.

40 Bumke, *Ueber Nervoese Entartung*, 62–7.

41 Ibid., 95; author's translation.

42 Kater, *Doctors under Hitler*, 128–32.

43 Roelcke, "Continuities or Ruptures?," 169–71.

44 Rilke, *Auguste Rodin*, 104; author's translation.

45 Binswanger, "Die Kriegshysterie," 45; author's translation.

46 Reichswehrministerium, Heeres-Sanitaetsinspektion. *Sanitaetsbericht ueber das deutsche Heer*, vol. 3, 46–53.

47 Crouthamel, *Invisible Traumas*, 103.

48 Eric Leed, *No Man's Land*, 110.

49 Ibid., 111.

50 Lerner, "Ein Sieg Deutschen Willens," 85–108.

51 Lerner, "Niedergang und Fall des Hermann Oppenheim," 16–22.

52 Blackshaw and Wieber, *Journeys into Madness*, 1–42.

53 Freud, "Ueber Kriegsneurosen, Elektrotherapie und Psychoanalyse," 939; author's translation.

54 Oppenheim, *Die traumatischen Neurosen*, 178.

55 Barwinski, "Trauma, Symbolisierungsschwaeche und Externalisierung," 24.

56 Oppenheim, *Die traumatischen Neurosen*, 178; author's translation.

57 Freud, "Einleitung," 5.

58 Freud, *Vorlesungen zur Einfuehrung in die Psychoanalyse*, 285.

59 Richards, *The Jewish World of Sigmund Freud*, 68; Leys, *Trauma: A Genealogy*, 18–20.

60 Weitz, *Weimar Germany*, 2–7.

61 See also Hau, *The Cult of Health and Beauty*, 102–24.

62 Sigmund Freud, *Letter* (21 September 1897) to Wilhelm Fliess, in Masson, *Sigmund Freud. Briefe an Wilhelm Fliess 1887–1904*, 283; author's translation.

63 Freud, *Meine Ansichten ueber die Rolle der Sexualitaet*, 152; Leys, *Trauma: A Genealogy*, 22–5.

64 Vogelsaenger, "Auf den Spuren der psychosomatischen Medizin," 255–71.

65 Oppenheim, "Der Krieg und die traumatischen Neurose," 257; author's translation.

66 Gocht later became the founding head of the department of orthopaedic surgery at the Berlin Charité. Gocht (1916), in Mollenhauer, "Bericht ueber die ausserordentliche Tagung der Deutschen Gesellschaft fuer Krueppelfuersorge," 74–88.

67 Ibid., 88; author's translation.

68 Remarque, *The Road Back*, 213.

69 Weitz, *Weimar Germany*, 32–4.

70 Alfred Hauptmann, *Letter* (28 December 1918) to Max Nonne, qtd from Peiffer, *Hirnforschung in Deutschland*, 399; author's translation (author's emphasis).

71 Max Nonne, *Letter* (4 December 1918) from the field to the neurologist Alfred Hauptmann, qtd from Peiffer, *Hirnforschung in Deutschland*, 399; author's translation.

72 Cf. Humphries and Kurschinski, *Rest, Relax, and Get Well*, 89–110; Kingsley Kent, *Aftershocks: Politics and Trauma in Britain, 1918–1933*, 10–34.

73 Eckart and Gradmann, *Die Medizin und der Erste Weltkrieg*, 1–7.

74 Tandler, "Zum Fall Wagner-Jauregg, Replik," columns 2045–89.

75 Becker, qtd from Crouthamel, *Invisible Traumas*, 103.

76 Weitz, *Weimar Germany*, 34–6.

77 In 1933, when the Nazis came to power in Germany, despite fifteen years of reparation payments, the Weimar Republic had only been able to pay back one eighth of its debt. Peukert, *The Weimar Republic*, 22–32.

78 Willi Meyer in *Berliner Tageblatt* (29 September 1920): n.p.; author's translation.

79 Linden and Jones, *German Battle Casualties*, 628.

80 Prussian State Assembly (28 March 1919).

81 Hartmann, 1919, 32–3, qtd from Crouthamel, *Invisible Traumas*, 103.

82 Ibid.

83 However, it shoud be pointed out that hardly any other view would be possible: rehabilitation and restitution to normal life remain the goal of similar efforts today, and are still regarded as amelioration of the patients' suffering and restoration of their ability to control their own lives. Cf. Weitz, *Weimar Germany*, 7–40.

84 Vogelsaenger, "Auf den Spuren der psychosomatischen Medizin," 255–71.

85 Hofer, *Nervenschwaeche und Krieg*, 13–42.

86 Freud, "Einleitung," 5.

87 Holdorff, "Ueber Max Lewandowskys Kriegsaufsatz," 61–6.

88 Stahnisch, "Sex and Human Behavior," 972–3.

89 Freud, "Einleitung," 5.

90 Abraham, "Erstes Korreferat," 35.

91 Freud, "Einleitung," 3.

92 Ibid., 3–8.

93 Freud, "Ueber Kriegsneurosen, Elektrotherapie und Psychoanalyse," 945.

94 Richards, *The Jewish World of Sigmund Freud*, 68.

95 Doeblin, *Unser Dasein*, 28; author's translation.

96 It is important in this respect to realize that the majority of the Weimar physicians were seriously opposed to social welfare programs, primarily after the massive doctors' strike (1923–24) – against political attempts to bring all physicians into state employment positions and thus out of their private practices and independent income – for what they understood as "the liberty of their profession." Eckart, *Man, Medicine and the State*, 73–87. For the Austrian situation see in Hofer, *Nervenschwaeche und Krieg*, 230–42.

97 Solbrig, Bundt, and Boehm, *Handbuecherei fuer Staatsmedizin*, 11–12; author's translation.

98 Ibid., 12–15.

99 For example, see the neurologist Alfred Hauptmann, *Letter* (1 November 1917) from the field, to Max Nonne, qtd from Peiffer, *Hirnforschung in Deutschland*, 871; author's translation.

100 Aschaffenburg, *Handbuch der Psychiatrie*, 4–6; author's translation.

101 Alfred Hauptmann, *Letter* (30 December, 1917) to Max Nonne in Hamburg, qtd from Peiffer, *Hirnforschung in Deutschland*, 394–5; author's translation.

102 Letter exchanges from October 1914 to January 1915 between Weil at the Western Front and Keibel in the Strasburg institute for anatomy. ADAS, AL 103 / No. 1200 / Pa. 254, Collection on the Medical Faculty, Department of Anatomy (January 1898–October 1918).

103 Wilhelm Erb, *Letter* (21 October 1921) to Adolf von Struempell in Leipzig, qtd from Peiffer, *Hirnforschung in Deutschland*, 410; author's translation.

104 Bumke, *Ueber Nervoese Entartung*, 74–105.

105 Roelcke, "Electrified Nerves," 177–97.

106 Von Weizsaecker, *Wahrnehmen und Bewegen. Die Taetigkeit des Nervensystems*, 30.

107 Harrington, *Reenchanted Science*, 103–39.

108 Von Weizsaecker, *Natur und Geist*, 54; author's translation.

109 Ibid., 60–5.

110 Janet, *L'automatisme psychologique*, 147; author's translation.

111 Freud, *Meine Ansichten ueber die Rolle der Sexualitaet* (1910), 149; author's translation.

112 Janet, *L'automatisme psychologique*, 148; author's translation.

113 Horn, "Erlebnis und Trauma," 135.

114 In a way, in this psychiatric service some type of holistic medicine continued in Germany even throughout the 1930s and 1940s, after Goldstein and members of his group had to flee Berlin. Yet in a similar way, because the overall therapeutic direction stood openly against the principles of emerging Nazi medical philosophy, von Weizsaecker encountered strong antagonism to his form of anthropological medicine from peer neurologists and psychiatrists early in the 1930s. Geisthoevel and Hitzer, *Auf der Suche nach einer anderen Medizin*, 146.

115 Friedrich Schultze, *Letter* (24 March 1934) to Max Nonne in Hamburg qtd from Peiffer, *Hirnforschung in Deutschland*, 501; author's translation (emphasis in original).

116 Carl Schneider, *Letter* (2 January 1935) to Ernst Ruedin in Munich qtd from Peiffer, *Hirnforschung in Deutschland*, 514; author's translation.

117 Majewsky and Sozańska, *Die Schlacht um Breslau*, 82–90.

118 Von Weizsaecker, *Soziale Krankheit und soziale Gesundung*, 31–75; author's translation.

119 (... *und dieser Fall ist politisch, ethisch und religiöes der Entscheidende*). Von Weizsaecker, "Vom Begriff der Therapie," 1169; author's translation.

120 Most notable is the recent biography by German historian of medicine Udo Benzenhoefer on Viktor von Weizsaecker. Benzenhoefer, *Der Arztphilosoph Viktor von Weizsaecker*, 161; author's translation.

121 Ibid., 162.

122 Ibid., 15–25.

123 Von Weizsaecker's type of medical theorizing can be perceived as something intrinsically "Weimar" in the form of a complementary conservative image that had its foundation in Christian traditions as well as social philosophy. This is what makes looking at anthropological medicine so promising, when the communities of Weimar brain psychiatrists and early neuroscientists are taken into account. While enriching the contemporary discourses about the mental and social pathologies, they drew inspiration for their work largely from social needs, political and religious backgrounds, and new technological advancements. Cf. Von Weizsaecker, "Soziologische Bedeutung der nervoesen Krankheiten," 295; author's translation.

124 Bielschowsky and Unger, "Die Ueberbrueckung grosser Nervenluecken," 309; author's translation.

125 Harrington, *Reenchanted Science*, 291–7; Dressler, "Viktor von Weizsaecker," 11–21.

126 Cf. Bronfen, Erdle, and Weigel, *Trauma*, 16–27; Harrington, ibid., 291–7.

127 Stahnisch and Nitsch, "Santiago Ramón y Cajal's Concept," 589–91.

128 Cf. Aschaffenburg, *Handbuch der Psychiatrie*, 5; Aschaffenburg, *Die Einteilung der Psychosen*, 7–15.

129 Paul Flechsig, *Letter* (13 August 1915) to Ludwig Edinger, qtd from Peiffer, *Hirnforschung in Deutschland*, 374; author's translation.

130 From an earlier manuscript draft of Constantin von Monakow and Raoul Mourge [b. 1847] for *Zeitschrift fuer Psychologie* 115, no. 4 (ca. 1921): 403–10, esp. 403. University of Zurich, Institute for Medical History and Museum, Archives; Monakow, Constantin von, Correspondence, Box 2.

131 Will, *Max Bielschowsky*, 130.

132 Ibid., 129–60.

133 Bielschowsky and Unger, "Die Ueberbrueckung grosser Nervenluecken," 309; author's translation.

134 Van Rahden, *Jews and Other Germans*, 21–63.

135 (*"Ueber einen Fall von Perityphlitis suppurativa mit Ausgang in Septico-Pyaemie"*). Kraepelin, *Memoirs*, 106–18.

136 The Bielschowsky method was essentially a derivative of Ramón y Cajal's famous gold-based staining method, which enabled microscopic views particularly of the finer endings of the nerve axon dendrites. Stahnisch, "Making the Brain Plastic," 415.

137 Alzheimer, "Ueber eine eigenartige Erkrankung der Hirnrinde," 146–8.

138 Dohm, *Geschichte der Histopathologie*, 302.

139 Stahnisch, "Making the Brain Plastic," 415.

140 Willibald Oscar Scholz (1889–1971); Richard Henneberg (1868–1962); Albert Dollinger (b. 1888); Stahnisch, "Zur Bedeutung der Konzepte der 'neuronalen De- und Regeneration,'" 243–69.

141 Holdorff, "Founding Years of Clinical Neurology in Berlin," 223–38.

142 Satzinger, *Die Geschichte der genetisch orientierten Hirnforschung*, 189–96.

143 Hagner, *Geniale Gehirne*, 288–302.

144 Will, "Max Bielschowsky," 130–1.

145 Burgmair and Weber, "Das Geld ist gut angelegt, und Du brauchst keine Reue haben," 343–78.

146 Deichmann and Mueller-Hill, *Biological Research at Universities*, 160–70.

147 The argument has been intriguingly made in Zimmerman, *Anthropology and Antihumanism*, 217–38.

148 Proctor, *The Nazi War on Cancer*, 15–57.

149 Schmiedebach, "The Public's View of Neurasthenia in Germany," 219–38.

150 Dohm, *Geschichte der Histopathologie*, 302.

151 Stahnisch, "Transforming the Lab," 46–8.

152 This research direction is prominently associated with Oskar Vogt's attempts to analyze a "genius brain," as represented in his histological investigation of Lenin's *cerebrum*. See Hagner, *Geniale Gehirne*, 54–81.

153 Max Bielschowsky, *Letter* (18 May 1933) to Julius Hallervorden (1882–1965) in Berlin, in which he informs the latter about the conflict with Mr V. Zirner, who was supported by Vogt, qtd from Peiffer, *Hirnforschung in Deutschland*, 394–5.

154 The guiding understanding was that an augmented morphology in the motor areas of the human cortex was, for example, associated with agricultural societies and augmentation of the strata of the occipital lobes and the sensorimotor cortex areas with industrialized surroundings. Satzinger, *Die Geschichte der genetisch orientierten Hirnforschung*, 91–5.

155 Bielschowsky, "Die Silberimpraegnation der Neurofibrillen," 169–70.

156 Marinesco, "L'hystérie après Babinski," 411–22.

157 Bielschowsky, "Entwurf eines Systems der Heredo-Degenerationen," 48–50; author's translation.

158 Engstrom, "Emil Kraepelin: Psychiatry and Public Affairs in Wilhelmine Germany," 111–32.

159 Hildebrandt, *The Anatomy of Murder*, 245.

160 Julius Hallervorden, *Letter* (18 December 1931) to Walther Spielmeyer in Munich, qtd from Peiffer, *Hirnforschung in Deutschland*, 462.

161 Will, *Max Bielschowsky*, 129–60.

162 Falk and Hauer, *Brandenburg-Goerden*, 10–98.

163 Max Reinhardt (1932), qtd from Weitz, *Weimar Germany*, 27.

164 Weitz, *Weimar Germany*, 32–6.

165 Ibid., 36–40.

166 Hobsbawm, *The Age of Extremes*, 468–9.

167 Geisthoevel and Hitzer, *Auf der Suche nach einer anderen Medizin*, 144–54.

168 Zuckermann, *Geschichte und Psychoanalyse*, 119–34.

169 Peiffer, *Hirnforschung in Deutschland*, 67–85.

CHAPTER FIVE

1 President Friedrich Ebert (1871–1925), *Rede zur Eroeffnung der Verfassungsgebenden Nationalversammlung* (6 February 1919), qtd from Weitz, *Weimar Germany*, 32.

2 Hauptmann, *Wanda*, 465; author's translation.

3 Cf. Marshall, *The German Naturalists and Gerhard Hauptmann*, 40; Delbrueck, "Gerhart Hauptmanns 'Vor Sonnenaufgang,'" 512–45; Dhuill, "Ein neues, maechtiges Volkstum," 405–22.

4 See also Roelcke, "Die Etablierung der psychiatrischen Genetik in Deutschland, Grossbritannien und den USA," 173–90; Hoff and Weber, "Sozialdarwinismus und die Psychiatrie im Nationalsozialismus," 1017–18.

5 As in Lorenz, "Proto-Eugenic Thought and Breeding Utopias in the United States before 1870," 67–90.

6 Winau, "Menschenzuechtung. Utopien und ethische Bewertung," 56; Lanzoni, "Diagnosing Modernity," 107–11.

7 Hilscher, *Gerhart Hauptmann*, 101.

8 Hass, *Gerhart Hauptmann*, 55.

9 Ploetz subsequently became the model for the literary figure of the alcohol prohibitionist "Alfred Loth" in Hauptmann's *Vor Sonnenaufgang*; and he also quoted him in this drama from Gustav von Bunge's (1844–1920) work *The Alcohol Question* (Germ. 1887).

10 Cowen, *Hauptmann. Kommentar zum dramatischen Werk*, 36; Sprengel, *Gerhart Hauptmann*, 254–66.

11 As in Weikart, *From Darwin to Hitler*, 86.

12 Qtd from Ehrenreich and English, *Complaints and Disorders*, 72.

13 Eden, *Socialism and Eugenics*, 9–10.

14 See, for example, Weber, "Ernst Ruedin, 1874–1952," 64–129.

15 Carl Hauptmann also became a significant writer and poet. Current themes of modern medicine and eugenics had been present in his publications since the 1890s; such as in Hauptmann, *Metaphysics in Modern Physiology*, 273–89 (*Metaphysik in der modernen Physiologie*).

16 Ringer, *The Decline of the German Mandarins*, 14–35.

17 Tschoertner, "Die Sieben," 70–1.

18 Kuechenhoff, "Der Psychiater Auguste Forel und seine Stellung zur Eugenik," 19–36.

19 See in Lenz, *Menschliche Auslese und Rassenhygiene*, 260.

20 The British minister and philosopher Thomas Robert Malthus (1766–1834). Forel, *Rueckblick auf mein Leben*, 156; author's translation.

21 Frank Wedekind was also the son of a physician, the Hannover gynaecologist Friedrich Wilhelm Wedekind (1816–1888), who after the failing bourgeois revolution of 1848 emigrated to San Francisco in California. As an introduction to Wedekind's personal pro-eugenic networks with writers and academics in the German-American context see Rothe, *Frank Wedekinds Dramen*, 76–80 and 93–8.

22 Becker, *Zur Geschichte der Rassenhygiene*, 61.

23 Hass, *Gerhart Hauptmann*, 1065; author's translation.

24 See Black, *War Against the Weak*, 261–2.

25 See, for example, in Hauptmann, *Atlantis*, 63–105 and 190–200; Weindling, *Health, Race and German Politics*, 68–9.

26 Ploetz, *Grundlinien einer Rassenhygiene*, 492; author's translation.

27 Ploetz, "Die Begriffe Rasse und Gesellschaft," 20.

28 Ibid., 17–19.

29 Stahnisch Eugenics, "The Early Eugenics Movement and Emerging Professional Psychiatry," 19–27.

30 Ploetz, "Die Begriffe Rasse und Gesellschaft," 15.

31 Lenz, "Eugenics in Germany," 223–31; author's translation (author's emphasis).

32 Cf. Weindling, *Health, Race and German Politics*, 155–69.

33 Kuehl, *The Nazi Connection*, 53–64.

34 Rissom, *Fritz Lenz und die Rassenhygiene*, 83–97; these exchanges often included the German émigré biologist Leo Loeb (1869–1959), with whom Charles B. Davenport corresponded on issues regarding funding for German brain psychiatry – on behalf of the Carnegie Institution of Washington and the Rockefeller Foundation in New York. Furthermore, Loeb, who held close contacts to eugenics researchers on both sides of the Atlantic, had an advisory member status on genetic issues at the Eugenics Record Office in Cold Spring Harbor. See, for example, Archives and Rare

Books Division of the Becker Library, WUSM (Loeb, Leo; FC0002; corr. C–Ha, box 2, n.p.).

35 Lenz, "Eugenics in Germany," 223.

36 Ibid., 224–6; author's translation (author's emphasis).

37 Cf. Reyer, *Eugenik und Paedagogik*, 54; Kraepelin, *Zur Entartungsfrage*, 745–51; Alzheimer, "Ist die Einrichtung einer psychiatrischen Abteilung im Reichsgesundheitsamt erstrebenswert," 242–46; Sommer, "Eine psychiatrische Abteilung des Reichsgesundheitsamtes," 295–8.

38 See Ploetz, "Die Begriffe Rasse und Gesellschaft," 2–3; author's translation.

39 Similar assumptions help to explain why some Jewish psychiatrists not only fostered proto-eugenic thought, but continued to hold racial hygienic ideas themselves. One interesting case, for instance, is the genetic psychiatrist Franz Joseph Kallmann, who worked closely together with Ruedin in Munich and decided to leave Germany only in 1939 – just before the outbreak of World War II. Cf. Mildenberger, "Auf der Spur des 'Scientific Pursuit,'" 183–200; Rainer, "Franz Kallmann's Views on Eugenics," 1361–2.

40 In 1942, Pauline Ruedin committed suicide in Switzerland under obscure conditions. Brinkschulte, "Weibliche Aerzte," 179–80.

41 See in Borck, "Mediating Philanthropy," 3; Weber, "Harnack-Prinzip oder Fuehrerprinzip?" 412.

42 Vom Brocke, *Bevoelkerungswissenschaft – Quo vadis?* 436.

43 Weiss, "The Race Hygiene Movement in Germany," 193–236.

44 Weindling, *Health, Race and German Politics*, 305–98.

45 Von Verschuer, "Alfred Ploetz," 69–72; Ruedin, "Ehrung von Prof. Dr. Alfred Ploetz," 473–4.

46 Rickman, *Rassenpflege im voelkischen Staat*, 331.

47 Kurbegović, *Eugenics in Comparative Perspective*, 53–9.

48 See in Dowbiggin, *Keeping America Sane*, 70–190.

49 Weikart, *From Darwin to Hitler*, 84.

50 See Buchholz and Wolbert, *Die Lebensreform*, 25–33.

51 Cf. Richardson, *Love and Eugenics in the Late Nineteenth Century*, 65–7.

52 Weikart, *From Darwin to Hitler*, 15; MacLennan, "Beyond the Asylum," 7–23.

53 Cf. Karenberg, "Klinische Neurologie in Deutschland," 20–9.

54 Schmiedebach, "The Public's View of Neurasthenia in Germany," 219–38; Eckart, "Die wachsende Nervositaet unserer Zeit," 9–38; Hofer, "War Neurosis and Viennese Psychiatry," 243–60.

55 Voss, "Die Anfaenge der Institutionalisierung der klinischen Neurologie in Muenchen," 210–18.

56 Erb, *Ueber die wachsende Nervositaet unserer Zeit*, 1.

57 In his own scientific work, Erb – like Alzheimer and Forel – had made important anatomical discoveries and introduced a number of clinical signs and symptoms into medical diagnostics and psychosomatic medicine. Zuerner, *Von der Hirnanatomie zur Eugenik*, 160, 280–81, and 292–7.

58 Radkau, *Das Zeitalter der Nervositaet*, 9–15.

59 Roelcke, "Electrified Nerves," 177–97.

60 Morel, *Traité des dégénérescences physiques, et intellectuelles et morales*, 1–7.

61 Ibid., 53–74.

62 Ibid., 57–78; Engstrom, *Clinical Psychiatry in Imperial Germany*, 194–8.

63 Fangerau and Mueller, *Das Standardwerk der Rassenhygiene*, 1039–46.

64 Ackerknecht, *A Short History of Psychiatry*; Roelcke, "*Wir ruecken Schritt vor Schritt dem Tolhause naeher*," 56–67; Stahnisch, *Transforming the Lab*, 41–54.

65 From an earlier manuscript draft of von Monakow and Mourge, *Zeitschrift fuer Psychologie* 115, no. 4 (1928), 403–4. Institute for Medical History and Museum, Archives; Monakow, Constantin von, Correspondence, Box 2.

66 Radkau, *Das Zeitalter der Nervositaet*, 263–353.

67 It is interesting to see that similar assumptions were also widespread in the American eugenics community, which saw the American Civil War as a pivotal point of deterioration, because of the casualties it sustained within the white American population. It was assumed by Davenport and his followers that the perceived degeneration of US society had devastating long-term effects for a broad range of public health issues. Cf. Allan, "The Ideology of Elimination," 13–39.

68 Kraepelin, *Zur Entartungsfrage*, 745–51.

69 Kraepelin, *Memoirs*, 132–64.

70 Weindling, *Health, Race and German Politics*, 20–5.

71 Lenz, "Eugenics in Germany," 226.

72 Gruber, *Die Erhaltung und Mehrung der deutschen Volkskraft*, 253.

73 Also, see Engstrom, *Clinical Psychiatry in Imperial Germany*, 88–120.

74 Steinberg, "Alfred Erich Hoche in der Psychiatrie seiner Zeit," 68–102.

75 In Binding and Hoche, *Die Freigabe der Vernichtung lebensunwerten Lebens*, 22–3; author's translation.

76 See Crouthamel, *Invisible Traumas*, 103.

77 Ploetz qtd from Lenz, "Eugenics in Germany," 224.

78 This neo-Malthusian critique of social welfare programs as meeting the needs of modern disease forms due to changing industrialized work

conditions is also pertinent to the western side of the Atlantic – for example in the polemics of Margaret Sanger. Drogin, *Margaret Saenger*, 11–29; Sanger, *The Pivot of Civilization*.

79 Ruedin in the beginning of this public health debate; compare for example: Ruedin, *Studien ueber Vererbung*, 254–5; author's translation.

80 The Ministry of Finance had initially set aside one billion, two hundred million marks, which later had to be raised to four billion, encompassing one-third of the Republic's annual budget. The Labour Ministry's Pension Offices administered financial support, the National Insurance System continued medical care, and the pension courts decided on respective medical cases. See Crouthamel, *Invisible Traumas*, 100–61.

81 Steinberg, "Oswald Bumke in Leipzig," 348–56.

82 This was largely promoted by Bumke's influential treatise *On Nervous Degeneration* (1912). Bumke, *Ueber Nervoese Entartung*, here 74–96.

83 See also Hau, *The Cult of Health and Beauty*, 102–24.

84 Ernst Ruedin, *Letter* (10 July 1928) to accompany his funding application for the KWG. Personal File Ruedin; Historisches Archiv des Max-Planck-Instituts fuer Psychiatrie, Div. I, Rep. IA; author's translation.

85 Kuehl, *The Nazi Connection*, 105–6.

86 Weber, "Die Deutsche Forschungsanstalt fuer Psychiatrie," 25–6.

87 Cf. Leys and Evans, *Defining American Psychology*, 39–57; Lamb, *Pathologist of the Mind*, 99–129.

88 For example, see Brown, *Friendship and Philanthropy*, 288–311.

89 Meyer, *Prospectus of the Summer School of Neurology and Psychiatry*, 24.

90 Swiss émigré psychiatrist Adolph Meyer also ranged high on Alan Gregg's important support list of US and Canadian brain science. With a very strong influence, Meyer managed to be engaged as consultant and referee in a great number of job-finding commissions for psychiatrists and neurologists throughout the US and Eastern Canada. See, for example, Archives and Rare Books Division of the Becker Library, WUSM (RG C15:2, Department of Neurology and Psychiatry, series 2, Gregg's List, Am Assoc. of Colleges Med. Schools – of 1936), n.p.

91 Among the aids given by the Rockefeller Foundation in support of German biomedicine after the war was the provision of eugenics literature. With the help of the Deutsche Forschungsgemeinschaft, German psychiatrists had asked, for example, for a complete set of the Galton Laboratory of National Eugenics – Lecture and Memoir Series. By means of the middleman Aber Pearce (1881–1960), "with whom you have had a conference recently in regard to the medical literature which we are sending in your care," the literature became distributed widely in the way of a "reading circle" so that

every German medical school could make carbon copies for their needs; see RAC, RF Archives, RG 1.1, series 717, box 11, folder 67, 6–8.

92 Rockefeller Foundation officer John V. Van Sickle (1862–1939) writing back to the New York headquarter, after having visited Frankfurt am Main on May 15, 1931. RAC, RF archives, series 1.1, RG 717A, box 12, folder 97, 1–2.

93 Von Schwerin, *Experimentalisierung des Menschen*, 247–328; Weber, "*Harnack-Prinzip oder Fuehrerprinzip?*, 410–18.

94 Brown, *Friendship and Philanthropy*, 288–311.

95 Oppenheimer, qtd from Penfield, *The Difficult Art of Giving*, 370.

96 To a limited degree, this also included Canada, for example with grants and travel fellowships given out to neurochemist J.B.S. Browne (b. 1873?), McGill University/Goettingen (Germany), or neurophysiologist Velyien E. Henderson (1877–1945), University of Alberta/Berlin (Germany).

97 Alan Gregg, *What Is Psychiatry?* (Ms. New York, 1941, 9 pp.). RAC, RF Archives, RG 1.1, series 717A, box 1.1/2, folder 19, 9.

98 Anon, *German Displaced Scholars* (Ms. New York, 1935–36, 46 pp.). RAC, RF Archives, KG 6.1, series 1.1, box, folder, 8f.

99 Ruedin, *Studien ueber Vererbung*, 254–5.

100 Alan Gregg, *Letter* (25 October 1937) to RF officer D.P. O'Brian. RAC, RF Archives, DFA Psych. Res. 1936–40, RG 1.1, series 717A, box 10, 58–9.

101 Kraepelin, *Memoirs*, 118–19.

102 Anon. *Project Proposal* (DFA Psych. Hist. Rec. 1925–28, 54 pp.). RAC, RD Archives, RG 1.1, series 717 A, box 9, 11; RAC (author's emphasis).

103 As Borck, *Mediating Philanthropy*, 3, has worked out for the RAC. These findings could be confirmed through archival material in the Historisches Archiv des Max-Planck-Instituts fuer Psychiatrie, such as RAC, RF 1.1, KWI for Psychiatry, Germany, Felix Plaut, Memo 6 / 21 / 35PCO53.

104 For example, see the letter exchanges of neurologist Richard Schmidt (1873–1945) of the University of Frankfurt medical school in the 1940s with both Deutsche Forschungsgemeinschaft and the chair of the committee on military medicine (*Fachgliederung Wehrmedizin*), Berlin surgeon Ferdinand Sauerbruch (1875–1951). BA KO, Collections on the *Deutsche Forschungsgemeinschaft* R 73 / 14414 / (Film 2950 K–R 73-010022001000161), 13/1. Also, see Mitscherlich and Mielke, *Medizin ohne Menschlichkeit*, 133–204.

105 Weber, *Ernst Ruedin*, 53–92.

106 Alan Gregg, *Letter* (8 November 1935) to the clinical psychiatrist and epidemiologist Roy Grinker (1900–1993) in Chicago, IL. RAC, RF Archives, AG (Germany), series 106.

107 Alan Gregg, *Diary Entry* (24 February 1950), DFA Psych. Res. 1945–48/50. RAC, RF Archives, RG 1.1, series 717, box 89, 10.
108 Cf. Brown, *Friendship and Philanthropy*, 288–311.
109 Walther Spielmeyer, *Letter* (27 November 1934) to Alan Gregg in New York City, RAC, RF Archives, RG 1.1, series 717, box 9, folder 56, 108; author's translation.
110 For further cases, see the example of the socialist eugenics and forced sterilization program in the northern US State of Minnesota that was advanced by German-speaking immigrant physicians: Holtan, "The Eitels and Their Hospital," 52–4; for a Canadian case consult Gibson, "Involuntary Sterilization of the Mentally Retarded," 59–63.
111 Doeleke, *Alfred Ploetz, Sozialdarwinist und Gesellschaftsbiologe*, 46.
112 This is explicitly addressed in: Alfred Ploetz, *Letter* (December 24, 1913) to Gerhard Hauptmann in Breslau, qtd from Luedecke, *Der 'Fall Saller' und die Rassenhygiene*, 49.
113 For a comparison see Harwood, *Styles of Scientific Thought*, 138–80.
114 Alfred Ploetz, *Letter* (24 December 1913) to Gerhard Hauptmann in Breslau, qtd from Luedecke, *Der 'Fall Saller' und die Rassenhygiene*, 49.
115 Kraepelin, *Psychiatry*, 68–9.
116 Hoche referred to them as "*die Entarteten* or *Personen mit Hirndegeneration.*" Hoche, *Handbuch der gerichtlichen Psychiatrie*, 429–31.
117 Harrington, *Reenchanted Science*, 178–96.

CHAPTER SIX

1 Arnold Zweig (1887–1968). Arnold Zweig in *Theater, Drama, Politik* (10 January, 1921), qtd from Weitz, *Weimar Germany*, 27 (author's emphasis).
2 Among many others, see Zimmerman, *Anthropology and Antihumanism*, 38–67; Sarkin, *Germany's Genocide of the Herero*, 205–25; Proctor, *Racial Hygiene*, 3; Kater, *Doctors under Hitler*, 189–248.
3 Cf. Noth, "Robert Wartenberg," 575; Focke, *William G. Niederland*, 142–223; Kumbier and Haack, "Alfred Hauptmann," 204–9.
4 Kuemmel, "Die Ausschaltung rassisch und politisch missliebiger Aerzte," 56–81.
5 Eckart, *Man, Medicine and the State*, 7–12.
6 Schmuhl, *Hirnforschung und Krankenmord*, 53–6; Aly, *Aktion T4 1939–1945*, 189–92.
7 Cf. Galison, Graubard, and Mendelsohn, *Science in Culture*, v–vii; Harwood, "Weimar Culture and Biological Theory," 347–77; Haraway, "A Game of Cat's Cradle," 59–71.

8   Weindling, *John W. Thompson*, 3–10; Nicosia and Huener, *Medicine and Medical Ethics in Nazi Germany*, 1–15.

9   Shevell, "Neurosciences in the Third Reich," 132–8; and Lilienthal, "Patientinnen und Patienten aus brandenburgischen Heil- und Pflegeanstalten," 303–18.

10 Proctor, *Racial Hygiene*, 3.

11 See, for example, Kroener, *Von der Rassenhygiene zur Humangenetik*, 14–37.

12 This is apparent from nearly one hundred grant applications during the 1920s and early 1930s sent to the German Research Council that pertained to the wider field of neuroscience research activities. Notgemeinschaft/DFG, Praesidium Minutes (no day or month given, 1920), BA KO, Collections on the Deutsche Forschungsgemeinschaft R 73/69, 63.

13 Hollingsworth, "Institutionalizing Excellence in Biomedical Research," 15–18.

14 Kuhn, *The Structure of Scientific Revolutions*, 2–9.

15 Collmann, "Georges Schaltenbrand (26.11.1897–24.10.1979)," 65–73.

16 Schaltenbrand soon enrolled with a number of party organizations, such as the NSDAP, NSDAeB, NS *Volkswohlfahrt* and the NS *Fliegerkorps*. Ibid., 73–8.

17 Cf. the 1938/9 infrastructure research grant (principle investigator: Georges Schaltenbrand) from the DFG in BA KO, collection on the DFG, R73 / 14224: "Etiology of Multiple Sclerosis" (title of original grant application in German).

18 Shevell, "Neurosciences in the Third Reich," 132–8.

19 Klee, *Auschwitz, die NS-Medizin und ihre Opfer*, 67–71.

20 Letters of Hans Conrad Julius Reiter to the Deutsche Forschungsgemeinschaft, 1935 in BA KO, collection on the Deutsche Forschungsgemeinschaft, R 73 / 12475.

21 Schaltenbrand, *Die Multiple Sklerose des Menschen*, 180–201; Steger and Schaltenbrand, "Das Myogramm bei der Katatonie," 183–207.

22 Shevell, "Neurosciences in the Third Reich," 132–8.

23 See the intriguing review provided by Innes and Kurland, "Is Multiple Sclerosis Caused by a Virus?" 574–85.

24 Shorter, *Partnership for Excellence*, 249–50.

25 It is interesting to note that since about ten years ago, the viral hypothesis of multiple sclerosis aetiology has again been supported by studies in neuroanatomy, neuroserology, and epidemiology, which used the available data from the 1940s as a starting point. Cf. Marie, "Sclérose en plaques," 287–9, 305–7, 349–51 and 365–6; Williamson, "The Early Pathological Changes," 373–9.

26 (*Uebertragungsversuche vom Affen auf den Menschen und vom Menschen auf den Affen*). Schaltenbrand, *Die Multiple Sklerose des Menschen*, 120–201.
27 Schaltenbrand, "Der uebertragbare Markscheidenschwund," 1066–77.
28 Reuland, *Menschenversuche in der Weimarer Republik*, 82–91 and 248–53.
29 Cf. Roelcke, "Wissenschaften zwischen Innovation und Entgrenzung," 92–109.
30 Binching and Hoche, *Die Freigabe der Vernichtung lebensunwerten Lebens*, 17. There have recently been attempts to highlight the research contributions of Schaltenbrand through Wuerzburg-based neurologists on grounds of oral history interviews with family members and former colleagues. However, the murderous human experiments performed by Schaltenbrand were not further addressed, while the gist of this literature leads instead into a retroactive legitimization of Schaltenbrand's outright unethical research without critique of the oral history-taking methodology. Furthermore, Schaltenbrand's own ideological stances to win over Nazi officials to receive instantaneous rewards for his research program are likewise not contextualized. Publications of this kind tend to downgrade Nazi doctors' inhuman treatment of psychiatric and neurological patients during World War II. See in: Collmann, "Georges Schaltenbrand (26.11.1897–24.10.1979)," 78–88.
31 Klee, *Auschwitz, die NS-Medizin und ihre Opfer*, 70–5.
32 Maehle, "Doctors in Court, Honour, and Professional Ethics," 61–79.
33 Cf. Bleker, "'Der Erfolg der Gleichschaltungsaktion kann als durchschlagend bezeichnet werden,'" 87–96.
34 BA KO R73/II *Individual and Scientific Funding Files, Part I.*, 14 224, Schaltenbrand, G. (Aetiology of MS); Clinical Department of Neurology and Psychiatry at the University of Wuerzburg.
35 Shevell, "Neurosciences in the Third Reich," 132–8.
36 Roelcke, "Funding the Scientific Foundations of Race Policies: Ernst Ruedin and the Impact of Career Resources on Psychiatric Genetics, ca. 1910–1945," 73–87.
37 Weber, *Ernst Ruedin*, 174–205.
38 Ploetz, *Grundlinien einer Rassenhygiene*, ii; author's translation.
39 Kuehl, *The Nazi Connection*, 77–84.
40 He participated in this international conference literally during the last days of peace before World War II broke out. Weber, *Ernst Ruedin*, 185–97.
41 Adams, Allen, and Weiss, "Human Heredity and Politics," 232.

42 Campbell, qtd from Kuehl, *The Nazi Connection*, 132–4.

43 Weber, *Ernst Ruedin*, 193–205.

44 Stahnisch, "Flexible Antworten – Offene Fragen," 56–8.

45 Weber, "Von Emil Kraepelin zu Ernst Ruedin," 419–35.

46 Weber, *Ernst Ruedin*, 191–3.

47 The Reichsuniversitaet Strassburg was established similar to the other Reichsuniversitaeten in the Ostmark of former Czechoslovakia and Poland (such as Prague, Posen, and Dorpat, and others) in a comprehensive education program to establish Nazi German ideologies, administration, and hegemony over the occupied territories. Wechsler, *La Faculté de Médecine*, 12–31.

48 Ibid., 52–3.

49 Steinberg and Angermeyer, *Two Hundred Years of Psychiatry at Leipzig University*, 253–4.

50 In individual cases, forced sterilizations have been documented in the department of psychiatry and neurology at the Reichsuniversitaet under Bostroem's headship. Wechsler, *La Faculté de Medécine*, 106–219. The complete extension of that program still needs to be further addressed, however.

51 See the grant applications for neuroscientific research projects to the Notgemeinschaft/DFG (First Part), BA KO, General Collection of the Deutsche Forschungsgemeinsichaft, for example, R 73/ 11940, n.p. The support for Nikolaus Jensch can be seen as aligned with the general concentration of the Deutsche Forschungsgemeinschaft program in its funding activities on particularly well known departments of physiology and anatomy, as well as a more-than-equal system of support for research projects that sided with institutes of the KWG or other major extra-university institutions. This organization of the funding support shows that the Deutsche Forschungsgemeinschaft concentrated its available funds on renowned research centres, while the Reichsuniversitaet Strassburg came back into particular focus in the early 1940s.

52 Wechsler, *La Faculté de Médecine*, 187–201.

53 In his preparations of the bodies of murdered inmates from concentration camp Natzweiler-Struthof, he was helped by Anton Kiesselbach (1907–1984). Dr Kiesselbach was his former doctoral student at the University of Frankfurt, who followed Hirt to teach introductory courses in macroscopic anatomy at the Strasburg medical faculty. Kieselbach's funding, however, came almost exclusively from the Foundation *Ahnenerbe* of the SS. He later had a prolific career as *Ordinarius* professor of anatomy at the Medical Academy of Dueseldorf during the

postwar period, being well funded by the regional industry and national West German funding agencies. Pátek, *Die Entwicklung der Anatomie in Duesseldorf*, 82–95.

54 Apart from advancing general neuroscientific knowledge about the autonomic nervous system, the Strasburg researchers also aimed at applicable knowledge for the *Wehrmacht*: Since Germany's attack on the Soviet Union on 21 June 1941, thousands of soldiers had suffered from the aftereffects of frostbite during the grim Russian winters. It was well known that deep freeze temperatures led to sympathetic blood vessel constrictions and accelerated the velocity, and the tissue damage of frostbite in extremities. The Strasburg group of researchers, Hirt among a number of others from various departments, had offered to study the anatomical, pathophysiological, and pharmacological mechanisms leading to sympathetic actions, such as vasoconstrictions. As with Hirt's intention to chum up with Nazi officials to receive support for racial anthropology through the creation of the skeleton collection from concentration camp inmates, the neuroscientific context can likewise be seen in an "applied impetus" of the research pursued at Strasburg. See, for example, Schuetz, *Die Wirksamkeit der Sympathikusinfiltration und lumbalen Sympathektomie im Vergleich zur konservativen Therapie bei Erfrierungen* (1944).

55 Lullies, *Vegetative Physiologie: Blutkreislauf, Atmung, Stoffwechsel, Verdauung u. Exkretion*, 13–27.

56 Lullies, *Aktionsstroeme und Fasergruppen im Extremitaetennerven von Maja squinado* (1936).

57 After his "de-Nazification process," Lullies became the founding dean of the medical faculty in Homburg an der Saar in 1947, later an *Ordinarius* professor at the University of Kiel. Buerger, "Lullies, Hans," 1436.

58 Kaiserling, "Die Ausbreitungsformen der Nierenlymphbahninfekte und die lymphogene Nephrose," 561–87.

59 Fischer had managed to keep his Jewish origins secret until the beginning of World War II and then fled from Nazi Germany and emigrated to North America. Kaiserling's nationalist convictions were also very prominently reflected in his political dispute with Eugen Gerstenmaier (1906–1986). As a theologist, Gerstenmaier was refused a university position during the 1940s, since he had criticized the influence of Nazi ideologies on the German university system. Gerstenmaier later became the first president of the Parliament in the Federal Republic of Germany. Compare with "Ich Dien. Schaden durch Entschaedigung," *Der Spiegel* 4 (1 January 1969), n.p.

60 Wechsler, *La Faculté de Médecine*, 242–5.

61 See further the file records on "Military Medical Research;" BA KO, Collections on the *Deutsche Forschungsgemeinschaft* R 73 / 314–16.

62 Proctor, *Racial Hygiene*, 219–21; Weindling, *Victims and Survivors of Nazi Human Experiments Science and Suffering in the Holocaust*, 80–5.

63 Hildebrandt, *The Anatomy of Murder*, 153–7.

64 Fleischmann also had a remarkable postwar career as a science administrator and renowned experimental physicist at the Universities of Hamburg and Erlangen-Nuernberg. Weiss, "Der Kernphysiker Rudolf Fleischmann," 107–18.

65 Wechsler, *La Faculté de Médecine*, 169–76.

66 Goudsmith, *Alsos*, 5–35.

67 Craig, Scholarship and Nation Building, 220–5.

68 Stahnisch, "Griesinger, Wilhelm," 582–3.

69 Todes, *Ivan Pavlov*, 99–103.

70 Schilder's life ended tragically in a traffic accident in front of the New York hospital, where his son was born a few days earlier, while Schilder was visiting his wife at her childbed. Wittels, "Paul Schilder," 13–34.

71 Bostroem moved on to become the founding curator of the Reichsuniversitaet in Strasburg. After he had to leave the position of curator at the Reichsuniversitaet in 1942, due to the internal rivalries among the Nazi leadership group in Strasburg, Bostroem later returned to his chair and continued his research work. With his consultant physician Werner Wagner (1904–1956), he pursued somatically oriented research in the Leipzig tradition on questions of encephalitis, genetic development and neurosyphilis. Richard Arwed Pfeifer, Report (7 May 1946) to the Soviet Military Administration. Leipzig 1946, Film 1339, UAL [University Archives Leipzig], Collection on the Human Resources Department PA 48 (Richard Arwed Pfeifer), 81–105.

72 Ibid., 81–105. For the involvement of Schroeder and other faculty members of the University of Leipzig, see Schmuhl, *Hirnforschung und Krankenmord*, 20–48. The Leipzig situation regarding the involvement of faculty and physicians in the hereditary health courts and the euthansia program is described in Steinberg and Angermeyer, *Two Hundred Years of Psychiatry at Leipzig University*, 245–52.

73 Pfeifer's silence about the role that he and other Leipzig psychiatrists played in the Nazi atrocities kept him out of the limelight of the new Soviet leadership and allowed him to continue his successful career as a psychiatrist during the founding years of the German Democratic Republic. Krause, *Alma Mater Lipsiensis*, 587.

74 Bay HStA, MK 8/I Ministry of Science, Education and Art, 70335 Denazification, n.p.

75 Steinberg, "Oswald Bumke in Leipzig," 348–56.

76 Richard Arwed Pfeifer, *Report* (7 May 1946) to the Soviet Military Administration. Leipzig 1946, Film 1339, UAL, Collection on the Human Resources Department PA 48 (Richard Arwed Pfeifer), 59; author's translation. Certain prudence, however, applies here in following Pfeifer's description, since Bumke undoubtedly understood neuropathological work to be of foundational value for modern psychiatry. As an important example, he invited the Munich neuroanatomist and pathologist Hugo Spatz to contribute central basic science chapters for his textbook, on "Senile, Presenile, and Arteriosclerotic Forms of Dementia" and on "Anatomico-Pathological Findings in Hereditary Imbecility," in Bumke, *Lehrbuch der Geisteskrankheiten*, 461–81 and 608–13, thereby showing that he strove for an integration of the basic and clinical neurosciences with psychiatry.

77 Angermeyer and Steinberg, *200 Jahre Psychiatrie*, 105–30.

78 Dean Werner Hueck, *Report* (15 November 1945) to the Soviet Military Government on the History and Current State of the Medical Faculty. Leipzig 1945, Film 1339, UAL, Collection on the Medical Faculty BI 39, 1–69.

79 The separation of "neurological surgery" from the clinical department of neurology and psychiatry was closely associated with the influence of its founding director (1946–1956), Georg Merrem (1908–1971), who emphasized that the specialized surgical approach "of our modern times" could no longer be carried out by traditional neurologists and internists. Educated at the universities of Tuebingen and Berlin, Merrem had written his MD thesis on "The Treatment of Multiple Sclerosis with Germanin" (*Die Behandlung der Multiplen Sklerose mit Germanin*) in 1933, which followed the pathophysiological concept of multiple sclerosis that Georges Schaltenbrand had developed. Schaltenbrand, one of the most prominent neuropathologists in Germany between the 1930s to the 1950s, was an intimate friend of Merrem's neurosurgical mentor Wilhelm Toennis. Arnold, *Neurochirurgie in Deutschland*, 124.

80 Similar to Merrem in the German Democratic Republic, his western *pendant*, the neurosurgeon Wilhelm Toennis at Cologne University, had pursued the recent differential diagnostics, operational practices, and clinical research approaches of the new field of neurological surgery as founded by Emil Heymann (1878–1936) at the Auguste Victoria Hospital in Berlin. While Heymann was ousted from his position as a Jewish scientist in 1933, the next generation of neurosurgical trainees rose as stars in German

neurosurgery after World War II. Their close association with Toennis was beneficial for other neurosurgeons of this group too: Merrem, for example, became a founder of the German Society for Neurosurgery and their German Democratic Republic delegate. In a way, Merrem assumed the same leadership status in East Germany as Toennis in the Federal Republic of Germany, while both continued their communication, before the physical separation of the two postwar Germanies. Furthermore, Toennis invited the neurologist and neuropathologist Klaus Joachim Zuelch to leave Hamburg and join him in Cologne after Toennis had become a scientific member of the KWG in 1948 and assumed a position in the newly founded Max Planck Gesellschaft. It resembled their earlier collaboration between 1936 and 1944 in Berlin; and thus transcended a research network from the German National Socialist period into the postwar Federal Republic of Germany. Juergen Peiffer, *Letter* (10 June 2005) to author; Stahnisch, *Georg Merrem*, 71–6.

81 Bleker, "'Der Erfolg der Gleichschaltungsaktion kann als durchschlagend bezeichnet werden," 87–96; Weindling, *John W. Thomson*, 3–10.
82 Kater, *Doctors Under Hitler*, 52–102.
83 Cf. Proctor, *Racial Hygiene*, 131–76; Nicosia and Huener, *Medicine and Medical Ethics in Nazi Germany*, 1–15; and Weindling, *Health, Race and German Politics*, 489–564.
84 Kater, "The Burden of the Past: Problems of a Modern Historiography of Physians and Medicine in Nazi Germany," 31–56.
85 Bleker, "'Der Erfolg der Gleichschaltungsaktion kann als durchschlagend bezeichnet werden," 87–96.
86 The *voelkisches Ideal* of the Nazi government, its inflammatory conception of Aryan race supremacy, and its increasing violence toward patients and the mentally handicapped in German society also symbolized the overall hatred for Weimar democratic society. The gist of this aggressive pursuit is perhaps best represented in the ninety-six members of the German parliament in the Reichstag who had been murdered in the torture cells of the Gestapo and in concentration camps. Mommsen, "The Reichstag Fire and Its Political Consequences," 129–222; Hohendorf and Magull-Seltenreich, *Von der Heilkunde zur Massentoetung. Medizin im Nationalsozialismus*, 143–6.
87 Herrn, *Magnus Hirschfeld*, 97–152.
88 Heberer-Rice and Matthaeus, *Atrocities on Trial*, 27.
89 For the influences on the universities, see: Kater, *Doctors under Hitler*, 103–56; Nicosia and Huener, *Medicine and Medical Ethics in Nazi Germany*, 1–15; and Weindling, *Health, Race and German Politics*, 489–564.

90 Bleker, "Der Erfolg der Gleichschaltungsaktion kann als durchschlagend bezeichnet werden," 87–96.

91 Medawar and Pyke, *Hitler's Gift*, 231–40.

92 Fischer, *Identification of Emigration-Induced Scientific Change*, 23–47; Niederland, *The Emigration of Jewish Academics*, 285–300.

93 Stahnisch, *How the Nerves Reached the Muscle*, 351–84.

94 Fischer, *Identification of Emigration-Induced Scientific Change*, 23–47.

95 Krohn, *Handbuch der deutschsprachigen Emigration 1933–1945*, vol. 3, 904–1048; Niederland, *The Emigration of Jewish Academics*, 285–300.

96 Archives and Rare Books Division of the Becker Library, WUSM (PCO53, records of the American Academy of Neurology, series 7, history committee files, box 3, folder: historical materials, 1948–1953, lists of the American Academy of Neurology-committees); see also Loewenau, "Between Resentment and Aid," 348–62.

97 Juette, *Die Emigration der deutschsprachigen 'Wissenschaft des Judentums,'* 17–122; Soellner, *Deutsche Politikwissenschaftler in der Emigration*, 134–96.

98 For this genre, see authors who, like Medawar and Pyke, *Hitler's Gift*, 231–40, argue that the emigration wave of Central European émigré scientists just resulted in "a transfusion of fresh intellectual blood" to other countries abroad. See also Koch, *Deemed Suspect*, 230–54. Most recently, Bernd Holdorff has drawn attention to the "brain loss" that the Berlin context incurred between 1933 and 1945, see Holdorff, *Die Neurologie in Berlin, 1840–1945*, 202–33.

99 In fact, the exodus of psychoanalysts such as the Vienna-trained founder of modern psychosomatic medicine Franz Gabriel Alexander (1891–1964), who came to the University of Chicago; Frankfurt neurologist Leo Alexander (1905–1985) at Tufts in Boston; Sandor Radó (1890–1972) from Budapest, who went to Columbia University, where he became the head of psychiatry; Helene Deutsch (1884–1982) from Vienna, who went to Boston and co-founded the Boston Psychoanalytic Institute); or the German émigré psychiatrist Charles Fischer (1902–1987), later at the New York Psychoanalytic Institute, probably shaped American psychiatry, neurology, and mental health in more ways than any other process related to forced migration. Grob, *Mental Illness and American Society*, 124–65.

100 Kalinowsky, "Forced Migration as Public Relations Process?" 385–417.

101 Stahnisch, *How the Nerves Reached the Muscle*, 351–84.

102 Magoun, *American Neuroscience*, 405–10.

103 Pressmann, *Last Resort*, 158–60.

104 Sakel, "The Origin and Nature of the Hypoglycemic Therapy of the Psychoses," 97–109.

105 This success story of insulin therapy was based on the work of Swiss psychiatrist Max Mueller (1894–1980), professor and chair of psychiatry at the University of Berne, who took over Sakel's procedure in his asylum in Muensingen as a type of an "active therapy" which opposed noninvasive approaches in psychiatry. Roelcke, "Continuities or Ruptures?" 169–71.

106 As also pointed out by Borck, *Hirnstroeme*, 248–9.

107 Grob, *Mental Illness and American Society*, 126–43.

108 Pressmann, *Last Resort*, 48–84.

109 It is important to recognize the influences of émigré doctors in the American and Canadian mental health care systems, through transfer processes from their preceding contributions in the medical, psychiatric, and neurological communities of Central Europe, comprising the former Habsburg Empire, along with Italy, Switzerland, the Scandinavian countries, and centrally Germany. Cf. Grob, *Mental Illness and American Society*, 126–43.

110 See for example the publications in the *Bulletin of the German Historical Institute, Washington, DC*, the *Leo Baeck Institute Yearbook*, *Political Psychology*, or *Fortschritte der Neurologie – Psychiatrie*.

111 Seidelman, "The Legacy of Academic Medicine," 325–34; Israel, "Science and the Jewish Question," 191–261; Brock and Harward, *The Culture of Biomedicine*, 10; Galison, Graubard, and Mendelsohn, *Science in Culture*, v–vii; Schmidgen, Geimer, and Dierig, *Kultur im Experiment*, 7–14; Argote, "Organizational Learning," 10–13; Ash, "Wissens- und Wissenschaftstransfer," 181–9.

112 I examine here the complex space of interdisciplinary exchanges in which new forms of research practices and divergent investigative styles emerged, which have recently become more apparent through the equivalent works of Peiffer, "Die Vertreibung deutscher Neuropathologen," 99–109; Peiffer, "Neuropathology in the Third Reich," 184–90; Roelcke, "Wissenschaften zwischen Innovation und Entgrenzung," 92–109.

113 Worden, Schmitt, Swazey, and Adelman, *The Neurosciences: Paths of Discovery*, 3–104. This view has been further sustained by a recent review publication of Cowan, Harter and Kandel, *The Emergence of Modern Neuroscience*, 323–91.

114 An earlier process-oriented perspective developed in the 1990s by a group of scholars at the Berliner Wissenschaftskolleg has opened promising paths for the study "of [the] intellectual and cultural change" through the forced migration of European scientific émigrés. The Austria- and

Germany-based historians Mitchell Ash, Alfons Soellner, and Klaus Fischer have provided useful models on emigration-induced scientific change, which began to include the relevant social accounts of the historical developments, cultural reception, and (re-)integration of German-speaking émigré-scientists. Ash and Soellner, *Introduction*, 1–19.

115 Kandel described his situation on arrival in the United States this way: "Arriving in the United States was like starting life anew. Although I lacked both the prescience and the language to say 'Free at last,' I felt it and I have ever felt it since ... [And also] my father was undeterred. He loved America. Like many other immigrants, he often referred to it as the *goldene Medina*, the land of gold that promised Jews safety and democracy. In Vienna he had read the novels of Karl May [1842–1912] which mythologized the conquest of the American West and the bravery of American Indians, and my father was in his own way possessed of the frontier spirit." Kandel, *In Search of Memory*, 33–5.

116 Taylor, *Strangers in Paradise*, 9.

117 Bramadat and Saydak, "Nursing on the Canadian Prairies," 105–17.

118 Igersheimer, *The Story of a Jewish Refugee from Nazi Germany Imprisoned in Britain and Canada during World War II*, 2005.

119 Mullaly, *Dr. Roddie, Dr. Gus and the Golden Age of Medicine on Prince Edward Island*.

120 Kushner, *The Persistence of Prejudice*.

121 See Ash, *Scientific Changes in Germany*, 329–54. Their thinking as much as their perceptions of the working conditions displayed contemporary cultural values, most obvious for instance in Hallier and DuBois-Reymond's creation of the metaphorical term of a "microbiological culture," which transformed the "peripheral" African colonies into "experimental laboratories" of tropical disease, as Christoph Gradmann has shown for the case of Koch: Gradmann, *Laboratory Disease*, 253–97.

122 See for example: Kreft, *Deutsch-Juedische Geschichte und Hirnforschung*, 206–50; Ash, *Gestalt Psychology in German Culture*, 325–404; Harrington, *Reenchanted Science*, 257–371.

123 Kloocke, Schmiedebach, and Priebe, "Psychological Injury in the Two World Wars," 43–60.

124 On the Goldstein group see, for example, Ash, *Gestalt Psychology in German Culture*, 263–83; for the Munich neurohistologists Weber, "Ein Forschungsinstitut fuer Psychiatrie," 74–89; and for the private clinicians in Berlin see Holdorff, "Die nervesaerztlichen Polikliniken in Berlin vor und nach 1900," 127–39.

125 An illustrative letter from the physician-brother of the neurohistologist Martin Silberberg (1895–1969) to the German-American experimental biologist Loeb, after his arrival in St. Louis, MO. Loeb, like many influential biologists, medical scientists, and clinical psychiatrists, who already held strong relations with US and Canadian colleagues, made intensive use of his influence to help his family members and émigré colleagues to settle in North America and to find a new position. Loeb was instrumental and highly active in the Emergency Committee in Aid of Displaced Foreign Physicians, based in New York City. Achives and Rare Books Division of the Becker Library, WUSM (FC0002, Leo Loeb, correspondence R–S, box 5, folder: Silberberg, Martin and Ruth and FC0002, Leo Loeb, correspondence C–Ha, box 2, folder: Emergency Committee in Aid of Displaced Foreign Physicians).

126 Cf. Stahnisch, *German-Speaking Émigré-Neuroscientists*, 36–68.

127 Ash and Soellner, "Introduction," 3; Shevell, "Neurosciences in the Third Reich," 132–8; Seeman, "Psychiatry in the Nazi Era," 218–23.

128 Hubenstorf, *Ende einer Tradition und Fortsetzung als Provinz*, 33–53; On the issue of the bilateral implications of the forced migration process of scientists and physicians from Central Europe, see also Frank, *Double Exile*, 13–20.

129 German philosopher of science Klaus Fischer has proposed that there would be four major levels of historiographical analysis (the first three being the personal level, the level of networks, and the institutional level) to evaluate emigration-induced scientific change. It is also important, he adds, to introduce the cultural contextual level into such a model, to realize transatlantic comparisons of the emerging field, as described here for the field of neuromorphology in the German-speaking countries before World War II. Fischer, "Identification of Emigration-Induced Scientific Change" in Ash and Soellner, *Forced Migration and Scientific Change*, 23; see also Kroener, "Die Emigration deutschsprachiger Mediziner," 1–35.

130 Suggestion of the term by Christian Fleck, "Emigration of Social Scientists' Schools from Austria" in Ash and Soellner, *Forced Migration and Scientific Change*, 198–223.

131 Hoch, *Migration and the Generation of New Scientific Ideas*, 209–37.

132 For an earlier view on this topic see, for example, Schlich, *Der Eintritt von Juden in das Bildungsbuergertum des 18. und 19. Jahrhunderts*, 129–42.

133 For the German context see Vom Bruch, *Kontinuitaeten und Diskontinuitaeten in der Wissenschaftsgeschichte*, 9–17 and 19–38.

134 Finger, *Minds Behind the Brain*, 259–80.

135 Loewi, *The Excitement of a Life in Science*, 119.

136 Cf. Kaufman, *Searching for Justice*, 3–73. Another one of the absurd consequences of the political dynamics was the internment of so many fleeing
Jews and forced migrant scientists as "enemy aliens." They had managed
to escape to the UK on the eve of World War II and were consecutively
shipped to Canada and Australia, because of latent fear that they could
be foreign spies or collaborators. This is intriguingly described in
Kaufman, *Searching for Justice*, 45–56.

137 Lang, "Spaete Reise zu den Erben," 18.

138 See, for instance, the recollections of the essayist and poet Lessie Sachs
(1897–1942), "Advice from the Midwest," 229–32; Grob, *Mental Illness
and American Society*, 243–65.

139 For the emigration-ways leading away from Ellis Island see Marinbach,
Galvaston; for the Peer 21-deportations see Bartrop, "No Northern
Option," 79–98; Spencer, *Hanna's Diary, 1938–1941*.

140 In this letter he brought up an opportunity at the Middlesex University,
MA. Martin Silberberg (St Louis), *Letter*, to Leo Loeb (staying at Woods
Hole) on 4 April 1938; Archives and Rare Books Division of the Becker
Library, WUSM (FC0002, Leo Loeb, correspondence R–S, box 5, folder:
Silberberg, Martin and Ruth).

141 Martin Silberberg, New York City. *Letter*, to Leo Loeb (St Louis) on
2 December 1943; Achives and Rare Books Division of the Becker
Library, WUSM (FC0002, Leo Loeb, correspondence R–S, box 5, folder:
Silberberg, Martin and Ruth).

142 Fischer, *Identification of Emigration-Induced Scientific Change*, 25.

143 This is described, for example, in Hans-Joerg Rheinberger's discussion
about the contribution of the Austro-American biochemist Erwin
Chargaff (1905–2002) to the development of protein synthesis;
Rheinberger, *Toward a History of Epistemic Things*, 28–31.

144 Sigerist, *American Medicine*, 1. See also Stern's account, *Pillar of Fire*,
219–76.

145 Strauss and Roeder, *International Biographical Dictionary of Central
European Emigrés*, article Pollak, "Ottakar Jaroslav," 916–17; Pollak
subsequently held limited-term appointments at various state hospitals
in Massachusetts, Delaware, and Pennsylvania, and won a prestigious
Lasker Award for his histological research. He later remigrated to Europe,
where he died in The Netherlands in 1974.

146 This unsigned letter (emphasis in original) was supposedly written by the
biological chemist Philip A. Shaffer, who was the dean of the Washington

University School of Medicine between 1937 and 1946; Archives and Rare Books Division of the Becker Library, WUSM (RG OIC, central administration records, subgroup 1: Office of the Dean, ser. 10 general files from Dean's Off., box 64, WUSM Departments – Psychiatry and Neurology, 1938–59, various dates from 1938–59).

147 Cf., the president of the Rockefeller Foundation George E. Vincent (1864–1941), *Report* (1 November 1937), entitled "The Strategy of our Program in Psychiatry" to the New York Headquarters; RAC, RF Archives, RG 3, series 906, box 2, folder 17, 6–10.

148 Schuering, *Minervas verstossene Kinder*, 331–50.

149 Weil's address to the Canadian Psychiatric Association in 1969; citation taken from his manuscript-typography from the folders on the Robert Weil Correspondence (Ms 2–750, call # 2003–47, box 6, file 15, 10 pp.) in the Dalhousie University Archives & Special Collections, Killam Memorial Library, Halifax, NS.

150 Ibid., 1 (emphases in the original). By "Masonic gathering," Weil meant the learned and professional Canadian Psychiatric Association's annual meeting.

151 Conot, *Justice at Nuremberg*, 284–99; see also Alexander, *Classified Reports for the Combined Intelligent Subcommittee Reports – CIOS*, rept. 250.

152 Kalinowsky, "Der Einfluss deutschsprachiger Psychiater und Neurologen in Nordamerika und England," 625–8.

153 Regarding the Rockefeller Foundation's interaction with the ECiAFDP [Emergency Committee in Aid for Displaced Foreign Physicians], such as through the prominent French vascular surgeon Alexis Carrell's (1873–1944), see Schneider, *Rockefeller Philanthropy and Modern Biomedicine*, 208–22. The aid of the Rockefeller Foundation appeared quite ambivalent, because on the one hand, Rockefeller Foundation officials wanted to know whether particular émigrés were "good investments" to be supported by their foundation. On the other hand, Rockefeller Foundation played a crucial role in helping former awardees in their struggle with the German authorities, an example being the neuroserologist Felix Plaut (1877–1940), granting them tightly policed funds to secure their financial outcome and research careers long after the Nazis had seized power. The Rockefeller Foundation established a prominent in-aid-program that granted allowances in America and the United Kingdom, before the émigré neuroscientists were able to sustain their professional life in university or other clinical positions. Stahnisch, "Offene Fragen – Flexible Antworten," 56–62.

154 It is particularly important to mention the contributions of Italian refugee from Fascim Rita Levi-Montalcini (1909–2012), who in 1986 received the Nobel prize for her groundbreaking work on experimental embryology and fibre-outgrowth phenomena in chicken conducted both in Italy and at Washington University in St Louis. See, for example: Kandel, *Cellular Basis of Behavior*, 45–66. Meyer, *Historical Aspects of Cerebral Anatomy*; Tower, *A Century of Neuronal and Neuroglial Interactions*, 3–17; Cowan, Harter, and Kandel, "The Emergence of Modern Neuroanatomy and Developmental Neurobiology," 413–26; Squire, *The History of Neuroscience in Autobiography* (2001–16); and a former MPI director, *Interview* (14 November 2003) with author; Bill Feindel, *Interview* (11 November 2006); and Alberto Aguayo, *Letter* (20 November 2006).

155 Deichmann, *Biologists under Hitler*, 9.

156 Using historiography as a description of the "thick dimension" of research, laboratory practices, and clinical approaches allows for a more adequate view of the historical processes, particularly the adaptation and integration of communities of neurologists, psychiatrists, and brain investigators into pre-existing American cultures. See the accounts in: Geertz, *The Interpretation of Cultures*, 7–43; Daniel, "Kulturgeschichte," 186–204.

157 See, for example: Hammerstein, *Wissenschaftssystem und Wissenschaftspolitik im Nationalsozialismus*, 219–24; Schuering, "Ein Dilemma der Kontinuitaet," 453–63.

CHAPTER SEVEN

1 Walter William Spencer Cook (1888–1962), director of the Institute of Fine Arts in New York, 1933. Cook, "Hitler Is My Best Friend," 380.

2 According to Kroener, *Die Emigration deutschsprachiger Mediziner*, 1–35.

3 Cf. Stahnisch, *Émigré Psychiatrists, Psychologists, and Cognitive Scientists in North America since the Second World War*, 17–38.

4 Recent publications that have focused on the forced migration of German-speaking physicians from an institutional history viewpoint are: Zimmermann, *Die Medizinische Fakultaet der Universitaet Jena*, 33–96; Aumueller, Grundmann, Kraehwinkel, Lauer, and Remschmidt, *Die Marburger Medizinische Fakultaet im Dritten Reich*, 123–303; Hofer, Gruen, and Leven, *Medizin und Nationalsozialsmus*, 161–88; Forsbach, *Die Medizinische Fakultaet der Universitaet Bonn im "Dritten Reich,"* 333–93; Peiffer, "Die Vertreibung deutscher Neuropathologen," 99–109;

Peiffer, "Zur Neurologie im 'Dritten Reich,'" 728–33; and Roelcke, "Wissenschaften zwischen Innovation und Entgrenzung," 92–109. For further methodological discussions of the concept of knowledge transfers, see Ash, "Von Vielschichtigkeiten und Verschraenkungen," 91–105.

5 While the outbreak of the war led to some relaxation in Canadian immigration policies, many of the undersupplied territories retained their own schemes under British administration as far back as 1948. This worked in favour of the most sought for physicians, but sometimes they were viewed as mere "competitors" by local medical doctors. Weindling, "Medical Refugees in Britain," 451–9.

6 Stahnisch, "Learning Soft Skills the Hard Way," 299–319.

7 Kalinowsky, "Der Einfluss deutschsprachiger Psychiater und Neurologen in Nordamerika und England," 625–8.

8 Tartokoff, "Grete L. Bibring," 293–5.

9 Ibid.

10 Grossmann, "German Women Doctors from Berlin to New York," 65–88.

11 Gerrens, Psychiater unter der NS-Diktatur, 330–9.

12 Focke, Begegnung, 110–13.

13 Kalinowsky, "Der Einfluss deutschsprachiger Psychiater und Neurologen in Nordamerika und England," 625–8.

14 Particularly, the exodus of psychoanalysts will not be further explored here, since the forced migration movement in this group has received substantial coverage in the scholarship. For one, this development, its impact on clinical psychiatry, and many of the after-effects of the exchanges with the American biomedical landscape have demonstrated how psychiatric theorizing in clinical medicine became dominated by psychoanalytic theories for half a century. Another area of research has concerned the instance that psychoanalytic concepts also provided platforms for public discourse about modern American lifestyles and their limits. See, for example: Lunbeck, The Psychiatric Persuasion; Schwartz, Cassandra's Daughter; Marinelli and Mayer, Dreaming by the Book; or recently Engel, American Therapy.

15 Cf. Pickenhain, "Die Neurowissenschaft," 241–6; anon., "In Praise of the 'Brain Drain,'" 231.

16 For the identification of this particular group of émigrés, I include neurologists, psychiatrists, neuroanatomists, and neurophysiologists with a medical background and clinical psychologists who graduated from medicine. For purposes of comparison with this postwar development, I follow the consensus on the subdisciplines contributing synthetically to the field of neuroscience, building on earlier studies such as: Ash, Gestalt Psychology

in German Culture, 326–412; Deichmann, *Biologists under Hitler*, 52; Mueller, *Von Charlottenburg zum Central Park West*, 96–184.

17 On the persecution of psychiatric and neurological patients in the "euthanasia program" see: Aly, *Aktion T4 1939–1945*, 189–92; Shevell, "Neurosciences in the Third Reich," 132–8; and Lilienthal, "Patientinnen und Patienten aus brandenburgischen Heil- und Pflegeanstalten," 303–18.

18 On the Nazis' interpretation of "Jewish Science": Kater, *Doctors under Hitler*, 111–26; Michael Hubenstorf, "Vertreibung und Verfolgung," 277–88.

19 On the heterogenous field of *Nervenheilkunde* in the early twentieth century see: Eulner, "Psychiatrie und Neurologie," 257–82; Schmiedebach, *Robert Remak*, 245–94.

20 This artificial situation of the exodus of laboratory scientists and medical doctors from German-speaking countries opens up for a quasi "laboratory-like situation." Salt, "A Comparative Overview of International Trends," 431–56; Rhode, *East-West Migration*, 15–33; Gratzer, "Review of Jean Medawar and David Pyke," 907–8; and the general research journal on forced migration: *Exilforschung. Ein internationales Jahrbuch* (1983–present).

21 US Chief Counsel for the Prosecution of Axis Criminality, ed. *Nazi Conspiracy and Aggression*. Vol. 3. Washington, DC: Government Printing Office, 1946 (Document 1397–PS), 981–6 (official translation of original document: *Gesetz zur Wiederherstellung des Berufsbeamtentums*).

22 Cf. Ash and Soellner, *Forced Migration and Scientific Change*, 1–19.

23 The peculiar constitution of the German university and public health system led to the dismissal of thousands of doctors and researchers, as they were employed as civil servants in the 1930s. Kater, *Hitler's Early Doctors*, 25–53.

24 Ibid.

25 Weindling, *Health, Race and German Politics*, 489–564.

26 Hepp, *Die Ausbuergerung deutscher Staatsangehoeriger 1933–1945*, 3 vols.

27 Gruettner and Kinas, "Die Vertreibung von Wissenschaftlern," 123–86.

28 Efron, Weitzman, and Lehmann, *The Jews: A History*, 194–7.

29 Peters, "Emigration deutscher Psychiater nach England," 161–7. See also the reports on the meetings of the Gesellschaft Deutscher Nervenaerzte (renamed in 1950 as Deutsche Gesellschaft fuer Neurologie, DGN), which used to be published in the organ of the society: DZfNhlk.

30 Lewy later changed his name into Frederick Henry Lew(e)y upon his arrival in North America and his naturalization as a US citizen.

31 Pross and Winau, *Das Krankenhaus Moabit*, 184–6.

32 See the Introduction, which also describes some of the conditions under which it was conceived: Goldstein, *Der Aufbau des Organismus*, 1–20.

33 Cf. Ulrich, "Kurt Goldstein," 15.

34 Goldstein himself made similar remarks to a reporter in a German language interview for Radio Bremen. Bach, *Interview* with Kurt Goldstein (June, 1958) in New York City, min. 93–min. 114.

35 This is pertinent in the cases of Kandel, Stern, and Weil, who definitely counted among the younger neuroscientist to arrive in America, pursuing the longest part of their medical careers overseas.

36 Goldstein, *Human Nature in the Light of Psychopathology*, i.

37 Belz, "Kurt Goldstein (1878–1965)," 11–31.

38 From the study of singular historical events in terms of *Ereignisgeschichte*, individual perspectives from politics and culture, such as the advent of German nationalism, anti-Semitism in the European academy, and racial policies, were taken into account. Cf. Haentzschel, "Der Exodus von Wissenschaftlerinnen," 43–53; or Somit and Tanenhaus, *The Development of American Political Science*, 42–89. For process history: Porter, "History as Process," 297–313; Bleker, "Der Erfolg der Gleichschaltungsaktion kann als durchschlagend bezeichnet werden," 87–96; Kater, *Hitler's Early Doctors*, 25–53; Hubenstorf, "Ende einer Tradition und Fortsetzung als Provinz," 33–53.

39 Terrall, "Biography as Cultural History of Science," 306–13.

40 "If a biography is also to be a work of history of science, it must analyze ideas, intellectual sources, training, controversies, calculations, experiments, and so on and put these elements into the life. This is not simply a matter of exploring the 'thought' of one man, though that is part of it, but, rather, of figuring out how books, ideas, and metaphysical or theoretical commitments." Ibid., 309.

41 See Black, *War Against the Weak*, 1–15.

42 Cornwell, *Hitler's Scientists*, 154.

43 Czech, "Von der 'Aktion T4' zur 'dezentralen Euthanasie.' Die niederoesterreichischen Heil- und Pflegeanstalten Gugging, Mauer-Oehling und Ybbs," 219–66.

44 Paul A.T.M. Eling, *Interview* (13 July 2017) with author.

45 Plaenkers, Laier, Otto, and Rothe, *Psychoanalyse in Frankfurt am Main*, 41–72.

46 Stahnisch, *Émigré Psychiatrists, Psychologists, and Cognitive Scientists in North America since the Second World War*, 17–38.

47 Ash, *Gestalt Psychology in German Culture, 1890–1967*, 263–75.

48 Noppeney, "Kurt Goldstein," 67–78.

49 Ulrich was well acquainted with Goldstein's philosophical work. Yet in addition, since 1929, he had also been married to the Swedish nurse and human rights activist Elsa Braendstroem (1888–1948). After their emigration to the United States in 1933, due to their socialist convictions, Braendstroem organized relief help for newly arriving refugees from Europe and in this capacity also met Goldstein and his young wife.

50 Ulrich, "Kurt Goldstein," 15.

51 These intellectual undercurrents were not just affected by the forced migration of many members of the group, but were tangible in their local working milieux in Frankfurt am Main and Berlin before. For instance, in the exchange relations on speech and behavioural questions with Landauer from the Frankfurt Psychoanalytical Institute, or with Bethe, who was an *Ordinarius* professor for physiology and thus a near colleague from the medical faculty on brain plasticity. Benzenhoefer and Kreft, "Bemerkungen zur Frankfurter Zeit," 31–40; Plaenkers, Laier, and Otto, *Psychoanalyse in Frankfurt am Main*, 41–72.

52 Geisthoevel and Hitzer, *Auf der Suche nach einer anderen Medizin. Psychosomatik im 20. Jahrhundert*, 149.

53 Cf. Magoun, *American Neuroscience*, xv–xviii.

54 "The maturity of the basic sciences and philosophy ('the new psychology') in Europe naturally attracted young Americans to undertake their doctoral and postdoctoral studies overseas, with gains in proficiency and research experience, as well as in teaching, for both sides. With the largest concentration of such figures in Germany, its universities became the mecca for those who could afford study sojourns abroad." Magoun, *American Neuroscience*, xvii.

55 Kandel, *In Search of Memory*, 106 (author's emphasis).

56 Such differences between the North America and European research styles had been noted by Louise H. Marshall in Magoun, *American Neuroscience*, xv–xviii; also Louise H. Marshall, *Interview* (5 June 2002) with author.

57 Cf. Furgusen, *Virtual History*, 42–7.

58 The term "medical diaspora" or "scientific diaspora" is increasingly used in scholarship of various forms on intellectual migration, whether instigated through economic, political, training, or other reasons. It is hence particularly well suited to reflect the diverse nature of the status and effects of exiled physicians and scientists in their receiving countries, a meaning in which it is used here as well. Fiddian-Qasmiyeh, Loescher, and Sigona, *The Oxford Handbook of Refugee & Forced Migration Studies*, 178–86.

59 The reason that the members of the Goldstein group are regarded as a related network is given in their earlier tight interplay as teachers, colleagues, pupils, and friends, which made the astounding milieux in Frankfurt and Berlin possible. This interconnection was also an essential ingredient for the development of a large-scale and highly visible clinical "research school." For the latter concept see Geison, *Scientific Change*, 20–40. They also engaged in mutual support efforts *en grande distance*: for example, when informing the British Academic Assistance Council about the fate of their fellow members, writing letters of support for émigré colleagues, or exchanging on questions of the recruitment of lab assistants with the Aid Committee of the Rockefeller Foundation in New York. Thus, actions that were taken in Amsterdam impinged on decisions taken in New York; letters written from Munich gave rise to researchers' support in Montreal; and cables sent from London were eagerly awaited in Pennsylvania for decisions about offering academic jobs to émigré neuroscientists who had landed on the western side of the Atlantic. Their formation as a network of like-minded researchers and physicians helps us understand the international context of the reception of people in specific places and their continued work efforts, even if they could not be attributed solely to individuals' decisions. On the network concept for the analysis of issues in international migration, see also Keck and Sikkink, *Activists beyond Borders*, 39–78.

60 Simmel, "Kurt Goldstein, 1868–1975," 9–10.

61 As, for instance, the Berlin neurohistologist Bielschowsky wrote back from his London exile: "I am as well as a man with my past could be in a very strange country. You know how much I love my home country. All the friendliness and kind offers of support by my colleagues, however, will never really substitute for what I had to leave behind." Max Bielschowsky, *Letter* (14 November 1933) to Julius Hallervorden at the KWI for Brain Research in Berlin-Buch, qtd from Peiffer, *Hirnforschung in Deutschland*, 496.

62 They continued their collaborative work regardless of the disrupted local contexts along the East Coast, mediated by letter exchanges, phone calls, and the still dense railway system in the 1950s, as well as the organization of mutual symposia. Stahnisch and Hoffmann, "Kurt Goldstein and the Neurology of Movement," 283–6.

63 Danzer, *Vom Konkreten zum Abstrakten*, 23–4.

64 Reilly, *Belsen: The Liberation of a Concentration Camp*, 33.

65 Goldstein, *Human Nature in the Light of Psychopathology*, 1–50.

66 For the members of this group and some of their interactions, see Belz, "Kurt Goldstein (1878–1965)," 1–23; Harrington, *Reenchanted Science*, 259–317.

67 Teuber, "Kurt Goldstein's Role," 301–2.

68 Cf. Danzer, *Vom Abstrakten zum Konkreten*, 9; Holdorff, "Founding Years of Clinical Neurology in Berlin," 223–38, Peiffer, "Die Vertreibung deutscher Neuropathologen," 99–109.

69 This emanates, for example, from a letter sent by the officer Daniel P. O'Brian (1894–1958) from the Rockefeller Foundation's European office in Paris to R. Alexander Lambert (b. 1863) in the New York Headquarters of the Rockefeller Foundation, as written on 27 September 1934: "Prof. Goldstein called today on his way to America. He leaves from Cherbourg by the 'Berengaria' on the 29th [September 1934]. I reviewed his whole situation with him. He feels there is practically no chance of an opportunity either in the University of Amsterdam or in practice in Holland, for himself as well as for other Germans. He has apparently gone into the matter in considerable detail, and arrived at this conclusion. He has consequently taken steps to go over to America to see if he can secure a post there. G[oldstein]. expects to call on you shortly after his arrival, and hopes he may have the chance of discussing with you any openings that might occur. He has been invited to stay with [Smith Ely] Jelliffe [1866–1945]." Rockefeller Foundation officer D.P. O'Brian in New York City, *Letter* (September 27, 1934) to R.A. Lambert. RAC, RF Archives, refugee scholars collection – Kurt Goldstein, RG 200, series 1.1, box 78, folder 939, 17.

70 For Stern's particular example of a young and rising neuropathologist and clinical psychiatrist, see his autobiographical book: Stern, *Pillar of Fire*, 249–76, as well as Birmingham, "Some Thoughts on the Fiftieth Anniversary," 151–5.

71 Such as in the *Who's Who in America* or in the more university-oriented version of *American Men of Science*.

72 Brief record of the rector of Columbia University in New York City, Nicholas Murray Butler (1862–1947), dated 6 November 1939, about a telephone conversation of Abraham Flexner at Princeton, NJ, with Kurt Goldstein in New York. RAC, RG 200 (Columbia University; Goldstein, Kurt – refugee scholar, neurology, 1937–1940), series 1.1, box 9, folder 939, 65–6.

73 Simmel, "Kurt Goldstein, 1878–1965," 10.

74 Feindel and Leblanc, *The Wounded Brain Healed*, 166 and 241.

75 Ted Sourkes, *Interview* (12 December 2006) with author.

76 Michael I. Shevell, *Interview* (27 May 2007) with author; Maurice Dongier, *Interview* (May 26, 2007) with author.

77 In a fascinating article, Canadian gerontologist David Hogan has pointed to the circumstance that émigré physicians both from the German-speaking countries and the UK were particularly successful in occupying niche disciplines in America, such as the emerging area of specialization in geriatrics, in which Stern was a major protagonist, who importantly helped building geriatric psychiatry in Canada. See Hogan, *History of Geriatrics in Canada*, 131–50. This change from being a versatile laboratory researcher to being a clinical psychiatrist is further explored in: Goldblatt, "Star: Karl Stern (1906–1975)," 279–82.

78 The cultural dimension of science shows not only the institutional patterns with their infrastructure but also the interplay of conceptual, personal, and research relations that created a fertile ground for interdisciplinary endeavours to which the émigrés contributed.

79 Simmel, "Kurt Goldstein 1878–1965," 9–10.

80 Goldstein, *Human Nature in the Light of Psychopathology*, 223–4.

81 See similar examples of French experimental physiologists of the late nineteenth century in: Williams, *The Physical and the Moral*, 196–232; or the German theoretical pathologists, following Rudolf Virchow, in: Wittern, "Die Politik ist weiter nichts, als Medicin im Grossen," 150–7.

82 In fact, Goldstein had alluded to this trope on a number of occasions; for an example see Goldstein, "Die Neuroregulation," 9–13, or: "Das psychophysische Problem in seiner Bedeutung fuer aerztliches Handeln," 1–11. In fact, an anticipation of the vicious sociopolitical developments in Germany and other European countries is strongly present in Goldstein's neurological and philosophical reflections.

83 Teuber, "Kurt Goldstein's Role," 308.

84 Goldstein, *Notes on the Development of My Concepts*, 11–12; Teuber, "Kurt Goldstein's Role," 303, further emphasizes that, although Goldstein's neurological thinking could hardly be integrated into the technological approaches in American neurology and that his "William James Lectures" were only marginally received in the medical community, Goldstein nevertheless was quite successful in teaching at Tufts in Boston, Columbia, and at the New School in New York, "where his influence spread primarily among clinical psychologists in the United States." See also Harrington, *Reenchanted Science*, 316–17.

85 RAC, RG 717, series 1.1, box 35, file: Diary Lambert, "Walter Riese," 135.

86 Riese, "Kurt Goldstein," 25–7.

87 See, for example, Riese, *The Conception of Disease*, 47–70. Riese's writings took chiefly a history-of-ideas approach and were centred around conceptions of disease throughout the ages, with particular reference to the factors contributing to the various notions in each culture, as if expressing his own experiences. Nevertheless, Riese pioneered studies in the history of neuroscience for example through his book *A History of Neurology* (1959). In fact, quite a number of notable émigrés supported the emerging field of the history of neuroscience in the US, including the Czech-born and German-trained neurologist Francis Schiller (1909–2003). See Finger, "Francis Schiller (1909–2003)," 353–7.

88 Fee and Brown, *Making Medical History*, 288–311.

89 For this historiographical concept, see Ash and Soellner, *Forced Migration and Scientific Change*, 3.

90 Pross and Winau, *Nicht Misshandeln*, 109–79.

91 Stern, *Flight from Women*, 77.

92 For the discourse on neurological holism in the Weimar period, consult: Harrington, *Re-Enchanted Science*, 221–58; for a case example regarding a transfer of the concept of neurodegeneration to the workbench of the neuroanatomy laboratory, see Stahnisch, *Zur Bedeutung der Konzepte der "neuronalen De- und Regeneration,"* 243–69.

93 Teuber, "Kurt Goldstein's Role," 299.

94 A more sympathetic interpretation sees this development rather as a shift from "holistic neurology" to experimental psychology: Ash, *Gestalt Psychology in German Culture*, 263–83.

95 The exodus of so many doctors and medical scientists also led to the transplantation of neuroscientific cultures, even if, for example, the Goldstein group fell from brilliance to mediocrity, when its cutting-edge neuroscientific research orientation of the 1920s and early 1930s is compared with the dislocated and spurious attempts to rebuild programs and units abroad. Frazzetto and Anker, *Neuroculture*, 815–21.

96 Peyenson, *"Who the Guys Were,"* 155–88; Shapin and Thackray, *Prosopography as a Research Tool in History of Science*, 1–28; or more recently Soederqvist, *Neurobiographies*, 38–48.

97 Teuber, "Kurt Goldstein's Role," 304.

98 Communication with the neurosurgeon Moshe Feinsod from Haifa about Goldstein's visit to Israel, 1958: Moshe Feinsod, *Interview* (22 June 2007) with author.

99 Exchanges with the University of California at San Francisco neurosurgeon Steve Dell regarding San Francisco and Maryland émigré neuroscientists, as well as with paediatric neurologist Michael I. Shevell and neurochemist

Allen Sherwin at McGill University in Montreal. Steve Dell, *Interview* (28 June 2007) with author; Michael I. Shevell, *Interview* (May 27, 2007) with author; and Allen Sherwin (†), *Interview* (27 March 2009) with author.

100 Stern, *Pillar of Fire*, 75.

101 Sigerist, *American Medicine*, 321–2.

102 See related historiographical approaches in psychology in: Ash, *Gestalt Psychology in German Culture*, 362–404; in biology: Harwood, *Styles of Scientific Thought*, 274–314; or in theoretical physics: Sigurdson, "Physics, Life and Contingency," 48–70.

103 Recent historiography of medicine and science has made us aware of the important cultural grounding of scientific and professional practices in their situational, local, and even national contexts. See: Brock and Harward, *The Culture of Biomedicine*; Galison, Graubard, and Mendelsohn, *Science in Culture*; Schmidgen, Geimer, and Dierig, *Kultur im Experiment*; or Erickson, *Science, Culture and Society*. Similarly, I have focused on early twentieth-century neuroscience for an in-depth investigation of the cultural aspects of scientific and clinical practice with respect to the interdisciplinary advances in brain science and some intriguing perspectives on the development of forced migration in this field.

104 This is demonstrated in many autobiographical accounts of exiled individuals, which emphasized the frequent suicide attempts, such as in the case of the Tuebingen neuro-ophthalmologist Caesar Hirsch [Hearst, 1880–1940], who took his life while in exile in Los Angeles – in May 1940 – since he had been desperately homesick and experienced deep distress over the loss of his native country. Lang, "Spaete Reise zu den Erben," 18.

105 Mildenberger, "Auf der Spur des 'Scientific Pursuit,'" 183–200.

106 Weber, *Ernst Ruedin*, 195–6.

107 Kallmann, *The Genetics of Schizophrenia*, 40–6.

108 Ibid., 1–3.

109 In the drastic case of Mengele, this research was later extended to concentration camps such as Auschwitz in occupied Poland. For further details, see Weindling, *From Clinic to Concentration Camp*, 28–9.

110 It was about two decades later that Kallmann's research was eventually confirmed by American and Scandinavian adoption studies. Slater, "A Review of Earlier Evidence," 15–26; Essen-Moeller, *Psychiatrische Untersuchungen*, 3–19.

111 Annual Reports of the National Institutes of Mental Health in Bethesda, 1954, 65–7.

112 Hugo Moser, *Letter* (21 November 2006) to author.

113 Grob, *Mental Illness and American Society*, 124–6.
114 Annual Reports of the National Institutes of Mental Health in Bethesda, 1954, 3 (author's emphasis).
115 Grob, *Mental Illness and American Society*, 243–65.
116 Ibid., 124–65.
117 Kuehl, *The Nazi Connection*, 3–12.
118 For the example of Kallmann, see also Mildenberger, "Auf der Spur des 'Scientific Pursuit,'" 183–200.
119 Robertson, *An Interview with Eric Kandel*, 743–5.
120 Kandel, *The Age of Insight*, 16–17.
121 Academics and researchers who could officially prove – on the basis of certificates and administrative letters – that they had taught previously at universities and colleges in German-speaking universities, had the prospect of finding new academic teaching positions in North America and could thus enter the United States freely. All other refugees could only enter the United States and Canada on the basis of so-called affidavits, which guaranteed that they would not become financial wards of the country, but could rely on the support of family members, colleagues, and research institutions. Fermi, *Illustrious Immigrants*, 60–75.
122 Of course, Kandel's autobiographical books are "ego-documents" with specific intentions and goals. They are nevertheless interesting and useful pieces of information, since they considerably overlap with similar views expressed by contemporary émigré neurologists and psychiatrists in diaries, letter exchanges, and lecture manuscripts. Peiffer, *Hirnforschung in Deutschland*, 67–85.
123 Kandel, *In Search of Memory*, 54–6.
124 Fermi, *Illustrious Immigrants*, 407–8.
125 Ibid., 57–60.
126 Magoun, *American Neuroscience*, 148.
127 Fermi, *Illustrious Immigrants*, 60–75.
128 Pearle, "Aerzteemigration nach 1933 in die USA," 112–37.
129 Through the National Institutes of Health's extramural program, approximately a hundred émigré researchers and clinicians received support during the same time period, ranging from neurochemistry and neuroanatomy to clinical psychoanalysis, and brain stimulation research in psycho- and neurosurgery. Altogether, twenty-two émigré neuroscientists could be identified as having worked in the intramural program of the National Institutes of Health between 1948 and 1962 – i.e., when Schmitt laid the groundwork for the Neuroscience Research Program at the Massachusetts Institute of Technology (MIT) in Cambridge, MA. Cf. Stahnisch, "The Essential Tension," 151–82.

130 Hollingsworth, "Institutionalizing Excellence in Biomedical Research," 15–18.

131 Alan N. Schechter, *Interview* (27 April 2007) with author; Don Tower, *Interview* (20 April 2007) with author.

132 Mildenberger, "Auf der Spur des 'Scientific Pursuit,'" 183–200.

133 Since my narrative is concerned with the period of the emerging interdisciplinary research field of neuromorphology in the German-speaking countries until World War II, it is not possible to go further into the meandering but highly interesting later development of Kandel's work biography. Interested readers are referred to Robertson, *An Interview with Eric Kandel*, 743–5.

134 Kandel, *In Search of Memory*, xv.

135 Ibid., 230–55.

136 Kandel, *In Search of Memory*, 12.

137 For the acceptance of émigré scientists and doctors in the United States in the 1930s and 1940s, see Geiger, "The Dynamics of University Research in the United States 1945–1990," 3–17; Rudy, *Total War and Twentieth-Century Higher Learning*, 66–73.

138 Emery and Emery, *A Young Man's Benefit*, 175–7.

139 Stern, *Flight from Women*, 77.

140 Magoun, *American Neuroscience*, 82.

141 Gay, *Freud. Eine Biographie fuer unsere Zeit*, 215–16 and 517–21.

142 Kurzweil, "Psychoanalytic Science," 143.

143 Binding and Hoche, *Die Freigabe der Vernichtung lebensunwerten Lebens*, 22–3.

144 Peiffer, "Die Vertreibung deutscher Neuropathologen," 99.

145 Hartmann, *Essays on Ego Psychology*, 19.

146 Young, *The Harmony of Illusions*, 15.

147 Kurzweil, "Psychoanalytic Science," 143.

148 The role of "the stranger" in creating innovative fields in new cultural environments is of pivotal importance. Just as the social need for comparison in the immigrant individual becomes a vital property in the new cultural surrounding, the ability to relate to pre-existing traditions assumes ample input from local cultural values, readily shaped interpretations of new observations, or acquired clinical skills. Rosen, *The Specialization of Medicine with Particular Reference to Ophthalmology*, 39, and for a sophisticated socioanthropological account, see Simmel, "The Stranger," 143–9; Hartmann, *Essays on Ego Psychology*, 131.

149 Stahnisch, "Zur Zwangsemigration deutschsprachiger Neurowissenschaftler," 441–72.

150 Niederland, *A Refugee's Life*, 150.

151 Anonymous patient, reported after Niederland, *"Denkerinnerungen"*; qtd from Focke, *William G. Niederland*, 30.

152 The Romanian-American writer and Holocaust activist Elie Wiesel (1928–2016) qtd after Niederland, *Die Psychologie des 20. Jahrhunderts; in Focke, Willam G. Niederland*, 202.

153 Grob, "Mental Health Policy in Late Twentieth-Century America," 232.

154 Selye, *From Dream to Discovery*, 199–262.

155 Milagros Salas-Prato, *Letter* (16 June 2011) to author.

156 For the general daily need and the assistance patterns of intellectual migration processes, see Fawcett, *Networks, Linkages, and Migration Systems*, 671–80.

157 Regarding his clinical experiences during the 1960s, see Niederland, *A Refugee's Life*, 423.

158 Cf. "Psychiatric Disorders among Persecution Victims," 458–73; or "Clinical Observations on the Survivor Syndrome," 313–15.

159 Niederland, "Clinical Observations on the Survivor Syndrome," 313.

160 Ibid., 131–2.

161 Niederland, *Die Psychologie des 20. Jahrhunderts*, 1055; author's translation.

162 Muehlleitner, "Federn, Paul," 135–6.

163 Hartmann, *Essays on Ego Psychology*, 131.

164 See Klibansky, Panofsky, and Saxl, *Saturn and Melancholy*, 67–123.

165 Mildenberger, "Auf der Spur des 'Scientific Pursuit,'" 183–200; Harrington, *Reenchanted Science*, 221–58; Stahnisch, "Zur Zwangsemigration deutschsprachiger Neurowissenschaftler," 442–6.

166 Lamb, *Pathologist of the Mind*, 59–98.

167 Lamb, "The Most Important Professorship in the English-Speaking Domain," 1061–6.

168 This included the support programs for psychosomatics research with the Carnegie Foundation in Washington, DC, and the Rockefeller Foundation in New York City. See, for example, in: Archives and Rare Books Division of the Becker Library, WUSM (1936): (RG IC15:2, Department of Neurology and Psychiatry, series 2, Gregg's List, Am. Assoc. of Colleges Med. Schools – of 1936), 2.

169 Leys and Evans, *Defining American Psychology*, 39–57; with an astounding velocity and energy, the Rockefeller Foundation officer in charge of the funding program for psychiatry and neurology, Alan Gregg, managed to be engaged as consultant with an exceedingly large number of committees all over the US and also in Canada. See, for example, Archives and Rare Books Division of the Becker Library, WUSM (RG IC15: 2, Department of Neurology and Psychiatry, Series 2, n.p.

170 Archives and Rare Books Division of the Becker Library, WUSM (RG ICI5: 2, Gregg's list, Am Assoc. of Colleges Med. Schools – of 1936), n.p.

171 Brown, *Friendship and Philanthropy*, 288–311.

172 From these relationships emerged a tight network of émigré neuroscientists with their peers in their new host countries, as well as science administrators, politicians, and lobbyists. Altogether, the archival lists from the headquarters of the Rockefeller Foundation record the names of the more than two hundred refugees in biomedicine who had fled from the horrors of the Third Reich and who strove to find new placements through the American funding agency. See also: Ash, *Gestalt Psychology in German Culture*, 276–83; Kumbier and Haack, *Alfred Hauptmann*, 204–9; Noth, *Robert Wartenberg*, 575; Faulkner and Menninger, *The Selected Correspondence of Karl A. Menninger, 1919–1945*.

173 Cf. Stahnisch, "Offene Fragen – Flexible Antworten," 56–62.

174 See Roazen, *Helene Deutsch*, 272–88.

175 Lamb, *Pathologist of the Mind*, 205–45.

176 Fischer, "Psychoanalytische Grundlagen der Psychotraumatologie," 343; author's translation.

177 Schwartz, *Cassandra's Daughter*, 71–4.

178 Assmann, *Trauma des Krieges und Literatur*, 95–6.

179 Freud, "Weitere Ratschlaege zur Technik der Psychoanalyse," 126–36.

180 Horn, "Krieg und Krise," 633.

181 Baglole, "Nos disparus – Le Dr Robert Weil," 64.

182 See, for example, Davie and Koenig, "Adjustment of Refugees," 159–65.

183 Robert Weil, *Letter* (7 June 1986) from Halifax, NS, to Charles A. Roberts (1918–1996) in Ottawa, ON; Weil Correspondence (Ms 2–750, call # 2003–47, box 8, file 15; 1) in the Dalhousie University Archives & Special Collections, Killam Memorial Library, Halifax, NS, 64.

184 170 Ibid.

185 The individual achievements were not always aligned with the earlier importance of many neuroscientists and their ranks in the former German-speaking universities. See, for example, Scholz and Heidel, *Sozialpolitik und Judentum*, 88–96.

186 Baglole, "Nos disparus – Le Dr Robert Weil," 64.

187 Duffin, "The Guru and the Godfather," 191–218.

188 Robert Weil Collection (Ms 2-750, call # 2003–47, accession report, 1, box 5, file 3 and box 6, file 11) in the Dalhousie University Archives & Special Collections, Killam Memorial Library, Halifax, NS.

189 For Weil's activities at Dalhousie University see, for example: Anonymous, "Accession Report, Biographical Sketch/Administrative History"; "Group for the Advancement of Psychiatry. Reports"; and "Dalhousie University.

Faculty of Medicine. Committee on Medical Education. Elective Programme"; materials from the folders of the Robert Weil Collection (Ms 2-750, call # 2003–47, accession report, 1, box 5, file 3 and box 6, file 11).

190 Citation taken from the manuscript of Robert Weil's 1969 address to the Canadian Psychiatric Association (emphasis in original). Typography from the folders on the Robert Weil Correspondence (Ms 2–750, call # 2003–47, box 6, file 15) in the Dalhousie University Archives & Special Collections, Killam Memorial Library, Halifax, NS.

191 Stortz, "'Rescue Our Family from a Living Death,'" 231–61.

192 Seidelman, "Medical Selection," 437–8; Holdorff, "Founding Years of Clinical Neurology in Berlin," 223–38.

193 Bilson, "Muscles and Health," 398–411.

194 Bill Seidelman, *Letter* (7 October 2010) to author.

195 Friedman, *Capitalism and Freedom*, 154.

196 Report of the Department of Public Health: *On the Survey of Health Facilities in Nova Scotia under the Federal Health Survey Grant 1949–1950*; Nova Scotia Archives and Records Management, Halifax, NS, (V/F V. 324 #1, 1, Articles 4, 8; 6, Articles 1, 2, 3; 10, Articles 1, 3; V/RA983 A4 N935 1951, Medical Archives).

197 At the time, Newfoundland was an autonomous territory under British rule. For many refugees trying to emigrate onward from Britain, it was attractive because of the relatively uncomplicated access into the country and in spite of Newfoundland's obvious lack of academic institutions and research opportunities. Macleod, "Migrant, Intern, Doctor – Spy?" 79–89.

198 The office of the British Assistance Council, qtd from Zimmerman, "Narrow-Minded People," 298.

199 Miller qtd from Zimmerman, ibid., 300–1.

200 Hill qtd from Zimmerman, ibid., 301–2.

201 Abella and Troper, *None Is Too Many*, 36–41.

202 Stoke, "Canada and an Academic Refugee from Nazi Germany," 160–2.

203 Ibid.

204 Martin Silberberg, *Letters* (Halifax, St. Louis, and New York) to Leo Loeb (1869–1959; St. Louis); Archives and Rare Books Division of the Becker Library, WUSM (FC0002, Leo Loeb, correspondence R–S, box 5, folder: Silberberg, Martin and Ruth).

205 Cf. Patrias, "Socialists, Jews, and the 1947 Saskatchewan Bill of Rights," 265–92.

206 Nova Scotia Archives and Record Management, Halifax, NS (Ms 13, MacKenzie Special Collection on History of Medicine of Nova Scotia, Folder: C2 a–i). Lazar and Sheva, *In the Beginning*, 91–108.

207 Johnston, "Canada's Ellis Island," 52–3.

208 Coser, *Refugee Scholars in America*, 45–7.

209 Weil, *Letter* (7 June 1986) from Halifax, NS, to Charles A. Roberts in Ottawa. Weil Correspondence (Ms 2–750, call # 2003–47, box 8, file 15, 1) in the Dalhousie University Archives & Special Collections, Killam Memorial Library, Halifax, NS, 64.

210 Dowbiggin, *Keeping America Sane*, 167–8.

211 Advancement of Psychiatry. Reports; Notes & Articles on "Interdisciplinary Research"; Weil Collection (Ms 2–750, call # 2003-47, accession report, box 2, file 5; box 5, file 3) in the Dalhousie University Archives & Special Collections, Killam Memorial Library, Halifax, NS.

212 Ibid.

213 It marked a time when the German-trained émigré historian of medicine and health systems specialist Henry Sigerist conducted an overview study of the health services in Saskatchewan for Tommy C. Douglas (1904–1986); see Duffin, "The Guru and the Godfather," 191–218.

214 Department of Public Health Report (Sept. 25, 1951); Nova Scotia Archives and Records Management, Halifax, NS ([V/F V. 324 #1, 1, Articles 4, 8; 6, Articles 1, 2, 3; 10, Articles 1, 3; V/RA983 A4 N935 1951, Medical Archives).

215 For the development of the American psychiatric context see Pickwren and Schneider, *Psychology and The National Institute of Mental Health*, 3–16.

216 See Weil's address to the Canadian Psychiatric Association in 1969; quoted from his manuscript–typography from the folders on the Weil Correspondence (Ms 2–750, call # 2003–47, box 6, file 15) in the Dalhousie University Archives & Special Collections, Killam Memorial Library, Halifax, NS.

217 Cf. Dowbiggin, *Keeping America Sane*, 70–190. For Weil's own address of the Canadian health care situation see, for example, Easton and Weil, *Culture and Mental Disorders*, 71.

218 Anonymous, "In Memoriam Robert Weil," 1.

219 Robert Weil's own publications in psychiatry and its related fields extended to a whole range of themes: Weil and Demay, "Thiamine Chloride Intrathecally," 545–6; idem., "Mental Health and Disasters"; idem., *Letter*, 239.

220 Materials from the Weil Collection (Ms 2–750, Call # 2003–47, Accession Report, box 5, file 3; box 6, file 11, 1) in the Dalhousie University Archives & Special Collections, Killam Memorial Library, Halifax, NS.

221 In terms of his religion, Weil had converted to Protestantism in his early adolescence, including all of his family, at the will of his father. The latter had been a local merchant and thought that the family could assimilate

better into German society if they could accept the Christian faith. Anon., *In Memoriam Robert Weil*, 1.

222 Weil, *Letter* (June 7, 1986) from Halifax, NS, to Charles A. Roberts in Ottawa, ON; Weil Correspondence (Ms 2–750, Call # 2003–47, Box 8, File 15, 1) in the Dalhousie University Archives & Special Collections, Killam Memorial Library, Halifax, NS, 64.

223 Ibid. N.B.: The original letter entailed all grammatical errors as given in this quote, and the wording resembled that of a telegram-style postcard, likely written in haste, while they were taking the train back from Russia to Central Europe.

224 Stahnisch, "Karl T. Neubuerger (1890–1972) – Pioneer in Neurology," 1493–5.

225 Archives and Rare Books Division of the Becker Library, WUSM (FC0002, Leo Loeb, correspondence R–S, box 5, folder: Silberberg, Martin and Ruth), n.p.

226 Goldblatt, "Star: Karl Stern (1906–1975)," 279–82.

227 See also in Stahnisch, "Ludwig Edinger (1855–1918)," 147–8.

228 One article resulting from the collaboration with Spielmeyer was: "Severe Dementia Associated with Bilateral Symmetrical Degeneration of the Thalamus," 157–67.

229 Stern, *Pillar of Fire*, 116.

230 Kreft, "Zwischen Goldstein und Kleist," 131–44.

231 Stern, *Pillar of Fire*, 85–6.

232 Simmel, "Kurt Goldstein 1878–1965," 3–11.

233 Weber, "Psychiatric Research and Science Policy in Germany," 235–58.

234 Spielmeyer got in contact with Penfield through letter communication with Otfrid Foerster. He was later invited by the Montreal neurosurgeon to visit the "Neuro" at McGill. Stahnisch, "Zur Zwangsemigration deutschsprachiger Neurowissenschaftler nach Nordamerika. Der historische Fall des Montreal Neurological Institute," 441–72.

235 Clinghorn, *The Emergence of Psychiatry at McGill*, 551–5.

236 This was the first geriatric unit to open in Canada. Birmingham, "Some Thoughts on the Fiftieth Anniversary," 151–5.

237 The immersion in Goldstein's "holist neurology" meant a direct extension to his own philosophical and anthropological leanings. See Goldstein, *Der Aufbau des Organismus*, 57–66.

238 Karl Gustav Jung (1875–1961). Birmingham, "Some Thoughts on the Fiftieth Anniversary," 155.

239 Stern, *Pillar of Fire*, 119–33 and 249–58.

240 Nitsch and Stahnisch, "Neuronal Mechanisms Recording the Stream of Consciousness," 3347–55.

241 Burston, *A Forgotten Freudian*, 69–96.

242 University Archives of Ottawa (Fonds 43 NB–3056, Karl Stern Fonds, Human Resources Files).

243 Even though frequent services were held by a local cantor in Stern's hometown, Cham, he did not receive a deep religious education. At one point, he even tried to return to his Jewish faith and, although he attended an orthodox synagogue in Munich, the impression of philosophical literature from his university studies first compelled him to become an agnostic and Zionist. Through the reading of Catholic spiritual literature, he later converted to Catholicism, since Christian eschatology also offered him a source of hope during the appalling experiences he had undergone when fleeing into exile. Neuhaus, "Jewish Conversion to the Catholic Church," 38–52.

244 Pieper, *Autobiographische Schriften*, 338–9.

245 Burston, *A Forgotten Freudian*, 86–95.

246 University Archives of Ottawa (Fonds 6 NB–9656.8, Karl Stern Fonds, Human Resources Files).

247 DesGroseillers, "L'histoire de la psychanalyse à Albert-Prévost," 6–37, esp. 15.

248 Feindel, "The Montreal Neurological Institute," 821–2.

249 Feindel, "The Contributions of Wilder Penfield," 347–58.

250 Askonas, "From Protein Synthesis to Antibody Formation and Cellular Immunity," 3–4.

251 Birmingham, "Some Thoughts on the Fiftieth Anniversary," 151.

252 Burston, *A Forgotten Freudian*, 115–16.

253 Lewy, "Paralysis Agitans," 920–3.

254 Schiller, "Fritz Lewy and His Bodies," 148–51.

255 Stahnisch, "Catalyzing Neurophysiology: Jacques Loeb (1859–1924), the Stazione Zoologica di Napoli, and a Growing Network of Brain Scientists, 1900s–1930," 1–14; Groeben and de Sio, "Nobel Laureates at the Stazione Zoologica Anton Dohrn," 376–95.

256 Holdorff, "Friedrich Heinrich Lewy," 19–28.

257 Holdorff, "Zwischen Hirnforschung, Neuropsychiatrie und Emanzipation," 157–74.

258 Cf. Scholz, Barth, Pappai, and Wacker, "Das Schicksal des Lehrkoerpers der Medizinischen Fakultaet Breslau nach der Vertreibung 1945/46," 497–533; Kreft, "Zwischen Goldstein und Kleist," 201–18.

259 Holdorff, *Die Neurologie in Berlin, 1840–1945*, 46–56.

260 Zimmerman, "The Society for the Protection of Science and Learning and the Politicization of British Science in the 1930s," 25–45.

261 Weindling, "The Impact of German Medical Scientists on British Medicine," 86–114.

262 Frederic Henry Lewy, *Letter* (24 July 24, 1933) to the Academic Assistance Council on 24 July 1933 in the box on Lewy from the collection on the "Society for the Protection of Learning and Science" in the Bodleian Libraries, Oxford University, qtd from Holdorff, "Friedrich Heinrich Lewy," 23.

263 Stahnisch and Tynedal, "Sir Ludwig Guttmann (1899–1980): Pioneer in Neurology," 1512–14.

264 Frederic Henry Lewy, *Letter* (5 June 1934) to the Emergency Committee in Aid of Displaced Foreign Physicians on 5 June 1934; ibid.

265 This built upon the non-permissive legislation the Canadian government had in place since the Quota Act of 1921 and the Immigration Act of 1924, whose reverberations were felt in the medical and scientific spheres as well. Cf. Kohler, "Relicensing Central European Refugee Physicians," 3–32; Seidelman, "Medical Selection," 437–8.

266 Stortz, "'Rescue Our Family From a Living Death'"; Zimmerman, "Narrow-Minded People."

267 On the Turkish situation and its integration of émigré neuroscientists after 1933, see Russell, "A Variation on Forced Migration: Wilhelm Peters (Prussia via Britain to Turkey) and Muzafer Sherif (Turkey to the United States)," 320–47.

268 Krohn, *Handbuch der deutschsprachigen Emigration 1933–1945*, vol. 3, 904–1048, lists forty-two physicians and biomedical researchers who emigrated to Canada. Although this might seem a small number in comparison with the US, it is still a quite impressive group, given the restrictions they faced in comparison with a number of South American countries such as Chile, Uruguay, and Paraguay, which barely received any refugee doctors from German-speaking countries. See Kugelmann and Reiche, *Nordamerika*, 178–80. Between 1933 and 1939, the general numbers of Jewish refugees in Canada, were a few hundred annually. An impressive number of 2,700 "enemy aliens" arrived later on British ships from internment camps in the UK in 1940. Igersheimer, *The Story of a Jewish Refugee from Nazi Germany Imprisoned in Britain and Canada during World War II*, 2005. Among those stranded on the Iberian Peninsula in 1941 were a number of neuroscientists such as Paul Schuster (1867–1940) from Berlin and Ludwig Guttmann from Breslau, as Else Bielschowsky, the wife of Max Bielschowsky, informed Lewy's wife in a letter on 29 August 1935; qtd from Peiffer, *Hirnforschung in Deutschland*, 528.

269 Abella and Troper, *None Is Too Many*, 349–75.
270 Ibid., 36.
271 Zimmerman, "The Society for the Protection of Science and Learning," 25–45.
272 Else Bielschowsky, *Letter* (27 February 1935) to Mrs Lewy, qtd from Peiffer, *Hirnforschung in Deutschland*, 519; author's translation.
273 In terms of Lewy's and his family's religion, he had continued to practise it rather for personal and general cultural reasons. The realization of being "Jewish" occurred to him only from the outside, when the Nazi administrators released the German race laws after 1933 and 1935. At that time, Lewy really thought of himself as a "cultural" Jew, which meant that he kept the traditions of the major Jewish religious holidays. His religious faith became reinforced only through his experience of escaping the Nazis and feeling gratitude for the support he received.
274 The British Academic Assistance Council had been called the "Society for the Protection of Science and Learning" after 1936. Medawar and Pyke, "Obituary: Esther Simpson," 1.
275 Frederic Henry Lewy, *Letter* (10 October 1943) to Ms Esther Simpson in the shelfmark (Ms. S.P.S.L. 396/1-10 on neurologists) regarding Lewy from the Society for the Protection of Science and Learning Collection in the Bodleian Libraries, Oxford University; qtd. from Holdorff, "Friedrich Heinrich Lewy," 23.
276 Holdorff, "Friedrich Heinrich Lewy," 19–28.
277 Immediately after the war, Lewy received further grants from the National Institute of Mental Health in Bethesda. As a consultant to the Veterans Administration, he had even become a member of the National Research Council in Aviation Medicine; Farreras, Hannaway, and Harden, *Mind, Brain, Body, and Behavior*, 312–13.
278 Lewy was quickly integrated into the American neurological community through his acquaintance with some of its core individuals such as the neurological surgeons William P. van Wagenen in Philadelphia and Percival Bailey (1892–1973) from Chicago, IL, as well as another refugee neurologist from Danzig, Robert Wartenberg at the University of California, San Francisco. Senior history of neuroscience book collector Bob Gordon, *Interview* (11 September 2007) with author.
279 Sweeney, Lloyd, and Daroff, "What's in a Name?" 629–30.
280 Quoted from Holdorff, "Friedrich Heinrich Lewy," 25. The archival collection on Lewy from the British Academic Assistance Council is kept as shelfmark (Ms. S.P.S.L. 396/1-10 on neurologists) at the Bodleian Libraries, Oxford University.

281 Holdorff, *Die Neurologie in Berlin, 1840–1945*, 46–56.

282 On the history of the International Brain Research Organization see Richter, "The Brain Commission of the International Association of Academies," 445–57.

283 Noth, *Robert Wartenberg*, 575. The membership list of the American Academy of Neurology, founded as an elitist neurological society, presents Lewy as a founding member in 1948. He later became a Fellow of the American Academy of Neurology and together with Wartenberg they were the only émigré neurologists among its thirteen associates on the board of trustees. Archives and Rare Books Division of the Becker Library, WUSM (PC053, records of the American Academy of Neurology, series 8, membership committee files, box 2).

284 Lewy died in 1950, five years after the war, but he was definitely one of the small number of émigrés who managed to assimilate very well, and even pursue his original work on degenerative diseases of the brain without disruptions. Lewy, "Historical Introduction," 1–20.

285 This question has not figured prominently on the agenda of medical historians. For an important step in this direction see Ritter and Roelcke, "Psychiatric Genetics in Munich and Basel between 1925 and 1945," 263–88.

286 Cf. Waltraud Strickhausen, "Kanada," and Claus-Dieter Krohn, "Vereinigte Staaten von Amerika," in Krohn, von zur Muehlen, Paul, and Winckler, *Handbuch der deutschsprachigen Emigration 1933–1945*, 284–97 and 446–66.

287 The resulting changes in research scope and neuroscientific topics, as well as in the very language of research publications (a strong shift toward English-language publications), is also represented in major history of neuroscience collections, such as the Mackie Family History of Neuroscience Collection at the University of Calgary (https://www.ucalgary.ca/neuro/about).

288 Neville, *The Royal Vic*, 103–27; Luescher, "Neuroscience at Penn State," 4–6; Flynn, *Dalhousie's Department of Psychiatry*.

289 The works of Gerhard Baader and Werner Friedrich Kuemmel, in particular, must be mentioned in this respect: Baader, "Politisch motivierte Emigration deutscher Aerzte," 67–84; Kuemmel, "Die Ausschaltung rassisch und politisch missliebiger Aerzte," 56–81.

290 Bach, *Interview* with Kurt Goldstein (June, 1958) in New York City, min. 93–min. 114.

291 Harrington, *Reenchanted Science*, 166; Bullemer, *"Die hiesigen Juden sind in Cham alteingesessen,"* 44–56.

292 The closure in 2001 was due to Berlin's repeated austerity measures in the public health sector. Pross and Winau, *Das Krankenhaus Moabit*, 184–6. As far as the author is aware, no plaque in honour of Goldstein commemorates his forced expulsion from Germany today.

293 Holdorff, "Friedrich Heinrich Lewy," 24–5.

294 See, for example, the letter exchanges between Else Bielschowsky and Lewy's wife in: Peiffer, *Hirnforschung in Deutschland*, 528.

295 Zeman and Klímek, *The Life of Edvard Benes 1884–1948*, 92–100.

296 German-Bohemian Heritage Society, *Newsletter* 8, no. 1 (1997), 6.

297 Schuering, *Minervas verstossene Kinder*, 331–50.

298 Lepsien and Lange, "Verfolgung, Emigration und Ermordung juedischer Aerzte," 42.

299 Some of the re-migrants at older ages included Dr Ruth Silberberg (to Zurich in Switzerland) or Dr Alice Ilian Botan (b. 1924 to Bad Oeyenhausen, Munich). See further in Peters, "Emigration deutscher Psychiater nach England," 161–7.

300 Kater, "Unresolved Questions of German Medicine and Medical History in the Past and Present," 407–23.

301 See: Archives and Rare Books Division of the Becker Library, WUSM (FC0002, Leo Loeb, correspondence R–S, box 5, folder: Silberberg, Martin and Ruth), n.p.

302 Holdorff, "Friedrich Heinrich Lewy," 24–5.

303 Hobsbawm, *The Age of Extremes*, 468–9.

304 The North American refugees were particularly important for the neurologists, psychiatrists, and psychoanalysts who created and worked in the new field of trauma research, which they advanced further in the US. Kurzweil, *Psychoanalytic Science*, 139–55; Mueller, *Von Charlottenburg zum Central Park West*, 185–245.

305 Niederland, *Folgen der Verfolgung*, 10.

306 Focke, *William G. Niederland*, 259–307.

307 Cf. Kuhn, *The Essential Tension*, 156–77.

CHAPTER EIGHT

1 Hauptmann, *Wanda (Der Daemon)*, 465; author's translation.

2 Cf. Sachse, 'Whitewash Culture', 373–99.

3 Vidal and Ortega, *Being Brains*, 105–27.

4 Cf. Harwood, *Styles of Scientific Thought*, 1–45; Zimmerman, *Anthropology and Antihumanism*, 86–107.

5 Bleker, "Der Erfolg der Gleichschaltungsaktion kann als durchschlagend bezeichnet werden," 87–96; Weindling, *Health, Race and German Politics*, 305–98.

6 This became also more relevant for the general character of research in other fields of biomedicine; see Stadler, *Assembling Life*, 137–98; Quirke and Gaudillère, "The Era of Biomedicine," 442.

7 Valuable and instructive exceptions are: Gaudillière, "Making Heredity in Mice and Men," 181–202; Krige and Pestre, *Science in the Twentieth Century*, 897–918; Timmermann, "Appropriating Risk Factors," 157–74.

8 Timmermann, "Americans and Pavlovians," 244–56. Historiographical perspectives on the Soviet Occupied Zone have been put forward by the Contemporary Working Group at the Institute for the History of Medicine in Berlin, see Schleiermacher, *Contested Spaces*, 175–204; Gaudillière and Rheinberger, *From Molecular Genetics to Genomics* (2004).

9 Timmermann, "Americans and Pavlovians," 244–65.

10 Quirke and Gaudillère, "The Era of Biomedicine," 441.

11 Cf. Ash, *Gestalt Psychology in German Culture*, 326–412; Baader, *Politisch motivierte Emigration deutscher Aerzte*, 67–84; Weindling, *Medical Refugees in Britain*, 451–9.

12 See also Stahnisch, "Des gens commes moi étaient désignés comme des 'psychiatres vétérinaires,'" 81–117.

13 Deichmann, *Emigration, Isolation and the Slow Start of Molecular Biology*, 449.

14 Fischer, *Licht und Leben*, 9–13.

15 Eigen, *Erinnerungen an Francis Otto Schmitt*, 35–7.

16 Kroen, *A Political History of the Consumer*, 709–36.

17 Hogan, *The Marshall Plan: America, Britain, and the Reconstruction of Western Europe, 1947–1952* (1987).

18 Fehling, *Die Forschungsfoerderung der amerikanischen Bundesregierung*, 1–32; Krige and Pestre, *Science in the Twentieth Century*, 795–819.

19 A former MPI director, *Interview* (14 November 2003) with author. The quotations given here are from the author's own English translations of original German interviews, when the interviews were conducted in German. English interview excerpts are transcribed, but not translated.

20 Vom Brocke, "Die Kaiser-Wilhelm-/Max-Planck-Gesellschaft," 1–32.

21 Brady, *Eisenhower and Adenauer*, 151–96.

22 Dulles, "U.S.-German Understandings on Cultural Exchange," 567–8.

23 Oral history interviews have been insightful sources, since they provide a more in-depth and lively insight into how young and up-and-coming

researchers looked back at the history of the emergence of the research field of neuroscience from its beginnings in the 1910s to the crises of World War I and World War II. Cf. Adelman, "The Neurosciences Research Program," 15–23.

24 A former MPI director, *Interview* (14 November 2003) with author; author's translation.

25 Globig, *Impulse geben, Wissen stiften*, 231.

26 German neurohistologist Walther Spielmeyer, *List of German Brain Researchers* (30 November 1935) to Rockefeller Foundation officer Alan Gregg. RAC, RG 717, series 1.1, box 9, file 56.

27 Cf. Richardson, "Philanthropy and the Internationality of Learning," 21–58; Hammerstein, *Die Deutsche Forschungsgemeinschaft in der Zeit der Weimarer Republik und im Dritten Reich*, 32–87.

28 Schneider, *Rockefeller Philanthropy and Modern Biomedicine*, 107–9.

29 Farreras, Hannaway, and Harden, *Mind, Brain, Body, and Behavior*, 312–13.

30 Alan N. Schechter at the National Institutes of Health, *Interview* (27 April 2007) with author.

31 US Information Agency, *A Republic of Science*, 4–5.

32 Magoun, *American Neuroscience*, 295–8.

33 A former MPI director, *Interview* (21 November 2003) with author; author's translation.

34 Ibid.

35 Stadler, *Assembling Life*, 199–247; Quirke and Gaudillère, "The Era of Biomedicine," 442; Rose, Abi-Rached, *Neuro*, 9–22.

36 Cf. Stahnisch, "Des gens commes moi étaient désignés comme des 'psychiatres vétérinaires,'" 81–117.

37 Katrin Amunts, *Interview* (15 June 2001) with author; Singer, *Auf dem Weg nach Innen*, 20–34. Professor Anton Kiesselbach, who had been August Hirt's assistant and an SS-funded anatomist at Strasburg during the Nazi period, emerged as a leading voice in identifying the Vogts' brain collection as "German scientific heritage." He seconded its transfer and reception to the Medical Academy of Duesseldorf, where a chair and later an institute were built around this early brain science collection. Pátek, *Die Entwicklung der Anatomie in Duesseldorf*, 82–95.

38 Topp and Peiffer, "Das MPI für Hirnforschung in Giessen: Institutskrise nach 1945, die Hypothek der NS-'Euthanasie' und das Schweigen der Fakultaet," 539–607.

39 Historian John Russell Taylor cunningly described this: "What first fascinated me, appropriately enough for a study that concerns itself in large

measure with the Hollywood dream-factory, was an image ... How did it
feel to be Thomas Mann or Bertold Brecht [1898–1956] or Arnold
Schoenberg [1874–1951] or Theodor Adorno [1903–1969] in Los Angeles
in the 1940s?" Taylor, *Strangers in Paradise*, 165–226, as well as 9
(emphasis in original) for the quotation.

40 A former MPI director, *Interview* (14 November 2003) with author;
author's translation.

41 The director of the medical program Andrew J. Warren (1886–1953?) to
the associate director of the International Health Department, George K.
Strode (1886–1958), in the Rockefeller Foundation's Paris Office, *Letter*
(8 April 1947). RAC, RF archives, RG 717A (postwar survey), series 1.1,
box 2, file 15, 1.

42 Seidelman, "Dissecting the History of Anatomy in the Third Reich – 1989–
2010: A Personal Account," 228–36; Waessle, "A Collection of Brain
Sections of 'Euthanasia' Victims, 166–75.

43 Schmuhl, *Hirnforschung und Krankenmord*, 20–48; Weindling, *Nazi
Medicine and the Nuremberg Trials*, 251–6.

44 List of European institutions that received Rockefeller Foundation funding
(31 December 1951) 717, series 1.1, box T37, 16.

45 Hogan, *The Marshall Plan: America, Britain, and the Reconstruction of
Western Europe, 1947–1952*, 430.

46 Mitscherlich and Mielke, *Medizin ohne Menschlichkeit*, 248–81.

47 RAC, RF 717, series 1.1, box 7, file 37, 50–1.

48 Walther Spielmeyer, *List of German Brain Researchers* (30 November
1935) to Rockefeller Foundation officer Alan Gregg. RAC, RG 717,
series 1.1, box 9, file 56.

49 Alan Gregg (Diary, 1929–1947), *Interviews* with American and German
psychiatrists and neurologists, Monday, 8 December 1947. RAC, RF
archives, RG 717, series 1.1, box T37, 144.

50 RAC, RF archives, RG 717, series 1.1, box 7, file 37: Diary Lambert,
"Walter Riese," 33–4 (emphasis in original).

51 Fehling, *Die Forschungsfoerderung der amerikanischen Bundesregierung*,
1–32.

52 See also Casper, "Atlantic Conjectures in Anglo-American Neurology,"
650.

53 Walther Spielmeyer, *List of German Brain Researchers* (30 November
1935) to Rockefeller Foundation officer Alan Gregg. RAC, RG 717,
series 1.1, box 9, file 56; Diary Lambert, "Walter Riese," 116.

54 Shevell, "Neurosciences in the Third Reich," 132–8.

55 Beddies and Schmiedebach, "'Euthanasie'-Opfer und Versuchsobjekte,"
165–96.

56 Topp, "Shifting Cultures of Memory," 147–82.

57 A former MPI director, *Interview* (14 November 2003) with author; author's translation.

58 Kandel, *In Search of Memory*, 106.

59 A senior scientific member of the Max Planck Gesellschaft, *Interview* (14 November 2003) with author; and a former MPI director, *Interview* (21 November 2003) with author.

60 See Bar-On, *The Role of the Weizmann Institute of Science in Normalizing Israeli-German Relations*, 215–33.

61 Ibid.; author's translation (author's emphasis).

62 Stahnisch, "Karl T. Neubuerger (1890–1972): Pioneer in Neurology," 1493–5.

63 See also: Schuering, *Minervas verstossene Kinder*, 331–47.

64 Cf. Stahnisch, "Zur Zwangsemigration deutschsprachiger Neurowissenschaftler," 442–3; and a former MPI director, *Interview* (21 November 2003) with author; author's translation.

65 Peiffer, *Hirnforschung in Deutschland*, 116–19.

66 Braese and Gross, *NS-Medizin und Oeffentlichkeit. Formen der Aufarbeitung nach 1945*, 323–8; Wolfgang Schuetz, "Der Umgang der oesterreichischen Aerzteschaft mit der NS-Vergangenheit," 213–16.

67 See the belated interest reflected in the series *Geschichte der KWG*, edited by Ruerup, Reinhard, and Wolfgang Schieder (Goettingen, Germany: Wallstein, 2000–05), 28 vols.

68 Stahnisch, "History of Neurology," 9–10.

69 Walter Zieglgaensberger, *Interview* (22 May 2017) with author.

70 A former MPI director, *Interview* (21 November 2003) with author; author's translation.

71 Brady, *Eisenhower and Adenauer*, 151–96.

72 The influences of the Minerva Foundation were also very important in fostering academic exchanges with Israel during the earlier postwar period. See Bar-On, *The Role of the Weizmann Institute of Science in Normalizing Israeli-German Relations*, 215–33.

73 Stahnisch, "History of Neurology: Bringing Back Neurology Following WWII," 9–10.

74 A former MPI director, *Interview* (21 November 2003) with author.

75 Adelman and Smith, "Francis Otto Schmitt," 7.

76 Neuburger, *The Historical Development of Experimental Brain and Spinal Cord Physiology before Flourens*, 40–3; Schmitt, *The Never-Ceasing Search*, 321 (emphasis in original).

77 "Acutely aware that the division of science into disciplinary pigeonholes was an arbitrary artifice, Frank was convinced that it did great harm by

creating barriers for heuristically futile communication. In particular, he fervently believed in the need for a cross-disciplinary perspective in order to find physical solutions to biological problems, and thus he became a leader in the effort to broaden and reformulate the nascent interdisciplinary field of biophysics." Adelman and Smith, "Francis Otto Schmitt," 7; Worden, Schmitt, Swazey, and Adelman, *The Neurosciences*, 3–4.

78 See, for example, Schmitt, *The Never-Ceasing Search*, 189–230; as well as Worden, Schmitt, Swazey, and Adelman, *The Neurosciences*, 3–104.

79 Adelman and Smith, "Francis Otto Schmitt," 1–14.

80 Worden, Schmitt, Swazey, and Adelman, *The Neurosciences*, 545 (author's emphasis).

81 Bechtel, "Cognitive Neuroscience," 82; Kay, "Conceptual Models and Analytical Tools," 207–46; Kay, "Rethinking Institutions," 283–93; Worden, Schmitt, Swazey, and Adelman, *The Neurosciences*, 3–4; Pickenhain, "Die Neurowissenschaft," 241–6.

82 Schmitt, *The Never-Ceasing Search*, 214–17.

83 Pickenhain, ibid., 243–4.

84 Kuhn, *The Structure of Scientific Revolutions*, 2–9.

85 Schmitt, *The Never-Ceasing Search*, 231–2.

86 Magoun, *American Neuroscience*, 165–92.

87 Schmitt, "Molecular Biology among the Neurosciences," 561–72; Marcus Raichle, *Interview* (12 July 2007) with author.

88 Schmitt, *The Never-Ceasing Search*, 214–17.

89 Anonymus, "Francis O. Schmitt," 5. He was one of the very few neuroscientists ever to appear on the frontpage of *Time Magazine*. Robert Sulivan, "Francis O. Schmitt, 91, Is Dead; Led Studies in Molecular Biology." *New York Times* 143 (7 October 1995), n.p.

90 Cf. Squire, *The History of Neuroscience in Autobiography*, vol. 1, i–vii.

91 See also Kreutzberg, "Vorwort," 35.

92 Schmitt's emphasis on large-scale group research projects is well reflected in his own autobiographical accounts, as well as in interviews with contemporaries. Squire, *The History of Neuroscience in Autobiography*, vol. 1.

93 The US National Research Council, inaugurated in 1916, was itself a funding institution modeled after the German system of regional academies and the KWG. It continued to transmit a new national style of research cooperation ("*Grossforschung*"), which is convincingly argued in Kevles, "Into Hostile Political Camps," 49–50.

94 On the "Harnack principle" of the KWG, see also Weber, "Harnack-Prinzip oder Fuehrerprinzip?," 410–18.

95 Schmitt, *The Never-Ceasing Search*, 80–4 and 226–7.

96 Cf. Peukert, *The Weimar Republic*, 21–46; Ash and Soellner, *Forced Migration and Scientific Change*, 1–22; Medawar and Pyke, *Hitler's Gift*, 231–40.

97 Ruerup and Schuering, *Schicksale und Karrieren*, 379–82.

98 Schmitt, *The Never-Ceasing Search*, 86–7. Manfred Eigen later won the Nobel Prize in Chemistry for his work on the physical chemistry of membrane ultrastructures in 1967. Mandel, *Manfred Eigen Festschrift*, 101–390.

99 See also the Reports and Agendas of the officers of the Rockefeller Foundation, which give intriguing insights into researchers' private relations and ways of communication at the time. Historisches Archiv des Max-Planck-Instituts fuer Psychiatrie, RAC, RF Collection International Finance Corporation, KWIBR, America's Great Depression, 27.

100 Schmitt, *The Never-Ceasing Search*, 202–7.

101 A senior scientific member of the Max Planck Gesellschaft, *Interview* (14 November 2003) with author.

102 Eigen, "Erinnerungen an Francis Otto Schmitt," 36.

103 A former MPI director, *Interview* (14 November 2003) with author.

104 See, for example, Harwood, *Styles of Scientific Thought*, 138–80.

105 A former MPI director, *Interview* (14 November 2003) with author.

106 The individual answers in the interviews in this chapter are not identified here; yet much background information was gained through interviews (formal and informal exchanges) with the following individuals: a former MPI director, *Interview* (14 November 2003) with author; a senior scientific member of the Max Planck Gesellschaft, *Interview* (14 November 2003) with author.

107 Schmitt, *The Never-Ceasing Search*, 92–3.

108 The number of resident scientists was just about forty all in all. A former MPI director, *Interview* (14 November 2003) with author, who stayed at the Massachusetts Institute of Technology's Department of Psychology from 1964 to 1965. Another MPI director visited the Austrian émigré neurobiologist Paul Weiss (1898–1989) at New York's Rockefeller University between 1967 and 1968; and he later worked with the German émigré neuropsychologist Hans-Lukas Teuber at the Massachusetts Institute of Technology. He even visited the ethology laboratory that Teuber established as the director of the primate centre in Tenerife, Spain; former MPI director, *Interview* (21 November 2003) with author. Both neuroscientists were among the residents of the Neuroscience Research Program, while vividly emphasizing the pragmatic set-up of the American program which constituted a luxurious atmosphere which they described as free of political prejudices.

109 Eigen, "Erinnerungen an Francis Otto Schmitt," 36.

110 This particularly included the opportunities that the program offered for postgraduate training of a new generation of German-speaking neuroscientists. Eigen also wrote many grant proposals to receive financial support from the Federal Republic of Germany, while eventually obtaining a strong engagement through the German Volkswagen Foundation in the mid-1960s. As a consequence of these sustained planning steps, German neuroscientists were enabled to participate in vigorous international exchanges with other participants in the Neuroscience Research Program. A former MPI director, *Interview* (14 November 2003) with author.

111 The setting and the scenery resembled very much the workshop locale that Schmitt had earlier encountered at Hahnenklee in the Harz mountains, when visiting Eigen in Goettingen several years before. Schmitt, *The Never-Ceasing Search*, 4 and 192–3.

112 The Boulder Meetings brought together two hundred biologists, chemists, physicists, psychologists, and engineers to attend formal lectures and informal workshops. "During term break they used to rent half the campus and the dormitories. It was a great meeting atmosphere and Manfred Eigen played music ... Everyone who did high quality research in neuroscience was there." A former MPI director, *Interview* (14 November 2003) with author.

113 See, for example, Schmitt and Warden, *The Neurosciences*, 305–10. The first edition of the foundational textbook (with its organization along many interdisciplinary topic areas) by Kandel, Schwartz, and Jessell, *Principles of Neural Science* (1981), can also be seen as having its origins in the discussion areas and the networking opportunity that the NRP had provided over the two decades before its first publication.

114 "Everyone knew each other, but the relationships were not as institutionalized as today." A senior scientific member of the Max Planck Gesellschaft, *Interview* (14 November 2003) with author.

115 A former MPI director, *Interview* with author (14 November 2003); author's translation.

116 A former MPI director, *Interview* (14 November 2003) with author. Only seven senior neuroscientists from German-speaking countries took active part in the early years of the Neuroscience Research Program: Leo de Maeyer (1927–2014); Richard Jung (1911–1986); Hans Georg Baumgarten (b. 1936); Manfred Eigen; Detlef Ploog (1920–2005); Hans Thoenen (1928–2012); and Werner Reichhardt (1924–1992). However, there had been a great number of junior scientists as participants, the

total being a staggering number of two thousand in the nearly fifteen years of its existence. Schmitt, *The Never-Ceasing Search*, 234–5.

117 Marcus Raichle, *Interview* (12 July 2007); Schmitt, "Molecular Biology among the Neurosciences," 561–72.

118 A former MPI director, *Interview* (14 November 2003) with author.

119 Alumni members, however, continued their relationships with Neuroscience Research Program as designated "Honorary Associates," such as De Maeyer, Eigen, Ploog, Thoenen, while Reichhardt continued as a permanent member until the Neuroscience Research Program was succeeded by the Society for Neuroscience. A senior scientific member of the Max Planck Gesellschaft, *Interview* (14 November 2003) with author.

120 Schmitt, *The Never-Ceasing Search*, 224–5.

121 They were aided by the help of assistant writers and Neuroscience Research Program staff members. A former MPI director, *Interview* (14 November 2003) with author.

122 A former MPI director, *Interview* (14 November 2003) with author.

123 Cf. Nitsch, *Zur cholinergen Innervation identifizierter Neurone*, 85–93.

124 Francis O. Schmitt et al., eds., *The Neuroscience Research (Program) Bulletin* (Cambridge, MA: MIT Press), 1964–82, 21 vols.

125 See the exchanges between the Deutsche Forschungsgemeinschaft and the RF during the Weimar period. RAC, RF Archives, RG 1.1, series 717, box 7, folder 36, as well as *Notgemeinschaft/Deutsche Forschungsgemeinschaft Bestand* (1921–1933), BA KO, Collections: R 56/68/70.

126 A former MPI director, *Interview* (21 November 2003) with author.

127 A former MPI director, *Interview* (14 November 2003) with author.

128 A former MPI director, *Interview* (21 November 2003) with author; author's translation.

129 Worden, Schmitt, Swazey, and Adelman, *The Neurosciences*, 545; Schmitt, *The Never-Ceasing Search*, 298–9.

130 A senior scientific member of the Max Planck Gesellschaft, *Interview* (14 November 2003) with author.

131 The number of early presidents among Neuroscience Research Program general members was even higher. Magoun, *American Neuroscience*, 165–240.

132 Adelman and Smith, "Francis Otto Schmitt," 354.

133 Barry Smith and George Adelman have stated that Schmitt had sought to create a "hybrid field" of research and continuous learning through both the Neuroscience Research Program's interdisciplinary organization and

its biophysics precursor, the Intensive Study Program. This intention is further emphasized by Schmitt's conviction that "on every level – neuroscience perspectives are equal." A former MPI director, *Interview* (14 November 2003) with author.

134 Cf. Latour, *Science in Action*, 125–95; Kuhn, *The Essential Tension*, 293–319; as well as Lakatos and Musgrave, *Criticism and the Growth of Knowledge*, 91–196.

135 Kuhn, *The Essential Tension*, 307–19.

136 Leibowitz and Held, "Hans-Lukas Teuber," 1–3.

137 See also in Barnes and Edge, *Science in Context*, 65–6.

138 Cf. Worden, Schmitt, Swazey, and Adelman, *The Neurosciences*, 3–4.

139 Kevles, "Into Hostile Political Camps," 47–60.

140 A former MPI director, *Interview* (14 November 2003) with author; author's translation.

141 Charpa and Deichmann, *Jews and Sciences in German Contexts*, 270–95.

142 Between 1999 to 2004, the Max Planck Society for the Advancement of Science had, for example, created a research program, facilitated by Professors Reinhard Ruerup (Berlin) and Carola Sachse (Vienna) – among others in the leadership team – on the ".The History of the Kaiser Wilhelm Society under National Socialism." It ended with a noteworthy public apology of then-Max Planck Society President, Professor Hubert Markl (1838–2015), at their Final Conference in 2001: "In truth, only those who are guilty can beg for pardon. Nevertheless, I ask you, the surviving victims, most sincerely to forgive those who, for whatever reason, have themselves failed to beg your pardon ... [And] The most honest form of apology lies in the disclosure of guilt." Hubert Markl qtd from Von Aretin, "Under the Watchful Gaze of Minerva: Traditions, Symbols and Dealing with the Past," p. 6.

143 Peiffer, "Die Vertreibung deutscher Neuropathologen," 99–109; Peiffer, "Zur Neurologie im 'Dritten Reich,'" 728–33.

144 Feldmann, *Historische Vergangenheitsbearbeitung*, 5–21.

145 Popper, *The Open Society and Its Enemies*, 265–70.

146 Cf. Sachse, '*Whitewash Culture*', 373–99.

147 Kandel, *In Search of Memory*, 33–5.

CONCLUSION

1 Statement by a former MPI director *Interview* (14 November 2003) with author.

2 See, for example: Harrington, *Reenchanted Science,* 103–39; Richter, *Das Kaiser-Wilhelm-Institut fuer Hirnforschung,* 352–72; Borck, *Hirnstroeme,* 85–140.

3 Radkau, *Das Zeitalter der Nervositaet,* 173–259.

4 Hofer, *Nervenschwaeche und Krieg,* 13–42; Hau, *The Cult of Health and Beauty,* 102–24.

5 Hofer, *Nervenschwaeche und Krieg,* 13–42; Turda, *The Biology of War,* 238–64.

6 Stahnisch, "Zur Bedeutung der Konzepte der 'neuronalen De- und Regeneration,'" 243–69.

7 Weindling, *Health, Race and German Politics,* 61–154, Nicosia and Huener, *Medicine and Medical Ethics in Nazi Germany,* 1–15; and Aly, *Aktion T4 1939–1945,* 189–92.

8 See, for example, Lawrence and Weisz, *Greater than the Parts,* 1–22.

9 Institutionally, this differentiation took off with the creation of the first independent clinical chair for neurology in Hamburg in 1913. Stahnisch and Koehler, "Three Twentieth-Century Multi-Authored Handbooks," 1067–75.

10 The latter had been earlier founded as Verein deutscher Irrenaerzte in 1864 under the presidency of Carl Friedrich Fleming (1799–1880), who was the chief of service of the mental asylum in Schwerin, Mecklenburg.

11 Karenberg, "Klinische Neurologie in Deutschland," 20–9.

12 In Binding and Hoche, *Die Freigabe der Vernichtung lebensunwerten Lebens,* 22–3; author's translation.

13 See in Greenblatt, Dagi, Epstein, *A History of Neurosurgery in Its Scientific and Professional Contexts,* 15–24.

14 Cf. Kuhn, *The Structure of Scientific Revolutions,* 2–9.

15 Efron, *Medicine and the German Jews,* 234–64.

16 Stahnisch, "Der 'Rosenthal'sche Versuch,'" 15.

17 Charpa and Deichmann, *Jews and Sciences in German Contexts,* 270–95.

18 Ringer, *The Decline of the German Mandarins,* 14–35.

19 Cf. Harwood, *Styles of Scientific Thought,* 195–226.

20 See also Stahnisch, "Psychiatrie und Hirnforschung," 76–81.

21 Holdorff, *Die Neurologie in Berlin, 1840–1945,* 155–77.

22 Stahnisch, "Der 'Rosenthal'sche Versuch,'" 15.

23 Huentelmann, "Ehrlich faerbt am laengsten," 354–80.

24 Dohm, *Geschichte der Histopathologie,* 302; Bielschowsky, "Die Silberimpraegnation der Neurofibrillen," 186–7.

25 Von Weizsaecker, *Wahrnehmen und Bewegen,* 30.

26 Von Weizsaecker, *Der Arzt und der Kranke*, 187; author's translation (emphasis in original).

27 Schierer, *Das Laboratorium der buergerlichen Welt*, 15–30.

28 Weindling, *Health, Race and German Politics*, 305–98.

29 Peiffer, "Zur Neurologie im 'Dritten Reich,'" 728–33; Roelcke, "Wissenschaften zwischen Innovation und Entgrenzung," 92–109; and Roelcke, "Programm und Praxis der psychiatrischen Genetik," 21–55.

30 Weindling, *Health, Race and German Politics*, 305–50.

31 Aly, *Aktion T4 1939–1945*, 134–9.

32 Proctor, *The Nazi War on Cancer*, 15–57.

33 Vom Brocke, *Die Kaiser-Wilhelm-/Max-Planck-Gesellschaft*, 1–32; Schmuhl, *Hirnforschung und Krankenmord*, 41–52.

34 Cf. Cottebrune, *Die Deutsche Forschungsgemeinschaft*, 354–78.

35 Schmuhl, *Hirnforschung und Krankenmord*, 53–6; Zimmermann, *Die Medizinische Fakultaet der Universitaet Jena waehrend der Zeit des Nationalsozialismus*, 82–3; Wechsler, *La Faculté de Médecine*, 12–31.

36 Richter, *Das Kaiser-Wilhelm-Institut fuer Hirnforschung*, 367–73.

37 Weindling, *Victims and Survivors of Nazi Human Experiments Science and Suffering in the Holocaust*, 36–56 and 92–102.

38 This has sometimes been implied in the early research literature on the subject. Cf. Kater, *Doctors under Hitler*, 12–34.

39 See some of the direct quotations from the contemporary brain researchers in: Peiffer, *Hirnforschung in Deutschland*, 44–59.

40 Nicosia and Huener, *Medicine and Medical Ethics in Nazi Germany*, 1–15.

41 Hildebrandt, *The Anatomy of Murder*, 44–69.

42 Schmuhl, *Die Gesellschaft Deutscher Neurologen und Psychiater im Nationalsozialismus*, 8–13.

43 Aly, *Aktion T4 1939–1945*, 189–92.

44 Ibid.

45 Nicosia and Huener, *Medicine and Medical Ethics in Nazi Germany*, 1–15; Cornwell, *Hitler's Scientists*, 71–90.

46 Cf. Kuehl, *The Nazi Connection*, 3–12.

47 Forel, *Alkohol, Vererbung und Sexualleben*, 1–20; Kleist, *Gehirnpathologie*, 1364–70.

48 Ruedin, *Studien ueber Vererbung*, 254–6. Among the standard therapies counted, for example, forms of electroconvulsive therapy, psychosurgery, and insulin shock therapies, pharmacotherapy (e.g. lithium, bromide, valproate, and sleep-inducers) as well as physical therapy.

49 Schmaltz, *Kampfstoff-Forschung im Nationalsozialismus*, 144–87.

50 See Black, *War Against the Weak*, 261–2.

51 Mitscherlich and Mielke, *Medizin ohne Menschlichkeit*, 19.
52 This assessment drew on archival research in, for example: Leipzig 1934, Film 443, UAL, Collection on the Medical Faculty, B III 1a/vol. 1 – Anatomy Chair (1849–1917), n.pag.; Strasburg 1898–1918, ADAS, AL 103 / No. 1200 / Pa. 254, Collection on the Medical Faculty, Department of Anatomy (January 1898–October 1918), n.p.
53 Adelman, "The Neurosciences Research Program," 15–23.
54 Satzinger, *Die Geschichte der genetisch orientierten Hirnforschung*, 65–95.
55 On the international influences from outside Germany and Austria, see also Richter, *Das Kaiser-Wilhelm-Institut fuer Hirnforschung*, 349–408.
56 Engstrom, *Clinical Psychiatry in Imperial Germany*, 194–203.
57 Fehling, *Die Forschungsfoerderung der amerikanischen Bundesregierung*, 1–32; Stahnisch, *Flexible Antworten – Offene Fragen*, 56–8.
58 Cf. Brock and Harward, *The Culture of Biomedicine*, 10.
59 This clearly led to a plethora of misunderstandings, irritations, and even the discontinuation of research by dozens of émigré neuroscientists when they landed on the western side of the Atlantic. See, for example, the archival materials (BA KO, Collections on the *Deutsche Forschungsgemeinschaft* R 73 / 69 /) from the Deutsche Forschungsgemeinschaft in Koblenz, the RAC in Sleepy Hollow and the NIH [National Institutes of Health] in Bethesda, MD.
60 Fehling, *Die Forschungsfoerderung der amerikanischen Bundesregierung*, 1–32.
61 The process of a "normalization" of research support and exchanges – both on a pragmatic and procedural level, as well as an ethical and moral level – is visibly put forward in: "The Problem of Germany is primarily a moral problem." Report by the Chicago physicist Robert J. Havigherst (RJH), 1900–1991. RAC, RF archives, record group report, RF 717, series 1.1, box 7, 57.
62 Timmermann, "Americans and Pavlovians," 244–56; Quirke and Gaudillière, "The Era of Biomedicine," 441.
63 Assmann, *Trauma des Krieges und Literatur*, 95–6; Schleiermacher, *Contested Spaces*, 175–204; Ash, "Von Vielschichtigkeiten und Verschraenkungen," 91–105.
64 Feindel and Leblanc, *The Wounded Brain Healed*, 193–238.
65 For the underlying philosophy of science foundations, which changed during this period as well, see Craver, *Explaining the Brain*, 228–71.
66 See for example the early works of Baader, "Politisch motivierte Emigration deutscher Aerzte," 67–84; Kuemmel, "Die Ausschaltung rassisch und politisch missliebiger Aerzte," 56–81.

67 Cf. Fleming and Bailyn, *The Intellectual Migration*, 3–10, 371–419 and
   420–45; Coser, *Refugee Scholars in America*, 45–7; Medawar and Pyke,
   Hitler's Gift, 231–40; Hunt, *Secret Agenda*, 217–39; Rose and Abi-Rached,
   Neuro, 23–4 and 232–4.
68 Stahnisch, *The "Brain Gain Thesis" Revisited*, 128–45.

Bibliography

ARCHIVAL SOURCES AND RESEARCH LIBRARY COLLECTIONS

Austria

Archives and Collections on the Medical Faculty; Obersteiner Collections; Medical University of Vienna, Vienna
History of Medicine Library; Institute for the History of Medicine; Josephinum, Medical University of Vienna, Vienna

Canada

Dalhousie University Archives & Special Collections; Robert Weil Correspondence; Killam Memorial Library, Halifax
Division des Archives Universitaires de l'Université de Montréal; Hans Selye Papers; Montreal
Library and Archives Canada; Collection on the Canadian Society for the Protection of Science and Learning and Collection on Passenger Lists to Halifax, 1865–1935; Ottawa
Library of the Montreal Neurological Institute; McGill University, Montreal
Mackie Family Collection for the History of Neuroscience; Calgary
MacKimmie Library; Special Collections; University of Calgary
National Library of Quebec; Collection on Immigration to Canada; Montreal
Nova Scotia Archives and Records Management; Department of Public Health Reports; Halifax
Osler Library for the History of Medicine; General Collection; Wilder Penfield Fonds; Collection on the Montreal Neurological Institute; Montreal

Pier 21 Memorial Museum; Collection on Immigration Records; Halifax

Provincial Archives; Collection on the Royal College of Physicians and
Surgeons of Nova Scotia; Halifax

Redpath Library; Special Collections and Journal Collections; McGill
University, Montreal

University Archives of McGill University; Human Resources Files and
Collection on the Allan Memorial Institute; Montreal

University Archives of the University of Alberta; Collection on the
Physiological Institute; Edmonton

University Archives of the University of Ottawa; Karl Stern Fonds, Human
Resources Files; Ottawa

University Library and the Special Collection of Medical History; Dalhousie
University, Halifax

France

Archives départementales [du Bas-Rhin] à Strasbourg; Collections on the
Medical Faculty and Collections on the Curator of the Kaiser Wilhelm
University; Strasburg

Archives universitaires de l'Université de Strasbourg (Pasteur); Collections on
the Medical Faculty; Strasburg

Bibliothèque de l'Université de Strasbourg (Pasteur); Collections on the
Medical Faculty; Strasburg

Bibliothèque nationale de France (BnF); Paris

Laboratoire d'épistemologie des sciences de la vie et de la santé; Collection on
the Institute of Pathology and Collection on the Institutes of Anatomy of
the Reichsuniversitaet and the Kaiser-Wilhelm-Universitaet Strassburg;
Université de Strasbourg, Strasburg

Germany

Archival Collections of the German Hygiene Museum in Dresden; Dresden

Archive for the History of Psychiatry; Collection on the Clinical Department
of Neurology and Psychiatry; University of Leipzig, Leipzig

Archives of the C. and O. Vogt Institute for Brain Research, Medical Faculty;
Photographical Collection on the Berlin Neurobiological Laboratory;
Heinrich Heine University Duesseldorf

Autograph Collection of the Library of the University of Leipzig, Leipzig

Bavarian State Library; Special Collections; Munich

Bavarian Main State Archive, Collection MK 8/I Ministry of Science, Education
and Art; Munich

Bundesarchiv Koblenz (BA KO); General Collections on the Deutsche Forschungsgemeinschaft (DFG) R 73 and Collections on Praesidium Minutes; Koblenz

Central Medical Library; Humboldt University (Charité); Berlin

External Historical Archive of the Max Planck Institute for Psychiatry; Collections on the Deutsche Forschungsanstalt fuer Psychiatrie; MPI for Psychiatry, Munich

Historical Archive of the Max Planck Gesellschaft; Collections on the Kaiser Wilhelm Society, KWI for Brain Research Fonds; Otto Warburg House, Berlin

Institute for the History and Ethics of Medicine; Collections on the Ludwig Edinger Institute; Johann Wolfgang Goethe University, Frankfurt am Main

Institute Library of the Clinical Department of Psychiatry; Friedrich Alexander University Erlangen-Nuernberg, Erlangen

Institute Library of the Department of Anatomy I; Friedrich Alexander University Erlangen-Nuernberg, Erlangen

Institute Library of the Department of Neurobiology; Institute for Anatomy; Charité Medical School, Humboldt University Berlin

Institute Library of the Institute for the History of Medicine; Humboldt University (Charité), Berlin

Institute Library of the Institute for the History and Ethics of Medicine; Friedrich Alexander University, Erlangen-Nuernberg

Institute Library of the Institute for the History of Medicine; Ludwigs Maximilians University, Wuerzburg

Institute Library of the Institute for the History and Ethics of Medicine; Eberhard Karls University, Heidelberg

Institute Library of the Institute for the History, Philosophy and Ethics of Medicine; Johannes Gutenberg University, Mainz

Institute Library of the Senckenberg Institute for the History and Ethics of Medicine; Johann Wolfgang Goethe University, Frankfurt am Main

Library of the Max Planck Institute for Brain Research; Report and Preprint Collection on the History of the Institute; MPI for Brain Research, Frankfurt am Main

Library of the Karl Sudhoff Institute for the History of Medicine and Science; Collection on the University of Leipzig Institutes and the Paul Flechsig Institute; University of Leipzig, Leipzig

Library of the Max Planck Institute for Neurobiology; Historical Collection; MPI for Neurobiology, Martinsried

Library of the Max Planck Institute for the History of Science; Berlin

Personal Collection of Juergen Peiffer; Collection of Letter Exchanges between Brain Researchers, 1910 to 1945; Tuebingen

Prussian State Library; Special Collections; Culture Forum, Berlin
Senckenberg Library Frankfurt; Collections on the University; Frankfurt am Main
University Archives of the Humboldt University of Berlin; Collections on the Medical Faculty and Human Resources Files; Humboldt University of Berlin, Berlin
University Archives of the Johann Wolfgang Goethe University of Frankfurt; Collections on the Medical Faculty and Collection on the "Edinger Commission"; Frankfurt am Main
University Archives of the University of Leipzig; Collections on the Medical Faculty, Collection on the Human Resources Department PA 48 and Special Collections, Medical Faculty; University of Leipzig, Leipzig
University Archives of the Ludwigs Maximilians University of Munich; Collections on the Medical Faculty, Munich
University Library; Eberhard Karls University; Tuebingen
University Library; Friedrich Alexander University, Erlangen-Nuernberg
University Library; Paul Moebius Papers; University of Leipzig, Leipzig

Hungary

University Archives of the Ignaz Semmelweis University; Collection on the Anatomical Institute; Ignaz Semmelweis University, Budapest

Poland

Archives of the Medical Faculty; Human Resources Files; University of Breslau, Wrocław
State Archives of Silesia; Collections on the Prussian Province of Silesia and Collections on the Friedrich Wilhelms University of Breslau; Wrocław
University Archives Breslau; Collections on the Medical Faculty; Wrocław

Switzerland

Archives of the Institute for Medical History and Museum; Monakow, Constantin von, Correspondence; University of Zurich, Zurich
University Library of the University of Zurich, Zurich

United Kingdom

Bodleian Libraries; Collection on the "Society for the Protection of Learning and Science"; Oxford

Library of the Wellcome Centre for the History of Medicine and Disease; Durham University, Durham
National Library of Scotland – Leabharlann Nàiseanta na h-Alba, Edinburgh
University Library of the University of Edinburgh, Edinburgh
Wellcome Library for the History and Understanding of Medicine; Ludwig Guttmann Papers; London

United States

Archives and Rare Books Division of the Becker Library; Faculty of Medicine, Central Administration, and Archival Collections on the American Academy of Neurology; Washington University School of Medicine; St Louis, Missouri
Archives of Columbia University; Kurt Goldstein Papers; Columbia University, New York City
Bancroft Library; Archival collections on the University of California; University of California at Berkeley, Berkeley, California
De Witt Institute for the History of Psychiatry; Diethelm Library for the History of Psychiatry; Cornell and Columbia Medical Center, New York City
Doe University Library; Special Collections; University of California at Berkeley, Berkeley, California
Harvard University Archives; Countway Library for the History of Medicine; Harvard Medical School, Boston, Massachusetts
Holocaust Center of Northern California; William G. Niederland Box, San Francisco, California
Library of the Leo-Baeck-Institute, New York City
National Archives of the United States of America; Field Intelligence Agency (technical) Records, Franz Boas Papers, Washington, DC
National Library of Medicine; Collection of the Annual Research Reports of the Intramural Program and Extramural Program of the National Institutes of Health, 1948–1960; National Institutes of Health, Bethesda, Maryland
Neuroscience History Archives; Oral History Interview Project and Collection on Caesar Hirsch; Louise M. Darling Library, University of California at Los Angeles, Los Angeles, California
Office of the History of Medicine; Archival Collections on the History of the National Institutes of Health; National Institutes of Health, Bethesda, Maryland
Office of the History of Science and Technoloy; Library; University of California at Berkeley, Berkeley, California
Rockefeller Archives Center; Collections on Alan Gregg; German Displaced Scholars; Germany; Kaiser Wilhelm Society in Germany; Rockefeller

Collection and Funding Program for Psychosomatics, Sleepy Hollow, New York
University Library; Johns Hopkins University, Baltimore, Maryland
University Library; Stanford University, Palo Alto, California
University Library; Adolf Wallenberg Collection; University of California at San Francisco, San Francisco, California

INTERVIEWS AND CORRESPONDENCE

Alberto Aguayo, *Letter*, 20 November 2006

Katrin Amunts, *Interview*, 15 June 2001

Ingo Bechmann, *Interview*, 19 February 2007

Volker Bigl (†), *Interview*, 15 September 2004

David Colman (†), *Interview*, 26 May 2007

Javier de Felipe, *Letter*, 18 November 2001

Steve Dell, *Interview*, 28 June 2007

Rolando del Maestro, *Interview*, 5 May 2005

Maurice Dongier (†), *Interview*, 26 May 2007

Karl Max Einhaeupl, *Interview*, 27 August 2001

Paul A.T.M. Eling, *Interview*, 13 July 2017

Bill Feindel (†), *Interview*, 11 November 2006

Moshe Feinsod, *Interview*, 22 June 2007

Bob Gordon, *Interview*, 11 September 2007

Hermann Handwerker, *Interview*, 13 June, 2003

Bernd Holdorff, *Interview*, 2 October 2007

Georg W. Kreutzberg (†), *Interviews*, 14 November 2003 and 18 May 2017

Wolfgang Kuehnel (†), *Letter*, 15 February 2002

Werner Friedrich Kuemmel, *Interview*, 17 October 2005

Winfried Neuhuber, *Interview*, 28 October 2004

Robert Nitsch, *Interview*, 29 November 2010

Ruediger Lorenz (†), *Interview*, 15 May 1999

Louise H. Marshall (†), *Interview*, 5 June 2002

Hugo Moser (†), *Letter*, 21 November 2006

Olaf Ninnemann, *Interview*, 14 June 2001

Leo Peichl, *Interview*, 26 April 2004

Juergen Peiffer (†), *Letter*, 10 June 2005

Lothar Pickenhain (†), *Letter*, 13 September 2004

Detlev Ploog (†), *Interview*, 21 November 2003

Marcus Raichle, *Interview*, 12 July 2007

Gebhard Reiss, *Interview*, 10 July 2002

Wolfram Richter (†), *Interview*, 27 July 2001
Bert Sakmann, *Interview*, 20 May 2017
Milagros Salas-Prato, *Letter*, 16 June 2011
Alan N. Schechter, *Interview*, 27 April 2007
Bill Seidelman, *Letter*, 7 October 2010
Allen Sherwin (†), *Interview*, 27 March 2009
Michael I. Shevell, *Interview*, 27 May 2007
Ted Sourkes (†), *Interview*, 12 December 2006
Hans Thoenen (†), *Interview*, 14 November 2003
Donald B. Tower (†), *Interview*, 20 April 2007
Hartmut Wekerle, *Interview*, 25 May 2017
Walter Zieglgaensberger, *Interview*, 22 May 2017
Karl Zilles, *Interview*, 6 March 2005

PUBLISHED SOURCES

Abella, Irving and Harold Troper. *None Is Too Many: Canada and the Jews of Europe: 1933–1948*. Toronto: University of Toronto Press, 1982.
Abraham, Karl. "Erstes Korreferat." *Zur Psychoanalyse der Kriegsneurosen. Internationale Psychoanalytische Bibliothek* 1, no. 1 (1919): 31–41.
Ackerknecht, Erwin H. *A Short History of Psychiatry*. New York: Hafner, 1968.
Adams, Annmarie. "Désigning Penfield: Inside the Montreal Neurological Institute." *Bulletin of the History of Medicine* 93, no. 2 (2019): 207–40.
Adams, Mark B., Garland E. Allen, and Sheila Faith, Weiss. "Human Heredity and Politics: A Comparative Institutional Study of the Eugenics Record Office at Cold Spring Harbor (United States), the Kaiser Wilhelm Institute for Anthropology, Human Heredity and Eugenics (Germany) and the Maxim Gorky Medical Genetics Institute (USSR)." *OSIRIS, 2nd Series* 20, no. 1 (2005): 232–62.
Adelman, George. "The Neurosciences Research Program at MIT and the Beginning of the Modern Field of Neuroscience." *Journal of the History of the Neurosciences* 19, no. 1 (2010): 15–23.
Adelman, George and Barry Smith. "Francis Otto Schmitt. November 23, 1903–October 3, 1995." *Biographical Memoirs of the National Academy of Science* 75, no. 3 (1998): 1–14.
Alexander, Leo. "Classified Reports for the Combined Intelligence Subcommittee Reports – CIOS." Partially published as *The Treatment of Shock from Prolonged Exposure to Cold, Especially in Water*, edited by US

Army Medical Corps, rept. 250. Washington, DC: Office of the Publication Board, Department of Commerce, 1946.

Allan, Garland E. "The Ideology of Elimination: American and German Eugenics, 1900–1945." In *Medicine and Medical Ethics in Nazi Germany: Origins, Practices, Legacies*, edited by Francis R. Nicosia and Jonathan Huener, 13–39. New York: Berghahn Books, 2002.

Aly, Goetz, ed. *Aktion T4 1939–1945. Die "Euthanasie-Zentrale" in der Tiergartenstrasse*. Berlin, Germany: Edition Hentrich, 1987.

Alzheimer, Alois. "Ueber eine eigenartige Erkrankung der Hirnrinde." *Allgemeine Zeitschrift fuer Psychiatrie und Psychisch-gerichtliche Medizin* 64, no. 1 (1907): 146–8.

– "Ist die Einrichtung einer psychiatrischen Abteilung im Reichsgesundheitsamt erstrebenswert?" *Zeitschrift fuer die gesamte Neurologie und Psychiatrie* 6, no. 1 (1911): 242–6.

Ammerer, Heinrich. "Seelenheilkunde und Wissenschaft im 'Goldenen Zeitalter der Psychiatrie': Richard von Krafft-Ebing (1840–1902)." PhD Diss., University of Salzburg, Austria, 2010.

Anctil, Michel. *Dawn of the Neuron: The Early Struggles to Trace the Origin of Nervous Systems*. Montreal and Kingston: McGill-Queen's University Press, 2015.

Angermeyer, Matthias C., and Holger Steinberg. *200 Jahre Psychiatrie an der Universitaet Leipzig. Personen und Konzepte*. Berlin, Germany: Springer, 2005.

Anon. "Ich Dien – Schaden durch Entschaedigung." *Der Spiegel*, 1 January 1969, 21.

– "Francis O. Schmitt, 91; Pioneer in Biological Research at MIT." *Boston Globe*, 5 October 1995, 1 and 5.

– "In Memoriam Robert Weil." *Dalhousie News*, 15 May 2002, 1.

– "In Praise of the 'Brain Drain' (Editorial)." *Nature* 446, no. 7133 (2007): 231.

Argote, Linda. *Organizational Learning: Creating, Retaining, and Transferring Knowledge*. Boston: Kluwer, 1999.

Arnold, Hans, ed. *Neurochirurgie in Deutschland: Geschichte und Gegenwart. 50 Jahre Deutsche Gesellschaft fuer Neurochirurgie*. Berlin, Germany: Blackwell, 2001.

Aschaffenburg, Gustav. *Handbuch der Psychiatrie*. 7 vols. Leipzig, Germany: Franz Deuticke, 1911–29.

– ed. *Die Einteilung der Psychosen*. Leipzig: Franz Deuticke, 1915.

Ash, Mitchell G. *Gestalt Psychology in German Culture, 1890–1967. Holism and the Quest for Objectivity*. Cambridge, MA: Cambridge University Press, 1995.

– "Scientific Changes in Germany 1933, 1945, 1990: Towards a Comparison." *Minerva* 37, no. 3 (1999): 329–54.

– "Wissens- und Wissenschaftstransfer – Einfuehrende Bemerkungen."
  Berichte zur Wissenschaftsgeschichte 29, no. 3 (2006): 181–3.
– "Von Vielschichtigkeiten und Verschraenkungen: 'Kulturen der Wissenschaft
  – Wissenschaften in der Kultur.'" *Berichte zur Wissenschaftsgeschichte* 30,
  no. 2 (2007): 91–105.
– "Wandlungen der Wissenschaftslandschaften im fruehen Kalten Krieg." In
  Die Akademien der Wissenschaften in Zentraleuropa im Kalten Krieg.
  Transformationsprozesse im Spannungsfeld von Abgrenzung und
  Annaeherung, edited by Johannes Feichtinger and Heidemarie Uhl, 29–65.
  Vienna, Austria: Austrian Academies of Sciences Press, 2018.
Ash, Mitchell G., and Alfons Soellner, eds. *Forced Migration and Scientific*
  Change: Émigré German-Speaking Scientists after 1933. Cambridge, UK:
  Cambridge University Press, 1996.
Ashwal, Stephen, ed. *The Founders of Child Neurology.* San Francisco:
  Norman Publishing, 1990.
Askonas, Brigitte A. "From Protein Synthesis to Antibody Formation and
  Cellular Immunity." In *The Excitement and Fascination of Science:*
  Reflections by Eminent Scientists, edited by George Holman Bishop and
  William Carelton Gibson, 493–511. Palo Alto, CA: Annual Reviews, 1965.
Assmann, Aleida. "Trauma des Krieges und Literatur." In *Trauma. Zwischen*
  Psychoanalyse und kulturellem Deutungsmuster, edited by Elisabeth Bronfen,
  Birgit Erdle, and Sigrid Weigel, 95–116. Cologne, Germany: Boehlau, 1999.
Auerbach, Siegmund. "Die Aufbrauchtheorie und das Gesetz der
  Laehmungstypen." *DZfNhlk* 53, no. 6 (1915): 449–63.
Aumueller, Gerhard, Kornelia Grundmann, Esther Kraehwinkel, Hans H.
  Lauer, and Helmut Remschmidt, eds. *Die Marburger Medizinische Fakultaet*
  im Dritten Reich. Munich, Germany: K.G. Saur, 2001.
B. B. "Duesseldorf erhaelt Hirnforschungsinstitut. Akademie gewann Wettlauf
  der Hochschulen – Neuer Lehrstuhl geplant." *Duesseldorfer Nachrichten,*
  16 April 1964, 9.
Baader, Gerhard. "Politisch motivierte Emigration deutscher Aerzte." *Berichte*
  zur Wissenschaftsgeschichte 7, no. 2 (1984): 67–84.
Bach, M[ichelle]. I. "Interview with Kurt Goldstein (June, 1958) in NYC." In
  Auszug des Geistes. Bericht ueber eine Sendereihe, edited by Lutz Besch,
  93–114. Bremen, Germany: B.C. Hege, 1962.
Baeumer, Beatrix. *Von der physiologischen Chemie zur fruehen biochemischen*
  Arzneimittelforschung. Der Apotheker und Chemiker Erwin Baumann
  (1846–1896) an den Universitaeten Strasburg, Berlin, Freiburg und in der
  pharmazeutischen Industrie. Cologne, Germany: Deutscher Apothekerverlag,
  1996.

Baglole, Tanya. "Nos disparus – Le Dr Robert Weil, un fondateur de l'APC, est décédé." *Canadian Psychiatric Association Bulletin* 34, no. 1 (2002): 64.

Bar-On, Hanan. "The Role of the Weizmann Institute of Science in Normalizing Israeli-German Relations." *Annals of the New York Academy of Sciences* 866, no. 2 (1998): 215–33.

Barnes, Barry and David Edge, eds. *Science in Context. Readings in the Sociology of Science.* Cambridge, MA: MIT Press, 1982.

Barwinski, Faeh R. "Trauma, Symbolisierungsschwaeche und Externalisierung im realen Feld." *Forum Psychoanalyse* 17, no. 1 (2001): 20–37.

Bauer, Karl Friedrich. "Das Reliefbild des Nervengewebes. Ein Beitrag zur Kenntnis der Struktur des Integrationsorganes nach Anwendung der Metallbeschattung." *Acta Anatomica* 13, no. 4 (1951): 351–70.

Bauer, Karl Friedrich and Erich Mueller. "Die Zellenlehre." In *Medizinische Grundlagenforschung*, edited by Karl Friedrich Bauer, 167–93. Vol. 2. Stuttgart, Germany: Thieme, 1959.

Beard, George Miller. *American Nervousness: Its Causes and Consequences: A Supplement to Nervous Exhaustion (Neurasthenia).* New York: Putnam, 1881.

Bechmann, Ingo, Robert Nitsch, Franz Pera, Andreas Winkelmann, and Frank W. Stahnisch. "Zentrales Nervensystem, Systema nervosum centrale, Gehirn, Encephalon, und Rueckenmark, Medulla spinalis." In *Waldeyer Anatomie des Menschen, 17. ed. (gen. revised. edition)*, edited by Jochen Fanghaenel, Franz Pera, Franz Anderhuber, and Robert Nitsch, 355–550. Berlin, Germany: DeGruyter, 2003.

Bechmann, Zarah. "Heinrich Obersteiner (1847–1922) – Leben und Werk." MD Diss., University of Tuebingen, Germany, 1999.

Bechtel, William. "Cognitive Neuroscience. Relating Neural Mechanisms and Cognition." In *Theory and Method in the Neurosciences*, edited by Peter K. Machamer, Rick Grush, and Peter McLaughlin, 81–111. Pittsburgh, PA: University of Pittsburgh Press, 2001.

Becker, Cornelia, Christine Feja, Wolfgang Schmidt, and Katharina Spanel-Borowski, eds. *Das Institut fuer Anatomie in Leipzig. Eine Geschichte in Bildern.* Beucha, Germany: Sax-Verlag, 2005.

Becker, Peter Emil. *Zur Geschichte der Rassenhygiene. Wege ins Dritte Reich.* Stuttgart, Germany: Thieme, 1988.

Beddies, Thomas and Heinz-Peter Schmiedebach. "'Euthanasie'-Opfer und Versuchsobjekte. Kranke und behinderte Kinder in Berlin waehrend des Zweiten Weltkriegs." *Medizinhistorisches Journal* 39, no. 2–3 (2004): 165–96.

Belz, Wolfram. "Kurt Goldstein (1878–1965). Lebens-und zeitgeschichtliche Hintergruende." In *Vom Abstrakten zum Konkreten. Leben und Werk Kurt Goldsteins (1878–1965)*, edited by Gerd Danzer, 11–70. Frankfurt am Main, Germany: VAS Verlag, 2006.

Benjamin, Walter. "On the Concept of History." In *Walter Benjamin: Selected Writings*, edited by Michael W. Jennings and Howard Eiland. Vol. 4, 389–400. Cambridge, MA, and London, UK: Harvard University Press, 2006.

Bennett, Max R. "The Early History of the Synapse: From Plato to Sherrington." *Brain Research Bulletin* 50, no. 2 (1999): 95–118.

Benzenhoefer, Udo. *Der Arztphilosoph Viktor von Weizsaecker. Leben und Werk im Ueberblick*. Goettingen, Germany: Vandenhoeck & Ruprecht, 2007.

Benzenhoefer, Udo and Gerald Kreft. "Bemerkungen zur Frankfurter Zeit (1917–1933) des juedischen Neurologen und Psychiaters Walther Riese." *SDGGN3*, no. 1 (1997): 31–40.

Berghahn, Volker R. "The Debate on 'Americanization' among Economic and Cultural Historians." *Historiographical Review* 10, no. 1 (2010): 107–30.

Bernard, Claude. *Einfuehrung in das Studium der experimentellen Medizin* (French 1865). Translated by Paul Szendroe and introduced by Karl E. Rothschuh. Leipzig: Johann Ambrosius Barth, 1960.

Bertelmez, George W. "Charles Judson Herrick." *Biographical Memoirs of the National Academy of Science* 43, no. 1 (1973): 77–108.

Bethe, Albrecht. "Neue Versuche ueber die Regeneration der Nervenfasern." *Pflueger's Archiv fuer die gesante Physiologie (Bonn)* 116, no. 7–9 (1907): 385–478.

Bielka, Heinz. *Die Medizinisch-Biologischen Institute Berlin-Buch: Beitraege zur Geschichte*. Berlin, Germany: Springer, 1997.

Bielschowsky, Max. "Ueber einen Fall von Perityphlitis suppurativa mit Ausgang in Septico-Pyaemie." PhD Diss., Senckenbergische Stiftungen Frankfurt am Main, 1893.

– "Die Silberimpraegnation der Neurofibrillen." *Journal fuer Psychologie und Neurologie* 3, no. 4 (1904): 169–88.

– "Ueber das Verhalten der Achsencylinder in Geschwuelsten des Nervensystems und in Kompressionsgebieten des Rueckenmarks." *Journal fuer Psychologie und Neurologie* 7, no. 1 (1906): 101–39.

– "Ueber Regenerationserscheinungen an Zentralen Nervenfasern." *Journal fuer Psychologie und Neurologie* 14, nos. 3–4 (1909): 131–49.

– "Entwurf eines Systems der Heredo-Degenerationen des Zentralnervensystems einschliesslich der zugehoerigen Striatumerkrankungen." *Journal fuer Psychologie und Neurologie* 24, no. 1 (1918): 48–50.

– *Nervengewebe, das peripherische Nervensystem, das Zentralnervensystem.* Berlin, Germany: Springer, 1928.

Bielschowsky, Max and Gerhard Unger. "Die Ueberbrueckung grosser Nervenluecken." *Journal fuer Psychologie und Neurologie* 22, no. 2 (1917): 267–314.

Bilson, Geoffrey. "'Muscles and Health': Health and the Canadian Immigrant." In *Health, Disease and Medicine*, edited by Charles G. Roland, 398–411. Toronto: The Hannah Institute for the History of Medicine, 1984.

Binding, Karl, and Alfred Hoche. *Die Freigabe der Vernichtung lebensunwerten Lebens. Ihr Mass und ihre Form.* Leipzig, Germany: Johann Ambrosius Barth, 1920.

Binswanger, Otto. "Die Kriegshysterie." In *Handbuch der Aerztlichen Erfahrungen im Weltkriege 1914–1918*, edited by Karl Bonhoeffer, 45–67. Vol. 4. Leipzig, Germany: Johann Ambrosius Barth, 1922.

Birmingham, Mary K. "Some Thoughts on the Fiftieth Anniversary." In *Building on a Proud Past: 50 Years of Psychiatry at McGill*, edited by Theodore L. Sourkes and Gilbert Pinard, 151–5. Montreal: McGill University, 1995.

Black, Edwin. *War Against the Weak: Eugenics and America's Campaign to Create a Master Race.* New York: Four Walls Eight Windows, 2003.

Blackshaw, Gemman, and Sabine Wieber, eds. *Journeys into Madness: Mapping Mental Illness in the Austro-Hungarian Empire.* New York: Berghahn Books, 2012.

Bleker, Johanna, and Christine Eckelmann. "'Der Erfolg der Gleichschaltung-saktion kann als durchschlagend bezeichnet werden.' Der Bund Deutscher Aerztinnen 1933–1936." In *Medizin im "Dritten Reich,"* edited by Johanna Bleker and Norbert Jachertz, 87–96. Cologne, Germany: Deutscher Aerz-teverlag, 1989.

Bliss, Michael. *The Making of Modern Medicine: Turning Points in the Treatment of Disease.* Toronto: University of Toronto Press, 2011.

Bohleber, Werner. "Die Entwicklung der Traumatheorie in der Psychoanalyse." *Psyche. Zeitschrift fuer Psychoanalyse und ihre Anwendungen* 54, no. 9–10 (2000): 797–839.

Bonah, Christian. *Les sciences physiologiques en Europe: Analyses comparées du XIX siècle.* Lyon, France: Librairie philosophique J. Vrin, 1995.

Borck, Cornelius. "Visualizing Nerve Cells and Psychic Mechanisms: The Rhetoric of Freud's Illustrations." In *Freud and the Neurosciences: From Brain Research to the Unconscious*, edited by Giselher Guttmann and Inge Scholz-Strasser, 75–86. Vienna, Austria: Oesterreichische Akademie der Wissenschaften, 1998.

- "Fuehlfaeden und Fangarme. Metaphern des Organischen als Dispositiv der Hirnforschung." In *Ecce cortex. Beitraege zur Geschichte des modernen Gehirns*, edited by Michael Hagner, 144–76. Goettingen, Germany: Wallstein, 1999.
- "Mediating Philanthropy in Changing Political Circumstances: The Rockefeller Foundation's Funding for Brain Research in Germany, 1930–1950." Rockefeller Archive Center Research Reports. Edited by RAC. Latest modified April 2001. Accessed 5 February 2018. http://www.rockarch.org/publications/resrep/borck.pdf.
- *Hirnstroeme. Eine Kulturgeschichte der Elektroenzephalographie*. Goettingen, Germany: Wallstein, 2005.

Bracegirdle, Brian. *A History of Microtechnique*. Ithaca, NY: Cornell University Press, 1978.

Brady, Steven J. *Eisenhower and Adenauer: Alliance Maintenance under Pressure, 1953–1960*. Lanham, MD: Lexington Books, 2010.

Braese, Stephan and Dominik Gross. *NS-Medizin und Oeffentlichkeit. Formen der Aufarbeitung nach 1945*. Frankfurt am Main and New York: Campus, 2015.

Braitenberg, Valentin. "Hirnforschung zwischen Lokalisationslehre und Systemanalyse." *Attempto* 35–6, no. 1 (1970): 47–8.

Bramadat, Ina J. and Marion I. Saydak, "Nursing on the canadian Prairies: Effects of Immigration." *Nursing History Review* 1, no. 1 (1993): 105–17.

Brazier, Mary A.B. *A History of Neurophysiology in the 19th Century*. New York: Raven Press, 1988.

Breidbach, Olaf. *Die Materialisierung des Ichs. Zur Geschichte der Hirnforschung im 19. und 20. Jahrhundert*. Frankfurt am Main, Germany: Suhrkamp Verlag, 1997.

Brinkschulte, Eva. *Weibliche Aerzte: Die Durchsetzung des Berufsbildes in Deutschland*. Berlin, Germany: Edition Hentrich, 1995.

Brock, D. Heward and Ann Harward, eds. *The Culture of Biomedicine*. Newark, DL: University of Delaware Press, 1984.

Brodmann, Korbinian. "Beitraege zur histologischen Lokalisation der Grosshirnrinde. I. Mitteilung: Die Regio Rolandica." *JfPN* 2, no. 1 (1903): 79–107.
- "Beitraege zur histologischen Lokalisation der Grosshirnrinde. VII. Mitteilung: Die cytoarchitektonische Cortexgliederung der Halbaffen (Lemuriden)." *JfPN*, Suppl. no. 10 (1908): 287–334.
- *Vergleichende Lokalisationslehre der Grosshirnrinde in ihren Prinzipien dargestellt auf Grund des Zellbaues*. Leipzig, Germany: Johann Ambrosius Barth, 1909.

Bronfen, Elisabeth, Birgit R. Erdle, and Sigrid Weigel. *Trauma. Zwischen Psychoanalyse und kulturellem Deutungsmuster*. Vienna, Austria: Boehlau, 1999.

Brosnan, Caragh and Mike Michael. "Enacting the 'Neuro' in Practice: Translational Research, Adhesion and the Promise of Porosity." *Social Studies of Science* 44, no. 5 (2014): 680–700.

Brown, Theodore M. "Friendship and Philanthropy: Henry Sigerist, Alan Gregg and the Rockefeller Foundation." In *Making Medical History: The Life and Time of Henry E. Sigerist*, edited by Elizabeth Fee and Theodore M. Brown, 288–311. Baltimore, MD: Johns Hopkins University Press, 1997.

Brunner, Jose. "Psychiatry, Psychoanalysis and Politics during the First World War." *Journal of the History of the Behavioral Sciences* 27, no. 4 (1991): 352–65.

Buchholz, Kai and Klaus Wolbert, eds. *Die Lebensreform. Entwuerfe zur Neugestaltung von Leben und Kunst um 1900*. Darmstadt, Germany: Haeusser-Media, 2001.

Buerger, Klaus. "Lullies, Hans." In *Altpreussische Biographie*, edited by Ernst Bahr, 1436. Marburg an der Lahn, Germany: Elwart 1995.

Bullemer, Timo. *"Die hiesigen Juden sind in Cham alteingesessen." Aus der Geschichte der juedischen Gemeinde vom Mittelalter bis zur Gegenwart*. Cham, Germany: City Archives of Cham, 2003.

Bumke, Oswald. "Ueber die gegenwaertigen Stroemungen in der klinischen Psychiatrie." *Zeitschrift fuer die gesamte Neurologie und Psychiatrie* 81, no. 3 (1924): 389–93.

– *Ueber Nervoese Entartung*. Berlin, Germany: Julius Springer, 1912.

– *Lehrbuch der Geisteskrankheiten* (1st ed. 1919). 4th ed. Munich. Germany: J.F. Bergmann, 1936.

– "Klinische Psychiatrie und Eugenik." *Allgemeine Zeitschrift fuer Psychiatrie und psychisch-gerichtliche Medizin* 80, nos. 1–3 (1927): 392–400.

Bumke, Oswald, and Otfrid Foerster, eds. *Handbuch der Neurologie*. 18 Vols. Berlin, Germany: Springer, 1935–7.

Burgmair, Wolfgang and Matthias M. Weber. "'Dass er selbst mit aller Energie gegen diese Hallucinationen ankaempfen muss.' Koenig Otto von Bayern und die Muenchner Psychiatrie um 1900." *Sudhoffs Archiv. Zeitschrift fuer Wissenschaftsgeschichte* 86, no. 1 (2002): 27–54.

– "'Das Geld ist gut angelegt, und Du brauchst keine Reue haben.' James Loeb, ein deutsch-amerikanischer Wissenschaftsmaezen zwischen Kaiserreich und Weimarer Republik." *Historische Zeitschrift* 277, no. 2 (2003): 343–78.

Burston, Daniel. *A Forgotten Freudian: The Passion of Karl Stern*. London, UK: Karnac Books, 2016.

Cajal, Santiago Ramón y. *Studien ueber Nervenregeneration*. Leipzig,
Germany: Johann Barth, 1908.
– *Degeneration and Regeneration of the Nervous System* (Spanish 1928).
Translated by Richard M. May. New York: Oxford University Press, 1991.
– *Recollections of My Life* (Spanish 1937). Translated by E. Horne Craigie.
Philadelphia, PA: American Philosophical Society, 1993.
Cambrosio, Alberto, Daniel Jacobi, and Peter Keating. "Phages, Antibodies and
'De-monstration.'" *History and Philosophy of the Life Sciences* 30, no. 2
(2008): 131–58.
Canguilhem, George. *The Normal and the Pathological* (French 1966).
Translated by Carolyn R. Fawcett and Robert S. Cohen. New York: Zone
Books, 1991.
Canning, Kathleen, Kerstin Barndt, and Kristin McGuire, eds. *Weimar Publics/
Weimar Subjects Rethinking the Political Culture of Germany in the 1920s*.
New York: Berghahn Books, 2010.
Casper, Stephen T. "Atlantic Conjectures in Anglo-American Neurology."
Bulletin of the History of Medicine 82, no. 3 (2008): 646–71.
– "One Hundred Members of the Association of British Neurologists: A
Collective Biography for 1933–1960." *Journal of the History of
Neuroscience* 20, no. 4 (2011): 338–56.
Casselman, Bill, Judith Dingwall, and Ronald Casselman, eds. *Dictionary of
Medical Derivations: The Real Meaning of Medical Terms*. Nashville, TN:
CRC Press, 1998.
Charpa, Ulrich, and Ute Deichman, eds. *Jews and Sciences in German Context:
Case Studies from the 19th and 20th Centuries*. Tuebingen, Germany: Mohr
Siebeck, 2007.
Choudhury, Suparna and Jan Slaby, eds. *Critical Neuroscience: A Handbook
of the Social and Cultural Contexts of Neuroscience*. Oxford, UK: Wiley-
Blackwell, 2011.
Churchill, Frederick B. "Regeneration, 1885–1901." In *A History of Regenera-
tion Research. Milestones in the Evolution of a Science*, edited by Charles E.
Dinsmore, 113–31. Cambridge, UK: Cambridge University Press, 1991.
Clark, Christopher. *The Sleepwalkers: How Europe Went to War in 1914*.
London, UK: Allen Lane, 2012.
Clarke, Edwin and L. Stephen Jacyna. *Nineteenth-Century Origins of
Neuroscience Concepts*. Berkeley, CA: University of California Press, 1987.
Clinghorn, Richard. "The Emergence of Psychiatry at McGill." *Canadian
Journal of Psychiatry* 29, no. 5 (1984): 551–6.
Collmann, Hartmut. "Georges Schaltenbrand (26.11.1897–24.10.1979)."
Wuerzburger medizinische Mitteilungen 27, no. 1 (2008): 64–92.

Conot, Robert E. *Justice at Nuremberg: The First Comprehensive Dramatic Account of the Trial of the Nazi Leaders*. New York: Harper & Row Publishers, 1983.

Cook, Walter. "Hitler Is My Best Friend" (ca. 1935). In *Meaning in the Visual Arts*, edited by Erwin Panowsky, 380–1. New York: Penguin, 1970.

Cornwell, John. *Hitler's Scientists: Science, War, and the Devil's Pact*. New York: Viking Press, 2003.

Coser, Lewis A. *Refugee Scholars in America: Their Impact and Their Experiences*. New Haven, CT: Yale University Press, 1984.

Cottebrune, Anne. "Die Deutsche Forschungsgemeinschaft, der NS-Staat und die Foerderung rassenhygienischer Forschung: 'Steuerbare' Forschung durch Gleichschaltung einer Selbstverwaltungsorganisation? " In *Zwischen Erziehung und Vernichtung. Zigeunerforschung und Zigeunerpolitik des 20. Jahrhunderts*, edited by Michael Zimmermann, 354–78. Stuttgart, Germany: Franz Steiner, 2007.

Cowan, W. Maxwell. "The Emergence of Modern Neuroanatomy and Developmental Neurobiology." *Neuron* 20, no. 3 (1998): 413–26.

Cowan, W. Maxwell, Derek H. Harter, and Eric Kandel. "The Emergence of Modern Neuroscience: Some Implications for Neurology and Psychiatry." *Annual Review of Neuroscience* 23, no. 3 (2000): 323–91.

Cowen, Roy C. *Hauptmann. Kommentar zum dramatischen Werk*. Munich, Germany: Winkler, 1980.

Craig, John, E. *Scholarship and Nation Building: The University of Strasbourg and Alsatian Society, 1870–1939*. Chicago, IL, and London, UK: University of Chicago Press, 1984.

Cranefield, Paul F. "The Organic Physics of 1847 and the Biophysics of Today." *Journal of the History of Medicine and Allied Sciences* 12, no. 10 (1957), 407–23.

Craver, Carl F. *Explaining the Brain: Mechanisms and the Mosaic Unity of Neurosciences*. Oxford, UK: Oxford University Press, 2009.

Crawford, Elisabeth, Josiane Olff-Nathan, Mark Walker, Léon Strauss, Burkhard Weiss, Françoise Olivier-Utard, and Christian Bonah, eds. *Sciences et cultures nationales. Les trois universités de Strasbourg, 1872–1945*. Strasbourg, France: Éditions de la Nuée Bleue, 1995.

Crome, Louis. "The Medical History of V.I. Lenin." *History of Medicine* 4, no. 1 (1972): 3–9 and 20–2.

Crouthamel, Jason. "Invisible Traumas: Psychological Wounds, World War I and German Society, 1914–1945." PhD Diss., Indiana University, Bloomington, IN, 2001.

– "War Neurosis versus Savings Psychosis: Working-class Politics and Psychological Trauma in Weimar Germany." *Journal of Contemporary History* 37, no. 2 (2002): 163–82.

Czech, Herwig. "Von der 'Aktion T4' zur 'dezentralen Euthanasie.' Die niederoesterreichischen Heil- und Pflegeanstalten Gugging, Mauer-Oehling und Ybbs." *Jahrbuch des Dokumentationsarchivs des oesterreichischen Widerstandes* 53, no. 1 (2016): 219–66.

Danek, Adrian and Jochen Rettig. "Korbinian Brodmann (1868–1918)." *Schweizer Archiv fuer Neurologie und Psychiatrie* 140, no. 6 (1989): 555–66.

Daniel, Ute. "Kulturgeschichte." In *Konzepte der Kulturwissenschaften. Theoretische Grundlagen – Ansaetze – Perspektiven*, edited by Ansgar Nuenning and Vera Nuenning, 186–204. Stuttgart, Germany: Boehlau, 2003.

Danzer, Georg, ed. *Vom Konkreten zum Abstrakten. Leben und Werk Kurt Goldsteins (1878–1965).* Frankfurt am Main, Germany: VAS-Verlag, 2006.

Da Solla Price, Derek. *Little Science, Big Science.* New York: Columbia University Press, 1963.

Daston, Lorraine. "The Moral Economy of Science." *OSIRIS, 2nd Series* 10, no. 1 (1995): 2–24.

Davie, Maurice R., and Samuel Koenig. "Adjustment of Refugees to American Life." *Annals of the American Academy of Political and Social Science* 262, no. 1 (1949), 159–65.

DeCyon, Elie. *Methodik der physiologischen Experimente und Vivisectionen.* St Petersburg, Russia: Carl Ricker, 1876.

Deichmann, Ute. *Biologists under Hitler.* Cambridge, MA: Harvard University Press, 1996.

– "Emigration, Isolation and the Slow Start of Molecular Biology in Germany." *Studies in History and Philosophy of Biological and Biomedical Sciences* 33, no. 3 (2002): 449–71.

Deichmann, Ute, and Benno Mueller-Hill. "Biological Research at Universities and Kaiser Wilhelm Institutes in Nazi Germany." In *Science, Technology, and National Socialism*, edited by Monika Renneberg and Mark Walker, 160–83. Cambridge, UK: Cambridge University Press, 1994.

Dejong, Russell N. "The Century of the National Hospital, Queen Square." *Neurology* 10, no. 7 (1960): 676–9.

Delbrueck, Hansgerd. "Gerhart Hauptmanns 'Vor Sonnenaufgang': Soziales Drama als Bil-dungskatastrophe." *Deutsche Vierteljahrsschrift fuer Literaturwissenschaft und Geistesgeschichte* 69, no. 3 (1995): 512–45.

Desgroseillers, Roger. "L'histoire de la psychoanalyse à Albert-Prévost." *Filigrane* 10, no. 1 (2001): 6–37.

[Deutscher] Reichstag. *Berichte des Kriegsbeschaedigten-Fuersorge-Ausschusses fuer das Jahr 1918*. Berlin, Germany: Deutscher Reichstag, 1918.

Dhúill, Caitriona Ní. "'Ein neues, maechtiges Volkstum': Eugenic Discourse and Its Impact on the Work of Gerhart Hauptmann." *German Life and Letters* 59, no. 3 (2006): 405–22.

Dickinson, Edward Ross. "Biopolitics, Fascism, Democracy: Some Reflections on Our Discourse about 'Modernity.'" *Central European History* 37, no. 1 (2004): 1–48.

Dierig, Sven. "Urbanization, Place of Experiment and How the Electric Fish Was Caught by Emil DuBois-Reymond." *Journal of the History of the Neurosciences* 9, no. 1 (2000): 5–13.

Dierig, Sven, Jens Lachmund, and J. Andrew Mendelsohn. "Introduction: Toward an Urban History of Science." *OSIRIS*, *2nd Series* 18, no. 1 (2003): 1–19.

Doeblin, Alfred. *Berlin Alexanderplatz*. Berlin, Germany: S. Fischer, 1929.

– *Unser Dasein*. Berlin, Germany: S. Fischer, 1933.

Doehl, Doerte. *Ludwig Hoffmann. Bauten fuer Berlin 1896–1924*. Tuebingen, Germany: Ernst Wasmuth, 2004.

Doeleke, Werner. "Alfred Ploetz, Sozialdarwinist und Gesellschaftsbiologe." MD Diss., University of Frankfurt, 1975.

Dohm, Georg. *Geschichte der Histopathologie*. Berlin, Germany: Springer, 2001.

Douglas, Mary. *How Institutions Think (Frank W. Abrams Lectures)*. New York: Syracuse University Press, 1986.

Dowbiggin, Ian Robert. *Keeping America Sane: Psychiatry and Eugenics in the United States and Canada, 1880–1940*. Ithaca, NY: Cornell University Press, 2003.

Dressler, Stephan. *Viktor von Weizsaecker. Medizinische Anthropologie und Philosophie*. Vienna, Dressler: Ueberreuter Wissenschaft, 1989.

Drogin, Elasah. *Margaret Saenger. Gruenderin der modernen Gesellschaft*. Abtsteinach, Germany: Aktion Leben, 2000.

Duffin, Jacalyn. "The Guru and the Godfather: Henry Sigerist, Hugh MacLean, and the Politics of Health Care Reform in 1940s Canada." *Canadian Bulletin of Medical History* 9, no. 2 (1992): 191–218.

Dulles, John Foster. "U.S.-German Understandings on Cultural Exchange." *Department of State Bulletin (United States of America)*, April 20, 1953, 567–8.

Dyck, Erika. *Facing Eugenics: Reproduction, Sterilization, and the Politics of Choice*. Baltimore, MD: Johns Hopkins University Press, 2012.

Easton, Joseph W. and Robert Weil. *Culture and Mental Disorders. A Comparative Study of the Hutterites and Other Populations.* Glencoe, IL: Free Press, 1955.

Eckart, Wolfgang U. "'Die wachsende Nervositaet unserer Zeit.' Medizin und Kultur im Fin de Siècle am Beispiel der Modekrankheit Neurasthenie." In *Psychiatrie um die Jahrhundertwende*, edited by Fritz Reimer. Heilbronn, Germany: Weinsberger Kolloquium, 1994, 9–38.

– ed. *Man, Medicine, and the State: The Human Body as an Object of Government-Sponsored Medical Research in the 20th Century.* Stuttgart, Germany: Franz Steiner, 2006.

Eckart, Wolfgang U., and Christoph Gradmann, eds. *Die Medizin und der Erste Weltkrieg.* Pfaffenweiler, Germany: Centaurus, 1996.

Eden, Paul. *Socialism and Eugenics.* Manchester, UK: National Labour Press, 1911.

Edinger, Ludwig. "Ueber die Schleimhaut des Fischdarmes nebst Bemerkungen zur Phylogenese der Druesen des Duenndarmes." *Archiv fuer mikroskopische Anatomie* 13, no. 3 (1877): 651–92.

– "Untersuchungen zur Physiologie und Pathologie des Magens" (*Habilitation*). PhD Diss., University of Giessen, Germany, 1881.

– *Vorlesungen ueber den Bau der nervoesen Zentralorgane des Menschen und der Tiere.* Vol. 1. Leipzig, Germany: Vogel, 1885.

– *The Anatomy of the Central Nervous System of Man and of Vertebrates in General* (Germ. 1885), Translated by Winfield S. Hall. Philadelphia, PA: F.A. Davis, 1885–99.

– "Ueber die Bedeutung der Hirnrinde im Anschluss an den Bericht ueber die Untersuchung eines Hundes dem Goltz das ganze Vorderhirn entfernt hatte." *Verhandlungen des XII. Internationalen Medicinischen Congresses* 12, no. 1 (1893): 350–8.

– "Studien ueber Nervenregeneration, uebersetzt von Dr. Johannes Bresler, mit 60 Abbildungen, Leipzig, Johann Ambrosius Barth, 1908, 196 S. 7,50 M, Ref. Edinger (Frankfurt a. M.), by S. Ramón y Cajal (Madrid)." *Deutsche Medizinische Wochenschrift* 29, no. 34 (1908): 1281.

– "Untersuchungen ueber die Neubildung des durchtrennten Nerven." *DZfNhlk.* 58, no. 1 (1908): 1–32.

– *Der Anteil der Funktion an der Entstehung von Nervenkrankheiten.* Wiesbaden, Germany: Bergmann, 1908.

– "The Relations of Comparative Anatomy to Comparative Psychology." *Journal of Comparative Neurology* 18, no. 5 (1908): 437–57.

– "Ueber die Regeneration des entarteten Nerven." *Deutsche Medizinische Wochenschrift* 43, no. 25 (1917): 769–70.

- "Aufbau und Funktion, Untergang und Neubildung der peripherischen Nerven." *DZfNhlk.* 59, no. 10 (1918): 10–32.
- *Mein Lebensgang. Erinnerungen eines Frankfurter Arztes und Hirnforschers* (1919), edited by Gerald Kreft, Werner Friedrich Kuemmel, Wolfgang Schlote, and Reiner Wiehl. Frankfurt am Main: Waldemar Kramer, 2005.

Edinger, Ludwig, and Bernhard Fischer. "Ein Mensch ohne Grosshirn." *Pfluegers Archiv fuer die gesamte Physiologie des Menschen und der Tiere* 152, nos. 11–12 (1913): 535–61.

Efron, John M. *Medicine and the German Jews: A History.* New Haven and London: Yale University Press, 2001.

Efron, John M., Steven Weitzman, and Matthias Lehmann. *The Jews: A History* (1st ed. 2008). 3rd ed. London: Pearson Education, 2018.

Ehrenreich, Barbara and Deirdre English. *Complaints and Disorders: The Sexual Politics of Sickness.* Old Westbury, NY: Glass Mountain Pamphlet, 1973.

Eigen, Manfred. "Erinnerungen an Francis Otto Schmitt (23.11.1903– 3.10.1995)." *Neuroforum* 2, no. 1 (1996): 35–7.

Eisenberg, Ulrike, Hartmut Collmann, and Daniel Dubinski. *Verraten – Vertrieben – Vergessen. Werk und Schicksal nach 1933 verfolgter deutscher Hirnchirurgen.* Berlin: Hentrich & Hentrich, 2017.

Emery, George, and J.C. Herbert Emery. *A Young Man's Benefit: The Independent Order of Odd Fellows and Sickness Insurance in the United States and Canada, 1860–1929.* Montreal and Kingston: McGill-Queen's University Press, 1999.

Emisch, Heidemarie. *Ludwig Edinger. Hirnanatomie und Psychologie.* Stuttgart: Gustav Fischer, 1991.

Engel, Jonathan. *American Therapy: The Rise of Psychotherapy in the United States.* New York: Gotham Books, 2008.

Engstrom, Eric J. *Clinical Psychiatry in Imperial Germany: A History of Psychiatric Practice.* Ithaca, NY: Cornell University Press, 2003.
- "Emil Kraepelin: Psychiatry and Public Affairs in Wilhelmine Germany." *History of Psychiatry* 2, no. 6 (1991): 111–32.

Erb, Wilhelm. *Ueber die wachsende Nervositaet unserer Zeit. Akademische Rede zum Geburtsfeste des hoechstseligen Grossherzogs Karl Friedrich am 22. November 1893 beim Vortrage des Jahresberichts und der Verkuendigung der akademischen Preise gehalten ...* Heidelberg, Germany: Universitaetsreden, 1893.

Erickson, Mark. *Science, Culture and Society: Understanding Science in the Twenty-First Century.* Cambridge, MA: Polity, 2005.

Esposito, Roberto. *Terms of the Political: Community, Immunity, Biopolitics.* Translated by Rhiannon Noel Welch. New York: Fordham University, 2013.

Essen-Moeller, Erik. *Psychiatrische Untersuchungen an einer Serie von Zwillingen.* Suppl. vol. 23. Munksgaard, Sweden: Acta Psychiatrica et Neurologica 200, no. 1 (1941): 7–10.

Eulenburg, Albert. "Catalepsy." In *Cyclopedia of the Practice of Medicine,* edited by Hugo von Ziemssen. Vol. XIV, 369–411. New York: William Wood, 1877.

Eulner, Heinrich H. "Psychiatrie und Neurologie." In *Die Entwicklung der medizinischen Spezialfaecher an den Universitaeten des deutschen Sprachgebietes,* edited by Heinrich H. Eulner, 257–82. Stuttgart, Germany: Enke, 1970.

Exilforschung. Ein internationales Jahrbuch. Munich, Germany: G. Saur, 1983–present.

Falk, Beatrice, and Friedrich Hauer, *Brandenburg-Goerden. Geschichte eines psychiatrischen Krankenhauses.* Bebra, Germany: Wissenschaftsverlag, 2007.

Fangerau, Heiner, and Irmgard Mueller. "Das Standardwerk der Rassenhygiene von Erwin Baur, Eugen Fischer und Fritz Lenz im Urteil der Psychiatrie und Neurologie 1921–1940." *Der Nervenarzt* 73, no. 11 (2002): 1039–46.

Farreras, Ingrid G., Caroline Hannaway, and Victoria A. Harden, eds. *Mind, Brain, Body, and Behavior: Foundations of Neuroscience and Behavioral Research at the National Institutes of Health.* Amsterdam, The Netherlands: IOS Press, 2004.

Faulkner, Howard J., and Karl A. Menninger. *The Selected Correspondence of Karl A. Menninger, 1919–1945.* New Haven, CT: Yale University Press, 1989.

Fawcett, John. "Networks, Linkages and Migration Systems." *International Migration Review* 23, no. 3 (1989): 671–80.

Fee, Elizabeth, and Theodore M. Brown, eds. *Making Medical History: The Life and Time of Henry E. Sigerist.* Baltimore, MD: Johns Hopkins University Press, 1997.

Fehling, August W. *Die Forschungsfoerderung der amerikanischen Bundesregierung und ihre Ruckwirkungen auf die Hochschulforschung.* Kiel, Germany: F. Hirt, 1954.

Feindel, William. "The Montreal Neurological Institute." *Journal of Neurosurgery* 75, no. 5 (1991): 821–2.

– "The Contributions of Wilder Penfield and the Montreal Neurological Institute to Canadian Neurosciences." In *Health, Disease and Medicine,* edited by Christopher C. Roland, 347–58. Toronto: Hannah Institute for the History of Medicine, 1984.

Feindel, William, and Richard Leblanc. *The Wounded Brain Healed: The Golden Age of the Montreal Neurological Institute, 1934–1984.* Montreal and Kingston: McGill-Queen's University Press, 2016.

Feldman, Gerald D. *Historische Vergangenheitsbearbeitung. Wirtschaft und Wissenschaft im Vergleich.* Berlin, Germany: Max Planck Institute for the History of Science, 2003.

Ferenczi, Sándor, and Sigmund Freud. *Zur Psychoanalyse der Kriegsneurosen: Diskussion gehalten auf dem V. Internationalen Psychoanalytischen Kongress in Budapest, 28. und 29. September 1918.* Vienna, Austria: Internationaler Psychoanalytischer Verlag, 1919.

Fergusen, Niall, ed. *Virtual History: Alternatives and Counterfactuals.* London, UK: Picador, 1997.

Fermi, Laura. *Illustrious Immigrants: The Intellectual Migration from Europe, 1930–41.* Chicago, IL: University of Chicago Press, 1968.

Fiddian-Qasmiyeh, Elena, Gil Loescher, and Nando Sigona, eds. *The Oxford Handbook of Refugee & Forced Migration Studies.* Oxford, UK: Oxford University Press, 2014.

Finger, Stanley. *Origins of Neuroscience. A History of Explorations into Brain Function.* New York: Oxford University Press, 1994.

– "Francis Schiller (1909–2003)." *Journal of the History of the Neurosciences* 13, no. 4 (2004a): 353–7.

– *Minds Behind the Brain: A History of the Pioneers and Their Discoveries.* Oxford, UK: Oxford University Press, 2004b.

Finkelstein, Gabriel. "Darwin and Neuroscience: The German Connection." *Frontiers in Neuroanatomy* 13, no. 1 (2019): 1–3.

– *Emil du Bois-Reymond: Neuroscience, Self, and Society in Nineteenth-Century Germany.* Cambridge, MA: MIT Press, 2013.

Fischer, Fritz. *From Kaiserreich to Third Reich: Elements of Continuity in German History,* transl. by Roger Fletcher. London, UK: Allen & Unwin, 1986.

Fischer, Gottfried. "Psychoanalytische Grundlagen der Psychotraumatologie: Aktueller Forschungsstand und Bedeutung fuer die Praxis." *Forum der Psychoanalyse* 22, no. 4 (2006): 342–57.

Fischer, Klaus. "Identification of Emigration-Induced Scientific Change." In *Forced Migration and Scientific Change: Émigré German-speaking Scientists and Scholars after 1933,* edited by Mitchell G. Ash and Alfons Soellner, 23–47. Washington, DC, 1996.

Fischer, Peter. *Licht und Leben: Ein Bericht ueber Max Delbrueck, den Wegbereiter der Molekularbiologie.* Konstanz, Germany: Universitaetsverlag, 1985.

Fitzgerald, Des, Melissa M. Littlefield, Kasper J. Knudson, James Tonks, and Martin J. Dietz. "Ambivalence, Equivocation and the Politics of Experimental Knowledge: A Transdisciplinary Neuroscience Encounter." *Social Studies of Science* 44, no. 5 (2014): 701–21.

Fix, Michael. "Leben und Werk des Gehirnanatomen Korbinian Brodmann (1868–1918)." MD Diss., University of Tuebingen, Germany, 1994.

Flechsig, Paul. *Die Irrenklinik der Universitaet Leipzig und ihre Wirksamkeit in den Jahren 1882–1886. Mit zwei Plaenen.* Leipzig, Germany: Verlag von Veit & Comp., 1888.

– *Die Localisation der geistigen Vorgaenge insbesondere der Empfindungen des Menschen. Vortrag gehalten auf der 68. Versammlung Deutscher Naturforscher und Aerzte zu Frankfurt a. M.* Leipzig, Germany: Verlag von Veit & Comp., 1896.

Fleck, Christian. "Emigration of Social Scientists' Schools from Austria." In Ash and Soellner, *Forced Migration and Scientific Change: Émigré German-Speaking Scientists after 1933*, 198–223.

Fleming, Donald and Bernard Bailyn, eds. *The Intellectual Migration: Germany and America, 1930–1960.* Cambridge, MA: Cambridge University Press, 1969.

Flexner, Abraham. "Medical Education in Europe: A Report to the Carnegie Foundation for the Advancement of Teaching." New York: Carnegie Foundation for the Advancement of Teaching, 1912.

Flynn, Patrick. *Dalhousie's Department of Psychiatry: A Historical Perspective.* Halifax: Dalhousie University, 1999.

Focke, Wenda. *William G. Niederland. Psychiater der Verfolgten, seine Zeit, sein Leben, sein Werk, ein Portraet.* Wuerzburg, Germany: Koenigshausen & Neumann, 1992.

– *Begegnung. Herta Seidemann. Psychiatrin-Neurologin 1900–1984.* Konstanz, Germany: Hartung-Gorre, 1986.

Foerster, Otfrid, and Wilder Penfield. "The Structural Basis of Traumatic Epilepsy and Results of Radical Operation." *Brain* 53, no. 2 (1930): 99–119.

Foley, Paul. *Encephalitis Lethargica: The Mind and Brain Virus.* New York: Springer, 2018.

Forel, Auguste. *Hygiene der Nerven und des Geistes im Gesunden und kranken Zustande.* Stuttgart, Germany: E. Moritz, 1905.

– *Alkohol, Vererbung und Sexualleben. Vortrag gehalten auf dem 10. Internationalen Kongress gegen Alkoholismus.* Berlin, Germany: J. Michaelis, 1907.

– *Rueckblick auf mein Leben.* Zurich, Switzerland: Europa Verlag, 1935.

Forsbach, Ralf. *Die Medizinische Fakultaet der Universitaet Bonn im "Dritten Reich."* Munich, Germany: Oldenbourg Verlag, 2006.

Fosdick, Raymond, B. *The Story of the Rockefeller Foundation. With a New Introduction by Stephen C. Wheatley.* Second Edition. New Brunswick, NJ: Transaction Publishers, 1989.

Foster, Lois R. "No Northern Option: Canada and Refugees from Nazism before the Second World War." In *False Havens: The British Empire and the Holocaust,* edited by Paul R. Bartrop, 79–98. Lanham, MD: University Press of America, 1995.

Frank, Tibor. *Double Exile. Migrations of Jewish-Hungarian Professionals through Germany to the United States, 1919–1945.* Frankfurt am Main, Germany: Peter Lang, 2009.

Frazzetto, Giovanni and Susan Anker. "Neuroculture." *Nature Review Neuroscience* 10, no. 11 (2009): 815–21.

Freemon, F. Roy. "American Neurology." In *Handbook of Clinical Neurology,* edited by Stanley Finger, François Boller, and Kenneth L. Tyler, 605–12. Edinburgh, UK: Elsevier B.V., 2010.

Freud, Sigmund. "Ueber das Rueckenmark niederer Fischarten." MD diss., University of Vienna, Austria, 1881.

– *Meine Ansichten ueber die Rolle der Sexualitaet in der Aetiologie der Neurosen* (1905). Collected Works of Sigmund Freud. 5th vol. Frankfurt am Main, Germany: Fischer, 1999, 147–57.

– "Weitere Ratschlaege zur Technik der Psychoanalyse (II): Erinnern, Wiederholen und Durcharbeiten." *Internationale Zeitschrift fuer aerztliche Psychoanalyse* 2, no. 1 (1914): 126–36.

– *Vorlesungen zur Einfuehrung in die Psychoanalyse* (1916/17). Collected Works of Sigmund Freud. 11th vol. Frankfurt am Main: Fischer, 1999, 282–95.

– "Einleitung." In *Zur Psychoanalyse der Kriegsneurosen,* edited by Sigmund Freud, Sándor Ferenczi, Karl Abraham, and Ernst Simmel. Vol. 1, 3–8. Leipzig, Germany: Internationale Psychoanalytische Bibliothek, 1919.

– "Ueber Kriegsneurosen, Elektrotherapie und Psychoanalyse (ein Auszug aus dem Protokoll des Untersuchungsverfahrens gegen Wagner-Jauregg im Oktober 1920)." *Psyche. Zeitschrift fuer Psychoanalyse* 26, no. 9 (1972): 939–51.

Friedman, Milton. *Capitalism and Freedom.* Chicago, IL: University of Chicago Press, 1962.

Fulton, John, ed. *Selected Readings in the History of Physiology,* completed by Leonard G. Wilson. Springfield, IL: C.C. Thomas, 1966.

Furgusen, Niall, ed. *Virtual History: Alternatives and Counterfactuals*. London, UK: Picador, 1997.

Galison, Peter. *Image and Logic. A Material Culture of Microphysics*. Chicago, IL: University of Chicago Press, 1997.

Galison, Peter, Stephen R. Graubard, and Everett Medelsohn, eds. *Science in Culture*. New Brunswick, NJ: Transaction Publishers, 2001.

Galton, Francis. *Inquiries into Human Faculty and Its Development*. London, UK: Macmillan and Co., 1883.

Ganesh, Aravind, and Frank W. Stahnisch. "The Gray Degeneration of the Brain and Spinal Cord: A Story of the Once Favored Diagnosis with Subsequent Vessel-Based Etiopathological Studies in Multiple Sclerosis." *Journal of Nervous and Mental Disease* 207, no. 6 (2019): 505–14.

Garey, Laurence J. *Brodmann's Localisation in the Cerebral Cortex*. London, UK: Smith-Gordon, 1994.

Gaudillière, Jean-Paul. "Making Heredity in Mice and Men: The Production and Uses of Animal Models in Postwar Human Genetics." In *Heredity and Infection: The History of Disease Transmission*, edited by Jean-Paul Gaudillière and Ilana Loewy, 181–202. London, UK: Routledge, 2001.

Gaudillière, Jean-Paul, and Hans-Joerg Rheinberger, eds. *From Molecular Genetics to Genomics: The Mapping Cultures of Twentieth-Century Genetics*. London, UK, and New York, 2004.

Gavrus, Delia. "Men of Dreams and Men of Action. Neurologists, Neurosurgeons, and the Performance of Professional Identity, 1920–1950." *Bulletin of the History of Medicine* 85, no. 1 (2011): 57–92.

Gavrus, Delia, and Stephen Casper, eds. *The History of the Brain and Mind Sciences: Technique, Technology, Therapy*. Rochester, NY: University of Rochester Press, 2017.

Gay, Peter. *Freud. Eine Biographie fuer unsere Zeit*. Frankfurt am Main: S. Fischer, 1989.

Geertz, Clifford. *The Interpretation of Cultures: Selected Essays*. New York: Basic Books, 1973.

Geiger, Roger L. "The Dynamics of University Research in the United States 1945–1990." In *Research and Higher Education: The United Kingdom and the United States*, edited by Thomas G. Whiston and Roger L. Geiger, 3–17. Suffolk, UK: The Society for Research into Higher Education, 1992.

Geison, Gerald L. "Scientific Change, Emerging Specialities, and Research Schools." *History of Science* 19, no. 1 (1981): 20–40.

Geisthoevel, Alexa, and Bettina Hitzer. *Auf der Suche nach einer anderen Medizin. Psychosomatik im 20. Jahrhundert*. Berlin, Germany: Suhrkamp Verlag, 2019.

Gelb, Adhémar, and Kurt Goldstein. *Psychologische Analysen hirnpathologischer Faelle auf Grund von Untersuchungen Hirnverletzter*. Berlin, Germany: Julius Springer, 1918.

Genty, Maurice. "Masson, Claude Laurent Pierre." *Archives biographiques françaises* 449, no. 2 (1972): 272–3.

German-Bohemian Heritage Society. Newsletter 8, no. 1, 1997, 6.

Geroulanos, Stefanos and Todd Meyers. *The Human Body in the Age of Catastrophe: Brittleness, Integration, Science, and the Great War*. Chicago, IL: University of Chicago Press, 2018.

Gerrens Uwe. "Psychiater unter der NS-Diktatur. Karl Bonhoeffers Einsatz fuer rassisch und politisch verfolgte Kolleginnen und Kollegen." *Fortschritte der Neurologie, Psychiatrie und ihrer Grenzgebiete* 67, no. 7 (2001): 330–9.

Gibson, David. "Involuntary Sterilization of the Mentally Retarded: A Western Canadian Phenomenon." *The Canadian Psychiatric Association Journal* 19, no. 1 (1974): 59–63.

Glees, Paul. "Ludwig Edinger (1855–1918)." *Journal of Neurophysiology* 15, no. 3 (1952): 251–5.

Gleichen, Alexander Wilhelm. *Die Theorie der modernen optischen Instrumente: ein Hilfs- und Uebungsbuch fuer Physiker und Konstrukteure optischer Werkstaetten, sowie fuer Ingenieure im Dienste des Heeres und der Marine*. Stuttgart, Germany: F. Enke, 1911.

Globig, Michael, ed. *Impulse geben, Wissen stiften. 40 Jahre Volkswagen Stiftung*. Goettingen, Germany: Vandenhoeck & Ruprecht, 2002.

Gocht, Hermann. "Bericht ueber die ausserordentliche Tagung der deutschen Gesellschaft fuer Krueppelfuersorge." *Zentralblatt fuer Chirurgische und Mechanische Orthopaedie* 10, no. 1 (1916): 74–81.

Goldblatt, Daniel. "Star: Karl Stern (1906–1975)." *Seminars in Neurology* 12, no. 3 (1992): 279–82.

Goldstein, Kurt. "Die Zusammensetzung der Hinterstraenge. Anatomische Beitraege und kritische Uebersicht." MD diss., University of Breslau, Germany, 1903.

– *Ueber Rassenhygiene*. Berlin, Germany: Julius Springer, 1913.

– *Die Behandlung, Fuersorge und Begutachtung der Hirnverletzten. Zugleich ein Beitrag zur Verwendung psychologischer Methoden in der Klinik*. Leipzig, Germany: Vogel, 1919.

– "Zum Problem der Angst: Angstund Furcht." *Allgemeine Aerztliche Zeitschrift fuer Psychotherapie* 2, no. 7 (1927): 409–37.

- "Die Neuroregulation. Referat." *Verhandlungen der Deutschen Gesellschaft fuer Innere Medizin* 43, no. 1 (1931): 9–13.
- *Der Aufbau des Organismus. Einfuehrung in die Biologie unter besonderer Beruecksichtigung der Erfahrungen am Kranken Menschen.* The Hague, The Netherlands: M. Nijhoff, 1934.
- *Human Nature in the Light of Psychopathology.* Cambridge, MA: Harvard University Press, 1940.
- *Selected Papers/Ausgewaehlte Schriften,* edited by Aaron Gurwitsch, Else M. Goldstein-Haudek, and William E. Haudek. The Hague, The Netherlands: Martinus Nijhoff, 1971.
- "Notes on the Development of My Concepts." In *Selected Papers/ Ausgewaehlte Schriften,* edited by Aron Gurwitsch, Else M. Goldstein-Haudek, and William E. Haudek, 1–12. The Hague, The Netherlands: Martinus Nijhoff, 1971.
- *Der Aufbau des Organismus. Einfuehrung in die Biologie unter besonderer Beruecksichtigung der Erfahrungen am kranken Menschen,* introduced and edited by Thomas Hoffmann and Frank W. Stahnisch. Series Uebergaenge, edited by Bernhard Waldenfels. Munich and Paderborn, Germany: Wilhelm Fink, 2014.
Goschler, Constantin, eds. *Wissenschaft und Oeffentlichkeit in Berlin, 1870–1930.* Stuttgart, Germany: Franz Steiner, 2000.
Goudsmith, Samuel Abraham. *Alsos: The Failure in German Science.* London, UK: Sigma, 1947.
Gradmann, Christoph. *Laboratory Disease: Robert Koch's Medical Bacteriology* (Germ. 2005). Transl. by Elborg Forster. Baltimore, MD: Johns Hopkins University Press, 2009.
Gratzer, Walter. Review of "Hitler's Gift: Scientists Who Fled Nazi Germany," by Jean Medawar and David Pyke. *Nature* 408, no. 6815 (2000): 907–8.
Greenblatt, Samuel H., T. Forcht Dagi, and Mel H. Epstein, eds. *A History of Neurosurgery in Its Scientific and Professional Contexts.* Park Ridge, IL: American Association of Neurological Surgeons, 1997.
Griesinger, Wilhelm. *Mental Pathology and Therapeutics* (1845). Translated by James Rutherford and C. Lockhart Robertson. London: New Sydenham Society, 1867.
Grob, Gerald N. *Mental Illness and American Society, 1875–1940.* Princeton, NJ: Princeton University Press, 1983.
- "Mental Health Policy in Late Twentieth-Century America." In *American Psychiatry after World War II (1944–1994),* edited by Roy W. Menninger and John C. Nemiah. Washington, DC: American Psychiatric Press, 2000.

Groeben, Christiane, and Fabio de Sio. "Nobel Laureates at the Stazione Zoologica Anton Dohrn: Phenomenology and Paths of Discovery in Neuroscience." *Journal of the History of the Neurosciences* 15, no. 4 (2006): 376–95.

Gruen, Bernd, Hans-Georg Hofer, and Karl-Heinz Leven, eds., *Medizin und Nationalsozialismus: die Freiburger Medizinische Fakultaet und das Klinikum in der Weimarer Republik und im "Dritten Reich."* Frankfurt am Main: Peter Lang, 2002.

Grossmann, Anita. "German Women Doctors from Berlin to New York: Maternity and Modernity in Weimar and in Exile." *Feminist Studies* 19, no. 1 (1993): 65–88.

Gruber, Max. *Die Erhaltung und Mehrung der deutschen Volkskraft.* Berlin, Germany: Zentralstelle fuer Volkswohlfahrt, 1916.

Gruber, Max, and Emil Kraepelin. *Wandtafeln zur Alkoholfrage. Erlaeuterungen nebst den 10 verkleinerten Tafeln in mehrfachem Farbendruck.* Munich, Germany: Lehmann, 1911.

Gruettner, Michael, and Sven Kinas. "Die Vertreibung von Wissenschaftlern aus den deutschen Universitaeten 1933–1945." *Vierteljahrshefte fuer Zeitgeschichte* 55, no. 1 (2007): 123–86.

Guttmann, Giselher, and Inge Scholz-Strasser, eds. *Freud and the Neurosciences: From Brain to the Unconscious.* Vienna, Austria: Verlag der Oesterreichischen Akademie der Wissenschaften, 1998.

Habermas, Juergen. *Erkenntnis und Interesse* (1962). Translated by Thomas Burger and Frederick Lawrence. Frankfurt am Main, Germany: Suhrkamp Verlag, 1968.

– *The Structural Transformation of the Public Sphere: An Inquiry into a Category of Bourgeois Society.* Cambridge, UK: Polity, 1989.

Haentzschel, Hiltrud. "Der Exodus von Wissenschaftlerinnen. 'Juedische' Studentinnen an der Muenchner Universitaet und was aus ihnen wurde." *Exil* 12, no. 2 (1992), 43–53.

Hagner, Michael. "Gehirnfuehrung. Zur Anatomie der geistigen Funktionen, 1870–1930." In *Ecce Cortex. Beitraege zur Geschichte des modernen Gehirns,* edited by Michael Hagner, 144–76. Goettingen, Germany: Wallstein, 1999.

– *Homo cerebralis. Der Wandel vom Seelenorgan zum Gehirn.* Frankfurt am Main, Germany: Insel, 2000.

– "Cultivating the Cortex in German Neuroanatomy." *Science in Context* 14, no. 4 (2001): 541–63.

– *Geniale Gehirne. Zur Geschichte der Elitegehirnforschung.* Goettingen, Germany: Wallstein, 2004.

Haines, Duane E. "Santiago Ramón y Cajal at Clark University, 1899: His Only Visit to the United States." *Brain Research Bulletin* 55, no. 2 (2007): 463–80.

Hammerstein, Notker. *Die Deutsche Forschungsgemeinschaft in der Zeit der Weimarer Repu-blik und im Dritten Reich. Wissenschaftspolitik in Republik und Diktatur.* Munich, Germany: C.H. Beck, 1999.

– "Wissenschaftssystem und Wissenschaftspolitik im Nationalsozialismus." In *Wissenschaften und Wissenschaftspolitik. Bestandsaufnahmen zu Formationen, Bruechen und Kontinuitaeten im Deutschland des 20. Jahrhunderts,* edited by Ruediger vom Bruch and Brigitte Kaderas, 219–24. Stuttgart, Germany: Franz Steiner, 2002.

– *Die Johann Wolfgang Goethe-Universitaet Frankfurt am Main. Von der Stiftungsuniversitaet zur Staatlichen Hochschule.* Vol. 1. Goettingen, Germany: Wallstein, 2012.

Hantke, Lydia. *Trauma und Dissoziation. Modelle der Verarbeitung traumatischer Erfahrungen.* Berlin: Wissenschaftliche Verlagsgesellschaft, 1999.

Haraway, Donna. "A Game of Cat's Cradle: Science Studies, Feminist Theory, Cultural Studies." *Configurations* 2, no. 1 (1994): 59–71.

Harrington, Anne. *Reenchanted Science: Holism in German Culture from Wilhelm II to Hitler.* Princeton, NJ: Princeton University Press, 1996.

Harrison, Ross G. "Experiments in Transplanting Limbs and their Bearings on the Problems of the Development of Nerves." *Journal of Experimental Zoology* 4, no. 2 (1907): 239–81.

Hartmann, Heinz. *Essays on Ego Psychology: Selected Papers in Psychoanalytic Theory.* New York: International Universities Press, 1964.

Harwood, Jonathan. *Styles of Scientific Thought: The German Genetics Community, 1900–1933.* Chicago, IL: University of Chicago Press, 1993.

– "Weimar Culture and Biological Theory: A Study of Richard Wolterede (1877–1944)." *History of Science* 24, no. 3 (1996): 347–77.

Hass, Hans-Egon, ed. *Gerhart Hauptmann. Saemtliche Werke.* 1st vol. Frankfurt am Main, Germany: Propylaeen Verlag, 1962.

Hau, Michael. *The Cult of Health and Beauty in Germany: A Social History, 1890–1930.* Chicago, IL: University of Chicago Press, 2003.

Hauptmann, Carl. *Die Metaphysik in der modernen Physiologie. Eine kritische Untersuchung.* Dresden, Germany: C. Ehlermann, 1893.

Hauptmann, Gerhart. *Vor Sonnenaufgang: Soziales Drama.* Berlin, Germany: C.F. Conrad, 1889.

– *Wanda (Der Daemon).* Berlin, Germany: S. Fischer, 1928.

– *Atlantis.* Berlin, Germany: S. Fischer, 1913.

Haymaker, Webb, and Francis Schiller, eds. *Founders of Neurology: One Hundred and Forty-Six Biographical Sketches by Eighty-Eight Authors.* 2nd edition. Springfield, IL: Charles C. Thomas, 1970.

Hayward, Rhodri. "Germany and the Making of 'English' Psychiatry: The Mandaley Hospital, 1908–1939." In *International Relations in Psychiatry. Britain, Germany, and the United States to World War II*, edited by Volker Roelcke, Paul J. Weindling, and Louise Westwood, 67–90. Rochester, NY: University of Rochester Press, 2010.

Heberer-Rice, Patricia, and Juergen Matthaeus. *Atrocities on Trial: The Politics of Prosecuting War Crimes in Historical Perspective.* Lincoln, NE: University of Nebraska Press, 2008.

Helmchen, Hanfried, ed. *Psychiater und Zeitgeist: Zur Geschichte der Psychiatrie in Berlin.* Berlin, Germany: Pabst Science Publisher, 2008.

Hepp, Michael, ed. *Die Ausbuergerung deutscher Staatsangehoeriger 1933– 1945 nach den im Reichsanzeiger veroeffentlichten Listen.* 3 Vols. Munich, Germany: G. Saur, 1985–8.

Herrick, Charles Judson. "Editorial Announcement." *Journal of Comparative Neurology and Psychology* 14, no. 1 (1904): 1.

Herrn, Rainer. "Magnus Hirschfeld, sein Institut für Sexualwissenschaft und die Buecherverbrennung." In *Verfemt und Verboten. Vorgeschichte und Folgen der Buecherverbrennungen 1933.* Hildesheim, Germany: Olms-Verlag, 2010, 97–152.

Heynen, Robert. *Degeneration and Revolution: Radical Cultural Politics and the Body in Weimar Germany.* New York: Haymarket Books, 2015.

Hildebrandt, Sabine. "The Women on Stieve's List: Victims of National Socialism Whose Bodies Were Used for Anatomical Research." *Clinical Anatomy* 26, no. 1 (2013): 3–21.

– *The Anatomy of Murder: Ethical Transgressions and Anatomical Science during the Third Reich.* New York: Berghahn Books, 2016.

Hilscher, Eberhard. *Gerhart Hauptmann. Leben und Werk.* Frankfurt am Main, Germany: Athenaeum Verlag, 1988.

His, Wilhelm. "Beschreibung eines Mikrotoms." *Archiv fuer mikroskopische Anatomie* 6, no. 1 (1870): 229–32.

Hobsbawm, Eric. *The Age of Extremes: The Short Twentieth Century, 1914– 1991.* London, UK: Michel Joseph, 1994.

Hoch, Paul K. "Migration and the Generation of New Scientific Ideas." *Minerva* 25, no. 3 (1987): 209–37.

Hoche, Alfred, ed. *Handbuch der gerichtlichen Psychiatrie.* 3rd ed. Compiled by Gustav Aschaffenburg. Berlin, Germany: Springer, 1934.

Hoeres, Peter. "Vor 'Mainhattan': Frankfurt am Main als amerikanische Stadt in der Weimarer Republik." In *Mythos USA*. *"Amerikanisierung" in Deutschland seit 1900*, edited by Frank Becker and Elke Reinhardt-Becker, 71–97. Frankfurt am Main, Germany: Campus, 2006.

Hofer, Hans-Georg. *Nervenschwaeche und Krieg. Modernitaetskritik und Krisenbewaeltigung in der oesterreichischen Psychiatrie (1880–1920)*. Vienna, Austria: Boehlau, 2004.

– "War Neurosis and Viennese Psychiatry in World War One." In *Uncovered Fields: Perspectives in First World War Studies*, edited by Jenny Macleod and Pierre Purseigle, 243–60. Amsterdam: Rodopi, 2004.

Hoff, Peter, and Matthias M. Weber. "Sozialdarwinismus und die Psychiatrie im Nationalsozialismus." *Der Nervenarzt* 73, no. 11 (2002): 1017–18.

Hogan, David. "History of Geriatrics in Canada." *Canadian Bulletin of Medical History* 24, no. 1 (2007): 131–50.

Hogan, Michael J. *The Marshall Plan: America, Britain, and the Reconstruction of Western Europe, 1947–1952*. Cambridge, UK: Cambridge University Press, 1987.

Hohendorf, Gerrit, and Achim Magull-Seltenreich, eds. *Von der Heilkunde zur Massentoetung. Medizin im Nationalsozialismus*. Heidelberg, Germany: Wunderhorn, 1990.

Holdorff, Bernd. *Die Neurologie in Berlin, 1840–1945*. Berlin, Germany: Hentrich & Hentrich, 2019.

– "Die nervenaerztlichen Polikliniken in Berlin vor und nach 1900." In *Geschichte der Neurologie in Berlin*, edited by Bernd Holdorff and Rolf Winau, 127–40. Berlin, Germany: DeGruyter, 2001.

– "Zwischen Hirnforschung, Neuropsychiatrie und Emanzipation." In *Geschichte der Neurologie in Berlin*, edited by Bernd Holdorff and Rolf Winau, 157–74. Berlin, Germany: DeGruyter, 2001.

– "Friedrich Heinrich Lewy (1885–1950) and his Work." *Journal of the History of the Neurosciences* 11, no. 1 (2002), 19–28.

– "Ueber Max Lewandowskys Kriegsaufsatz (1915) zur Internationalitaet der Wissenschaft." *SDGGN* 9, no. 1 (2003): 61–6.

– "Founding Years of Clinical Neurology in Berlin until 1933." *Journal of the History of the Neurosciences* 13, no. 3 (2004): 223–38.

Holdorff, Bernd and Manfred Wolter. "Ueber die Kontroversen Oskar Vogts in der Berliner Gesellschaft fuer Psychiatrie und Nervenkrankheiten (BGPN) in den Jahren 1911 und 1913 und die Folgen." *SDGGN* 13, no. 1 (2007): 413–27.

Holdorff, Bernd and Rolf Winau, eds. *Geschichte der Neurologie in Berlin*. Berlin, Germany: Walter DeGruyter, 2001.

Hollingsworth, J. Roger. "Institutionalizing Excellence in Biomedical Research." In *Creating a Tradition of Biomedical Research*, edited by Darwin H. Stapleton, 15–18. New York: Rockefeller University Press, 2004.

Holloway, David. "Totalitarianism and Science: The Nazi and the Soviet Experience." In *Totalitarian Societies and Democratic Transition: Essays in Memory of Victor Zaslavsky*, 231–50, edited by Tommaso Piffer and Vladislav Zubok. Budapest, Hungary: Central European University, 2017.

Holmes, Emily, Ata Ghaderi, Catherine Harmer, Paul G. Ramchandani, Pim Cuijpers, Anthony P. Morrison, Jonathan P. Roisen, Claudi L.H. Bockting, Rosy C. O'Connor, Roz Shafran, Michelle L. Moulds, and Michelle G. Oraske. "The Lancet Psychiatry Commission on Psychological Treatments Research in Tomorrow's Science." *The Lancet Psychiatry* 5, no. 3 (2018): 237–86.

Holmes, Frederic L. *Hans Krebs: Architect of Intermediary Metabolism, 1933–1937*. Oxford, UK: Oxford University Press, 1991.

– *Hans Krebs: The Formation of a Scientific Life, 1900–1933*. Oxford, UK: Oxford University Press, 1993.

Holtan, Neal Ross. "The Eitels and Their Hospital." *Minnesota Medicine* 36, no. 1 (2003): 52–4.

Horn, Eva. "Krieg und Krise. Zur anthropologischen Figur des Ersten Weltkriegs." In *Konzepte der Moderne. DFG-Symposion 1999*, edited by Gerhart von Graevenitz, 633–55. Stuttgart, Germany: Metzler, 1999.

– "Erlebnis und Trauma. Die narrative Konstruktion des Ereignisses in Psychiatrie und Kriegsroman." In *Modernitaet und Trauma*, edited by Inka Muelder-Bach, 131–62. Vienna, Austra: Universitaetsverlag, 2000.

Hossfeld, Uwe and Lennart Olsson. "The Road from Haeckel: The Jena Tradition in Evolutionary Morphology and the Origins of 'Evo-Devo.'" *Biology and Philosophy* 18, no. 2 (2003): 285–307.

Hubenstorf, Michael. "Ende einer Tradition und Fortsetzung als Provinz. Die Medizinischen Fakultaeten der Universitaeten Berlin und Wien 1925–1950." In *Medizin, Naturwissenschaft, Technik und Nationalsozialismus: Kontinuitaeten und Diskontinuitaeten*, edited by Christoph Meinel and Peter Voswinckel, 33–53. Stuttgart, Germany: Franz Steiner, 1994.

– "Vertreibung und Verfolgung. Zur Geschichte der oesterreichischen Medizin im 20. Jahrhundert." *Das Juedische Echo* 50, no. 1 (2001), 277–88.

Huentelmann, Axel C. "'Ehrlich faerbt am laengsten.' Sichtbarmachung bei Paul Ehrlich." *Berichte zur Wissenschaftsgeschichte* 36, no. 4 (2013): 354–80.

Hughes, Jeff. *The Manhattan Project: Big Science and the Atomic Bomb*. New York: Columbia University Press, 2002.

Hughlings-Jackson, John. "Gulstonian Lectures on Certain Points in the Study and Classification of the Diseases of the Nervous System. Lecture II." *British Medical Journal* 427, no. 1 (1869): 210 and 236.

Humphries, Mark and Kellen Kurschinski. "'Rest, Relax, and Get Well: Re-Conceptualising Great War Shell Shock Treatment.'" *War & Society (Australia)* 27, no. 2 (2008): 89–110.

Hunt, Linda. *Secret Agenda: The United States Government, Nazi Scientists, and Project Paperclip, 1945 to 1990.* New York: St Martin's Press, 1991.

Igersheimer, Walther W. *Blatant Injustice: The Story of a Jewish Refugee from Nazi Germany Imprisoned in Britain and Canada during World War II,* ed. and foreword by Ian Darrach. Montreal and Kingston: McGill-Queen's University Press, 2005.

Innes, John R.M., and Leonard T. Kurland. "Is Multiple Sclerosis Caused by a Virus?" *American Journal of Medicine* 12, no. 5 (1952): 574–85.

Israel, Giorgi. "Science and the Jewish Question in the Twentieth Century: The Case of Italy and What It Shows." *Aleph: Historical Studies in Science and Judaism* 4, no. 1 (2004): 191–261.

Jacob, François. *The Statue Within: An Autobiography.* New York: Basic Books, 1988.

Jacobson, Marcus. *Foundations of Neuroscience.* New York: Springer, 1993.

Jacyna, L. Steven. *Medicine and Modernism: A Biography of Sir Henry Head.* London, UK: Chatto & Pickering, 2008.

Janet, Pierre. *L'automatisme psychologique. Essai de psychologie expérimentale sur les formes inférieures de l'activité humaine.* Paris, France: Félix Alcan, 1889.

Jelliffe, Smith Ely, Arthur S. Link, and Lilly M. Mendelson, eds. *Fifty Years of American Neurology: An Historical Perspective.* Winston-Salem, UK: Stratford Books, 1998.

Johnston, Penelope. "Canada's Ellis Island." *The Beaver,* February–March 2009, 52–3.

Juette, Robert. *Die Emigration der deutschsprachigen "Wissenschaft des Judentums." Die Auswanderung juedischer Historiker nach Palaestina 1933–1945.* Stuttgart, Germany: Franz Steiner, 1991.

Jung, Richard. "Ueber eine Nachuntersuchung des Falles Schn. von Goldstein und Gelb." *Psychiatrie, Neurologie und medizinische Psychologie* 1, no. 3 (1949): 353–58.

Kaestner, Ingrid. "'… wurde Leipzig zu einer der Hauptstaetten neurologischer Forschung.' Neurologie an der Universitaet Leipzig von den Anfaengen bis zur Gegenwart." *SDGGN* 12, no. 1 (2006): 81–100.

Kaestner, Ingrid, and Christina Schroeder. *Sigmund Freud (1856–1939).*
Hirnforscher, Neurologe, Psychotherapeut. Ausgewaehlte Texte. Leipzig,
Germany: Barth, 1989.

Kaiserling, Helmut. "Die Ausbreitungsformen der Nierenlymphbahninfekte
und die lymphogene Nephrose. (Experimentelle, chemisch-physiologische
und morphologische Untersuchungen)." *Virchows Archiv fuer pathologische
Anatomie* 309, no. 2 (1942): 561–87.

Kalinowsky, Lothar B. "Der Einfluss deutschsprachiger Psychiater und
Neurologen in Nordamerika und England." *Fortschritte der Neurologie,
Psychiatrie und ihrer Genzgebiete* 46, no. 11 (1978): 625–8.

Kallmann, Franz Joseph. *The Genetics of Schizophrenia: A Study of Heredity
and Reproduction in the Families of 1,087 Schizophrenics.* New York: J.J.
Augustin, 1938.

Kandel, Eric. R. *Cellular Basis of Behavior: An Introduction to Behavioral
Neurobiology.* New York: W.H. Freeman, 1976.

– *In Search of Memory: The Emergence of a New Science of Mind.* London:
W.W. Norton & Company, 2006.

– *The Age of Insight: The Quest to Understand the Unconscious in Art, Mind,
and Brain, from Vienna 1900 to the Present.* New York: Random House,
2012.

Kandel, Eric R., James H. Schwartz, and Thomas M. Jessell, *Principles of
Neural Science.* New York: McGraw-Hill, 1981.

Karenberg, Axel. "Klinische Neurologie in Deutschland bis zum Ersten
Weltkrieg. Die Begruender des Faches und der Fachgesellschaft." In *100
Jahre Deutsche Gesellschaft fuer Neurologie,* edited by Detlef Koempf,
20–9. Berlin, Germany: Deutsche Gesellschaft fuer Neurologie, 2007.

Kater, Michael. "The Burden of the Past: Problems of a Modern
Historiography of Physians and Medicine in Nazi Germany." *German
Studies Review* 10, no. 1 (1987): 31–56.

– "Hitler's Early Doctors: Nazi Physicians in Pre-Depression Germany."
Journal of Modern History 95, no. 1 (1987): 25–52.

– *Doctors Under Hitler.* Chapell Hill, NC: University of North Carolina Press,
1989.

– "Unresolved Questions of German Medicine and Medical History in the
Past and Present." *Central European History* 25, no. 4 (1992), 407–23.

Kaufman, Fred. *Searching for Justice: An Autobiography.* Toronto: University
of Toronto Press, 2005.

Kaufmann, Doris. "Science as Cultural Practice: Psychiatry in the First World
War and Weimar Germany." *Journal of Contemporary History* 34, no. 1
(1999): 125–44.

Kay, Lilly E. "Conceptual Models and Analytical Tools: The Biology of
Physicist Max Delbrueck." *Journal of the History of Biology* 18, no. 2
(1985): 207–46.
– "Molecular Biology and Pauling's Immunochemistry: A Neglected
Dimension." *History and Philosophy of the Life Sciences* 11, no. 2 (1989):
211–19.
– "Rethinking Institutions: Philanthropy as an Historiographic Problem of
Knowledge and Power." *Minerva* 35, no. 3 (1997): 283–93.
Keck, Margaret E., and Kathryn Sikkink. *Activists beyond Borders: Advocacy
Networks in International Politics*. Ithaca, NY: Cornell University Press,
1998.
Keshishian, Haig. "Ross Harrison's 'The Outgrowth of the Nerve Fiber as a
Mode of Protoplasmatic Movement.'" *Journal of Experimental Zoology*
301A, no. 3 (2004): 201–3.
Kevles, Daniel J. "'Into Hostile Political Camps': The Reorganization of
International Science in World War I." *ISIS* 62, no. 1 (1971): 47–60.
Killen, Andreas. *Berlin Electropolis: Shock, Nerves, and German Modernity*.
Berkeley, CA: University of California Press, 2006.
Kingsley Kent, Susan. *Aftershocks: Politics and Trauma in Britain, 1918–1933*.
New York: Springer, 2009.
Klahre, Andrea S. "Die Psychiatrie profitiert von der Hirnforschung:
Weltkongress fuer Psychiatrie in Hamburg. Schere zwischen Erkenntnissen
der Forschung und ihrer Umsetzung in der Praxis." *Die Welt*, 9 August 1999,
n.p.
Klatzo, Igor. *Cécile and Oskar Vogt: The Visionaries of Modern Neuroscience*.
Vienna, Austria: Springer, 2002.
Klausewitz, Wolfgang. *175 Jahre Senckenbergische Naturforschende
Gesellschaft*. Frankfurt am Main, Germany: Kramer, 1992.
Klee, Ernst. *Das Personenlexikon zum Dritten Reich. Wer war was vor und
nach 1945*. Frankfurt am Main, Germany: Fischer Taschenbuch Verlag, 2003.
– *Auschwitz, die NS-Medizin und ihre Opfer*. Frankfurt am Main, Germany:
S. Fischer, 1997.
Kleist, Karl. *Gehirnpathologie, vornehmlich auf Grund der Kriegserfahrungen*.
Leipzig, Germany: Johann Ambrosius Barth, 1934.
Klibansky, Raymond, Erwin Panofsky, and Fritz Saxl. *Saturn and Melancholy:
Studies in the History of Natural Philosophy, Religion, and Art*. New York:
Basic Books, 1964.
Kloocke, Ruth, Heinz-Peter Schmiedebach, and Stefan Priebe. "Psychological
Injury in the Two World Wars: Changing Concepts and Terms in German
Psychiatry." *History of Psychiatry* 16, no. 1 (2005): 43–60.

Knorr-Cetina, Karin. "Das naturwissenschaftliche Labor als Ort der 'Verdichtung von Gesellschaft.'" *Zeitschrift fuer Soziologie* 17, no. 2 (1988): 85–101.

– *Epistemic Cultures: How the Sciences Make Knowledge.* Cambridge, MA: Harvard University Press, 1999.

Koch, Eric. *Deemed Suspect: A Wartime Blunder.* Toronto: Methuen, 1980.

Koenig, Tricia. "A Detour or a Shortcut? Pathological Laboratories in Cancer Treatment Centers." In *Transferring Public Health, Medical Knowledge and Science in the 19th and 20th Century*, edited by Astri Andresen and Tore Grønlie, 47–65. Bergen, Norway: Stein Rokkan Senteret, 2007.

Koetter, Rudolf, and Philipp Balsiger. "Interdisciplinarity and Transdisciplinarity: A Constant Challenge to the Sciences." *Issues in Integrative Studies* 17, no. 1 (1999): 87–120.

Kohler, Eric D. "Relicensing Central European Refugee Physicians in the United States, 1933–1945." *Simon Wiesenthal Center Annual White Plains N.Y.* 6, no. 1 (1989): 3–32.

Kohring, Rolf, and Gerald Kreft, eds. *Tilly Edinger. Leben und Werk einer juedischen Wissenschaftlerin.* Stuttgart: E. Schweizerbart'sche Verlagsbuchhandlung, 2003.

Kraepelin, Emil. "Zur Entartungsfrage." *zblNP* 31, no. 19 N.F. (1908): 745–51.

– *Psychiatrie. Ein Lehrbuch fuer Studierende und Aerzte.* Vol. 7. Leipzig, Germany: Johann Ambrosius Barth, 1899.

– *Psychiatrie. Ein Lehrbuch fuer Studierende und Aerzte.* Vol. 8. Leipzig, Germany: Johann Ambrosius Barth, 1915.

– *Memoirs* (1920). Translated by Cheryl Wooding-Deane. Berlin, Germany: Springer, 1987.

– *Psychiatry. A Textbook for Students and Physicians* (1899). Translated by Jacques M. Quen. Canton, MA: Science History Publications, 1990.

– "Psychiatric Observations on Contemporary Issues" (1919). Translated by Eric J. Engstrom. *History of Psychiatry* 3, no. 2 (1992): 256–69.

Krause, Konrad. *Alma Mater Lipsiensis. Geschichte der Universitaet Leipzig von 1409 bis zur Gegenwart.* Leipzig, Germany: Universitaetsverlag, 2003.

Kreft, Gerald. "Zwischen Goldstein und Kleist. Zum Verhaeltnis von Neurologie und Psychiatrie im Frankfurt am Main der 1920er Jahre." *SDGGN* 3, no. 1 (1997): 131–44.

– *Deutsch-juedische Geschichte der Hirnforschung. Ludwig Edingers Neurologisches Institut in Frankfurt am Main.* Frankfurt am Main, Germany: Mabuse-Verlag, 2005.

Kreft, Gerald, Gerald G. Kovacs, Till Voigtlaender, Christine Haberler, Johannes A. Hainfellner, Hubert Bernheimer, and Herbert Budka. "125th Anniversary of the Institute of Neurology (Obersteiner Institute) in Vienna: 'Germ Cell' of Interdisciplinary Neuroscience." *Clinical Neuropathology* 27, no. 6 (2008): 439–43.

Kreutzberg, Georg W. "Interview." *Neuroforum* 14, no. 3 (2008): 244–7.

Krige, John, and Dominique Pestre, ed. *Science in the Twentieth Century.* London, UK: Routledge, 2013.

Kroen, Sherryl. "A Political History of the Consumer." *The Historical Journal* 74, no. 3 (2004): 709–36.

Kroener, Hans-Peter. "*Die Emigration deutschsprachiger Mediziner im Nationalsozialismus.*" *Berichte zur Wissenschaftsgeschichte 12, no. 1 (1989),* 1–35.

– *Von der Rassenhygiene zur Humangenetik.* Stuttgart, Germany: Gustav Fischer, 1998.

Krohn, Claus-Dieter, Patrick von zur Muehlen, Gerhard Paul, and Lutz Winckler, eds. *Handbuch der deutschsprachigen Emigration 1933–1945.* Vol. 3. Darmstadt, Germany: Wissenschaftliche Verlagsbuchhandlung, 1998.

Krohn, Claus-Dieter, and Lutz Winckler, eds. *Exilforschung. Ein internationales Jahrbuch.* Munich, Germany: Saur 1983–Present.

Kruecke, Wilhelm, and Hugo Spatz. "Aus den Erinnerungen von Ludwig Edinger." In *Ludwig Edinger 1855–1918*, edited by Hugo Spatz, 35–41. Frankfurt am Main, Germany: Schriften der Wissenschaftlichen Gesellschaft an der Johann Wolfgang Goethe Universitaet, 1959.

Kuechenhoff, Bernhard. "Der Psychiater Auguste Forel und seine Stellung zur Eugenik." In *Eugenik und Erinnerungskultur*, edited by Anton Leist, 19–36. Zurich, Switzerland: Hochschulverlag, 2006.

Kuehl, Stefan. *The Nazi Connection: Eugenics, American Racism, and German National Socialism.* Oxford, UK: Oxford University Press, 1994.

Kuemmel, Werner Friedrich. "Die Ausschaltung rassisch und politisch missliebiger Aerzte." In *Aezte im Nationalsozialismus*, edited by Friedrich Kudlien, 56–81. Cologne, Germany: Deutscher Apothekerverlag, 1985.

Kugelmann, Cilly and Juergen Reiche. "Nordamerika." In *Heimat und Exil. Emigration der deutschen Juden nach 1933*, edited by Stiftung Juedisches Museum Berlin und Stiftung Haus der Geschichte der Bundesrepublik Deutschland, 178–80. Frankfurt am Main, Germany: Dumont, 2006.

Kuhn, Thomas S. *The Structure of Scientific Revolutions.* Chicago, IL: University of Chicago Press, 1962.

– *The Essential Tension: Selected Studies in Scientific Tradition and Change*. Chicago, IL: University of Chicago Press, 1977.

Kumbier, Ekkehardt, and Katrin Haack. "Alfred Hauptmann. Schicksal eines deutsch-juedischen Neurologen." *Fortschritte der Neurologie – Psychiatrie* 70, no. 4 (2002): 204–09.

Kurbegović, Erna. "Eugenics in Comparative Perspective: Explaining Manitoba and Alberta's Divergence on Eugenics Policy, 1910s to the 1930s." PhD Diss., University of Calgary, 2019.

Kurzweil, Edith. "Psychoanalytic Science: From Oedipus to Culture." In *Forced Migration and Scientific Change: Émigré German-Speaking Scientists and Scholars after 1933*, edited by Mitchell Ash and Alfons Soellner, 139–55. Cambridge, UK: Cambridge University Press, 1996.

Kushner, Tony. *The Persistence of Prejudice: Anti-Semitism in British Society during the Second World War*. Manchester, UK: Manchester University Press, 1989.

Lakatos, Imre, and Allen Musgrave, eds. *Criticizm and the Growth of Knowledge*. Cambridge, UK: Cambridge University Press, 1970.

Lamb, Susan D. "The Most Important Professorship in the English-Speaking Domain: Adolph Meyer and the Beginnings of Cinical Psychiatry in the United States." *Journal of Nervous and Mental Diseases* 200, no. 12 (2012): 1061–6.

– *Pathologist of the Mind: Adolf Meyer and the Origins of American Psychiatry*. Baltimore, MD: Johns Hopkins University Press, 2014.

Lang, Hans-Joachim. "Spaete Reise zu den Erben. Universitaetsbibliothek Tuebingen gibt nach 63 Jahren Privatbibliothek zurueck." *Aufbau. Juedisches Leben* 13, no. 6 (21 June 2001): 18.

Lanzoni, Susan. "Diagnosing Modernity: Mania and Authenticity in the Existential Genre." *Configurations* 12, no. 1 (2004): 107–31.

Latour, Bruno. *Science in Action: How to Follow Scientists and Engineers through Society*. Cambridge, MA: Harvard University Press, 1987.

– "One More Turn after the Sociological Turn." In *The Science Studies Reader*, edited by Mario Biagioli, 272–92. London, UK: Routledge, 1999.

Latour, Bruno, Philippe Mauguin, and Geneviève Teil. "A Note on Sociotechnical Graphs." *Social Studies of Science* 22, no. 1 (1992): 33–59 and 91–4.

Laudan, Larry. *Progress and Its Problems: Towards a Theory of Scientific Growth*. Berkeley, CA: University of California Press, 1977.

Lawrence, Christopher and George Weisz, eds. *Greater than the Parts: Holism in Biomedicine, 1920–1950*. Oxford, UK: Oxford University Press, 1998.

Lazar, Morty M., and Medjuc Sheva. "In the Beginning: A Brief History of Jews in Atlantic Canada." *Canadian Jewish Historical Society Journal* 5, no. 2 (1981): 91–108.

Leed, Eric. *No Man's Land: Combat and Identity in World War I.* Cambridge, UK: Cambridge University Press, 1979.

Lehmann, Georg. "Zur Casuistik des Inducirten Irreseins (Folie à deux)." *Archiv fuer Psychiatrie und Nervenkrankheiten* 14, no. 1 (1883): 145–54.

Lehrer, Jonah. "How the Brain Reacts to Financial Bubbles." *New York Times, Sunday Magazine,* 31 October 2010, MM24.

Leibowitz, Herschel, and Richard Held. "Hans-Lukas Teuber, 1916–1977." *Psychological Research* 40, no. 1 (1978): 1–3.

Lenoir, Timothy. *Instituting Science: The Cultural Production of Scientific Disciplines.* Stanford, CA: Stanford University Press, 1997.

Lenz, Fritz. *Menschliche Auslese und Rassenhygiene (Eugenik).* Munich, Germany: Lehmann, 1921.

– "Eugenics in Germany." *The Journal of Heredity* 15, no. 3 (1924): 223–31.

Lepenies, Wolf. "Toward an Interdisciplinary History of Science." *International Journal of Sociology* 8, no. 1–2 (1978): 45–69.

Lepsien, Katharina, and Wolfgang Lange. "Verfolgung, Emigration und Ermordung juedischer Aerzte." In *Dienstbare Medizin. Aerzte betrachten ihr Fach im Nationalsozialismus*, edited by Hannes Friedrich and Wolfgang Matzow, 32–43. Goettingen, Germany: Vandenhoeck & Ruprecht, 1992.

Lerner, Paul. "'Nieder mit der traumatischen Neurose, hoch die Hysterie': Niedergang und Fall des Hermann Oppenheim (1889–1919)." *Psychotherapie* 2, no. 1 (1997): 16–22.

– *Hysterical Men: War, Psychiatry, and the Politics of Trauma in Germany, 1890–1930.* Ithaca, NY: Cornell University Press.

– "Ein Sieg Deutschen Willens: Wille und Gemeinschaft in der deutschen Kriegspsychiatrie." In *Die Medizin und der Erste Weltkrieg*, edited by Wolfgang U. Eckart and Christoph Gradmann, 85–107. Pfaffenweiler, Germany: Centaurus, 1996.

Lethen, Helmut. "Lob der Kaelte. Ein Motiv der historischen Avantgarden." In *Die unvollendete Vernunft. Moderne vs. Postmoderne*, edited by Dietmar Kamper and Willem Van Reijen, 282–324. Frankfurt am Main, Germany: Suhrkamp Verlag, 1987.

Lewy, Frederic Henry. "Historical Introduction: The Basal Ganglia and Their Diseases." In *The Diseases of the Basal Ganglia*, edited by Research Publication of the Association for Research in Nervous and Mental Disease. Baltimore, MD: Johns Hopkins University Press, 1942, 1–20.

Lewy, Friedrich Heinrich. "Paralysis agitans. I Pathologische Anatomie." In *Handbuch der Neurologie*, edited by Max Lewandowsky, Oswald Bumke, and Otfrid Foerster, et al., 920–23. Berlin: Springer, 1912.

Ley, Astrid. "Bauer, Karl-Friedrich 1947–1974." In *Die Professoren und Dozenten der Friedrich-Alexander-Universitaet Erlangen: 1743–1960*, edited by Renate Wittern, 8–9. Erlangen, Germany: Universitaetsbund Erlangen-Nuernberg e. V., 1999.

Leys, Ruth. *Trauma: A Genealogy*. Chicago, IL: University of Chicago Press, 2000.

Leys, Ruth, and Rand B. Evans. *Defining American Psychology: The Correspondence Between Adolf Meyer and Edward Bradford Titchener*. Baltimore, MD: Johns Hopkins University, 1990.

Lilienthal, Georg. "Patientinnen und Patienten aus brandenburgischen Heil- und Pflegeanstalten als Opfer der NS-'Euthanasie'-Verbrechen in Hadamar." In *Brandenburgische Heil- und Pflegeanstalten in der NS-Zeit*, edited by Christina Huebener and Martin Heinze, 303–18. Berlin, Germany: Bebra Wissenschaftsverlag, 2002.

Linden, Stefanie Caroline, and Edgar Jones. "German Battle Casualties: The Treatment of Functional Somatic Disorders during World War I." *Journal of the History of Medicine and Allied Sciences* 68, no. 4 (2013): 627–58.

Loetsch, Gerhard. *Christian Roller und Ernst Fink. Die Anfaenge von Illenau*. Achern, Germany: Acheron Verlag, 1996.

Loewenau, Aleksandra. "Between Resentment and Aid: German and Austrian Psychiatrist and Neurologist Refugees in Great Britain since 1933." *Journal of the History of the Neurosciences* 25, no. 3 (2016): 348–62.

Loewi, Otto. "The Excitement of a Life in Science." In *A Dozen Doctors: Autobiographical Sketches*, edited by Dwight J. Ingle, 109–26. Chicago, IL: University of Chicago Press, 1963.

Loewy, Ilana. "The Strength of Loose Concepts – Boundary Concepts, Federative Experimental Strategies and Disciplinary Growth: The Case of Immunology." *History of Science* 30, no. 4 (1992): 371–96.

López-Muñoz, Francisco, Jesus Boya, and Alamo Cecilio. "Neuron Theory: The Cornerstone of Neuroscience, on the Centenary of the Nobel Prize Award to Santiago Ramón y Cajal." *Brain Research Bulletin* 70, no. 4–6 (2006): 391–405.

Lorenz, Maren. "Proto-Eugenic Thought and Breeding Utopias in the United States before 1870." *Bulletin of the German Historical Institute* 43, no. 2 (2008): 67–90.

Lovejoy, Arthur Oncken. "The Meaning of Vitalism." *Science* 851, no. 33 (1911): 610–14.

Luedecke, Andreas. *Der 'Fall Saller' und die Rassenhygiene. Eine Goettinger Fallstudie zu den Widerspruechen sozialbiologischer Ideologiebildung.* Marburg, Germany: Tectum Verlag, 1995.

Luers, Thea. *Geheimnisse des Gehirns. Weg und Werk des Hirnforscherehepaares Cécile und Oskar Vogt* (typoscript, 148 pages, ca. 1950), HAMPG, KWIBR fonds.

Luescher, Bernhard. "Neuroscience at Penn State." *Science Journal* 25, no. 2 (2006), 4–6.

Lullies, Hans. *Vegetative Physiologie: Blutkreislauf, Atmung, Stoffwechsel, Verdauung u. Exkretion*, Cologne, Germany: Troponwerke, 1958.

– "Aktionsstroeme und Fasergruppen im Extremitaetennerven von Maja squinado." *Pfluegers Archiv fuer die gesamte Physiologie des Menschen und der Tiere* 233, no. 1 (1934), 584–606.

Lunbeck, Elizabeth. *The Psychiatric Persuasion: Knowledge, Gender, and Power in Modern America.* Princeton, NJ: Princeton University Press, 1995.

Machamer, Peter, Peter McLaughlin, and Rick Grush, eds. *Theory and Method in the Neurosciences.* Pittsburgh, PA: University of Pittsburgh Press, 2001.

MacLennan, David. "Beyond the Asylum: Professionalization and the Mental Hygiene Movement in Canada, 1914–1928." *Canadian Bulletin of Medical History* 4, no. 1 (1987): 7–23.

Macleod, Malcolm. "Migrant, Intern, Doctor – Spy? Dr. Eric Wermuth in Second World War Newfoundland." *Newfoundland and Labrador Studies* 13, no. 1 (1997), 79–89.

MacMillan, Margaret. *The War That Ended Peace: How Europe Abandoned Peace for the First World War.* London, UK: Profile Books, 2013.

Maehle, Andreas-Holger. "Doctors in Court, Honour, and Professional Ethics: Two Scandals in Imperial Germany." *Gesnerus* 68, no. 1 (2011): 61–79.

Magoun, Horace Winchell. *American Neuroscience in the Twentieth Century: Confluence of the Neural, Behavioral, and Communicative Streams.* Edited and annotated by Louise H. Marshall. Lisse, The Netherlands: A.A. Balkema Publishers, 2003.

Majewsky, Ryszard, and Teresa Sozańska. *Die Schlacht um Breslau.* Berlin: Union Verlag, 1979.

Mandel, Michael. *Manfred Eigen Festschrift. Special Issue Dedicated to Professor Manfred Eigen on the Occasion of His 60th Birthday.* 26: A Supplement Volume to Biophysical Chemistry, Edinburgh, UK: Elsevier, 1987, 101–390.

Mann, Gunther G. "Senckenbergs Stiftung und die Frankfurter Republik der Aerzte im 19. Jahrhundert. *Medizinhistorisches Journal* 7, no. 4 (1972): 244–63.

Marie, Pierre, "Sclérose en plaque et maladies infectieuses." *Progrés de Medécine* 12, no. 2–3 (1884): 287–9, 305–7, and 365–6.

Marinbach, Bernard. *Galveston: Ellis Island of the West*. New York: Albany State University of New York Press, 1983.

Marinelli, Lydia, and Andreas Mayer. *Dreaming by the Book: Freud's "The Interpretation of Dreams" and the History of the Psychoanalytic Movement*. London, UK: The Other Press, 2003.

Marinesco, Gheorghe. "L'hystérie après Babinski. Contribution à l'étude du méchanisme physio-pathologique de l'hystérie." *Journal de médecine de Lyon* 17, no. 4 (1936): 411–22.

Marshall, Alan. *The German Naturalists and Gerhard Hauptmann: Reception and Influences*. Frankfurt am Main, Germany: Lang, 1982.

Masson, Jeffrey M., and Michael Schroeder, eds. *Sigmund Freud. Briefe an Wilhelm Fliess 1887–1904. Ungekuerzte Ausgabe*. Frankfurt am Main, Germany: Fischer, 1986.

Medawar, Jean and David Pyke. "Obituary: Esther Simpson." *The Independent*, 24 December 1996, 8.

– *Hitler's Gift: The True Story of the Scientists Expelled by the Nazi Regime*. New York: Arkade Publishing, 2001.

Mendelsohn, Everett. *Human Aspects of Biomedical Innovation*. Cambridge, MA: Harvard University Press, 1974.

Merrem, Georg. *Die Behandlung der Multiplen Sklerose mit Germanin*. Berlin, Germany: Pfau, 1934.

Meyer, Adolph. *Prospectus of the Summer School of Neurology and Psychiatry*. Kankakee, IL: State Board of Health Illinois, 1894.

Meyer, Alfred. *Historical Aspects of Cerebral Anatomy*. London, UK: Oxford University Press, 1971.

Meyers, Todd, and Stefanos Geroulanos. *Experimente im Individuum. Kurt Goldstein und die Frage des Organismus*. Cologne, Germany: August Verlag, 2014.

Mildenberger, Florian. "Auf der Spur des 'Scientific Pursuit' Franz Josef Kallmann (1897–1965) und die rassenhygienische Forschung." *Medizinhistorisches Journal* 37, no. 2 (2002): 183–200.

Millett, David. "Hans Berger: From Psychic Energy to the EEG." *Perspectives in Biology and Medicine* 44, no. 4 (2001): 522–42.

Mitscherlich, Alexander, and Fred Mielke. *Medizin ohne Menschlichkeit. Dokumente des Nuernberger Aerzteprozesses* (1st ed. 1947). 2nd ed. (paperback ed.). Heidelberg, Germany: Fischer, 1960.

Mollenhauer, Paul. "Bericht ueber die ausserordentliche Tagung der Deutschen Gesellschaft fuer Krueppelfuersorge." *Zentralblatt fuer chirurgische und mechanische Orthopaedie* 10, no. 3 (1916): 74–88.

Mommsen, Hans. "The Reichstag Fire and Its Political Consequences." In *From Republic to Reich: The Making of the Nazi Revolution*, edited by Hajo Holborn, 129–222. New York: Pantheon Books, 1972.

Mommsen, Wolfgang, eds. *Imperial Germany, 1867–1918*. Oxford, UK: Oxford University Press, 2008.

Morel, Bénédict Augustin. *Traité des dégénérescences physiques, et intellectuelles et morales de l'espèce humaine et de ces causes qui produisent ces variétiés maladives*. 2 vols. Paris, France: Baillière, 1857-8.

Moulin, Thierry, François Clarac, Henri Petit, and Emmanuel Broussolle. "Neurology Outside Paris Following Charcot." In *Following Charcot: A Forgotten History of Neurology and Psychiatry*, edited by Julien Bogousslavsky. Vol. 29, 170–86. Basel, Switzerland: Karger, 2011.

Muehlleitner, Elke. "Federn, Paul." In *Personallexikon der Psychotherapie*, edited by Gerhard Stumm, Alfred Pritz, Paul Gumhalter, Nora Nemeskeri, and Martin Voracek. Part 6, 135–6. Vienna, Austria: Martin Voracek, 2005.

Mueller, Thomas. *Von Charlottenburg zum Central Park West. Henry Lowenfeld und die Psychoanalyse in Berlin, Prag und New York*. Frankfurt am Main, Germany: Édition Déjà-Vu, 2000.

Mullaly, Sasha. "Dr. Roddie, Dr. Gus and the Golden Age of Medicine on Prince Edward Island." MA diss., University of Ottawa, ON, 1994.

Musil, Robert. *Der Mann ohne Eigenschaften*. 2 vols. Hamburg, Germany: Rowolth, 1930.

Nagel, Thomas. *The View from Nowhere*. Oxford, UK: Oxford University Press, 1986.

Neuburger, Max. *The Historical Development of Experimental Brain and Spinal Cord Physiology before Flourens*. Baltimore, MD: Johns Hopkins University, 1983.

Neuhaus, David M. "Jewish Conversion to the Catholic Church." *Pastoral Psychology* 37, no. 1 (1988): 38–52.

Neumaerker, Klaus J. and Andreas Joachim Bartsch. "Karl Kleist (1879–1960): A Pioneer of Neuropsychiatry." *History of Psychiatry* 14, no. 4 (2003): 411–58.

Neville, Terry. *The Royal Vic: The Story of Montreal's Royal Victoria Hospital*. Montreal: McGill-Queen's University Press, 1994.

Nicolas, Serge and Ludovic Ferrand. "Wundt's Laboratory at Leipzig in 1891." *History of Psychology* 2, no. 3 (1999): 194–203.

Nicosia, Francis R., and Jonathan Huener, eds. *Medicine and Medical Ethics in Nazi Germany: Origins, Practices, Legacies*. New York: Basic Books, 2002.

Niederland, Doron. "The Emigration of Jewish Academics and Professionals from Germany in the First Years of Nazi Rule." *Leo Baeck Institute Yearbook* 33, no. 1 (1988): 285–300.

Niederland, Wilhelm G. "Denkerinnerungen." *Monatsschrift Psychiatrie-Neurologie* 1 (1989), 163–64.

– "Psychiatric Disorders among Persecution Victims," *Journal of Nervous and Mental Disease* 193, no. 4 (1964): 458–73.

– "Clinical Observations on the Survivor Syndrome." *International Journal of Psychoanalysis* 49, no. 2 (1968): 313–15.

– *A Refugee's Life: The First Year* (San Francisco: typescript with annotations in handwriting, ca. 1968). Holocaust Center of Northern California, San Francisco, CA, Niederland box.

– *Folgen der Verfolgung. Das Ueberlebenden-Syndrom, Seelenmord.* Frankfurt am Main, Germany: Suhrkamp Verlag, 1980.

– *Die Psychologie des 20. Jahrhunderts. Sonderdruck aus dem fuenfzehn-baendigen Informationswerk: Die Psychologie des 20. Jahrhunderts* (Zurich, Switzerland: typescript, 1988, 1055–67). Holocaust Center of Northern California, San Francisco, CA Niederland box.

Niessl von Meyendorff, Erwin. *Die aphasischen Symptome und ihre corticale Lokalisation. Mit 51 Figuren und VII Tafeln.* Leipzig, Germany: Verlag von Wilhelm Engelmann, 1911.

– *Ueber die Prinzipien der Gehirnmechanik. Antrittsvorlesung gehalten am 5 Juni 1926 in der Aula der Universitaet Leipzig.* Stuttgart, Germany: Enke, 1926.

Nipperdey, Thomas. *Deutsche Geschichte 1866–1918. Machtstaat vor der Demokratie.* Vol. 2. Munich, Germany: Beck, 1992.

Nitsch, Robert. "Zur cholinergen Innervation identifizierter Neurone im Hippocampus der Ratte." MD diss., University of Frankfurt, Germany, 1989.

Nitsch, Robert and Frank W. Stahnisch. "Neuronal Mechanisms Recording the Stream of Consciousness: A Reappraisal of Wilder Penfield's (1891–1976) Concept of Experiential Phenomena Elicited by Electrical Stimulation of the Human Cortex." *Cerebral Cortex* 28, no. 9 (2018): 3347–55.

Noppeney, Ute. "Kurt Goldstein: A Philosophical Scientist." *Journal of the History of the Neurosciences* 10, no. 1 (2001): 67–78.

Noth, Johannes. "Robert Wartenberg. (1887–1956)." *Der Nervenarzt* 73, no. 6 (2002): 575.

Nyhart, Lynn. *Biology Takes Form: Animal Morphology and the German Universities, 1800–1900.* Chicago, IL: University of Chicago Press, 1995.

Obersteiner, Heinrich. *Beitraege zur Kenntnis vom feineren Bau der Kleinhirnrinde. Mit besonderer Beruecksichtigung der Entwicklung.* Vienna, Austria: Sitzungsberichte der Akademie der Wissenschaften, 1869.

Oppenheim, Hermann. *Die traumatischen Neurosen nach den in der Nervenklinik der Charité in den letzten 5 Jahren gesammelten Beobachtungen.* Berlin, Germany: Hirschwald, 1889.

– "Der Krieg und die traumatischen Neurose." *Berliner Klinische Wochenschrift* 52, no. 2 (1915): 257–68.

Parnes, Ohad. "'Trouble from Within': Allergy, Autoimmunity, and Pathology in the First Half of the Twentieth Century." *Studies in History and Philosophy of Biological and Biomedical Sciences* 34, no. 3 (2003): 425–54.

Pátek, Philipp. "Die Entwicklung der Anatomie in Duesseldorf. Von der Akademie fuer Praktische Medizin zur Universitaet Duesseldorf." MD diss., Heinrich Heine University, Duesseldorf, Germany, 2010.

Patrias, Carmela. "Socialists, Jews, and the 1947 Saskatchewan Bill of Rights." *Canadian Historical Review* 87, no. 2 (2006), 265–92.

Pearle, Kathleen M. "Aerzteemigration nach 1933 in die USA. Der Fall New York." *Medizinhistorisches Journal* 19, no. 1 (1984): 112–37.

Pearson, Ruth. "U.N. Cries 'Uncle.'" *Bulletin of the Atomic Scientists* 35, no. 8 (1988): 36–9.

Peiffer, Juergen. "Die Vertreibung deutscher Neuropathologen 1933–1939." *Der Nervenarzt* 69, no. 2 (1998): 99–109.

– "Zur Neurologie im 'Dritten Reich' und ihren Nachwirkungen." *Der Nervenarzt* 69, no. 8 (1998): 728–33.

– "Neuropathology in the Third Reich." *Epidemiologia e prevenzione* 22, no. 2 (1998): 184–90.

– *Hirnforschung in Deutschland 1849 bis 1974. Briefe zur Entwicklung von Psychiatrie und Neurowissenschaften sowie zum Einfluss des politischen Umfeldes auf Wissenschaftler.* Berlin, Germany: Springer, 2004.

Penfield, Wilder. *The Significance of the Montreal Neurological Institute* (The Foundation Volume Which Was Published for the Staff of the Montreal Neurological Institute of McGill University on 27 September 1934). Montreal: McGill University (Reprint from *Neurological Biographies & Addresses*, Vol. 68), 1934.

– *The Difficult Art of Giving: The Epic of Alan Gregg.* Boston, MA: Little, Brown and Company, 1967.

– *No Man Alone: A Neurosurgeon's Life.* Boston, MA: Little, Brown and Company, 1977.

Perry, Heather R. *Recycling the Disabled: Army, Medicine, and Society in World War I Germany.* Manchester, UK: Manchester University Press, 2014.

Peters, Uwe-Hendrik. "Emigration deutscher Psychiater nach England. (Teil 1)." *Fortschritte der Neurologie und Psychiatrie* 64, no. 5 (1996): 161–7.

Peukert, Detlev. *The Weimar Republic: The Crisis of Classical Modernity* (Germ. 1987). Translated by Richard Deveson. New York: Hill and Wang, 1992.

Peyenson, Lewis L. "'Who the Guys Were': Prosopography in the History of Science." *History of Science* 15, no. 3 (1977): 155–88.

Pickenhain, Lothar. "Die Neurowissenschaft – ein interdisziplinaeres und integratives Wissensgebiet." *SDGGN* 8, no. 1 (2002): 241–6.

Pickering, Andrew, ed. *Science as Practice and Culture.* Chicago, IL: University of Chicago Press, 1994.

Pickwren, Wade E., and Stanley F. Schneider, eds. *Psychology and The National Institute of Mental Health: Historical Analysis of Science, Practice, and Policy.* Washington, DC: National Institutes of Health, 2004.

Pieper, Josef. *Autobiographische Schriften. Ergebnisband 2.* Hamburg, Germany: Felix Meiner, 2003.

Plaenkers, Thomas, Michael Laier, Hans Heinrich Otto, Hans-Joachim Rothe, and Helmut Siefert, eds. *Psychoanalyse in Frankfurt am Main. Zerstoerte Anfaenge. Wiederannaehrung. Entwicklungen.* Tuebingen, Germany: Edition Diskord, 1996.

Ploetz, Alfred. *Grundlinien einer Rassenhygiene.* Vol. 1. Berlin, Germany: Prognos, 1895.

– *Die Tuechtigkeit unserer Rasse und der Schutz der Schwachen. Ein Versuch ueber Rassenhygiene und ihr Verhaeltnis zu den humanen Idealen, besonders zum Socialismus.* Frankfurt am Main, Germany: S. Fischer, 1895.

– "Die Begriffe Rasse und Gesellschaft und die davon abgeleiteten Disziplinen." *Archiv fuer Rassen- und Gesellschaftsbiologie* 1, no. 1 (1904): 2–26.

Popper, Karl. *The Open Society and Its Enemies.* Vol. 2. London, UK: Routledge, 1945.

Porter, Dale H. "History as Process." *History and Theory* 14 (1975): 297–313.

Pressmann, Jack. *Last Resort: Psychosurgery and the Limits of Medicine.* Cambridge, UK: Cambridge University Press, 1998.

Proctor, Robert N. *Racial Hygiene: Medicine under the Nazis.* Cambridge, MA: Harvard University Press, 1988.

– *The Nazi War on Cancer.* Princeton, NJ: Princeton University Press, 1999.

Pross, Christian and Rolf Winau, eds. *Das Krankenhaus Moabit 1920–1933. Ein Zentrum juedischer Aerzte in Berlin. 1933–1945. Verfolgung – Widerstand – Zerstoerung.* Berlin, Germany: Edition Hendrik, 1984.

Quirke, Vivian, and Jean-Paul Gaudillière. "The Era of Biomedicine: Science, Medicine and Public Health in Britain and France after the Second World War." *Medical History* 52, no. 4 (2008): 441–52.

Radkau, Joachim. *Das Zeitalter der Nervositaet. Deutschland zwischen Bismarck und Hitler.* Munich, Germany: Fink, 1998.

– "The Neurasthenic Experience in Imperial Germany: Expeditions into Patient Records and Side-Looks upon General History." In *Cultures of Neurasthenia: From Beard to the First World War,* edited by Marijke Gijswijt and Roy Porter, 199–217. Amsterdam, The Netherlands: Rodopi, 2001.

Rainer, John D. "Franz Kallmann's Views on Eugenics." *American Journal of Psychiatry* 146, no. 10 (1989): 1361–62.

Rasmussen, Nicolas. *Picture Control. The Electron Microscope and the Transformation of Biology in America, 1940–1960*. Stanford, CA: Stanford University Press, 1997.

Reichswehrministerium, Heeres-Sanitaetsinspektion. *Sanitaetsbericht ueber das deutsche Heer, (Deutsches Feld- und Besatzungsheer), im Weltkriege 1914–1918*, Vol. 3. Berlin, Germany: E.S. Mittler, 1934.

Reilly, Joanne. *Belsen: The Liberation of a Concentration Camp*. London, UK: Routledge, 1998.

Reisner, Steven. "Trauma: The Seductive Hypothesis." *Journal of the American Psychoanalytical Association* 51, no. 2 (2003): 381–414.

Remarque, Erich Maria. *The Road Back*. Translated by Arthur Wesley Wheen. Boston, MA: Little Brown & Company, 1931.

Reuland, Andreas Jens. *Menschenversuche in der Weimarer Republik*. Norderstedt, Germany: Books on Demand, 2004.

Rheinberger, Hans-Joerg. *Toward a History of Epistemic Things: Synthesizing Proteins in the Test Tube*. Stanford, CA: Stanford University Press, 1997.

Rhode, Barbara. *East-West Migration/Brain Drain: Mapping the Available Knowledge and Recommendations for a European Research Programme*. Brussels, Belgium: COST Social Sciences, EC Commission, 1991.

Richards, Arnold D., eds. *The Jewish World of Sigmund Freud: Essays on Cultural Roots and Problems of Religious Identity*. University Park, PA: Pennsylvania State University Press, 2009.

Richardson, Angelique. *Love and Eugenics in the Late Nineteenth Century: Rational Reproduction and the New Woman*. Oxford, UK: Oxford University Press, 2003.

Richardson, Malcom. "Philanthropy and the Internationality of Learning: The Rockefeller Foundation and National Socialist Germany." *Minerva* 28, no. 1 (1990): 21–58.

Richter, Jochen. "Das Kaiser-Wilhelm-Institut fuer Hirnforschung und die Topographie der Grosshirnhemisphaeren. Ein Beitrag zur Institutsgeschichte der Kaiser-Wilhelm-Gesellschaft und zur Geschichte der architektonischen Hirnforschung." In *Die Kaiser-Wilhelm-/Max-Planck-Gesellschaft und ihre Institute. Studien zu ihrer Geschichte: Das Harnack-Prinzip*, edited by Bernhard vom Brocke and Hubert Laitko, 349–408. Berlin, Germany: DeGruyter, 1996.

– "The Brain Commission of the International Association of Academies: The First International Society of Neurosciences." *Brain Research Bulletin* 52, no. 6 (2000): 445–57.

Rickman, Anahid S. "Rassenpflege im voelkischen Staat. Vom Verhaeltnis der
Rassenhygiene zur nationalsozialistischen Politik." PhD diss., University of
Bonn, Germany, 2002.

Riese, Walter. *The Conception of Disease*. New York: Philosophical Library, 1953.

– *A History of Neurology*, Springfield, IL: Thomas, 1959.

– "Kurt Goldstein – The Man and His Work." In *The Reach of Mind*, edited
by Marianne L. Simmel, 25–7. New York: Springer, 1968.

Rilke, Rainer Maria. *Auguste Rodin*. Berlin, Germany: Insel, 1919.

Ringer, Fritz. *The Decline of the German Mandarins: The German Academic
Community, 1890–1933*. Cambridge, MA: Harvard University Press, 1969.

– *Fields of Knowledge: French Academic Culture in Comparative Perspective
1890–1920*. Cambridge, UK: Cambridge University Press, 1992.

– *Toward a Social History of Knowledge: Collected Essays*. Oxford, UK:
Berghahn Books, 2001.

Rissom, Renate. *Fritz Lenz und die Rassenhygiene*. Husum, Germany:
Matthiesen Verlag, 1983.

Roazen, Paul. *Helene Deutsch: A Psychoanalyst's Life*. New Brunswick:
Transaction Publishers, 1985.

Robertson, Brian. "An Interview with Eric Kandel." *Journal of Physiology* 588,
no. 5 (2010): 743–45.

Roelcke, Volker. "Wir ruecken Schritt vor Schritt dem Tolhause naeher ...: Das
moderne Leben und die Nervenkrankheiten bei Johann Christian Reil
(1759–1813)." *Sudhoffs Archiv. Zeitschrift fuer Wissenschaftsgeschichte* 80,
no. 1 (1996): 56–67.

– "Electrified Nerves, Degenerated Bodies: Medical Discourses in
Neurasthenia in Germany; ca. 1990–1914." In *Cultures of Neurasthenia:
From Beard to the First World War*, edited by Marijke Gijswijt-Hofstra,
177–97. Amsterdam, The Netherlands: Rodopi, 2001.

– "Programm und Praxis der psychiatrischen Genetik an der Deutschen
Forschungsanstalt fuer Psychiatrie unter Ernst Ruedin: Zum Verhaeltnis
von Wissenschaft, Politik und Rasse-Begriff vor und nach 1933."
Medizinhistorisches Journal 37, no. 1 (2002): 21–55.

– Wissenschaften zwischen Innovation und Entgrenzung: Biomedizinische
Forschung an den Kaiser-Wilhelm-Instituten, 1911–1945. In
*Sozialdarwinismus, Genetik und Euthanasie. Menschenbilder in der
Psychiatrie*, edited by Martin Bruene and Theo R. Payk, 92–109. Stuttgart,
Germany: Wissenschaftliche Verlagsgesellschaft, 2004.

– "Continuities or Ruptures? Concepts, Institutions and Context of
Twentieth-Century German Psychiatry and Mental Health Care." In

Psychiatric Cultures Compared: Psychiatry and Mental Health Care in the Twentieth Century, edited by Marijke Gijswijt-Hofstra, Harry Oosterhuis, Joost Vijselaar, and Hugh Freeman, 162–82. Amsterdam, The Netherlands: Amsterdam University Press, 2005.

– "Funding the Scientific Foundations of Race Policies: Ernst Ruedin and the Impact of Career Resources on Psychiatric Genetics, ca. 1910–1945." In *Man, Medicine, and the State: The Human Body as an Object of Government Sponsored Medical Research in the 20th Century*, edited by Wolfgang U. Eckart, 73–87. Stuttgart, Germany: Franz Steiner, 2006.

– "Die Etablierung der psychiatrischen Genetik in Deutschland, Grossbritannien und den USA, ca. 1910–1960. Zur untrennbaren Geschichte von Eugenik und Humangenetik." *Acta Historica Leopoldina* 48, no. 1 (2007): 173–90.

Roelcke, Volker and Eric Engstrom. "Die 'alte Psychiatrie'? Zur Geschichte und Aktualitaet der Psychiatrie im 19. Jahrhundert." In *Psychiatrie im 19. Jahrhundert: Forschungen zur Geschichte von psychiatrischen Institutionen, Debatten und Praktiken im deutschen Sprachraum*, edited by Eric J. Engstrom and Volker Roelcke, 9–25. Basel, Switzerland: Schwabe, 2003.

Roscher, Stephan: *Die Kaiser-Wilhelms-Universitaet Strassburg 1872–1902*. Frankfurt am Main, Germany: Lang, 2006.

Rose, Nikolas and Joelle Abi-Rached. *Neuro: The New Brain Sciences and the Management of the Mind*. Princeton, NJ: Princeton University Press, 2013.

Rosen, George. *The Specialization of Medicine with Particular Reference to Ophthalmology*. New York: Froben Press, 1944.

Rothe, Friedrich. *Frank Wedekinds Dramen: Jugendstil und Lebensphilosophie*. Stuttgart, Germany: J.B. Metzlersche Verlagsbuchhandlung, 1968.

Rotzoll, Maike, Volker Roelcke, and Gerritt Hohendorf. "Carl Schneiders 'Forschungsabteilung' an der Heidelberger Psychiatrischen Universitaetsklinik 1943/44." *Heidelberg. Jahrbuch zur Geschichte der Stadt* 16, no.1 (2012): 113–22.

Rudy, Willis. *Total War and Twentieth-Century Higher Learning: Universities of the Western World in the First and Second World Wars*. London, UK: Associated University Press, 1991.

Ruedin, Ernst. "Ueber den Zusammenhang zwischen Geisteskrankheit und Kultur." *Archiv fuer Rassen- und Gesellschaftsbiologie* 7, no. 1 (1910): 722–48.

– *Zur Vererbung und Neuentstehung der Dementia praecox. Studien ueber Vererbung und Entstehung geistiger Stoerungen*. Berlin, Germany: Springer, 1916.

- "Ehrung von Prof. Dr. Alfred Ploetz." *Archiv fuer Rassenhygiene und Gesellschaftsbiologie* 32, no. 4 (1938): 473–4.

Ruerup, Reinhard and Wolfgang Schieder, eds. *Geschichte der Kaiser-Wilhelm-Gesellschaft.* 28 vols. Goettingen, Germany: Wallstein, 2000–05.

Ruerup, Reinhard and Michael Schuering. *Schicksale und Karrieren. Gedenkbuch fuer die von den Nationalsozialisten aus der Kaiser-Wilhelm-Gesellschaft vertriebenen Forscherinnen und Forscher.* Goettingen, Germany: Wallstein, 2008.

Russell, Guel. "A Variation on Forced Migration: Wilhelm Peters (Prussia via Britain to Turkey) and Muzafer Sherif (Turkey to the United States)." *Journal of the History of the Neurosciences* 25, no. 3 (2016): 320–47.

Sachs, Lessie. "Advice from the Midwest." In *Hitler's Exiles: Personal Stories of the Fight from Nazi Germany to America*, edited by Mark M. Anderson, 229–32. New York: New Press, 1998.

Sachse, Carola. "'Whitewash Culture': How the Kaiser Wilhelm/Max Planck Society Dealt with the Nazi Past." In *The Kaiser Wilhelm Society under National Socialism*, edited by Susanne Heim, Carola Sachse, and Mark Walker, 373–99. Cambridge, UK: Cambridge University Press, 2009.

Sakel, Manfred. "The Origin and Nature of the Hypoglycemic Therapy of the Psychoses." *Bulletin of the New York Academy of Medicine* 13, no. 3 (1937): 97–109.

Salt, John. "A Comparative Overview of International Trends and Types 1950–80." *International Migration Review* 23, no. 3 (1989): 431–56.

Sammet, Kai. *Ueber Irrenanstalten und deren Weiterentwicklung in Deutschland: Wilhelm Griesinger im Streit mit der konservativen Anstaltspsychiatrie 1865–1868.* Hamburg, Germany: LIT-Press, 1997.

Sanger, Margaret. *The Pivot of Civilization.* New York: Brentanos, 1922.

Saretzki, Thomas. *Reichsgesundheitsrat und Preußischer Landesgesundheitsrat in der Weimarer Republik.* Berlin, Germany: Weissensee Verlag, 2000.

Sarkin, Jeremy. *Germany's Genocide of the Herero: Kaiser Wilhelm II, His General, His Settlers, His Soldiers.* Rochester, NY: Boydell & Brewer, 2011.

Satzinger, Helga H. *Die Geschichte der genetisch orientierten Hirnforschung von Cécile und Oskar Vogt (1875–1962, 1870–1959) in der Zeit von 1895 bis ca. 1927.* Stuttgart, Germany. Deutscher Apotheker Verlag, 1998.

Schaltenbrand, Georges. "Der uebertragbare Markscheidenschwund." *Deutsche Medizinische Wochenschrift* 67, no. 39 (1941): 1066–70.

- *Die Multiple Sklerose des Menschen.* Leipzig, Germany: Thieme, 1943.

Schierer, Pierangelo. *Laboratorium der buergerlichen Welt. Deutsche Wissenschaft im 20. Jahrhundert.* Frankfurt am Main, Germany: Suhrkamp Verlag, 1992.

Schiller, Francis. "Fritz Lewy and His Bodies." *Journal of the History of the Neurosciences* 9, no. 2 (2000), 148–51.

Schleiermacher, Sabine. "Contested Spaces: Rival Models of Public Health in Post-War Germany." In *Shifting Boundaries of Public Health. Europe in the Twentieth Century*, edited by Susan Gross Solomon, Lion Murard, and Patrick Zylberman, 175–204. Rochester, NY: University of Rochester Press, 2008.

Schlich, Thomas. "Der Eintritt von Juden in das Bildungsbuergertum des 18. und 19. Jahrhunderts: die christlich-juedische Arztfamilie Speyer." *Medizinhistorisches Journal* 25, nos. 1–2 (1990): 129–42.

Schmaltz, Florian. *Kampfstoff-Forschung im Nationalsozialismus. Zur Kooperation von Kaiser-Wilhelm-Instituten, Militaer und Industrie*. Goettingen, Germany: Wallstein, 2005.

Schmidgen, Henning, Peter Geimer, and Sven Dierig, eds. *Kultur im Experiment*. Berlin, Germany: Cadmos, 2004.

Schmiedebach, Heinz-Peter. *Robert Remak (1815–1865): Ein juedischer Arzt im Spannungsfeld von Wissenschaft und Politik*. Stuttgart, Germany: G. Fischer, 1995.

– "The Public's View of Neurasthenia in Germany: Looking for a New Rhythm of Life." In *Cultures of Neurasthenia.: From Beard to the First World War*, edited by Marijke Gijswijt and Roy Porter, 219–38. Amsterdam, The Netherlands: Rodopi, 2001.

– "Post-Traumatic Neurosis in Nineteenth-Century Germany: A Disease in Political, Juridical and Professional Context." *History of Psychiatry* 10, no. 1 (1999), 27–57.

Schmitt, Francis O. "Molecular Biology Among the Neurosciences." *JAMA Neurology* 17, no. 6 (1968): 561–72.

– *The Never-Ceasing Search*. Philadelphia, PA: The American Philosophical Society, 1990.

Schmitt, Francis O., and Frederic Worden. *The Neurosciences. Third Study Program*. Cambridge, MA: MIT Press, 1974.

Schmitt, Francis O., et al., eds. *The Neuroscience Research (Program) Bulletin*. Cambridge, MA: Massachusetts Institute of Technology Press, 1964–82, 21 vols.

Schmuhl, Hans-Walter. *Hirnforschung und Krankenmord. Das Kaiser-Wilhelm-Institut fuer Hirnforschung 1937–1945*. Berlin, Germany: Max-Planck-Gesellschaft, 2000.

– *Die Gesellschaft Deutscher Neurologen und Psychiater im Nationalsozialismus*. Berlin: Springer, 2016.

Schneider, William H. *Rockefeller Philanthropy and Modern Biomedicine: International Initiatives from World War I to Cold War*. Bloomington, IN: Indiana University Press, 2002.

Scholz, Albrecht, and Caris-Petra Heidel, eds. *Sozialpolitik und Judentum.* Dresden, Germany: Union Druckerei, 2000.

Scholz, Albrecht, Thomas Barth, Anna-Sophia Pappai, and Axel Wacker. "Das Schicksal des Lehrkoerpers der Medizinischen Fakultaet Breslau nach der Vertreibung 1945/46." *Wuerzburger medizinhistorische Mitteilungen* 24, no. 1 (2005): 497–533.

Schuering, Michael. "Ein Dilemma der Kontinuitaet. Das Selbstverstaendnis der Max-Planck-Gesellschaft und der Umgang mit Emigranten in den 50er Jahren." In *Wissenschaften und Wissenschaftspolitik. Bestandsaufnahmen zu Formationen, Bruechen und Kontinuitaeten im Deutschland des 20. Jahrhunderts,* edited by Ruediger vom Bruch and Brigitte Kaderas, 453–63. Stuttgart, Germany: Franz Steiner, 2002.

– *Minervas verstossene Kinder. Vertriebene Wissenschaftler und die Vergangenheitspolitik der Max-Planck-Gesellschaft.* Goettingen, Germany: Wallstein, 2006.

Schuetz, Siegfried. "Die Wirksamkeit der Sympathikusinfiltration und lumbalen Sympathektomie im Vergleich zur konservativen Therapie bei Erfrierungen." MD Diss., University of Strasburg, Germany, 1944.

Schuetz, Wolfgang. "Der Umgang der oesterreichischen Aerzteschaft mit der NS-Vergangenheit." *Jahrbuch des Dokumentationsarchivs des oesterreichischen Widerstandes* 54, no. 1 (2017): 211–20.

Schulze, Heinz A.F. "Hirnlokalisationsforschung in Berlin." In *Geschichte der Neurologie in Berlin,* edited by Bernd Holdorff und Rolf Winau, 55–70. Berlin, Germany: DeGruyter, 2001.

– "Persoenliche Erinnerungen an Cécile und Oskar Vogt." *SDGGN* 10, no. 1 (2004): 397–405.

Schwartz, Joseph. *Cassandra's Daughter: A History of Psychoanalysis.* London, UK: Karnac 2003.

Seeman, Mary V. "Psychiatry in the Nazi Era." *Canadian Journal of Psychiatry* 50, no. 4 (2005): 218–25.

Seidelman, William. "Medical Selection: Auschwitz Antecedents and Effluent." *Holocaust and Genocide Studies* 4, no. 4 (1989), 437–48.

– "The Legacy of Academic Medicine and Human Exploitation in the Third Reich." *Perspectives in Biology and Medicine* 43, no. 3 (2000): 325–34.

– "Dissecting the History of Anatomy in the Third Reich – 1989–2010: A Personal Account." *Annals of Anatomy* 194, no. 3 (2012): 228–36.

Selye, Hans. *From Dream to Discovery: On Being a Scientist.* New York: McGraw-Hill, 1964.

Shapin, Steven, and Arnold Thackery. "Prosopography as a Research Tool in History of Science: The British Scientific Community, 1700–1900." *History of Science* 12, no. 1 (1974): 1–28.

Shepard, Gordon M. *Foundations of the Neuron Doctrine.* New York: Oxford University Press, 1991.

Shevell, Michael I. "Neurosciences in the Third Reich: From Ivory Tower to Death Camps." *Canadian Journal for Neurological Sciences* 26, no. 2 (1999): 132–8.

Shorter, Edward. *Partnership for Excellence: Medicine at the University of Toronto and Academic Hospitals.* Toronto: University of Toronto Press, 2013.

Siefert, Helmut. "'Den Kranken dem Leben zurueckgeben.' Zur Geschichte der Psychiatrie in Frankfurt am Main." In *In waldig laendlicher Umgebung. Das Waldkrankenhaus Koeppern. Von der agrikolen Kolonie der Stadt Frankfurt zum Zentrum f. Soziale Psychiatrie Hochtaunus*, edited by Christina Vanja and Helmut Siefert, 20–35. Kassel, Germany: Euregioverlag, 2001.

Sieg, Ulrich. "Strukturwandel der Wissenschaft im Nationalsozialismus." *Berichte zur Wissenschaftsgeschichte* 24, no. 4 (2001): 255–70.

Sigerist, Henry. *American Medicine* (Germ. 1933). New York: Norton, 1934.

Sigurdson, Skulí. "Physics, Life and Contingency: Born, Schroedinger and Weyl in Exile." In *Forced-Migration and Scientific Change: Emigré German-Speaking Scientists and Scholars after 1933*, edited by Mitchell G. Ash and Alfons Soellner, 48–70. Cambridge, UK: Cambridge University Press, 1996.

Simmel, Ernst. *Zur Psychoanalyse der Kriegsneurosen. Diskussion gehalten auf dem V. Internationalen Psychoanalytischen Kongress in Budapest 28. und 29. September, 1918.* Leipzig, Germany: Psychoanalytischer Verlag, 1919.

Simmel, Georg. "The Stranger." In *Individuality and Social Forms*, edited by Donald Levine, 143–49. Chicago, IL: University of Chicago Press, 1971.

Simmel, Marianne L. "Kurt Goldstein 1878–1965." In *The Reach of Mind: Essays in Memory of Kurt Goldstein*, edited by Marianne L. Simmel, 3–11. New York: Springer, 1968.

Simmer, Hans. *Der Berliner Pathologe Ludwig Pick (1868–1944). Leben und Werk eines juedischen Deutschen.* Husum, Germany: Matthiesen, 2000.

Singer, Wolf. "Auf dem Weg nach Innen. 50 Jahre Hirnforschung in der Max-Planck-Gesellschaft." In *Forschung an den Grenzen des Wissens. 50 Jahre Max-Planck-Gesellschaft 1948–1998. Dokumentation des wissenschaftlichen Festkolloquiums und der Festveranstaltung zum 50jaehrigen Gruendungsjubilaeum am 26. Februar 1998 in Goettingen*, edited by Max Planck Society, 20–34. Goettingen, Germany: Vandenhoeck & Ruprecht, 1998.

Slater, Eliot. "A Review of Earlier Evidence on Genetic Factors in Schizophrenia." In *The Transmission of Schizophrenia*, edited by David Rosenthal and Seymour Kety, 15–26. New York: Pergamon Press, 1968.

Soederqvist, Thomas. "Neurobiographies: Writing Lives in the History of Neurology and the Neurosciences." *Journal of the History of the Neurosciences* 11, no. 1 (2002): 38–48.

Soellner, Alfons. *Deutsche Politikwissenschaftler in der Emigration. Ihre Akkulturation und Wirkungsgeschichte, samt einer Bibliographie*. Opladen, Germany: VS Verlag, 1996.

Solbrig, Otto, Gustav Bundt, and Willi Boehm. *Handbuecherei fuer Staatsmedizin*. Vol. 1. Berlin, Germany: C. Heymanns, 1928.

Somit, Albert, and Joseph Tanenhaus. *The Development of American Political Science. From Burgess to Behavioralism*. Boston, MA: Allyn and Bacon, 1967.

Sommer, Robert. "Eine psychiatrische Abteilung des Reichsgesundheitsamtes." *Psychiatrisch-Neurologische Wochenschrift* 12, no. 2 (1910): 295–8.

Spencer, Hann. *Hanna's Diary, 1938–1941: Czechoslovakia to Canada*. Montreal: McGill-Queen's University Press, 2001.

Sprengel, Peter. *Gerhart Hauptmann. Buergerlichkeit und grosser Traum – Eine Biographie*. Munich, Germany: C.H. Beck, 2012.

Sprung, Helga, and Lothar Sprung. "Wilhelm Maximilian Wundt. Vater der experimentellen Psychologie." In *Wunderblock. Eine Geschichte der modernen Seele*, edited by Jean Clair, Cathrin Pichler, and Wolfgang Pircher, 343–50. Vienna, Austria: Loecker, 1989.

Squire, Larry R. *The History of Neuroscience in Autobiography*. San Diego, CA: Academic Press, 1996–2012.

Stadler, Max. "Assembling Life: Models, the Cell, and the Reformations of Biological Science, 1920–1960." PhD diss., Imperial College London, UK, 2009.

Stahnisch, Frank W. "Zur Bedeutung der Konzepte der 'neuronalen De- und Regeneration' sowie der 'Pathoarchitektonik der Hirnrinde' in den neurohistologischen Arbeiten Max Bielschowskys (1869–1940)." *SDGGN* 9, no. 1 (2003): 243–69.

– "Making the Brain Plastic: Early Neuroanatomical Staining Techniques and the Pursuit of Structural Plasticity, 1910–1970." *Journal of the History of the Neurosciences* 12, no. 4 (2003): 413–35.

– "Timoféeff-Ressovsky, Nicolai Vladimirovich (*1900 Moskau, †1981 Obninsk bei Moskau)." In *Aerzte-Lexikon. Von der Antike bis zum 20. Jahrhundert*, edited by Wolfgang U. Eckart and Christoph Gradmann, 323–4. Heidelberg, Germany: Springer, 2006.

– "Griesinger, Wilhelm (1817–1869)." In *Dictionary of Medical Biography*, edited by William F. Bynum and Helen Bynum. Vol. 2, 582–3. London, UK: Greenwood, 2006.

– "His, Wilhelm, the Elder (1831–1904)." In *Dictionary of Medical Biography*, edited by William F. Bynum and Helen Bynum. Vol. 3, 653–4. London, UK: Greenwood, 2006.

- "Mind the Gap: Synapsen oder keine Synapsen? – Bildkontrolle, Wortwechsel und Glaubenssaetze im Diskurs der morphologischen Hirnforschung." In *Bild und Gestalt. Wie formen Medienpraktiken das Wissen in Medizin und Humanwissenschaften?* edited by Frank W. Stahnisch and Heijko Bauer, 101–24. Muenster, Germany: LIT Press, 2007.
- "Ludwig Edinger (1855–1918): Pioneer in Neurology." *Journal of Neurology* 255, no. 1 (2008): 147–8.
- "Psychiatrie und Hirnforschung. Zu den interstitiellen Uebergaengen des staedtischen Wissenschaftsraums im Labor der Berliner Metropole – Oskar und Cécile Vogt, Korbinian Brodmann, Kurt Goldstein." In *Psychiater und Zeitgeist. Zur Geschichte der Psychiatrie in Berlin*, edited by Hanfried Helmchen, 76–93. Berlin, Germany: Pabst Science Publisher, 2008.
- "Zur Zwangsemigration deutschsprachiger Neurowissenschaftler nach Nordamerika: Der historische Fall des Montreal Neurological Institute." *SDGGN* 14, no. 1 (2008): 441–72.
- "Georg Merrem. Zum 100. Geburtstag am 21. September 2008 – Der Gruendungsdirektor der Neurochirurgischen Klinik der Universitaet Leipzig." In *Jubilaeen 2008. Personen und Ereignisse: 21 Kalenderblaetter zu Jubilaeen von Personen und Ereignissen der Universitaet Leipzig im Jahr 2008*, edited by Franz Haeuser, 71–6. Leipzig, Germany: University of Leipzig Press, 2008.
- "Transforming the Lab: Technological and Societal Concerns in the Pursuit of De- and Regeneration in the German Morphological Neurosciences, 1910–1930." *Medicine Studies: An International Journal for History, Philosophy, and Ethics of Medicine & Allied Sciences* 1, no. 1 (2009): 41–54.
- "'Abwehr,' 'Widerstand' und 'kulturelle Neuorientierung': Zu Konfigurationen der Traumaforschung bei zwangsemigrierten deutschsprachigen Neurologen und Psychiatern." In *Trauma und Wissenschaft*, edited by André Karger, 29–60. Goettingen, Germany, and Zurich, Switzerland: Vandenhoeck & Ruprecht, 2009.
- "German-Speaking Émigré-Neuroscientists in North America after 1933: Critical Reflections on Emigration-Induced Scientific Change." *Oesterreichische Zeitschrift fuer Geschichtswissenschaften (Vienna)* 21, no. 3 (2010): 36–68.
- "'Der Rosenthal'sche Versuch' oder: Ueber den Ort produktiver Forschung. Zur Exkursion des physiologischen Experimentallabors von Isidor Rosenthal (1836–1915) von der Stadt aufs Land." *Sudhoffs Archiv. Zeitschrift fuer Wissenschaftsgeschichte* 94, no. 1 (2010): 1–30.
- "Flexible Antworten – Offene Fragen: Zu den Foerderungsstrategien der Rockefellerstiftung fuer die deutsche Hirnforschung im Nationalsozialismus."

Journal fuer Neurologie, Neurochirurgie und Psychiatrie 12, no. 1 (2011): 56–62.

– "Sex and Human Behavior in the Thought of Freud." In *World History Encyclopedia, Era 7: The Age of Revolutions, 1750–1914*, edited by James H. Overfield, 972–3. Santa Barbara, CA: ABC-Clio/Greenwood, 2011.

– "The Essential Tension: On Ethical and Historical Conundrums in the Trajectories of Deep Brain Stimulation." In *Implanted Minds: The Neuroethics of Intracerebral Stem Cell Transplantation and Deep Brain Stimulation*, edited by Heiner Fangerau, Joerg M. Fegert, and Thorsten Trapp, 151–82. Bielefeld, Germany: Transcript, 2011.

– "The Emergence of Nervennahrung: Nerves, Mind and Metabolism in the Long Eighteenth Century." *Studies in the History and Philosophy of Biological and Biomedical Sciences* 43, no. 2 (2012): 405–17.

– *Medicine, Life and Function. Experimental Strategies and Medical Modernity at the Intersection of Pathology and Physiology*. Bochum, Germany: Projektverlag, 2012.

– "The Early Eugenics Movement and Emerging Professional Psychiatry: Conceptual Transfers and Personal Relationships between Germany and North America, 1880s to 1930s." *Canadian Bulletin of Medical History* 31, no. 1 (2014): 17–40.

– "Learning Soft Skills the Hard Way: Historiographical Considerations on the Cultural Adjustment Process of German-Speaking Émigré Neuroscientists in Canada, 1933 to 1963." *Journal of the History of the Neurosciences* 25, no. 3 (2016): 299–319.

– "Die Neurowissenschaften in Strassburg zwischen 1872 und 1945. Forschungsaktivitaeten zwischen politischen und kulturellen Zaesuren." *Sudhoffs Archiv. Zeitschrift fuer Wissenschaftsgeschichte* 100, no. 2 (2016): 227–62.

– "Forced Migration as Public Relations Process? Lothar B. Kalinowsky and the Trans-Atlantic Transfer of Electroconvulsive Therapy." *Canadian Bulletin of Medical History* 33, no. 2 (2016): 385–417.

– "How the Nerves Reached the Muscle: Bernard Katz, Stephen W. Kuffler and John C. Eccles – Certain Implications of Exile for the Development of 20th-Century Neurophysiology." *Journal of the History of the Neurosciences* 26, no. 4 (2017): 351–84.

– "History of Neurology: Bringing Back Neurology Following WWII." *World Neurology* 32, no. 6 (2017): 9–10.

– "The 'Brain Gain Thesis' Revisited: German-Speaking Émigré Neuroscientists and Psychiatrists in North America." In *Global Transformations in the Life Sciences, 1945–1980*, edited by Patrick

Manning and Mat Savelli, 128–45. Pittsburgh, PA: University of Pittsburgh Press, 2018.

– ed. *Émigré Psychiatrists, Psychologists, and Cognitive Scientists in North America since the Second World War*. Berlin, Germany: Max Planck Institute for the History of Science, 2018.

– "Karl T. Neubuerger (1890–1972): Pioneer in Neurology." *Journal of Neurology* 265, no. 6 (2018): 1493–95.

– "Catalyzing Neurophysiology: Jacques Loeb (1859–1924), the Stazione Zoologica di Napoli, and a Growing Network of Brain Scientists, 1900s–1930," *Frontiers in Neuroanatomy* 13, no. 1 (2019): 1–14.

– "Des gens comme moi étaient désignés comme des 'psychiatres vétérinaires': Les relations germano-américaines en recherche biomédicale dans la période de l'immédiat après-guerre, 1948-1973." In *Neuroscience et Psychiatrie*, edited by Claude Debru and Mireille Delbraccio, 81–117. Paris, France: Éditions Hermann, 2019.

Stahnisch, Frank W., and Andrew G.M. Bulloch. "Mihály (Michael von) Lenhossék (1863–1937)." *Journal of Neurology* 258, no. 10 (2011): 1901–03.

Stahnisch, Frank W., and Thomas Hoffmann. "Kurt Goldstein and the Neurology of Movement during the Interwar Years: Physiological Experimentation, Clinical Psychology and Early Rehabilitation." In *Was bewegt uns? Menschen im Spannungsfeld zwischen Mobilitaet und Beschleunigung*, edited by Christian Hoffstadt, Franz Peschke, and Andreas Schulz-Buchta, 283–311. Bochum, Germany: Projektverlag, 2010.

Stahnisch, Frank W., and Peter J. Koehler. "Three Twentieth-Century Multi-Authored Handbooks Serving as Vital Catalyzers of an Emerging Specialization: A Case Study from the History of Neurology and Psychiatry." *Journal of Mental and Nervous Diseases* 200, no. 12 (2012): 1067–75.

Stahnisch, Frank W., and Erna Kurbegović, eds. *Psychiatry and the Legacies of Eugenics: Historical Perspectives on Alberta and Beyond*. Edmonton: Athabasca University Press, 2020 (forthcoming).

Stahnisch, Frank W., and Robert Nitsch. "Santiago Ramón y Cajal's Concept of Neuronal Plasticity: The Ambiguity Lives On." *Trends in Neurosciences* 25, no. 11 (2002): 589–91.

Stahnisch, Frank W., and Guel Russell, eds. *Forced Migration in the History of 20th-Century Neuroscience and Psychiatry: New Perspectives*. London, UK: Routledge, 2017.

Stahnisch, Frank W., and Jeremy Tynedal. "Sir Ludwig Guttmann (1899–1980): Pioneer in Neurology." *Journal of Neurology* 259, no. 7 (2012): 1512–14.

Steger, Juergen and Georges Schaltenbrand. "Das Myogramm bei der Katatonie." *Zeitschrift fuer die gesamte Neurologie und Psychiatrie* 169, no. 1 (1940): 183–207.

Steinberg, Holger. "Alfred Erich Hoche in der Psychiatrie seiner Zeit vor dem Hintergrund der Schrift 'Die Freigabe der Vernichtung lebensunwerten Lebens.'" In *Die Freigabe der Vernichtung lebensunwerten Lebens. Beitraege des Symposiums ueber Karl Binding und Alfred Hoche am 2. Dezember 2004 in Leipzig*, edited by Ortrun Riha, 68–102. Aachen, Germany: Shaker, 2005.

– "Oswald Bumke in Leipzig." *Der Nervenarzt* 79, no. 3 (2008): 348–56.

Steinberg, Holger and Matthias C. Angermeyer. "Two Hundred Years of Psychiatry at Leipzig University: An Overview." *History of Psychiatry* 13, no. 3 (2002): 267–83.

Stern, Karl. *The Pillar of Fire*. New York: Harcourt Brace, 1951.

– *The Flight from Women*. New York: Paragon House Publishers, 1965.

Stern, Karl and Walter Spielmeyer. "Severe Dementia Associated with Bilateral Symmetrical Degeneration of the Thalamus." *Brain* 62, no. 1 (1939): 157–67.

Stichweh, Rudolf. *Zur Entstehung des modernen Systems wissenschaftlicher Disziplinen. Physik in Deutschland 1740–1890*. Frankfurt am Main, Germany: Suhrkamp Verlag, 1984.

Stoke, Lawrence D. "Canada and an Academic Refugee from Nazi Germany: The Case of Gerhard Herzberg." *Canadian Historical Review* 75, no. 2 (1976): 150–70.

Stortz, Paul, "'Rescue Our Family From a Living Death': Refugee Professors and the Canadian Society for the Protection of Science and Learning at the University of Toronto, 1935–1946." *Journal of the Canadian Historical Association* 14, no. 1 (2003): 231–61.

Strasser, Bruno. "Institutionalizing Molecular Biology in Post-War Europe: A Comparative Study." *Studies in the History of the Biological and Biomedical Sciences* 33, no. 4 (2002): 533–64.

Strauss, Herbert A., and Werner Roeder, eds. *International Biographical Dictionary of Central European Émigrés 1933–1945: The Arts, Sciences, and Literature*. 2 vols. Munich, Germany: K.G. Saur, 1983.

Strickhausen, Waltraud. "Kanada." In *Handbuch der deutschsprachigen Emigration 1933–1945*, edited by Claus-Dieter Krohn. Vol. 3, col. 293–5. Darmstadt, Germany: Wissenschaftliche Verlagsbuchhandlung, 1998.

Strippel, Andreas. *NS-Volkstumspolitik und die Neuordnung Europas. Rassenpolitische Selektion der Einwandererzentralstelle des Chefs der*

Sicherheitspolizei und des SD (1939–1945). Paderborn, Germany: Ferdinand Schoeningh Verlag, 2011.

Stroesser, Wolfgang. "Deutsche Gesellschaft fuer Neuropathologie und Neuroanatomie e.V. 1950–1992. Eine Untersuchung zur Entwicklung der Gesellschaft und zur Foerderung des Faches Neuropathologie in Deutschland." MD diss., Free University of Berlin, Germany: Deutsche Gesellschaft fuer Neuropathologie und Neuroanatomie e.V., 1993.

Sullivan, Robert. "Francis O. Schmitt, 91, Is Dead: Led Studies in Molecular Biology." *New York Times*, 7 October 1995, n.p.

Sulloway, Frank J. *Freud, Biologist of the Mind: Beyond the Psychoanalytic Legend*. New York: Basic Books, 1979.

Sweeney, Patrick J., Marc F. Lloyd, and Robert B. Daroff. "What's in a Name? Dr. Lewy and the Lewy Body." *Neurology* 49, no. 2 (1997): 629–30.

Tandler, Julius. "Zum Fall Wagner-Jauregg. Replik." *Muenchner Medizinische Wochenschrift* 70, no. 2 (1920): columns 2045–189.

Tartokoff, Helen H. "Grete L. Bibring, M.D. 1899–1977." *Psychoanalytic Quarterly* 47, no. 2 (1978): 293–5.

Taylor, Charles. *Grandeur et misère de la modernité*. Montreal: Bellarmin, 1991.

Taylor, John Russell. *Strangers in Paradise: The Hollywood Émigrés 1933–1950*. New York: Holt Rinehart and Winston, 1983.

Terrall, Mary. "Biography as Cultural History of Science." *ISIS* 97, no. 2 (2006): 306–13.

Teuber, Hans L. "Kurt Goldstein's Role in the Development of Neuropsychology." *Neuropsychologia* 4, no. 4 (1966): 299–310.

Thompson Klein, Julie. *Interdisciplinarity: History, Theory, and Practice*. Detroit, IL: Wayne State University Press, 1990.

Timmermann, Carsten. "Americans and Pavlovians: The Central Institute for Cardiovascular Research at the East German Academy of Sciences and Its Precursor Institutions as a Case Study of Biomedical Research in a Country of the Soviet Bloc (c. 1950–80)." In *Medicine, the Market and the Mass Media*, edited by Virginia Berridge and Kerry Loughlin, 244–56. London, UK: Routledge, 2005.

– "Appropriating Risk Factors: The Reception of an American Approach to Chronic Disease in the two German States, c. 1950–1990." *Social History of Medicine* 25, no. 1 (2012): 157–74.

Todes, Daniel. *Pavlov's Physiology Factory: Experiment, Interpretation, Laboratory Enterprise*. Baltimore, MD: Johns Hopkins University Press, 2002.

– *Ivan Pavlov: A Russian Life in Science*. Oxford, UK: Oxford University Press, 2014.

Topp, Sascha. "Shifting Cultures of Memory: The German Society of Pediatrics in Confrontation with Its Nazi Past." In *Silence, Scapegoats, Self-Reflection: The Shadow of Nazi Medical Crimes on Medicine and Bioethics*, edited by Volker Roelcke, Etienne Lepicard, and Sascha Topp, 147–82. Goettingen, Germany: V&R Unipress, 2014.

Topp, Sascha and Juergen Peiffer (†). "Das MPI fuer Hirnforschung in Giessen: Institutskrise nach 1945, die Hypothek der NS-'Euthanasie' und das Schweigen der Fakultaet." In *Die Medizinische Fakultaet der Universitaet Giessen im Nationalsozialismus und in der Nachkriegszeit. Personen und Institutionen, Umbrueche und Kontinuitaeten*, edited by Sigrid Oehler-Klein, 539–607. Stuttgart, Germany: Steiner, 2007.

Tower, Donald Bayley. "A Century of Neuronal and Neuroglial Interactions, and Their Pathological Implications: An Overview." *Progress in Brain Research* 94, no. 1 (1992): 3–17.

Troehler, Ulrich. "Theodor Kocher und die neurotopographische Diagnostik: Angewandte Forschung mit grundlegendem Ergebnis um 1900." *Gesnerus* 40, no. 1–2 (1983): 203–14.

Tschoertner, Heinz Dieter. "Die Sieben. Gerhart Hauptmann und die Ikarier." *Schlesischer Kulturspiegel* 38, no. 4 (October to December, 2003): 70–1.

Tubbs, R. Shane, Loukas Marios, E. George Salter, and Jerry Oakes. "Wilhelm Erb and Erb's Point." *Clinical Anatomy* 20, no. 5 (2007): 486–8.

Turda, Marius. "The Biology of War: Eugenics in Hungary, 1914–1918." *Austrian Historical Yearbook* 40, no. 1 (2009): 238–64.

Tutté, Juan C. "The Concept of Psychoanalytical Trauma: A Bridge in Interdisciplinary Space." *The International Journal for Psychoanalysis* 85, no. 4 (2004): 897–921.

Ulrich, Robert. "Kurt Goldstein." In *The Reach of Mind: Essays in the Memory of Kurt Goldstein*, edited by Marianne L. Simmel, 13–15. New York: Springer, 1968.

United States Chief Counsel for the Prosecution of Axis Criminality, ed. *Nazi Conspiracy and Aggression*. Vol. 3. Washington, DC: Government Printing Office, 1946 (document 1397–PS), 981–3 (official translation from German sources).

United States Information Agency. *A Republic of Science*. Washington, DC: Public Affairs/Information Resource Centers, 1997.

Universitaet Muenchen, *Personen und Vorlesungsverzeichnis. Verzeichnis der Vorlesungen im Sommerhalbjahr*. Munich, Germany: Ludwigs-Maximilians-Universitaet, 1913.

University College London. *Eugenics Laboratory Lecture Series.* 12 Vols. London, UK: Galton Laboratory for National Eugenics, 1909–27.

Van Rahden, Till. *Jews and Other Germans: Civil Society, Religious Diversity, and Urban Politics in Breslau, 1860–1925.* Madison, WI: University of Wisconsin Press, 2008.

Vein, Ala A., and Marion L.C. Maat-Schieman. "Famous Russian Brains: Historical Attempts to Understand Intelligence." *Brain* 131, no. 2 (2008): 583–90.

Vidal, Fernando. "Brains, Bodies, Selves, and Science: Anthropologies of Identity and the Resurrection of the Body." *Critical Inquiry* 28, no. 4 (2002): 930–74.

Vidal, Fernando, and Francisco Ortega. *Being Brains: Making the Cerebral Subject.* New York: Fordham University Press, 2017.

Vogelsaenger, Peter. "Auf den Spuren der psychosomatischen Medizin." In *Psychiater und Zeitgeist. Zur Geschichte der Psychiatrie in Berlin*, edited by Hanfried Helmchen, 255–71. Berlin, Germany: Pabst Science Publisher, 2008.

Vogt, Oskar. *Die Neurobiologischen Arbeiten.* Vol. 1. Jena, Germany: G. Fischer, 1904.

Vom Brocke, Bernhard. "Die Kaiser-Wilhelm-/Max-Planck-Gesellschaft und ihre Institute zwischen Universitaet und Akademie. Strukturprobleme und Historiographie." In *Die Kaiser-Wilhelm-/Max-Planck-Gesellschaft und ihre Institute. Das Harnack-Prinzip*, edited by Bernhard vom Brocke and Hubert Laitko, 1–32. Berlin, Germany: Walter DeGruyter, 1996.

– *Bevoelkerungswissenschaft – Quo vadis? Moeglichkeiten und Probleme einer Geschichte der Bevoelkerungswissenschaft in Deutschland.* Opladen, Germany: Leske & Budrich, 1998.

– "Schmidt-Ott, Friedrich Gustav Adolf Eduard Ludwig." *Neue Deutsche Biographie* 23, no. 1 (2007): 165–7.

Vom Bruch, Ruediger. *Kontinuitaeten und Diskontinuitaeten in der Wissenschaftsgeschichte im 20. Jahrhundert.* Stuttgart, Germany: Franz Steiner Press, 2005.

Von Aretin, Felicitas. "Under the Watchful Gaze of Minerva: Traditions, Symbols and Dealing with the Past." In *Denkorte. Max-Planck-Gesellschaft and Kaiser-Wilhelm-Gesellschaft (1911–2011): Success Stories in Research*, edited by Juergen Renn and Horst Kant, 1–6. Dresden, Germany: Sandstein, 2011.

Von Bunge, Gustav. *The Alcohol Question* (Germ. 1887). Translated by Florence A. Starling and edited by Ernest H. Starling. Westerville, OH: American Issue Publisher, 1907.

Von Lenhossék. "Die Nervenendigungen in den Endknospen der Mundschleimhaut der Fische." *Verhandlungen der naturforschenden Gesellschaft in Basel* 10, no. 1 (1892): 92–100.

- "Der feinere Bau und die Nervenendigungen in den Geschmacksknospen."
  AA 8, no. 4 (1893): 121–6.

Von Monakow, Constantin and Raoul Mourge. "Introduction Biologique à
l'Étude de la Neurologie et de la Psychopathologie. Intégration et désintégra-
tion de la fonction." *Zeitschrift fuer Psychologie* 115, no. 4 (1928): 403–10.

Von Rindfleisch, Georg Eduard. *Lehrbuch der pathologischen
Gewebelehre*. Leipzig, Germany: W. Engelmann, 1867–69.

Von Schwerin, Alexander. *Experimentalisierung des Menschen: Der Genetiker
Hans Nachtsheim und die Erbpathologie, 1920–1945*. Goettingen,
Germany: Wallstein, 2004.

Von Verschuer, Otmar. "Alfred Ploetz." *Der Erbarzt* 8, no. 6 (1940): 69–72.

Von Weizsaecker, Victor. *Der Arzt und der Kranke. Stuecke einer medizinischen
Anthropologie* (1926). Collected Works. Vol. 5. Frankfurt am Main,
Germany: Suhrkamp Verlag, 1987.

- *Soziale Krankheit und soziale Gesundung*. Berlin, Germany: Julius Springer,
  1930.
- "Vom Begriff der Therapie." *Deutsche Medizinische Wochenschrift* 59,
  no. 30 (1933): 1168–70.
- "Soziologische Bedeutung der nervoesen Krankheiten und der
  Psychotherapie." *Zentralblatt fuer Psychotherapie und ihre Grenzgebiete* 8,
  no. 5 (1935): 295–304.
- *Wahrnehmen und Bewegen. Die Taetigkeit des Nervensystems* (1941).
  Collected Works of Viktor von Weizsaecker. Vol. 3. Frankfurt am Main,
  Germany: Suhrkamp Verlag, 1990.
- *Natur und Geist: Erinnerungen eines Arztes*. Goettingen, Germany:
  Vandenhoeck & Ruprecht, 1954.

Voss, Peter. "Die Anfaenge der Institutionalisierung der klinischen Neurologie
in Muenchen (1913–1933)." *Der Nervenarzt* 86, no. 2 (2015): 210–18.

Waessle, Heinz. "A Collection of Brain Sections of 'Euthanasia' Victims: The
Series H of Julius Hallervorden." *Endeavour* 41, no. 4 (2017): 166–75.

Wagner, Armin, and Holger Steinberg. *Neurologie an der Universitaet Leipzig.
Beitraege zur Entwicklung des klinischen Fachgebietes von 1880 bis 1985*.
Leipzig, Germany: Leipziger Universitaetsverlag, 2015.

Wahren, Wilfried. "Oskar Vogt. 6.4.1870–31.7.1959." *DZfNhlk*. 180, no. 4
(1960): 361–80.

Wallenberg, Adolf. "Ludwig Edinger zum 60. Geburtstage." *Archiv fuer
Psychiatrie und Nervenkrankheiten* 55, no. 3 (1915): 997–1008.

Weber, Matthias M. "'Ein Forschungsinstitut fuer Psychiatrie …'. Die
Entwicklung der Deutschen Forschungsanstalt fuer Psychiatrie in Muenchen
zwischen 1917 und 1945." *Sudhoffs Archiv. Zeitschrift fuer
Wissenschaftsgeschichte* 75, no. 1 (1991): 74–89.

- "Die Deutsche Forschungsanstalt fuer Psychiatrie." In *75 Jahre Max-Planck-Institut fuer Psychiatrie*, edited by *Max-Planck-Gesellschaft*, 11–33. Munich, Germany: Max-Planck-Gesellschaft, 1992.
- *Ernst Ruedin: Eine kritische Biographie*. Berlin, Germany: Springer, 1993.
- "Harnack-Prinzip oder Fuehrerprinzip? Erbbiologie unter Ernst Ruedin an der Deutschen Forschungsanstalt fuer Psychiatrie (Kaiser-Wilhelm-Institut) in Muenchen." In *Die Kaiser-Wilhelm-Max-Planck-Gesellschaft und ihre Institute*, edited by Vom Brocke, Bernhard and Hubert Laitko, 409–22. Berlin, Germany: DeGruyter, 1996.
- "Von Emil Kraepelin zu Ernst Ruedin: Die Deutsche Forschungsanstalt fuer Psychiatrie 1917–1945." *Schriftenreihe der Deutschen Gesellschaft fuer Geschichte der Nervenheilkunde* 2, no. 1 (1997): 419–35.
- "Psychiatric Research and Science Policy in Germany: The History of the Deutsche Forschungsanstalt fuer Psychiatrie in Munich from 1917 to 1945." *History of Psychiatry* 11, no. 43 (2000): 235–58.
- "Ernst Ruedin, 1874–1952: A German Psychiatrist and Geneticist." *American Journal of Medical Genetics* 26, no. 3 (2007): 323–31.
Wechsler, Patrick. "La Faculté de Médecine de la Reichsuniversitaet Strassburg (1941–1945) à l'heure national-socialiste." MD diss., Université Louis Pasteur, Strasbourg, France, 1991.
Weigert, Carl. "Zwei Faelle von Missbildung eines Ureters und einer Samenblase mit Bemerkungen ueber einfache Nabelarterien (1886)." *Virchows Archiv fuer pathologische Anatomie und Physiologie* 104, no. 1 (1886): 10–20.
Weikart, Richard. *From Darwin to Hitler: Evolutionary Ethics, Eugenics, and Racism in Germany*. New York: Palgrave Macmillan, 2004.
Weil, Robert. "Mental Health and Disasters." In *Symposium in Human Problems in the Utilization of Fallout Shelters*, edited by George W. Baker and John H. Rohrer, 11–17. Washington, DC: National Institutes of Health, 1960.
Weil, Robert, and Maurice Demay. "Thiamine Chloride Intrathecally." *Canadian Medical Association Journal* 56, no. 5 (1947): 545–6.
Weinberg, Alvin. *Reflexions on Big Science*. Cambridge, MA: MIT Press, 1967.
Weindling, Paul. *Health, Race and German Politics between National Unification and Nazism, 1870–1945*. Cambridge, UK: Cambridge University Press, 1989.
- "The Impact of German Medical Scientists on British Medicine: A Case Study of Oxford, 1933–45." In *Forced Migration and Scientific Change: Émigré German-speaking Scientists after 1933*, edited by Mitchel Ash and Alfons Soellner, 86–114. Cambridge, UK: Cambridge University Press, 1996.

– *Nazi Medicine and the Nuremberg Trials: From Medical War Crimes to
Informed Consent.* Houndmills, Basingstoke, UK: Palgrave, 2004, 251–6.
– "Medical Refugees in Britain and the Wider World, 1930–1960:
Introduction." *Social History of Medicine* 22, no. 3 (2009), 451–9.
– *John W. Thompson: Psychiatrist in the Shadow of the Holocaust.* Rochester,
NY: University of Rochester Press, 2010.
– *Victims and Survivors of Nazi Human Experiments: Science and Suffering in
the Holocaust.* London, UK: Bloomsbury, 2015.
– ed. *From Clinic to Concentration Camp: Reassessing Nazi Medical and
Racial Research, 1933–1945.* London, UK: Routledge, 2017.
Weingart, Peter, Juergen Kroll, and Kurt Bayertz. *Rasse, Blut und Gene.
Geschichte der Eugenik und Rassenhygiene in Deutschland.* Frankfurt am
Main, Germany: Suhrkamp Verlag, 1988.
Weiss, Burkhardt. "Der Kernphysiker Rudolf Fleischmann und die Medizin an
der Reichsuniversitaet Strassburg (1941–1944)." *NTM* 14, no. 2 (2006):
107–18.
Weiss, Sheila Faith. "The Race Hygiene Movement in Germany." *OSIRIS, 2nd
series* 3, no. 1 (1987): 193–236.
Weisz, George. "The Development of Medical Specialization in Nineteenth-
Century Paris." In *French Medical Culture in the Nineteenth Century,* edited
by Anne La Berge and Moshe Feingold, 149–87. Amsterdam, The
Netherlands: Rodopi, 1994.
– *The Medical Mandarins: The French Academy of Medicine in the 19th
and Early 20th Centuries.* Oxford, UK: Oxford University Press, 1995.
Weitz, Eric D. *Weimar Germany: Promise and Tragedy.* Princeton, NJ:
Princeton University Press, 2007.
Wells, Herbert George. *The War that will end War.* London, UK: Frank &
Cecil Palmer, 1914.
Werner, Sylwia, Claus Zittel, and Frank W. Stahnisch, eds. *Ludwik Fleck:
Denkstile und Tatsachen. Gesammelte Schriften und Zeugnisse.* Berlin,
Germany: Suhrkamp Verlag, 2011.
Will, Markus. "Max Bielschowsky. Eine Bioergographie." MD diss., University
of Muenster, Germany, 2000.
Williams, Elizabeth A. *The Physical and the Moral: Anthropology, Physiology,
and Philosophical Medicine in France, 1750–1850.* Cambridge, UK:
Cambridge University Press, 1994.
Williamson, Richard Thomas. "The Early Pathological Changes in
Disseminated Sclerosis." *Medical Chronicle of Manchester* 19, no. 3 (1894):
373–9.
Winau, Rolf. *Medizin in Berlin.* Berlin, Germany: Walter DeGruyter, 1987.

- "Menschenzuechtung. Utopien und ethische Bewertung." In *Machbarkeitsphantasien*, edited by Alfred Schaefer and Michael Wimmer, 55–65. Opladen, Germany: VS Verlag, 2003.

Winkelmann, Andreas. "Wilhelm von Waldeyer-Hartz (1836–1921): An Anatomist Who Left His Mark." *Clinical Anatomy* 20, no. 3 (2007): 231–4.

Winkelmann, Andreas, and Udo Schagen. "Hermann Stieve's Clinical-Anatomical Research on Executed Women during the 'Third Reich.'" *Clinical Anatomy* 22, no. 2 (2009): 163–71.

Wittels, Fritz. "Paul Schilder, 1886–1940." *Psychoanalytic Quarterly* 10, no. 1 (1941): 131–4.

Wittern, Renate. "Die Politik ist weiter nichts, als Medicin im Grossen." Rudolf Virchow und seine Bedeutung fuer die Entwicklung der Sozialmedizin." *Verhandlungen der Deutschen Gesellschaft fuer Pathologie* 87, no. 2 (2003): 150–7.

Wollenberg, Robert. "Ich gedenke mit Wehmut und Ruehrung (1906)." In *Als Student in Koenigsberg. Erinnerungen bekannter Korporierter*, edited by Kurt U. Bertrams, 100–10. Hilden, Germany: WJK Verlag, 2006.

Worden, Frederic G., Francis O. Schmitt, Judith P. Swazey, and George Adelman. *The Neurosciences: Paths of Discovery.* Cambridge, MA: MIT Press, 1975.

Wundt, Wilhelm. *Grundzuege der physiologischen Psychologie.* 3 Vols. Leipzig, Germany: W. Engelmann, 1859–62.

Yeung, Andy Wai Kan, Tazuko K. Goto, and Keung W. Leung. "The Changing Landscape of Neuroscience Research, 2006–2015: A Bibliometric Study." *Frontiers in Neuroscience* 11, no. 3 (2017): 1–10.

Young, Allen. *The Harmony of Illusions: Inventing Posttraumatic Stress Disorder.* Princeton, NJ: Princeton University Press, 1995.

- "W.H.R. Rivers and the War Neuroses." *Journal of the History of Behavioral Science* 35, no. 4 (1999): 359–78.

Zeman, Zbyněk, and Antonín Klímek. *The Life of Edvard Benes 1884–1948: Czechoslovakia in Peace and War.* Oxford, UK: Oxford University Press, 1997.

Zierold, Kurt. *Forschungsfoerderung in drei Epochen. Deutsche Forschungsgemeinschaft: Geschichte, Arbeitsweise, Kommentar.* Stuttgart, Germany: Franz Steiner, 1968.

Zilles, Karl. "Brodmann: A Pioneer of Human Brain Mapping – His Impact on Concepts of Cortical Organization." *Brain* 141, no. 11 (2018): 3262–78.

Zimmerman, Andrew. *Anthropology and Antihumanism in Imperial Germany.* Chicago, IL: University of Chicago Press, 2001.

Zimmerman, David. "The Society for the Protection of Science and Learning and the Politicization of British Science in the 1930s." *Minerva* 44, no. 1 (2006), 25–45.

– "'Narrow-Minded People': Canadian Universities and the Academic Refugee Crises, 1933–1941." *Canadian Historical Review* 88, no. 2 (2007), 291–315.

Zimmermann, Susanne. *Die Medizinische Fakultaet der Universitaet Jena waehrend der Zeit des Nationalsozialismus.* Berlin, Germany: VWB Verlag, 2000.

Zuckermann, Moshe, ed. *Geschichte und Psychoanalyse.* Goettingen, Germany: Wallstein, 2004.

Zuerner, Peter. "Von der Hirnanatomie zur Eugenik. Die Suche nach den biologischen Ursachen der Geisteskrankheiten. Eine Untersuchung am Beispiel des Werkes von August Forel (1848–1931)." MD diss., University of Mainz, Germany, 1983.

Zweig, Arnold. *Erziehung vor Verdun.* Amsterdam, The Netherlands: Querido, 1935.

Index